Medical and Psychosocial Aspects of

Chronic Illness and Disability

FOURTH EDITION

Donna R. Falvo, PhD, RN, CRC

Professor
Rehabilitation Counseling and Psychology
Allied Health Sciences
School of Medicine
The University of North Carolina at Chapel Hill
Chapel Hill, North Carolina

JONES AND BARTLETT PUBLISHERS
Sudbury, Massachusetts
BOSTON   TORONTO   LONDON   SINGAPORE

World Headquarters
Jones and Bartlett Publishers
40 Tall Pine Drive
Sudbury, MA 01776
978-443-5000
info@jbpub.com
www.jbpub.com

Jones and Bartlett Publishers
Canada
6339 Ormindale Way
Mississauga, Ontario L5V 1J2
Canada

Jones and Bartlett Publishers
International
Barb House, Barb Mews
London W6 7PA
United Kingdom

Jones and Bartlett's books and products are available through most bookstores and online booksellers. To contact Jones and Bartlett Publishers directly, call 800-832-0034, fax 978-443-8000, or visit our website www .jbpub.com.

Substantial discounts on bulk quantities of Jones and Bartlett's publications are available to corporations, professional associations, and other qualified organizations. For details and specific discount information, contact the special sales department at Jones and Bartlett via the above contact information or send an email to specialsales@jbpub.com.

The authors, editor, and publisher have made every effort to provide accurate information. However, they are not responsible for errors, omissions, or for any outcomes related to the use of the contents of this book and take no responsibility for the use of the products and procedures described. Treatments and side effects described in this book may not be applicable to all people; likewise, some people may require a dose or experience a side effect that is not described herein. Drugs and medical devices are discussed that may have limited availability controlled by the Food and Drug Administration (FDA) for use only in a research study or clinical trial. Research, clinical practice, and government regulations often change the accepted standard in this field. When consideration is being given to use of any drug in the clinical setting, the health care provider or reader is responsible for determining FDA status of the drug, reading the package insert, and reviewing prescribing information for the most up-to-date recommendations on dose, precautions, and contraindications, and determining the appropriate usage for the product. This is especially important in the case of drugs that are new or seldom used.

Library of Congress Cataloging-in-Publication Data
Falvo, Donna R.
  Medical and psychosocial aspects of chronic illness and disability / Donna Falvo. -- 4th ed.
    p. ; cm.
  Includes bibliographical references and index.
  ISBN-13: 978-0-7637-4461-8 (alk. paper)
  ISBN-10: 0-7637-4461-1 (alk. paper)
  1. Chronic diseases. 2. Chronically ill--Rehabilitation. 3. Chronic diseases--Social aspects.
  4. Chronic diseases--Psychological aspects. I. Title.
  [DNLM: 1. Chronic Disease. 2. Disabled Persons--psychology. 3. Disabled Persons--rehabilitation. 4. Social Adjustment. WT 500 F197m 2009]
RC108.F35 2009
616'.044--dc22

                  2007048895

6048

Production Credits
Publisher: Kevin Sullivan
Aquisitions Editor: Emily Ekle
Aquisitions Editor: Amy Sibley
Editorial Assistant: Patricia Donnelly
Editorial Assistant: Rachel Shuster
Associate Production Editor: Amanda Clerkin
Associate Marketing Manager: Rebecca Wasley

Manufacturing and Inventory Control Supervisor: Amy Bacus
Composition: MacPS
Cover Design: Brian Moore
Cover Image Credit: © Photos.com
Printing and Binding: Malloy, Inc.
Cover Printing: Malloy, Inc.

Printed in the United States of America
12 11 10 09 08   10 9 8 7 6 5 4 3 2

Dedication

This book is dedicated to the memory of

K.V. Talkington

A man of grace and humor,
compassion and understanding.
Whose love of learning touched and influenced the lives of many.

"All things considered, he would rather be in Chicago"

Contents

About the Author

Donna Falvo, PhD, RN, CRC, is Clinical Professor at The University of North Carolina at Chapel Hill School of Medicine, Division of Rehabilitation Psychology and Counseling, Allied Health Sciences. She is a registered nurse, licensed psychologist, and certified rehabilitation counselor. She has over 30 years of experience as a teacher, clinician, and researcher. Prior to moving to North Carolina she was Professor and Coordinator of Rehabilitation Counseling at the Rehabilitation Institute, Southern Illinois University, as well as Director of Behavioral Science, Family and Community Medicine in the School of Medicine. She is a former Mary Switzer Scholar and was elected to Sigma XI National Scientific Research Society in 1995. She is a past president of the American Rehabilitation Counseling Association and currently serves on the editorial board of the *Rehabilitation Counseling Bulletin*. She also served as a dimension expert with the National Research Corporation/Picker Institute from 2005–2008 and currently serves as expert faculty with the Patient Centered Care Institute. She is author of over 40 articles and book chapters and, in addition to authoring the three previous editions of *Medical and Psychosocial Aspects of Chronic Illness and Disability*, she is also author of the book *Effective Patient Education: A Guide to Increased Compliance*, currently in its third edition.

Acknowledgments

Richard L. Buck, MD, MPH, FACPM
Health Care Strategist
Picker Institute Patient-Centered Dimension
  Expert
St. Louis, Missouri

Sujata C. Buck, MD, MPH, FAAP, FACPM
St. Louis, Missouri

Eileen Burker, PhD, CRC
Associate Professor
Division of Rehabilitation Counseling and
  Psychology
Allied Health Sciences
School of Medicine
The University of North Carolina at Chapel
  Hill
Chapel Hill, North Carolina

Catherine T. Calvert, PhD, CRC
Rehabilitation Counselor
North Carolina Jaycee Burn Center
University of North Carolina Hospitals
Chapel Hill, North Carolina

Bruce Cairns, MD
Medical Director
North Carolina Jaycee Burn Center
University of North Carolina Hospitals
Chapel Hill, North Carolina

Richard E. Falvo, PhD
Adjunct Professor
Cell and Molecular Biology
School of Medicine
The University of North Carolina at Chapel
  Hill
Chapel Hill, North Carolina

Lloyd Goodwin, PhD, LPC, CRC-MAC, LCAS, CCS, ACS
Director & Professor
Substance Abuse & Clinical Counseling
  Education Program
Department of Rehabilitation Studies
School of Allied Health Sciences
East Carolina University
Greenville, North Carolina

Tammy Koger, MS
Executive Director
North Carolina Assistive Technology Program
Raleigh, North Carolina

Sandra Hamel, MS, CRC
Sacramento, California

Katie Horstmann
Case Management Supervisor
HIV/STD Community Program
Wake County Human Services
Raleigh, North Carolina

Kelly Kazukaukas, PhD, CVE, CRC
Assistant Professor
Division of Rehabilitation Counseling and
Psychology
Allied Health Sciences
School of Medicine
The University of North Carolina at Chapel
  Hill
Chapel Hill, North Carolina

Moe R. Lim, MD
Assistant Professor
Orthopaedics
School of Medicine
The University of North Carolina at Chapel
  Hill
Chapel Hill, North Carolina

Greg Olley, PhD
Professor
Clinical Center for the Study of Development
  and Learning
The University of North Carolina at Chapel
  Hill
Chapel Hill, North Carolina

Mark Stebnicki, PhD, CRC, LPC, CCM
Professor & Director Graduate Program in
  Rehabilitation Counseling
Department of Rehabilitation Studies
School of Allied Health Sciences
East Carolina University
Greenville, North Carolina

Robert McClure, MD
Assistant Professor
Department of Psychiatry
School of Medicine
The University of North Carolina at Chapel
  Hill
Chapel Hill, North Carolina

Nancy McKenna, AuD, CCC-A
Clinical Assistant Professor
Division of Speech and Hearing Sciences
School of Medicine
The University of North Carolina at Chapel
  Hill
Chapel Hill, North Carolina

Steve Murphy, MS, CRC
Division of Services for the Blind
Raleigh, North Carolina

Clara D. Neyhart, RN, BSN, CNN
University of North Carolina Kidney Center
Division of Nephrology and Hypertension
School of Medicine
The University of North Carolina at Chapel
  Hill
Chapel Hill, North Carolina

Patricia Porter, PhD
Professor
Department of Allied Health Sciences
Associate Director
Center for Literacy and Disability Studies
School of Medicine
The University of North Carolina at Chapel
  Hill
Chapel Hill, North Carolina

William Primack, MD
Professor
University of North Carolina Kidney Center
School of Medicine
The University of North Carolina at Chapel
  Hill
Chapel Hill, North Carolina

Dianne Rawdanowicz, MS
Rehabilitation Counselor
North Carolina Division Vocational Rehabili-
  tation Services
Department of Health and Human Services
Raleigh, North Carolina

Mary Sugioka, MD
Retired Clinical Associate Professor
School of Medicine
The University of North Carolina at Chapel
  Hill
Chapel Hill, North Carolina

And special thanks to others who assisted:
Franklin Lamm
Dick Henderson, MD
and
Graduate Students: Lennie Moore and Keith
Goodman

Special Acknowledgment

Illustrations for the fourth edition of *Medical and Psychosocial Aspects of Chronic Illness and Disability* were created by painter **Jane Lamm, BFA**, Chapel Hill, North Carolina.

The following figures are © Jane Lamm, 2007: Figure 3-1; Figure 3-2; Figure 3-3; Figure 4-1; Figure 4-2; Figure 4-3; Figure 4-4; Figure 5-1; Figure 6-1; Figure 6-2; Figure 10-1; Figure 11-1; Figure 12-1; Figure 12-2; Figure 12-3; Figure 13-1; Figure 14-1; Figure 14-2; Figure 15-1; Figure 15-2; Figure 15-3; Figure 15-4; Figure 15-5; Figure 15-6; Figure 16-1; Figure 16-2; Figure 16-3; Figure 16-4; Figure 16-5; Figure 16-6; Figure 17-1; Figure 17-2; Figure 17-3; Figure 18-1.

Contributor

Michael D. Landry, PT, PhD
Adjunct Assistant Professor
Department of Health Policy and Administration
School of Public Health
The University of North Carolina at Chapel Hill
Chapel Hill, North Carolina

Preface

This book, like the previous three editions, is designed as a reference for non-medical professionals and as a text for students who have little prior medical knowledge, but who work with individuals with chronic illness and disability and need to have an understanding of what the conditions entail. This fourth edition of *Medical and Psychosocial Aspects of Chronic Illness and Disability* has been revised and updated, but the format has also been changed to reflect an approach more consistent with the philosophical underpinnings of the International Classification of Functioning, Disability and Health (ICF). New chapters on Conceptualizing Chronic Illness and Disability, Intellectual Disability; and Financing Rehabilitation have been added. In addition, chapters on Psychiatric Disability, Substance Use, and Conditions of the Blood and Immune System have been expanded.

The experience of chronic illness and disability is individualized. No two people experience the same chronic illness and disability in the same way. Consequences of chronic illness and disability are related to a multitude of factors separate from the condition itself.

The impact chronic illness and disability have on the individual is related not only to the condition itself, but to attitudes, social and environmental barriers, and prejudices, apart from characteristics of the condition and associated functional capabilities. The condition, in this respect, is not as important as how the individual's activities and participation are affected by contextual factors.

In the past, chronic illness and disability have been defined in terms of diagnosis and impairment; pathology to be cured or treated; limitation of ability; and threat to productive activity. The major focus has been on the diagnosis rather than the person in the context of his or her perceptions, goals, abilities, life circumstances, and individual environment. Although this book still addresses changes in anatomical structure or physiological function as the result of a variety of conditions, the focus is on functional ability from an individual and societal perspective in the context of activities and participation in all areas of the individual's life and varying life situations.

DRF

Chapter 1

Conceptualizing Chronic Illness and Disability

The relationship between cultural belief systems and societal attitudes toward individuals with disability is well known and has been studied extensively (Mallory, 1993). The culture and society that one inhabits significantly influence the context in which disability is viewed. Individuals with disability are found in every country and every culture of the world. The way disability is viewed and the extent to which individuals with disability are included or excluded in their environment is in the context of their particular culture and society. As countries and cultures undergo change, beliefs about disability also change, and those changes have direct consequences for individuals with disability.

In the United States for many years, understanding of chronic illness and disability has been delineated by the *medical model* (Smart, 2001). This model emphasizes pathology, or cause of chronic illness and disability; has objective, standardized measures to define and characterize the condition; and focuses on treatment and prognosis. (Fowler & Wadsworth, 1991). From this perspective, efforts are made to diagnose, treat, and theoretically "cure" the pathology, so the individual can return to the idealized "norm" (Longmore, 1995; McCarthy, 1993). The ideal consequence from this point of view would be a world in which chronic illness or disability is eliminated. Hence, given the premise of this "ideal,"

it follows that any deviation from the "norm" would be viewed as "abnormal" and, essentially, "undesirable."

The underlying philosophy of the medical model can have significant implications for individuals with chronic illness or disability. From this perspective, pathology and associated problems related to the chronic illness or disability lie within the individual. If individuals are unable to be "cured," the implication is that that they are "abnormal" or "dysfunctional" and, consequently, are passive recipients of treatment having little or no control or choice related to the treatment they receive. Conceptualization of chronic illness and disability from the standpoint of the medical model largely ignored the individual's role and function within the broader context of society and the environment. From this viewpoint, alteration of the individual's role and function from the societal expected norm results in social reactions and social comparisons that devalue or stigmatize individuals with chronic illness and disability, often making them objects of prejudice.

The way individuals with chronic illness and disability are viewed in society is, however, changing. Disability is not a consequence of biological forces or societal conceptualization alone, but rather the result of a complex interaction of factors. Rather than being solely a physical or mental condition, disability is an *experience* in which body, behavior, and society are intertwined (Imrie, 2004). The medical model emphasizes the diagnosis and any corresponding limitation or functional capacity relative to the societal norm (Stucki, Cieza, & Melvin, 2007), but individuals do not exist in isolation. Diagnostic labels alone neither predict nor describe actual functional capacity of the individual within the context of his or her daily life. The social and physical environments within which individuals live and interact can either enhance their ability to function or can exaggerate a disability. Consequently, social and physical environments can determine the extent and type of disability experience. Defining disability in terms of functional capacity rather than medical diagnosis permits a greater understanding of the individual's subjective experience of the disability.

The term "experience" implies that how individuals perceive disability is not only the result of the condition itself, but also the result of limitations, barriers, or circumstances they encounter within their social and physical environments. Social environments exist at many levels, extending from the insular level of family and friends, to the larger social environment of community and work, and finally to the broader level that encompasses cultural, economic, and political environments. Physical environments include not only physical barriers within the immediate environment, but also other factors such as climate, weather, housing, and transportation.

The experience of disability is dynamic and varies in different life stages and in different environments. Developmental factors affect individuals' experience of disability. Specifically, the experience of disability is different for each age group. As individuals pass through various life stages, they face new challenges associated with a particular stage of life, which would occur whether or not they had a disability. These life stage challenges, in turn, influence individuals' experience with disability. For

instance, the experience of chronic illness and disability during childhood is different from the experience of the same condition during adulthood. The experience of chronic illness and disability in adolescence is different from what would be experienced by an individual with the same disability in the later years of life.

How individuals experience chronic illness or disability also varies within different environments. For instance, the experience of disability at home may be different from the experience of disability in the workplace. The experience of disability in the grocery store may be quite different from the experience of disability at the beach. In short, there is a dynamic interaction between individuals' functioning and disability within a given context.

■ THE INTERNATIONAL CLASSIFICATION OF FUNCTIONING, DISABILITY, AND HEALTH

The need to view chronic illness and disability from a broader perspective has gradually been recognized. As a result there has been increased awareness of the need for a new model to conceptualize functioning, disability, and health. In 2001, the *World Health Organization (WHO)* adopted a new classification system of function in relationship to diagnostic information utilized in health services. This classification system, called the *International Classification of Functioning, Disability, and Health (ICF),* is an international standard for describing and measuring health and disability and is a universal classification of functional status associated with a number of health conditions (Peterson & Rosenthal, 2005a; Peterson, 2005). The classification system serves not only as a tool for standardizing concepts related to functional impact of disability, but also as a tool for measuring efficiency and effectiveness of rehabilitation services (Üstün, Okawa, Bickenbach, Kastanjsek, & Schneider, 2003).

The ICF grew out of another classification system, the *International Classification of Impairments, Disabilities and Handicaps (ICIDH)* (WHO, 1980), which was based on the medical model. The ICIDH was revised and updated to become the current ICF. The new ICF de-emphasizes consequences of disease and instead focuses on health. It places health on a continuum so that people both with and without disability are included. This view of health acknowledges that everyone has the potential to experience a decline in health with some degree of disability. Thus the ICF, which is much broader than the medical model, promotes the concept of disability not as a "problem" within the person, but rather as the result of assets or barriers found within the social or physical environment (Peterson & Kosciulek, 2005).

The ICF provides a standard language and framework for conceptualizing health and a variety of health conditions by providing a specific and complete evaluation of health and function in terms of individuals' daily lives (Bryuére & Peterson, 2005). Using this classification system, disability is viewed as more than a medical diagnosis or a medical or biological dysfunction, but rather as a part of the health continuum as it affects function. Consequently, health and disability are viewed on the continuum and as a universal human experience with an emphasis on both the psychosocial and environmental aspects of chronic illness and disability.

■ PHILOSOPHICAL APPLICATIONS

Although the ICF provides a systematic coding scheme that can be valuable in research, education, and practice, perhaps more important is its philosophical underpinnings, which present a different way of viewing chronic illness and disability. In the past, diagnostic labels often overshadowed individual potential and abilities, focusing only on deficits and limitations. Rather than viewing chronic illness and

disability from the perspective of the medical model, which emphasizes diagnosis, and the biomedical aspects of function, the ICF broadens the perspective, placing emphasis on the integration of biomedical, personal, societal, and environmental factors with a positive focus on function and health. Rather than viewing disability as a personal attribute, the ICF provides a wider framework for addressing human experience in the context of function and disability by considering disability as a social construct, which reflects the interaction between the individual and the environment (WHO, 2001).

■ FUNCTION AND STRUCTURE; ACTIVITY AND PARTICIPATION

The ICF addresses more than disability. It also classifies health and health-related states with or without disability because the emphasis is on function and health conditions, both of which may be on a continuum. The *experience* of disability focuses on the individual and his or her personal resources, health condition, and individual environment. Health, as portrayed by the ICF, is a dynamic interaction between function and disability within the context of the individual's environment and personal factors (Stucki & Melvin, 2007).

The core structure of the ICF is divided into two parts, each with two components (see Figure 1-1). The first part, *Function and Disability*, is divided into two components: *body function and structure* and *activity and participation*. In the first component, *body function* refers to physiological functioning of body systems, such as mental function, sensory function, function of the heart, or function of the immune system; and *body structure* refers to anatomical components of the body, such as the structure of the nervous system or the structure of the cardiovascular system. The second component, *activity and participation*, is conceptualized by qualifiers of *capacity and performance*. *Activity* refers to tasks or actions that individuals carry out in daily life, such as reading, writing, managing daily routines, dressing, and bathing. *Participation* refers to the individual's involvement in activities of daily life or of society. It includes the individual's ability to fully participate in activities in the broader social system, such as going to school, having a job, engaging in recreational activities, or being integrated into the community.

The qualifier *capacity* refers to the individual's *actual ability*, or level of function to perform a task or action, whereas *performance* refers to what the individual *actually does* in his or her current environment. For instance, an individual may have the capacity to walk from the front porch to the mailbox, but does not do so because a neighbor brings the mail to the individual's door each day.

The second part of the core structure of the ICF, *contextual factors*, consists of two components: *environmental factors* and *personal factors*. Both components include factors that can be either *facilitators* or *barriers* in helping individuals acquire full participation.

The first component, *environmental factors*, refers to more than the physical environment, such as accessibility of buildings or the availability of accessible transportation. It also includes products and technology (such as telephones or computers), climate (such as dry, humid, hot, or cold), and factors in the social environment (such as social attitudes, norms, services, and political systems). In this context, environmental factors are divided into three levels:

- Individual level: individual systems of support; support network
- Services level: services and resources available
- Cultural/legal systems level: societal and cultural attitudes; political and legal factors (Peterson & Rosenthal, 2005b)

The second component, *personal factors*, is recognized as an important interactive component in defining function, but is not coded in the ICF because of the complexity and highly individualized nature of these factors. Personal factors include gender, race, education, occupation, and hard-to-quantify human factors, such as past personal experiences, individual temperament, and other intrinsic characteristics, such as state of mind. Although these factors are not coded, they are considered and recognized as contributing to the overall function of the individual.

The core structure of the ICF provides a perspective on health conditions from the standpoint of function. It offers a perspective on how body structure and function affect individuals' ability to function in the context of their particular social and physical environment as well as the direct impact of the social and physical environment on function. The ICF focuses on the dynamic and interactive nature of biological, social, personal, and environmental factors in determining individuals' functional capacity.

Part I. Function and Disability
  A. Body functions and structures
  B. Activities and participation

Part II. Contextual Factors
  A. Environmental factors
  B. Personal factors

Figure 1–1   Core structure of the International Classification of Functioning, Disability, and Health

ACHIEVING OPTIMAL VERSUS MAXIMUM FUNCTIONAL CAPACITY

For individuals to achieve full functional capacity, there must be an awareness not only of the functional implications of various chronic illness and disability, but also the implications of the strengths and barriers that are found in the social and physical environment. Emphasis is on building and strengthening personal resources with the goal of helping individuals achieve *optimal functioning* and full *inclusion* and *participation* in all aspects of life. In this context, both strengths and limitations must be identified.

It is commonly assumed that achieving *maximum function* is the ideal goal; however, *optimal function* rather than *maximum function* is emphasized. Although "maximum" refers to the greatest degree of function possible, maximum function for an individual may not be optimal. *Maximum function* is based on an objective viewpoint, while *optimal function* is based on the subjective viewpoint of the individual and derived from his or her own goals and experience. Optimizing function requires a comprehensive understanding of individuals within the context of their environment and within their own frame of reference.

HEALTH, FUNCTIONING, AND DISABILITY

The focus of the new 2001 ICF is on *health* and *function* as they relate to disability, rather than on *impairment* and *handicap*. The latter terms appeared and were defined in the 1980 ICF (WHO, 1980). The current ICF defines these terms as follows:

- **Health** refers to *components of health* (physical or psychological function) and *components of well-being* (capacity to function within the environment).

- **Function** refers to all body functions, activities, and participation in society.
- **Disability** refers to any impairment, activity limitations, or participation restrictions that result from the health condition or from personal, societal, or environmental factors in the individual's life.
- **Impairment** refers to a deviation from certain generally accepted population standards of function (WHO, 2001).

Although impairments associated with a number of health conditions cause some degree of disability in most people (e.g., spinal cord injury), the degree to which an impairment results in disability is also determined by individuals' unique circumstances. What may appear to be a relatively minor disruption of function may actually have major consequences for the life of the individual affected. For example, loss of an index finger would be more disabling for a baseball pitcher than it would be for a heavy-equipment operator. Spinal cord injury resulting in paraplegia has a different impact for someone who is an accountant than it would have for someone who is a construction worker. Rather than imposing preconceived ideas about the extent of disability associated with a particular health condition, determining the extent of disability requires that consideration be given to the condition in the context of the individual's life, particular circumstances, and goals.

A health condition that results in a disability for one individual may not result in a disability for another individual with the same health condition. Therefore, the degree of disability an individual experiences as a result of a health condition depends on the individual's goals as well as those facilitators or barriers that are present in the physical and social environment.

The ICF emphasizes functional capacity in the individual's natural environment. Evaluation and assessment of an individual's functional capacity in a laboratory or testing environment may not be an accurate reflection of his or her level of function. What individuals are able to do in a standardized environment may be quite different from what they are able to do in their natural environment. For example, an individual, after stroke resulting in hemiplegia, may be able to ambulate to the bathroom in a laboratory setting; however, at home, with no indoor plumbing and only outdoor facilities, the same person may be unable to perform this task. Without assessing function in the context of the individual's everyday life, a realistic view of function may not be obtained. Likewise, there may be a discrepancy between the individual's capacity to function and his or her actual performance. Individuals may have the capacity to perform a task but may lack the motivation or social support to carry it out. For instance, an individual with emphysema may have the ability to carry out household chores, but because of overprotective family members may be discouraged from doing so. Function is more complex than merely having the ability to carry out a task or action.

■ CONCLUSIONS

Reconceptualizing chronic illness and disability in the context of the continuum of health and function helps to decrease the stigmatization and isolation that have been associated with chronic illness and disability in the past. By emphasizing functional capacity rather than deficits, and by focusing on personal goals and the ability to perform in the context of the environment, optimal function can be achieved. Greater understanding of chronic illness and disability as an experience rather than as a medical condition can help to decrease the discrimination and prejudice that too often accompany chronic illness and disability and that too often are the major barriers to achievement of optimal activity and participation in the broader community, social, and vocational environments.

■ REFERENCES

Bruyére, S. M., & Peterson, D. B. (2005). Introduction to the special section on the International Classification of Functioning, Disability and Health (ICF): Implications for rehabilitation psychology. *Rehabilitation Psychology, 50*, 103–104.

Fowler, C. A., & Wadsworth, J. S. (1991). Individualism and equity: Critical values in North American culture and the impact on disability. *Journal of Applied Rehabilitation Counseling, 22*, 19–23.

Imrie, R. (2004). Demystifying disability: A review of the International Classification of Functioning, Disability and Health. *Sociology of Health and Illness, 26*, 287–305.

Longmore, P. K. (1995). Medical decision-making and people with disabilities: A clash of cultures. *Journal of Law, Medicine, and Ethics, 23*, 82–87.

Mallory, B. L. (1993). Changing beliefs about disability in developing countries: Historical factors and socio-cultural variables. In B. L. Mallory, R. W. Nichols, J. I. Charlton, & K. Marfo, *Traditional and changing views of disability in developing societies: Causes, consequences, cautions* (pp. 1–24). Durham, NII: The International Exchange of Experts and Information in Rehabilitation.

McCarthy, H. (1993). Learning with Beatrice A. Wright: A breath of fresh air that uncovers the unique virtues and human flaws in us all. *Rehabilitation Education, 10*, 149–166.

Peterson, D. B. (2005). International Classification of Functioning, Disability and Health (ICF): An introduction for rehabilitation psychologists. *Rehabilitation Psychology, 50*, 105–112.

Peterson, D. B., & Kosciulek, J. F. (2005). Introduction to the special issue of *Rehabilitation Education:* The International Classification of Functioning, Disability and Health (ICF). *Rehabilitation Education, 19*(2 & 3), 75–80.

Peterson, D. B., & Rosenthal, D. (2005a). The ICF as an historical allegory for history in rehabilitation education. *Rehabilitation Education, 19*, 95–104.

Peterson, D. B., & Rosenthal, D. A. (2005b). The International Classification of Functioning, Disability and Health (ICF): A primer for rehabilitation educators. *Rehabilitation Education, 19*(2 & 3), 81–94.

Smart, J. F. (2001). *Disability, society and the individual.* Austin, TX; Pro-Ed.

Stucki, G., Cieza, A., & Melvin, J. (2007). The International Classification of Functioning, Disability and Health: A unifying model for the conceptual description of the rehabilitation strategy. *Journal of Rehabilitation Medicine, 39,* 279–285.

Stucki, G., & Melvin, J. (2007). The International Classification of Functioning, Disability and Health: A unifying model for the conceptual description of physical and rehabilitation medicine. *Journal of Rehabilitation Medicine, 39,* 286–292.

Üstün, S., Okawa, Y., Bickenbach, J., Kastanjsek, N., & Schnieder, M. (2003). The International Classification of Functioning, Disability and Health: A new tool for understanding disability and health. *Disability and Rehabilitation, 25,* 565–571.

World Health Organization. (1980). *International classification of impairments, disabilities, and handicaps* (ICIDH). Geneva: Author.

World Health Organization. (2001). *ICF: International classification of functioning, disability and health.* Geneva: Author.

Chapter 2

Psychosocial and Functional Aspects of Chronic Illness and Disability

■ THE EXPERIENCE OF CHRONIC ILLNESS AND DISABILITY

The way individuals experience chronic illness or disability encompasses many different areas and is influenced by numerous factors, including the following:

- Personal factors (such as gender, race, age, coping styles, and past experience)
- Social and family relationships and social support
- Socioeconomic status
- Culture
- Environment (physical, social, and political)
- Activities (including those related to daily living, recreation, school, and work)
- Goals of the individual

The extent to which a health condition is disabling depends on the interplay between the individual's health condition and these factors. Limitations that individuals experience may not be so much a function of their health condition as a function of elements in their environment. Individual reactions to chronic illness and disability vary considerably. The individual with a health condition that has associated limitations may not place as much importance on the condition and its associated features as do members of society. Social groups establish their own standards with regard to idealized physical and emotional traits, roles, and responsibilities. Individuals with chronic illness or disability who do not fit the societal determined "norm" may find that, regardless of their strengths and abilities, society as a whole focuses more on the limitations associated with the condition than on what they are actually able to do.

People vary in terms of their personal resources such as tolerance to symptoms, functional capacity, general ability to cope, and social supports. Consequently, each individual must be considered in the context of all aspects of his or her life, and specifically in terms of the individual's capacity to function within his or her environment.

Functional capacity goes beyond specific tasks and activities. It also includes significant events and relationships with family, friends, employers, and casual acquaintances. No relationship exists in isolation. Just as individuals' reactions to illness or disability influence the reactions of others, so the reactions of others affect individuals' self-concept and perception of their own strengths and abilities.

Participation in family, social, and work activities assumes interaction and the capacity to perform a variety of activities. As interactions or capacities change, or as they become limited or restricted, alterations in roles and relationships also occur. Although some changes and adjustments may be made with relative ease, other changes can have repercussions in many areas of daily life. The meaning and importance that individuals and their families attribute to these associated changes influence their ability to accept the condition and to make necessary adjustments. The health condition itself is only one factor that determines individuals' ability to function effectively.

Disease and Illness

Words are powerful conveyers of concepts. Using a standard definition of terms facilitates communication and understanding of what each term implies. The term *disease* is derived from the medical model, which refers directly to changes in structure or function of body systems. The *medical model* focuses on treatment and elimination of symptoms. The term *illness* refers to individuals' perception of their symptoms and how they and their families respond to symptoms they are experiencing (Morof, Lubkin, & Larson, 2002). It is important to understand both concepts.

Professionals working with individuals with chronic illness or disability must understand symptoms, functional ability, and progression of a condition so that they can understand individuals' experience, and facilitate their ability to achieve optimal functional capacity. Insight into the nature of the individuals' health condition helps guide professionals in assessments and interventions as well as in understanding each individual's functional capacity and general experience (Dudgeon, 2002). It is also important for professionals to have insights into individuals' perception of their condition, the personal relevance and meaning it has for them, and their goals so that interventions can be directed toward meeting specific needs and goals (Shaw, Segal, Polatajko, & Harburn, 2002).

There must be an understanding of the individual's strengths, resources, and abilities, as well as how these will affect functional capacity. Professionals also need an understanding of clients' personal factors, activities, and social and physical environments to effectively assess how the condition will affect an individual's daily life and goals in relationship to functional capacity at home, at work, and in the community.

Medical Terms Related to Chronic Illness and Disability

Although understanding the experience of the individual in regard to his or her health condition is crucial, understanding terms and concepts utilized by the medical community as a whole is also important to facilitate communication and avoid misinterpretation. Two key terms that influence the treatment of a health condition by medical personnel are concepts of *acute* and *chronic*. Acute refers to sudden onset of symptoms that are short term and affect functional capacity on a short-term basis. Chronic refers to symptoms that last indefinitely and are attributed to a cause that may or may not be able to be identified. Some conditions begin acutely but are not resolved, thus becoming ongoing and chronic.

When health conditions are chronic, depending on the nature of the condition and the circumstances, *activities and participation* may be affected and changes in activities may be needed to accommodate manifestations of the condition. In some instances, if symptoms of the condition progress or as other personal, social, or environmental factors change, accommodations may be needed to manage the condition. The course of an illness over time, plus actions taken by individuals and their families to manage or shape the course of the condition, is called a *trajectory* (Corbin, 2001). This concept is important to professionals working with individuals with chronic illness and disability because it implies a continuum and emphasizes the social and environmental effects of the condition.

The *course* of the condition refers to the nature or stages of the chronic illness or disability. Some conditions are classified as *stable*, meaning that the condition is being managed, symptoms are not progressing, and the health status of the individual is not deteriorating. In other instances, conditions are known as *progressive*, meaning that symptoms continue to progress and health and/or functional capacity continue to decline. Other conditions are classified as *episodic*, meaning that symptoms may not always be present, but flare up occasionally. The term *degenerative* refers to conditions in which there is continuing breakdown of structure or function. Some conditions have periods of *exacerbations* (periods when symptoms become worse) and periods of *remissions* (periods of time when symptoms remain stable or do not progress).

The course of chronic illness or disability can have a major influence on individuals' experience of the condition as well as on their functional capacity. For instance, individuals who have a progressive condition have continuing adaptation and adjustment as their health and function continue to decline, whereas individuals with a stable condition may have an initial period of adjustment but no ongoing functional loss.

■ STRESS IN CHRONIC ILLNESS AND DISABILITY

Change is an unavoidable part of life. Change of job, change of home, change of family composition, or changes brought about through the normal aging process are all events that everyone experiences. Depending on individuals' perceptions and the circumstances involved, change may be positive or negative. Whether positive or negative, change requires some adjustment or adaptation, which produces a certain degree of stress.

Chronic illness and disability produce significant change and consequently stress associated with both physical imbalance and psychological turmoil as individuals must deal with a change of customary lifestyle, loss of control, disruption of physiological processes, pain or discomfort, and potential loss of role, status, independence, and financial stability. When individuals have confidence in their ability to maintain control over their destiny, and when they believe that changes—although inevitable—are manageable, stress is less pronounced. When individuals perceive the changes associated with chronic illness or disability as insurmountable or beyond their ability to cope, stress can be overwhelming.

The degree of stress associated with chronic illness or disability is often related to the degree of threat it represents to individuals. Potential threats posed by chronic illness or disability include the following:

- Threats to life and physical well-being
- Threats to body integrity and comfort as a result of the illness or disability itself, diagnostic procedures, or treatment
- Threats to independence, privacy, autonomy, and control
- Threats to self-concept and fulfillment of customary roles
- Threats to life goals and future plans
- Threats to relationships with family, friends, and colleagues
- Threats to the ability to remain in familiar surroundings
- Threats to economic well-being

In addition to threats associated with chronic illness or disability, another consideration is the individual's perception of the meaning or purpose of life itself. Although a chronic illness or disability may still produce stress if individuals feel that their life has no meaning or that they have already fulfilled their purpose in life, the stress experienced may be quite different from that experienced by individuals who believe that they still have a significant purpose to fulfill.

Responses to stresses imposed by threat of chronic illness or disability depend on individuals' perceptions of the impact the condition has on various areas of life as well as on individuals' capacity to cope. Stress cannot be easily quantified, but it can be interpreted in relationship to behaviors exhibited by individuals who are experiencing chronic illness or disability. When demands exceed psychological, social, or financial resources, stress may be manifested in a variety of ways, such as noncompliance with recommended treatment, self-destructive behaviors such as substance abuse, behavioral consequences such as irritability or hostility, or inward manifestations such as depression.

Individuals in the same situation do not necessarily experience the same degree of stress, and the amount of change or adjustment required is not necessarily an indicator of the amount of stress perceived. Individuals who are able to adapt and cope effectively and mobilize resources are more successful in managing stress and achieving more stable outcomes.

Coping

Coping is a constellation of many acts rather than a single act, is constantly changing, and is highly individualized. Coping mechanisms are learned and developed over time. Individuals use them to manage, tolerate, or reduce stress associated with significant life events and to attempt to restore psychological equilibrium after a stressful or traumatic event. Everyone has a variety of coping mechanisms developed through life experiences, although each individual relies on a predominant coping style to reduce anxiety and restore equilibrium when confronted with a stressful situation. Coping is manifested through behavior. Coping behavior is *effective* and *adaptive* when it helps individuals reduce stress and enhance attainment of their fullest potential. It is *ineffective*

and *maladaptive* when it inhibits growth and potential or contributes to physical or mental deterioration. Coping may be required not only for dealing with the initial diagnosis, but also for managing subsequent events. Conditions that are progressive with compounding limitations necessitate ongoing coping and adjustment to incorporate additional changes into daily life.

Individuals cope with illness and disability in different ways. Some actively confront their condition, learning new skills or actively engaging in treatment to control or manage the condition. Others defend themselves from stress and the realities of the diagnosis by denying its seriousness, ignoring treatment recommendations, or refusing to learn new skills or behaviors associated with the condition. Still others cope by engaging in self-destructive behavior, actively continuing behavior that has detrimental effects on their physical condition.

Effective coping must be viewed in the context of each individual's personal background and experiences, life situation, and perception of his or her own circumstances. Individuals tend to use coping strategies that have worked successfully for them in the past. When old strategies are no longer effective or are not appropriate to the new situation, new coping strategies must be implemented to neutralize events surrounding the chronic illness or disability and to adjust to any associated limitations. Effective coping enables individuals to attain emotional equilibrium, to achieve a positive mental outlook, and to avoid incapacitation from fear, anxiety, anger, or depression.

Coping, however, does not occur in a vacuum. The social environment in which individuals find themselves can facilitate or discourage effective coping. In general, an environment that helps individuals gain a sense of control through active participation in decision making and take responsibility for their own destiny as much as possible best equips them to cope effectively with chronic illness and disability.

Coping Strategies

Coping strategies are subconscious mechanisms that individuals use to cope with stress. All individuals have predominant coping strategies that they use to reduce anxiety and restore equilibrium when they are confronted with stress. The coping strategies that individuals used in the past are often those employed when individuals are confronted with the stress of chronic illness or disability. Use of coping strategies reduces anxiety, helping individuals to achieve balance and productivity in their lives. Although coping strategies can be helpful, their overuse can also be detrimental.

Denial

Diagnosis of chronic illness or disability and the associated implications can be devastating and provoke anxiety. *Denial* is a coping strategy individuals use to negate the reality of a situation. In the case of chronic illness or disability, individuals may deny that they have the condition by avoiding recommended treatment or by denying the implications of the condition. In the early stages of adjustment, denial may be beneficial in that it enables individuals to adjust to the reality of their situation at their own pace, preventing excessive anxiety. When denial continues, however, it can prevent individuals from following medical recommendations or learning new skills that would help them reach their optimum potential.

Denial of the chronic illness or disability can have far-reaching effects on others as well if, by denying the condition, the affected individual places others at risk. For example, proper precautions can greatly reduce the spread of some contagious diseases, such as tuberculosis or HIV infection. Individuals in active denial of their condition or its ramifications may

neglect to take anti-tuberculosis medications regularly or may have unprotected sex in the case of HIV, putting others in jeopardy. Some individuals may put others at risk by denying their limitations, such as individuals who are legally blind but continue to drive even though driving has been prohibited.

Regression

In *regression*, individuals revert to an earlier stage of development, so that they become more dependent, behave more passively, or exhibit more emotionality than would normally be expected at their developmental level. In the early stages of chronic illness or disability, returning to a state of dependency experienced in an earlier stage of development can be therapeutic, especially if treatment of the condition requires rest and inactivity. When individuals remain in a regressive mode, however, it can interfere with their adjustment and attainment of a level of independence that allows individuals to reach their optimal functional capacity. For example, after a myocardial infarction (heart attack), individuals may be encouraged to walk several miles each day to increase their strength and endurance; some, however, may continue to stay in bed, asking that family members wait on them.

Compensation

Individuals using *compensation* as a coping strategy learn to counteract limitations in one area by becoming stronger or more proficient in another area. When function is lost in one area, individuals may find ways to excel in another sphere. Compensatory behavior is generally highly constructive when new behaviors are directed toward positive goals and outcomes. For example, individuals who are unable to maintain their level of activity because of physical limitations associated with their condition may turn to creative writing or other means of self-expression. Compensation as a coping strategy can be detrimental, however, if the new behaviors used in compensating for limitations are self-destructive or socially unacceptable. For example, an individual who experiences disfigurement as a result of a disability may become promiscuous as a way of compensating for his or her perception of physical unattractiveness.

Rationalization

As a coping strategy, *rationalization* enables individuals to find socially acceptable reasons for their behavior or to excuse themselves for not reaching goals or not accomplishing tasks. Although rationalization can soften the disappointment of dreams unrealized or goals not reached, it can also produce negative effects if it becomes a barrier to adjustment, prevents individuals from reaching their full potential, or interferes with effective management of the medical condition itself. For example, an individual with visual impairment who is a student may rationalize that he or she failed the test because of the difficulty with vision, rather than admitting that he or she failed the test because they went to the beach with friends rather than studying for the test.

Diversion of Feelings

One of the most positive and constructive of all coping strategies can be the *diversion* of unacceptable feelings or ideas into socially acceptable behaviors. Individuals with chronic illness or disability may have particularly strong feelings of anger or hostility about their diagnosis or the circumstances surrounding their condition. If their emotional energy can be redefined and diverted into positive activity, the results can be beneficial, making virtue out of necessity and transforming deficit into gain. As with all coping strategies, diversion of feelings can have negative effects if feelings of anger or hostility are channeled into negative behaviors or socially unacceptable activities. For example, an individual with diabetes may have neglected to follow foot care precautions, which resulted in lower leg amputation.

Rather than acknowledging self-anger, the individual may instead express hostility and blame toward family members.

Emotional Reactions to Chronic Illness or Disability

Sudden, unexpected, or life-threatening chronic illness or disability engenders a variety of reactions. How individuals view their condition, its causes, and its consequences greatly affects what they do in the face of it. They may view their condition as a challenge, an enemy to be fought, a punishment, a sign of weakness, a relief, a strategy for gaining attention, an irreparable loss, or an uplifting spiritual experience. Although the emotional reactions of individuals experiencing chronic illness or disability vary both in type and in intensity, the following reactions are common. Although each emotional reaction is discussed individually, it is important to note that reactions are often experienced simultaneously.

Grief

Grief is a normal reaction to loss. Individuals with chronic illness and disability may experience loss of a body part; loss of function, role, or social status; or other perceived losses that result in a reaction of grief. Although the grieving and the progression through stages of grief vary from person to person, a common initial reaction to chronic illness or disability is shock, disbelief, or numbness with the diagnosis or its seriousness being denied or disputed. As individuals acknowledge the reality of the situation, the grief reaction may be more pronounced.

After repeated confrontations with elements of loss, normal adaptation results in gradual change in emphasis and focus that enables individuals to accept the loss emotionally and to make adjustments and adaptations that are necessary to reestablish their place within the everyday world. When the grief reaction is prolonged, individuals may develop a pathological grief reaction, which may become more disabling than the chronic illness or disability itself.

Fear and Anxiety

Individuals normally become anxious when confronted with a threat. The presence of a chronic illness or disability can pose a threat because of the potential loss of function, loss of love, loss of independence, or loss of financial security. Threats cause anxiety. Some individuals fear the unknown or unpredictability of the condition, which provokes anxiety. For others, hospitalizations that immerse them in a strange and unfamiliar environment away from home, family, and the security of routine produces anxiety. When conditions are life-threatening, fear and anxiety may be associated not only with loss of function, but also with loss of life. Fear and anxiety associated with chronic illness or disability can place individuals in a state of panic, rendering them psychologically immobile and unable to act.

Assisting individuals to regain a sense of control over their situation through information and shared decision making can be an important step in reducing anxiety and facilitating rehabilitation. It is important to note that fear experienced by individuals may have both rational and irrational aspects. Fear and anxiety are oftentimes future oriented, having to do with perceptions of what could occur rather than based on what is actually known in the present.

Anger

Individuals with chronic illness or disability may experience anger at themselves or others for perceived injustices or loss associated with their condition. They may believe that their chronic illness or disability was caused by negligence or that their condition was avoidable. If they perceive themselves as victims, their anger may be directed toward the persons or circumstances they blame for the condition or situation. If they believe that their own actions

were partly to blame for the chronic illness or disability, the anger may be directed inward.

Anger can also be the result of frustration. Individuals may vent their frustration and anger by displacing hostility toward others, even when those parties have no relationship to the development of the chronic illness or disability and no influence over its outcome. Anger may also be an expression of the realization of the seriousness of the situation and associated feelings of helplessness. At times, anger may not be openly expressed but rather hidden in quarreling, arguing, complaining, or being excessively demanding, in an attempt to gain some control. Helping individuals express anger in appropriate ways and enabling them to regain a sense of control over their situation can help to resolve anger that would otherwise be detrimental to successful rehabilitation.

Depression

With the realization of the reality, seriousness, and implications of the chronic illness or disability, individuals may experience feelings of depression, helplessness and hopelessness, apathy, and/or feelings of dejection and discouragement. Signs of depression include sleep disturbances, changes in appetite, difficulty concentrating, and withdrawal from activity. Not all individuals with chronic illness or disability experience significant depression and, in those who do, depression may not be prolonged. The extent to which depression is experienced varies from person to person. Prolonged or unresolved depression can result in self-destructive behaviors, such as substance abuse or attempted suicide. Individuals with prolonged depression should be referred for mental health evaluation and treatment.

Guilt

Guilt can be described as self-criticism or blame. Individuals or family members may feel guilt if they believe they contributed to, or in some way caused, the chronic illness or disability. For instance, individuals who develop lung cancer or emphysema after years of tobacco use, or those who experienced a spinal cord injury owing to an accident that occurred because they were driving while intoxicated, may experience guilt because of the role they played in the development of their chronic illness and disability. In other instances, they may experience guilt because they believe their chronic illness or disability places a burden on their family, or because they are unable to fulfill former roles. Still other scenarios of guilt include the concept of *survivor guilt*, in which an individual survives a situation when others in the same situation did not. For example, an individual who, although sustaining severe injuries, survives a tornado when none of his or her family members did may experience intense guilt, questioning why he or she survived when other family members perished.

Family members may also experience guilt because of feelings of anger or resentment they have toward the individual. Guilt may also be associated with blame if family members believe the individual is actively to blame for his or her chronic illness or disability. For instance, if an individual develops cirrhosis of the liver due to heavy drinking, but had been told previously to cut down on alcohol consumption because of impending liver failure, family members may actively blame the individual for his or her condition, causing the person to experience more guilt.

Guilt may be expressed or unexpressed and can occur in varying dimensions. It can be an obstacle to the successful adjustment to the condition and its limitations. Self-blame or blame ascribed by others is detrimental not only to the individual's self-concept, but also to rehabilitative efforts as a whole. Guilt that affects rehabilitation potential or well-being is an indication that referral to appropriate professionals for evaluation and treatment may be appropriate.

■ CHRONIC ILLNESS AND DISABILITY THROUGH THE LIFE CYCLE

Development is not static or finite but rather a continual process from infancy to old age and death. Each developmental stage is associated with certain age-appropriate behaviors, skills, and developmental tasks, which allow for psychological and cognitive transitions from one stage to another. Individuals' age and developmental stage influence their reactions to chronic illness or disability and the problems and consequences they experience.

Each developmental stage of life has its own particular stresses or demands, apart from those experienced as a result of illness or disability. Chronic illness and disability at various stages of development can influence the independence and self-control associated with the developmental stages and can impede development of qualities and life skills associated with different developmental stages. The needs, responsibilities, and resources of adults differ from those of children; as a consequence, the impact of chronic illness or disability in later years is different from the impact of chronic illness or disability experienced in young adulthood.

Family members and others generally adjust their behavior to accommodate and appropriately interact with individuals as they pass from one developmental stage to the next. When individuals experience chronic illness or disability, however, others may modify expectations of age-appropriate behavior. These modified expectations may then interfere with the individual's mastery of the normal skills required to meet the challenges of future developmental stages.

All aspects of development are related, so each developmental stage must be understood within the context of the individual's past and current experiences. Individuals with chronic illness or disability must be considered in the context of their particular developmental stage and the way in which the changes and limitations associated with their condition influence attitudes, perceptions, actions, and behaviors characteristic of stage of development. Individuals' stage of development serves as a guideline not only in assessing their functional capacity, but also in determining potential stressors and reactions.

Problems and stresses at different developmental stages are similar whether individuals do or do not have a chronic illness or disability. Although there are no clear lines of demarcation between life stages and all individuals certainly develop at different rates, there are some commonalities associated with different life stages.

Ideally, those with chronic illness or disability should be encouraged to progress through each stage of development as normally as possible, despite their condition. Individuals whose emotional, social, educational, or occupational development has been thwarted may be more handicapped by their inability to cope with the subsequent challenges of life than by any limitations experienced because of illness or disability per se.

Chronic Illness or Disability in Childhood

Although the majority of children with chronic illness or disability and their families adapt successfully, children with chronic illness or disability are at increased risk of emotional and behavioral disorders (Gledhill, Rangel, & Garralda, 2000). In early life, children develop a sense of trust in others, a sense of autonomy, and an awareness and mastery of their environment. During these years, they begin to learn communication and social skills that enable them to interact effectively with others. They also learn that limits are set on their explorations, expressions of autonomy, and behaviors. Important to their development is a balance between encouraging initiative and setting limits consistently.

Chronic illness or disability can impede attainment of normal developmental goals. Repeated or prolonged hospitalizations may deprive children of nurturing by a consistent and loving caregiver. Physical limitations associated with the condition or treatment may prevent normal activities, socialization, and exploration of the environment. In some cases, overly protective family members may restrict activities or prohibit the child from displaying normal emotional expression. In other instances, overly sympathetic parents may condone inappropriate behaviors rather than correct them.

Conditions affecting development of communication skills may also affect children's interaction with the environment as well as their future development. Developmental disabilities (conditions present at birth or occurring during childhood) require adjustments throughout individuals' development. Limitations associated with such a developmental disability must be confronted and compensated for with every new aspect of normal development. Maintaining awareness of normal developmental needs and facilitating of experiences that foster normal development will enhance children's ability to reach their full potential.

For most children, entering school expands their world beyond the scope of their family. Before children attend school, the values, rules, and expectations that they experience are, for the most part, largely those expressed within the family. When they enter school, however, they are exposed to a larger social environment. Not only do they learn social relationships and cooperative interactions, but they also begin to develop a sense of initiative and industry. Children gradually become aware of their special strengths. As new skills begin to develop, school-aged children gain the capacity for sustained effort that eventually results in the ability to follow through with tasks to completion. The approval and encouragement of others and acceptance by their peers help children to build self-confidence, further enhancing development.

When children with chronic illness or disability enter school, they may not need specific special education placement, but they may require coordinated school interventions to maximize attendance and facilitate educational and social growth. Children with chronic illness or disability may experience school-related problems reflected in their psychological well-being, interactions with other children, or academic performance. When physical or cognitive limitations affect children's ability to perform skills normally valued at this developmental stage, acceptance by peers may be affected. School attendance may be disrupted by the need for repeated absences, resulting in an inability to interact on a consistent basis within the peer group, which in turn may diminish social interactions.

In an attempt to shield the child from hurt and emotional pain, family members may further isolate the child from social interactions, creating the potential for reduced self-confidence. Reluctance of sympathetic family members to allow the child to participate in activities in which the child may experience failure can interfere with the child's ability to accurately evaluate his or her potential. Encouragement of social interactions and activities to the greatest degree possible allows the child the opportunity to develop the skills and abilities that are needed for later integration into the larger world.

Chronic Illness or Disability in Adolescence

Perceptions of and interactions with peers become increasingly important as adolescents further define their identity apart from membership in their family. With the need to establish independence, adolescents begin to emancipate themselves from their parents and may rebel against authority of parents or others. Physical maturation brings a strong preoccupation with the body and appearance. Adolescents' need to identify themselves as a person attractive to others often becomes paramount. Awareness of and experimentation with sexual feelings present a new dimension with which the adolescent must learn to cope. Dating and expression of sexuality are important aspects of maturation. Any alteration in physical appearance caused by the condition can influence adolescents' perception of body image and self-concept, thwarting expression of sexual feelings.

Adolescents with physical disabilities may be at risk for secondary disabilities associated with psychosocial factors. Illness or disability during adolescence can disrupt relationships with peers, resulting in delayed social and emotional development. Limitations experienced because of the condition, its treatment, or sympathetic and protective reactions by family members may become barriers to the adolescent's attainment of independence and individual identity. Parents may be overprotective to the point of infantilizing the adolescent, decreasing self-esteem and self-confidence.

In the attempt to become independent, characteristics of normal adolescent development, such as rebellion against authority or the need to be accepted by a peer group, may sometimes interfere with treatment necessitated by chronic illness or disability. If adolescents deny limitations associated with their disability or ignore treatment recommendations, there can be further detrimental effects on physical and functional capacity.

Chronic Illness or Disability in Young Adulthood

In young adulthood, individuals establish themselves as productive members of society, integrating vocational goals, developing the capacity for intimate relationships, and accepting social responsibility. When chronic illness or disability occur during this stage of the life cycle, associated limitations—rather than interests or abilities of individuals—may define social, vocational, and occupational goals.

Physical limitations may also inhibit individuals' efforts to build intimate relationships or to maintain relationships that they have already established. At this developmental stage, established relationships are likely to be recent, and the level of commitment and willingness to make necessary sacrifices may be variable. Depending on the nature of the condition, procreation may be difficult or impossible. If the individual already has young children, childcare issues may be the source of additional concerns in light of the functional limitations inherent in a specific chronic illness or disability. Young adults who had not yet fully gained independence or left their family of origin at the time of the onset of chronic illness or disability may find gaining independence more difficult. In some cases, the family's overprotectiveness may prevent individuals from having experiences appropriate to their own age group.

Chronic Illness or Disability in Middle Age

Individuals in middle age are generally established in their careers, have committed relationships, and are often providing guidance to their own children as they leave the family to establish their own careers and families. At the same time, middle-aged individuals may be assuming greater responsibility for their own aging parents, who may be becoming increasingly fragile and dependent. During middle age, individuals may begin to reassess their goals and relationships as they begin to recognize their own mortality and limited remaining time.

Illness or disability during middle age can interfere with further occupational development and may even result in early retirement. Such changes can have a significant impact on the economic well-being of individuals and their families, as well as on their identity, self-concept, and self-esteem. It may be necessary to alter established roles and associated responsibilities within the family. At the same time, individuals' partners, even when the relationship is a long-term one, may be reevaluating their own life goals. They may perceive chronic illness or disability as a violation of their own well-being and may choose to leave the relationship. Responsibilities for children and aging parents add more financial and emotional stress to that experienced as a result of illness or disability.

Chronic Illness or Disability in Older Adulthood

Ideally, older adults have adapted to the triumphs and disappointments of life and have accepted their own life and imminent death. Although physical limitations associated with normal aging are variable, older adults often experience diminished physical strength and stamina, as well as losses of visual and hearing acuity. Illness or disability during older adulthood can impose physical or cognitive limitations in addition to those caused by aging. The spouse or significant others of the same age group may also have decreased physical stamina, making physical care of individuals with chronic illness or disability more difficult. When older adults with chronic illness or disability are unable to attend to their own needs or when care in the home is unmanageable, they may find it necessary to surrender their own lifestyle and move to another environment for care and supervision. Many individuals in the older age group live on fixed retirement incomes, so the additional expenses associated with chronic illness or disability may place a significant strain on an already tight budget. Not all older individuals, of course, have retirement benefits, savings, or other resources to draw on in time of financial need.

■ MULTICULTURAL ISSUES IN CHRONIC ILLNESS AND DISABILITY

Adjustment and adaptation to chronic illness and disability are also related to a variety of cultural aspects, including race, gender, ethnicity, spiritual/religious beliefs, and sexual orientation. Cultural factors shape individuals' perception of self as well as define views of chronic illness and disability and their meaning in the context of culture. Concepts about causes of and reasons for various health conditions, values, and accepted ways of managing a condition are all cultural variables that determine attitude, adjustment, expectations, and outcomes related to chronic illness and disability.

■ OTHER ISSUES IN CHRONIC ILLNESS AND DISABILITY

Self-Concept, Self-Esteem, and Social Identity

Self-concept is tied to self-esteem and personal identity, and includes individuals' perceptions and beliefs about their own strengths and weaknesses, as well as others' perceptions

of them. *Self-esteem* can be defined as "the evaluative component of an individual's self-concept" (Corwyn, 2000, p. 357). It is often thought of as individuals' assessment of their own self-worth with regard to attained qualities and performance (Gledhill, Rangel, & Garralda, 2000).

Self-concept influences the perceptions of others about an individual. A negative self-concept can produce negative responses in others, just as a positive self-concept can increase the likelihood that others will react in a positive manner. Individuals' self-esteem is related to their self-concept and how others respond to them. Consequently, self-concept has a significant impact on interactions with others and the psychological well-being of the individual.

Social identity is a term that refers to an individual's self-concept that is derived from perceived membership in a social group (Tajfel & Turner, 1986). Depending on the social context, individuals may have different social identities at different levels according to their internalized perception of group membership. For example, an individual may identify himself or herself as a medical student, but may also identify himself or herself as a member of the Young Republicans or Young Democrats, or according to an ethnic group, such as Native American. Group membership involves defining the self in terms of characteristics of the group rather than as an individual. Group membership can be an aspect of self-concept and can provide grounds for group comparisons. The more individuals view group membership as central to their self-definition, the stronger their social identity with the group (Haslam, 2001).

Social identity can influence how individuals think, act, and feel based on their perception of group inclusion or exclusion. If an individual views a group positively, his or her perception of inclusion in the group can boost self-esteem. Perceptions of exclusion from the group can, however, have the opposite effect. Likewise, if an individual perceives a group negatively but identifies as part of the group, the person's self-esteem can be negatively affected.

Body Image

Body image, which is an important part of self-concept, involves individuals' mental view of their body with regard to appearance, sexuality, and ability to perform various physical tasks. It is influenced by bodily sensations, social and cultural expectations, and reactions of and experiences with others (White, 2000). Body image is influenced by each individual's personal conception of attractiveness, which is also determined by social and cultural influences and is related to both self-concept and self-esteem.

Body image is influenced by biological, cultural, social, and historical factors. It changes over time as alteration of appearance, capabilities, functional status, and social role occurs over the life cycle. Individuals' perceptions of their body are associated with more than cosmetic concerns; they also influence individuals' general health, personal relationships and intimacy, and general well-being (Biordi et al., 2002).

Chronic illness or disability may modify body image by requiring an alteration of self-view to accommodate the associated changes. The following factors influence the degree of alteration:

- Visibility of the change
- Functional significance of the change
- Speed with which the change occurred
- Importance of the physical change or associated functional limitations to the individual
- Reactions of others (Moore, Franzep, Hennessey, Kunz, Ferrando, & Rabkin, 2000)

Body image is a reflection of individuals' image of themselves as well as how they believe others see them. Individuals' feelings and thoughts about their body image influence not only social relationships, but also psychological characteristics and perceptions of the world. The degree to which the alteration of self-view is perceived by the individual in a negative way influences social and intrapersonal interactions, functional capacity, and success or failure in the workplace (Cusack, 2000).

The extent to which individuals incorporate change into their body image also depends on the meaning and significance of the change to the particular individual. The degree of physical change or disfigurement is not always proportional to the reaction it provokes. A change considered minimal by one individual may be considered catastrophic by another person.

Changes do not have to be visible to alter body image. Burn scars on parts of the body normally covered by clothing or the introduction of an artificial opening or stoma such as with colostomy may cause significant alteration in body image even though physical changes are not readily apparent to others.

The concept of body image is complex and individually determined. Body image is not only the way individuals perceive themselves, but also the way they perceive others as seeing them. Negative views of body image can be a barrier to psychological well-being, social interactions, functional capacity, and workplace adjustment. Consequently, the ultimate goal is to help individuals adapt to changes brought about by chronic illness or disability, integrating changes into a restructured body image that can be assimilated and incorporated into daily life.

Stigma

Stigma is a socially constructed concept that is a universal phenomenon and has evolved throughout history. The concept is generally associated with individual feelings of shame due to disapproval of others and guilt resulting from being discredited or devalued by others. Stigma is something that precludes an individual's full social acceptance. The degree of stigma varies from setting to setting, and from person to person. Although the concept of stigma is universal, it is socially constructed. As a consequence, a number of factors within different societies as well as within different cultures may modify what is considered stigmatizing.

Overall, stigma is related to what a certain society considers to be deviations from the norm in a number of different areas. These areas are defined by societally determined categories, which include those attributes, characteristics, and behaviors that individuals exhibit in each category. Because these categories are based on the expectations of the "majority," they define what is considered acceptable or "the norm" based on majority standards. Categories may include age, race, gender, ethnic background or nationality, religion, occupation, or social roles. Individuals who meet the expectations of the majority regarding appearance, behavior, or group association are generally accepted and valued. Individuals who deviate from the expectations of the majority regarding what is acceptable in these categories are labeled as different from the majority and, therefore, less desirable. Thus individuals deviating from these expectations are often stigmatized. Because stigma is socially defined, it can vary from setting to setting, depending on the views of the majority. What is stigmatizing in one setting may not be stigmatizing in another venue.

Most stigmas are viewed as anxiety provoking and threatening to others. For example, older adults are often stigmatized because aging is a reminder of mortality and vulnerability. Individuals from different ethnic backgrounds, nationalities, or religions may be stigmatized because of lack of understanding by the majority of the meanings of traditions or beliefs in different groups. Individuals with HIV/AIDS are often stigmatized based on moral judgments. Likewise, individuals with chronic illness or disability often experience stigma owing to negative value judgments. Stigma results in discrimination, social isolation, disregard, depreciation, devaluation, and, in some instances, threats to safety and well-being.

The power of stigma may overshadow the positive characteristics of individuals who experience the stigma. Individuals who are stigmatized may find it difficult to overcome the social reactions of others regardless of their positive attributes. For example, individuals with psychiatric disability may face continued stereotypes and prejudices regarding psychiatric disability regardless of their level of success in the workplace or community (Lyons & Ziviani, 1995).

Individuals with chronic illness and disability continue to experience stigma. Modern society's emphasis on youth, attractiveness, self-sufficiency, and productivity contribute to the tendency to devalue those who are perceived as deviating from these valued characteristics (Saylor, Yoder, & Mann, 2002). Stigma can have a profound effect on the ability to regain and maintain functional capacity and on the individual's acceptance of his or her illness or disability. Gender and race or ethnic background may be secondary sources of prejudice and subsequent stigma, causing additional stress and creating additional barriers to effective functioning (Nosek & Hughes, 2003).

Stigma affects not only the individual, but also members of his or her family. Family members may experience social isolation and prejudice because of their association with the individual. Family members' ability to cope with their family member's chronic illness or disability may be severely compromised by societal stigma. If there are unresolved family problems, societal stigma may merely exacerbate the shame and guilt they may already feel.

Stigma has an impact on individuals' self-concept and self-esteem, and can produce barriers that prohibit affected persons from reaching their full potential. In an effort to avoid stigma, individuals may deny, minimize, or ignore their condition or treatment recommendations. If the condition is not readily discernable, hiding the disability may be more easily accomplished. As time goes by and the individual's attempt to hide the chronic illness or disability becomes reinforced, they may become proficient in concealing the condition so as to reduce the associated stigma. Although stigma may be reduced in this way, pretending not to have the condition can become detrimental. Not only may denial interfere with needed treatment, but it may also delay acceptance of and adjustment to the condition (Saylor, Yoder, & Mann, 2002).

Although efforts to reduce or obliterate stigma in society should continue, stigma is most likely to be overcome through positive interactions with individuals. It is possible to reduce the negative implications of societal stigma by helping individuals establish a sense of their own intrinsic worth.

The Impact of Uncertainty

Uncertainty in the lives of individuals with chronic illness and disability can exist for a variety of reasons, but is often related to concerns about an unknown future, the erratic nature of symptoms, the unpredictability of progression of the disease, or the ambiguity of symptoms. Some chronic illnesses and disabilities have immediate and permanent effects on functional capacity; in other cases, the course of the illness or disability is more variable. Deterioration may occur slowly over the span of several years or rapidly within months. Some conditions have periods of remission, when symptoms become less noticeable or almost nonexistent, only to be followed by periods of unpredictable exacerbation, when symptoms become worse. In some cases, the same condition progresses at different rates for different individuals—progressing rapidly for some, but slowly for others. With some conditions, it is difficult to determine when or if the condition will reach the point of severe disability or whether a dramatic change of functional capacity will take place.

Uncertainty of prognosis or progression of the condition can make planning and prediction of the future difficult and can sometimes render an individual immobile. The unpredictability of chronic illness or disability can be frustrating for both affected individuals and those around them. There may be reluctance to plan for the future at all, so that inability to predict the future becomes more disabling than the actual physical consequences of the condition itself. In other instances, given the unpredictability of their condition, individuals may elect to follow a different life course than they would have otherwise chosen. Decisions not to have children, to cut down on the number of hours spent in the work environment, or to suddenly relocate to a different part of the country may be misinterpreted by those unaware of the individual's condition or its associated unpredictability. For those conditions in which symptoms or residual effects are unapparent to others, such decisions may be met with misunderstanding or criticism. Criticisms of such decisions may be particularly distressing to individuals who do not wish to disclose or share intimate details of their condition with the casual observer.

Insecurity about the course of the condition may also be reflected by the attitude of those closest to the individual who, in an attempt to protect the person from potential future loss, withdraw emotional interactions or support. Uncertainty of progression of a condition imposes particular challenges for individuals and their families and can be a source of stress. Emphasizing the importance of living in the present, rather than dwelling on events that may or may not occur, can help to reduce the amount of stress and anxiety experienced as well as enhance the quality of life currently experienced.

Invisible Disabilities

Some chronic illnesses or disabilities have associated physical changes that can be objectively assessed by others or have functional limitations that necessitate the use of adaptive devices. The *visibility* of a condition has often been associated with stigmatization and marginality (Livneh & Wilson, 2003). Some conditions, such as diabetes or cardiac conditions, have no outward signs that alert casual observers to individuals' condition. The term *invisible disability* refers to these latter conditions. Because there are no outward physical signs or other cues to indicate limitations associated with chronic illness or disability, others have no basis on which to alter expectations with regard to individuals' functional capacity. Although this lack of reaction can be positive (in the sense that it prevents actions by others that are based on prejudice or stereotypes), it can also be negative in the sense that it can enable individuals to deny or avoid acceptance of their condition and its associated implications.

The degree to which a condition remains invisible may be a function of the closeness of the observer's association with the individual. Although casual acquaintances may not notice the limitations, those more closely involved with the individual in day-to-day activities may more readily observe them. Other conditions under normal circumstances may offer no visible signs or cues, no matter how close the association with the individual.

The unapparent aspect of the limitation in invisible disability may be a unique element related to individuals' adjustment and acceptance of their limitation. Without environmental feedback to create a tangible reality of the condition, individuals with invisible disability may postpone adaptation or ignore medical treatment or recommendations necessary for control of the condition and prevention of further disability.

Sexuality

Human sexuality is more than genital acts or sexual function. It is intrinsic to a person's sense of self (Hordern & Currow, 2003). It is an ever-changing, lived experience, affecting the way individuals view themselves and their bodies (Hordern, 2000). Sexuality encompasses the whole person and is reflected in all that individuals say and do. It is an important part of identity, self-image, and self-concept. Each person is a sexual being with a need for intimacy, physical contact, and love. The effects of chronic illness or disability on sexuality are multifactorial and can affect all phases of sexual response (McInnes, 2003).

Expression of sexual urges is one form of sexuality. Chronic illness or disability can affect sexual expression through physical limitations, depression, lack of energy, pain, alterations in self-image, or the reactions of others. In some conditions, the main barrier to sexual expression may be problems with self-concept and bodyimage; with other conditions, physical changes may present physical barriers, which affect sexual function directly. In other instances, attitudes of others or of society as a whole can be a major barrier to sexual expression. For example, although there has been increased acceptance of expression of sexuality by adults with intellectual disability, sexual expression that includes marriage or desire to start a family remains contentious (Cuskelly & Bryde, 2004).

Regardless of the types of limitations associated with chronic illness or disability, sexual expression remains an important part of function that should be addressed (McBride & Rines, 2000). In some instances, it may be necessary to help individuals overcome their own misperceptions and fears to establish a means for sexual expression. In other instances, individuals may need assistance to overcome barriers or to learn methods of sexual expression different from those used previously. In any case, sexual adjustment is a significant element in the restoration of an individual's optimal functional capacity.

Family Adaptation to Chronic Illness and Disability

Family is the social network from which individuals derive identity and with which individuals feel strong psychological bonds. Family has different meanings for different people and is not always related by blood or law. Family provides protection, socialization, physical care, support, and love. Each individual within the family structure plays some role that is incorporated into everyday family function.

Chronic illness or disability has both emotional and economic impacts on families as well as on individuals. Family reactions to chronic illness and disability may be similar to those experienced by the individual and may include shock, denial, anger, guilt, anxiety, and depression. Families must make adaptations, adjustments, and role changes both as a unit and as individual family members. The way in which families react and adapt to chronic illness and disability will influence affected individuals' subsequent adjustment. Whether families foster independence or dependence, show acceptance or rejection, or encourage or sabotage compliance with restrictions and recommended treatments has profound effects on individuals' ultimate functional capacity.

Specific issues for families when a family member develops chronic illness or disability are loss related to normal family functioning and loss related to functioning of the individual. There may be a strong desire to be a "normal" family again. Family members' prior expectations for the individual's future or

"what might have been" may lead them to experience anger, resentment, or disappointment if they see chronic illness or disability as interfering with achievement of their expectations.

Family members can also act as advocates for the individual. They may need to become more involved with health professionals and service agencies or become increasingly assertive to obtain necessary services. If individuals with chronic illness or disability require significant care or therapies to be administered at home, family members may become fatigued because of the extra responsibility and tasks required, especially if respite services are limited.

Families, like individuals, have differing resources, depending on life circumstances, previous experiences, and the personalities involved. Individual family members may be called upon to provide not only emotional support, but also physical care, supervision, transportation, or a variety of other services necessitated by the individual's condition. In addition, changes of roles or financial circumstances due to chronic illness or disability may alter goals and plans of other family members, such as college plans of a sibling or early retirement plans of a parent. The amount of care and attention required by individuals with chronic illness or disability may create emotional strain among family members, resulting in feelings of resentment, antagonism, and frustration. Role change and ambiguity may make it necessary to redefine family relationships as new and unaccustomed duties and responsibilities arise.

Quality of Life

Successful rehabilitation means more than assisting individuals to reach their optimal functional capacity; it also means assisting individuals to achieve and enhance quality of life. *Quality of life* is subjective in nature with no universal meaning. No two people define the term in quite the same way. Although quality of life may be viewed by some as optimal functioning at the highest level of independence, others may place greater emphasis on life itself, regardless of level of function. Only the individual can determine the personal meaning of the quality of life. Individual value systems, cultural backgrounds, spiritual perspectives, and the attitudes and reactions of those within the environment all influence the interpretation of quality of life.

Each individual's situation and experience are unique. Perceptions of the same condition and its impact vary from individual to individual (Burker, Carels, Thompson, Rodgers, & Egan, 2000; Crews, Jefferson, Broshek, Barth, & Robbins, 2000). People with similar conditions, symptoms, and limitations may perceive their condition in totally different manners.

The perception of chronic illness or disability depends on characteristics of the condition and treatment, age and developmental stage of the individual, the degree of limitation and the extent of disability experienced, and the manner in which characteristics of the condition affect the individual's definition of quality of life. Symptoms or limitations that one individual accepts and to which he or she adapts may be perceived as overwhelming and intolerable to another individual. The impact of chronic illness or disability on the overall quality of life often determines daily choices and day-to-day management of the condition.

Assessment of quality of life is made difficult by the ambiguous nature of the concept. Attempts to discover and accurately measure quality of life have caused considerable confusion and resulted in the development of multiple indicators. Indicators of quality of life have ranged from physiologic parameters, to the ability to return to work, to the ability to participate in social activities, to the number of psychological problems experienced by the individual. In addition, studies of quality of life have often identified discrepancies between the judgment of service providers and that of consumers regarding quality-of-life outcomes (Leplege & Hunt, 1997).

Individuals' perception of quality of life is among the main determinants of demand for services, compliance with treatment, and satisfaction with treatment and services provided. How some individuals assess the impact of their condition on their quality of life is determined by the degree to which they feel they have control over their life circumstances or destiny. Accurate knowledge about their condition and treatment, together with active participation in decision making about the management of the condition, can enable individuals with chronic illness and disability to make judgments that will enable them to enhance quality of life in terms of their own needs, goals, and circumstances.

Adherence to Prescribed Treatment and Recommendations

Most chronic illnesses or disabling conditions require ongoing treatment, medical supervision, or restrictions on activity to control the condition or to prevent complications. However, many individuals with chronic illness or disability fail to follow the recommendations prescribed, potentially imperiling their own well-being (Graham, 2003; Dunbar-Jacob, Erlen, Schlenk, Ryan, Sereika, & Doswell, 2000). Neglecting to take medications as prescribed, resisting restriction of activities, or engaging in behaviors that are likely to cause complications of chronic illness or disability can significantly influence individuals' medical prognosis and functional capacity (Dolder, Lacro, Leckband, & Jeste, 2003; Vergouwen, Bakker, Katon, Verheij, & Koerselman, 2003; Zygmunt, Olfson, Boyer, & Mechanic, 2002; Schmaling, Afari, & Blume, 2000). The best rehabilitation plan is of little value if individuals do not follow the treatments designed to manage their symptoms or condition or to prevent complications or progression (Loghman-Adham, 2003; Kovac, Patel, Peterson, & Kimmel, 2002).

Although individuals who purposely behave in a way that makes their condition worse seem irrational, there are a number of explanations for nonadherent behavior. Illness or disability elicits many responses from individuals and their families. Different reactions, experiences, and motives direct behavior and can help or hinder adherence to treatment recommendations.

Individuals' lives are guided by a set of norms and values—expressed and unexpressed. Each individual has a personal, unique perspective on health, illness, and medical care itself. There is a remarkable difference in perceptions of and reactions to apparently similar medical conditions. The meaning of illness and the consequences ascribed to adherence to recommendations are based mainly on individuals' perceptions of the condition and its associated limitations as well as their perceptions of treatment recommendations and their implications. While some individuals react mildly to a condition that may devastate another, others display considerable emotional and physical discomfort with conditions that most people consider minor. Obviously, various psychosocial factors determine individuals' reactions to illness and, consequently, their reactions to the recommendations and advice given.

Chronic illness or disability disrupts the way individuals view themselves and the world, and it can produce distortions in thinking. Most individuals initially experience a feeling of vulnerability and a shattering of the magical belief that they are immune from illness, injury, or even death. With this realization, they may lose their sense of security and cohesiveness. Life may seem a maze of inconveniences, hazards, and restrictions. Nonadherence to recommendations may be an attempt to exert self-determination, to regain a sense of autonomy and control, and to claim some mastery over individual destiny. In other instances, resistance to treatment recommendations may be a denial of the condition itself.

Nonadherence can also be a reflection of individuals' feelings about their life circumstances. For some individuals, having a chronic illness or disability is not a positive role; for others, it may be far preferable to the social role that they held previously. Some persons may vacillate between the wish to be independent and the wish to remain dependent. Chronic illness or disability can be a means of legitimizing dependency as well as a means of increasing the amount of attention received. Subsequently, individuals may be reluctant to return to their former roles and obligations. The motivation to retain the sick role is at times greater than the motivation to gain optimal function. As a result, ultimate rehabilitation is hampered.

Failure to adhere to recommendations is sometimes a response to guilt that has been incorporated into the reaction to or beliefs about illness or disability. If health and well-being are perceived as rewards for a life well lived, illness or disability may be viewed as punishment for real or imagined actions of the past. Adherence to medical advice may be perceived as interference with a punishment believed to be deserved. In other instances, individuals may feel guilty because they believe that the illness or disability is a direct result of their own negligence or overt actions.

Guilt or shame at being different may also hinder adherence to treatment recommendations. Some individuals may attempt to hide their condition from others and, therefore, fail to follow recommendations that they fear may call attention to their condition.

The impact of chronic illness or disability on an individual's general economic well-being can also affect his or her ability and willingness to follow treatment recommendations. While many occupations offer fringe benefits, such as paid sick days or even time off with pay in which to seek medical care, other occupations provide no such benefits. In the latter instances, days taken off from work because of illness or medical appointments can decrease income. The economic consequences of chronic illness or disability may also cause the opposite reaction. If an individual is receiving disability benefits and has little opportunity for satisfactory employment, he or she may not follow recommendations that would increase their ability to return to work, thereby decreasing or eliminating benefits.

Finally, quality of life is a relative concept, uniquely defined by each individual. If treatment recommendations, or side effects of treatment, result in pain, discomfort, or inconvenience greater than the benefit perceived by the individual in terms of his or her own subjective definition of the quality of life, compliance with prescribed recommendations may not be perceived as worth the psychological, social, or physical cost. Treatment can sometimes—but not always—be adjusted to make adhering to recommendations more palatable. Individuals' right to self-determination must be carefully balanced with assurance that the choice of nonadherence is based on information and full understanding of the consequences.

Some individuals readily adjust to the challenges, limitations, and associated behavioral changes necessitated by chronic illness or disability. Many individuals, however, actively sabotage treatment and recommendations, to their own detriment. In such instances, professionals' goals should be to attempt to understand the underlying problems and motivations of individuals and to help them make the necessary adjustments and adaptations to maximize their functional

outcomes. Rather than criticizing individuals with chronic illness or disability for disinterest, a lack of motivation, or failure to follow recommendations, it is important to identify the barriers that inhibit adherence and to recognize that such reactions may indicate difficulty in accepting the condition or adapting recommendations into the individual's own unique way of life. The best way to achieve adherence is to consider the individual's perceptions, goals, and environment and lifestyle, and to tailor recommendations to best meet those needs (Falvo, 2004).

Client and Family Education (Patient Education)

Although medical care, support, and auxiliary services are important aspects of helping individuals reach their optimal potential, successful management of chronic disease or disability requires considerable individual and family effort. Regardless of the complexity of the condition, many individuals are now expected to carry out treatments in their home rather than depend on medical personnel in healthcare settings. Individuals' understanding of their condition and treatment is one of the basic components of self-determination and responsible care. Not only must they understand how to integrate these regimens into their daily routines and how to carry out daily care activities, but they must also understand preventive healthcare measures to help them retain function and prevent further disability or health problems (Falvo, 2004).

Because of increasing public awareness of the need for individuals to accept this greater role of responsibility and self-determination, a number of programs and counseling services have been established to help clients and their families reach this goal. Client and family education can take place individually or in a group setting, can be formal or informal, and can include ongoing counseling or referral to resources for self-directed learning. Regardless of the type of setting in which educational services are delivered, the most effective client education will be that which considers the specific circumstances and goals of the individual (Falvo, 2004).

Stages of Adaptation and Adjustment

A host of personal, social, and environmental experiences, demands, supports and resources, and coping strategies interact to influence adaptation outcomes (Livneh, 2001). The process of adjustment includes a search for meaning in the experience and an attempt to regain control and self-determination over the events that affect one's life. Most individuals with chronic illness and disability experience some form of loss—either a direct physical loss or a more indirect loss of the ability to participate in some previously performed activity. Regardless of the nature of the loss, a variety of reactions may take place while individuals attempt to make necessary adaptations and changes.

Stages of adjustment are individual and varied. The shock of diagnosis and its consequent implications may have a numbing effect, so initially individuals may demonstrate little emotional reaction. As the reality of the situation becomes clear, individuals may experience a sense of hopelessness and despair, mourning for a self, a role, or a function that is lost. They may also experience feelings of anger, which alternate with depression. Many individuals go through a period of mourning and bereavement similar to that experienced when a loved one is lost. Mourning is a natural reaction to loss and allows time for reflection and reestablishment of emotional equilibrium. As individuals begin to appraise their condition realistically, examine the limitations that it imposes, and adjust to the associated losses, they may gradually seek alternatives and adaptations to achieve their integration into a broader world.

The ultimate outcome of adjustment is acceptance of the condition and its associated limitations, along with a realistic appraisal and implementation of strengths. Acceptance does not mean passivity regarding implications of the condition, but rather that individuals are ready to move toward reaching optimal functional capacity. The amount of time that individuals need to reach acceptance is dependent on personality, reactions of family and significant others, life circumstances, available resources, and the types of challenges that confront each individual. Some individuals never reach acceptance. Maladjustment and nonacceptance are characterized by immobility, marked dependency, continued anger and hostility, prolonged mourning, or participation in detrimental or self-destructive activities. Just as coping mechanisms are vital parts of human nature, serving to protect against stress, reduce anxiety, and facilitate adjustment, so overuse or maladaptive use of coping mechanisms can postpone or inhibit adjustment.

■ FUNCTIONAL ASPECTS OF CHRONIC ILLNESS AND DISABILITY

Functional effects of chronic illness or disability are many and varied. Each individual has different needs, abilities, and circumstances that determine how chronic illness or disability affects his or her functional capacity. The extent to which the individual experiences disability as a result of the condition depends to a great extent on his or her goals and perception of the condition, the environment, and the reactions of family, friends, and the societal and political environment. The severity of the condition as measured by diagnostic tests is not always an indication of functional capacity. Also, individuals' ability to function is not always directly correlated with the severity of the condition itself. Rather, function is determined by an interaction of factors related to the person and his or her environment. Individuals' reactions may differ even though they have similar chronic illness or disability.

Professionals working with individuals with chronic illness or disability need an understanding of the potential limitations or restrictions associated with a specific condition or treatment to help individuals and their families make appropriate changes to gain optimal functional capacity. The effects of chronic illness and disability are far-reaching and include psychological, social, and vocational effects as well as changes and adjustments in both general lifestyle and activities of daily living. The medical diagnosis per se is not as important as the individual's goals and the degree to which function in each area of the individual's life is affected. The interactive nature of function between each of the areas determines the extent to which individuals can reach their optimal potential. A focus on any one area without full consideration of the impact of chronic illness or disability on all other areas can dilute the effectiveness of the total rehabilitative efforts. Understanding and working effectively with individuals who have a chronic illness or disability requires a broad outlook that goes beyond medical diagnosis; it requires recognition that the most important factor is the individuals' ability to function with the condition within their environment and all areas of their life.

Personal and Psychological Issues in Chronic Illness and Disability

Individuals react both cognitively and emotionally to events that involve them. These reactions, in turn, affect the later course of those events. Personal and psychological factors are ever present in all aspects of chronic illness and disability, and they influence individuals' response to the illness or disability. Sometimes psychological factors are part of the symptoms of the condition itself. These factors affect not only individuals' adjustment and subsequent functional capacity, but also their outcome and prognosis.

Lifestyle Activities Issues in Chronic Illness and Disability

Life activities consist of the daily tasks and activities of daily living within an individual's environment. They include the ability to perform tasks related to grooming, housekeeping, and preparing meals. They also include activities related to transportation, daily schedules, need for rest or activity, recreation, sexuality, and privacy. At times, limitations in performing the activities of daily living may result from environmental considerations that serve as barriers to effective functioning. Modifications such as widening doorways to permit the passage of a wheelchair, placing handrails in a bathroom, or installing more effective lighting may be required to increase functional capacity. Other modifications may be necessary because of the additional tasks and time commitments related to medical treatment of a specific condition. In some instances, restrictions of diet or activity, continued treatments, medical appointments, and related activities may require significant alteration of the individual's daily schedule.

Social Participation Issues in Chronic Illness and Disability

The social environment can be defined as individuals' perceived involvement in personal, family, group, and community relationships and activities. Social well-being is based on emotionally satisfying experiences in social activities involving those within the individual's social group. Chronic illness and disability often lead to changes in social status. Individuals with chronic illness or disability may find themselves in a socially devalued role. As a result, they may experience changes in social relationships or interactions, or limit the number of social activities; any of these changes can result in social isolation. Even when individuals with chronic illness or disability attempt to remain socially active, they may have difficulty entering community facilities because of environmental barriers or because of prejudice or stereotyping. Many factors contribute to an individual's adaptation or adjustment to any social limitations associated with a particular medical condition.

Individuals' perception or misperception of the reactions of others in social groups may determine the level of acceptance that they receive. The degree to which individuals are able to adapt, accept, and adjust to their condition are determined in part by their interactions with others in their environment as well as by their interpretation of the reactions of others.

Vocational Issues in Chronic Illness and Disability

The significance of work in the rehabilitation of people with chronic illness and disability has been well documented (Cunningham, Wolbert, & Brockmeier, 2000). Work involves more than remuneration for services rendered and does not necessarily include only activity related to financial incentives. Work provides a sense of contribution, accomplishment, and meaning to life (Ben-Shlomo, Canfield, & Warner, 2002; Corrigan, Bogner, Mysiw, Clinchot, & Fugate, 2001; Bond, Resnick, Bebout, Drake, Xie, & McHugo, 2001). Consequently, loss of ability to work extends beyond financial considerations to social and psychological well-being. Loss of ability to work means more than the loss of income; it also means the loss of a socially valued role. For many individuals,

work is not merely a major part of their identity, but a source of social interaction, structure, and purpose in life.

The degree to which chronic illness and disability affect individuals' ability and willingness to work depends on a variety of factors in addition to the limitations imposed by the illness or disability itself (Young & Murphy, 2002). These factors include the nature of the work, the physical environment of the work setting, and the attitudes of employers and co-workers. Psychosocial variables may also complicate functional capacity and, therefore, the rehabilitation process. At times, individuals with chronic illness or disability may continue to perform the same work they performed before the onset of the condition. At other times, certain work tasks, environmental conditions, or work schedules must be modified to accommodate limitations associated with the chronic illness or disability. If modifications cannot be made in these cases, individuals must change employment. Some individuals must assume disability status because appropriate modifications cannot be made or because their limitations are severe. Job stress or attitudes of employers or co-workers can also significantly interfere with individuals' ability to return to the workforce. Problems with transportation to and from work because of limitations associated with chronic illness or disability may make a return to work more difficult. In other instances, time required to carry out treatment recommendations related to the condition may make completing a full day at work virtually impossible.

Individuals' capacity to function at a job can depend on cognitive, psychomotor, and attitudinal factors as well as on the physical aspects of illness or disability. Accurate assessment of individuals' capacity to return to work consists of more than evaluation of physical factors alone. Success or failure at work is often determined by factors other than physical skill or ability. Individuals' fear of reinjury, vocational dissatisfaction, or legal issues can hamper return to work. Individuals' ability to relate to and interact with others within the work environment must also be considered. Interests, aptitudes, and abilities are always pivotal factors in determining vocational success, regardless of limitations. Effective rehabilitation that enables individuals to function effectively in their job often involves interdisciplinary efforts of many types of medical and nonmedical professionals to conduct assessment, evaluation, therapy, and vocational guidance.

■ REFERENCES

Anderson, E. M., & Klarke, L. (1982). *Disability in adolescence*. London: Methuen.

Ben-Shlomo, Y., Canfield, L., & Warner, T. (2002). What are the determinants of quality of life in people with cervical dystonia? *Journal of Neurology and Neurosurgical Psychiatry, 72*, 608–614.

Biordi, D. L., Boville, D., King, D. S., Knapik, G., Warner, A., Zartman, K. A., & Zwick D. M. (2002). In I. M. Lubkin & P. D. Larsen (Eds.), *Chronic illness: Impact and interventions* (5th ed., pp. 261–277). Sudbury, MA: Jones and Bartlett.

Bond, G. R., Resnick, S. G., Bebout, R. R., Drake, R. E., Xie, H., & McHugo, G. J. (2001). Does competitive employment improve nonvocational outcomes for people with severe mental illness? *Journal of Consulting Clinical Psychology, 69*, 489–501.

Burker, E. J., Carels, R. A., Thompson, L. F., Rodgers, L., & Egan, T. (2000). Quality of life in patients awaiting lung transplant: Cystic fibrosis versus other end-stage lung diseases. *Pediatric Pulmonology, 30*, 453–460.

Corbin, J. (2001). Introduction and overview of chronic illness and nursing. In R. Hyman & J. Corbin (Eds.), *Chronic illness: Research and theory for nursing practice* (pp. 1–15). New York: Springer.

Corrigan, J. D., Bogner, J. A., Mysiw, J. W., Clinchot, D., & Fugate, L. (2001). Life satisfaction after traumatic brain injury. *Journal of Head Trauma Rehabilitation, 16*, 543–555.

Corwyn, R. F. (2000). The factor structure of global self esteem among adolescents and adults. *Journal of Research and Personality, 34*, 357–379.

Crews, W., Jefferson, A., Broshek, D., Barth, J., & Robbins, M . (2000). Neuropsychological sequelae in a series of patients with end-stage cystic fibrosis: Lung transplant evaluation. *Archives of Clinical Neuropsychology, 15*, 59–70.

Cunningham, K., Wolbert, R., & Brockmeier, M. B. (2000). Moving beyond the illness: Factors contributing to gaining and maintaining employment. *American Journal of Community Psychology, 28*(4), 481–493.

Cusack, L. (2000). Perceptions of body image: Implications for the workplace. *Employee Assistance Quarterly, 15*(3), 23–29.

Cuskelly, M., & Bryde, R. (2004). Attitudes toward the sexuality of adults with an intellectual disability: Parents, support staff and a community sample. *Journal of Intellectual and Developmental Disability, 29*(3), 255–264.

Dolder, C. R., Lacro, J. P., Leckband, S., & Jeste, D. V. (2003). Interventions to improve antipsychotic medication adherence: Review of recent literature. *Journal of Clinical Psychopharmacology, 23*(4), 389–399.

Dudgeon, B. J. (2002) Physical disability and the experience of chronic pain. *Archives of Physical Medicine and Rehabilitation, 83*(2), 229–235.

Dunbar-Jacob, J., Erlen, J. A., Schlenk, E. A., Ryan, C. M., Sereika, S. M., & Doswell, W. M. (2000). Adherence in chronic disease. *Annual Review of Nursing Research, 18*, 48–90.

Falvo, D. R. (2004). *Effective patient education: A guide to increased compliance* Boston: Jones and Bartlett.

Gledhill, J., Rangel, L., & Garralda, E. (2000). Surviving chronic physical illness: Psychosocial outcomes in adult life. *Archives of Disease in Childhood, 83*(2), 104–110.

Graham, H. (2003). A conceptual map for studying long-term exercise adherence in a cardiac population. *Rehabilitation Nursing, 28*(3), 80–86.

Haslam, A. S. (2001). *Psychology in organizations: The social identity approach*. London: Sage.

Hordern, A. J. & Currow, D. C. (2003). A patient-centered approach to sexuality in the face of life-limiting illness. *Medical Journal of Australia, 179*(6 suppl), S8–11.

Kovac, J. A., Patel, S. S., Peterson, R. A., & Kimmel, P. L. (2002). Patient satisfaction with care and behavioral compliance in end-stage renal disease patients treated with hemodialysis. *American Journal of Kidney Disease, 39*(6), 1236–1244.

Leplege, A., & Hunt, S. (1997). The problem of quality of life in medicine. *Journal of the American Medical Association, 278*(1), 47–50.

Livneh, H. (2001). Psychosocial adaptation to chronic illness and disability: A conceptual framework. *Rehabilitation Counseling Bulletin, 44*(3), 150–160.

Livneh, H., & Wilson, L. M. (2003). Coping strategies as predictors and mediators of disability-related variables and psychosocial adaptation: An exploratory investigation. *Rehabilitation Counseling Bulletin, 46*(4), 194–208.

Loghman-Adham, M. (2003). Medication noncompliance in patients with chronic disease: Issues in dialysis and renal transplantation. *American Journal of Managed Care, 9*(2), 155–171.

Lyons, M., & Ziviani, H. (1995). Stereotypes, stigma, and mental illness: Learning from fieldwork experiences. *American Journal of Occupational Therapy, 49*(10), 1002–1008.

McBride, K. E., & Rines, B. (2000). Sexuality and spinal cord injury: A road map for nurses. *SCI Nursing, 17*(1), 8–13.

McInnes R. A. (2003). Chronic illness and sexuality. *Medical Journal of Australia, 179*(5), 263–266.

Moore, G. M., Hennessey, P., Kunz, N. M., Ferrando, S., & Rabkin, J. G. (2000). Kaposi's sarcoma: The scarlet letter of AIDS. The psychological effects of a skin disease. *Psychosomatics, 41*(4), 360–363.

Morof, I., Lubkin, P. D., & Larsen, P. (2002). *Chronic illness: Impact and interventions* Boston: Jones and Bartlett.

Nosek, M. A., & Hughes, R. B. (2003). Psychosocial issues of women with physical disabilities: The continuing gender debate. *Rehabilitation Counseling Bulletin, 46*(4), 224–233.

Saylor, C., Yoder, M., & Mann, R. J. (2002). Stigma. In I. M. Lubkin & P. D. Larsen (Eds.), *Chronic illness: Impact and interventions* (pp. 53–76). Sudbury, MA; Jones and Bartlett.

Schmaling, K. B., Afari, N., & Blume, A. W. (2000). Assessment of psychological factors associated with adherence to medication regimens among adult patients with asthma. *Journal of Asthma, 37*(4), 335–343.

Shaw, L., Segal, R., Polatajkos, H., & Harburn, K. (2002). Understanding return to work behaviors: Promoting the importance of individual perceptions in the study of return to work. *Disability & Rehabilitation, 24*(4), 185–195.

Tajfel, H., & Turner, J. C. (1986). The social identity theory of inter-group behavior. In S. Worchel & L. W. Austin (Eds.), *Psychology of intergroup relations.*, Chiucago: Nelson-Hall, Chicago, 129–152.

Vergouwen, A. C., Bakker, A., Katon, W. J., Verheij, T. J., & Koerselman, F. (2003). Improving adherence to antidepressants: A systematic review of interventions. *Journal of Clinical Psychiatry, 64*(12), 1415–1420.

White, C. A. (2000). Body image dimensions and cancer: A heuristic cognitive behavioural model. *Psych-Oncology, 9,* 183–192.

Young, A., & Murphy, G. A. (2002). A social psychology approach to measuring vocational rehabilitation intervention effectiveness. *Journal of Occupational Rehabilitation, 12,* 175–189.

Zygmunt, A., Olfson, M., Boyer, C. A., & Mechanic, D. (2002). Interventions to improve medication adherence in schizophrenia. *American Journal of Psychiatry, 159*(10), 1653–1654.

Chapter 3

Conditions of the Nervous System
Part I. Conditions of the Brain

■ STRUCTURE AND FUNCTION OF THE NERVOUS SYSTEM

The nervous system is a complex regulatory system that, along with the endocrine system (see Chapter 11), controls and coordinates activities and functions throughout the body, internally and externally, by sending, receiving, and sorting electrical impulses. Disruption of any part of the nervous system affects body function in some way, either internally or externally.

The nervous system consists of the *central nervous system*, which includes the *brain* and *spinal cord*, and the *peripheral nervous system*, which includes *nerve fibers* extending from the brain and spinal cord that carry information between the central nervous system and the rest of the body. The peripheral nervous system is further divided into two parts: *the afferent system*, which carries messages from other parts of the body *to* the central nervous system, and the *efferent system*, which carries messages *from* the central nervous system to other parts of the body (see Table 3-1).

Functions of the nervous system include the following:

- Organizing and directing motor responses of the *voluntary muscle system*, enabling the body to move more effectively as a whole and to achieve purposeful movement. This coordination of voluntary muscles makes possible complex activities, such as walking, running, playing a piano, and using a computer, as well as simple activities, such as maintaining muscle tone and posture while at rest.

Table 3-1   The Nervous System

I. Central nervous system
   A. Brain
   B. Spinal cord
II. Peripheral nervous system
   A. Afferent (sensory)
   B. Efferent (motor)
      1. Somatic nervous system
      2. Autonomic nervous system
         a. Sympathetic nervous system
         b. Parasympathetic nervous system

- Monitoring and recognizing stimuli (and information) within the environment, and then directing an appropriate response to the stimuli. This function makes possible reflex actions, such as pulling away one's hand from a hot surface, as well as perceiving music being played in the next room.

- Monitoring and coordinating internal body states so that internal organs function as a unit, internal body constancy is maintained, and protective action is taken. For example, in response to a lack of oxygen, more rapid breathing occurs; the body shivers in response to cold; and when threat or danger is encountered, the heart beats more rapidly.

Other functions, such as display of personality traits, language, speech, learning, remembering, feeling emotion, reasoning, and generating and relaying thoughts, are also controlled by the nervous system—specifically, by the brain.

Nerve Cells

Specialized cells called **neurons** are the functional units of the nervous system. Neurons transmit messages to and from the brain. They consist of a cell body and processes (*nerve fibers*) that extend beyond the cell body. In most cases, a single long nerve fiber called an *axon* conducts nerve impulses (and information) away from the cell body to other neurons. Smaller, shorter nerve fibers called **dendrites** conduct nerve impulses toward the cell body after receiving information from other neurons. Fibers that carry information from parts of the body to the brain are called **afferent neurons** (sensory neurons). Fibers that carry information from the brain to other parts of the body are called **efferent neurons** (motor neurons).

Surrounding neurons is a fatty sheath called **myelin,** which, much like the covering of electrical cords, provides insulation, ensuring that electrical impulses are able to flow smoothly and reliably. Information is passed from neuron to neuron by both electrical and chemical impulses. The electrical impulse, which has been picked up by the dendrites, is passed through the cell body to the axon. The electrical impulse then moves down the full length of the axon until it reaches its tip. At the tip of the axon are tiny processes, which release chemicals known as **neurotransmitters.** Neurotransmitters, through chemical means, transfer the impulse from one neuron to another across a space between the two neurons called the **synapse.** The electrical impulse, through the vehicle of neurotransmitters, then moves to the next neuron's dendrites and the process begins again (see Figure 3-1). After neurotransmitters are released, they are either taken up again by the neuron or destroyed.

Longer axons are generally grouped in bundles. When they are transmitting impulses within the central nervous system, these bundles are referred to as *tracts*. Those bundles located outside the central nervous system are referred to as *nerves*.

The Central Nervous System

The *central nervous system* is made up of the brain and spinal cord. Bony coverings protect both the brain and the spinal cord. On the interior of these bony coverings are three membranes (**meninges**) that provide additional protection:

- The **dura mater** is the outer membrane, lying closest to the bony covering of the brain and spinal cord.
- The **arachnoid membrane** is the middle membrane, a cobweb-appearing membrane.
- The **pia mater** is the inner membrane, which lies next to the brain and spinal cord.

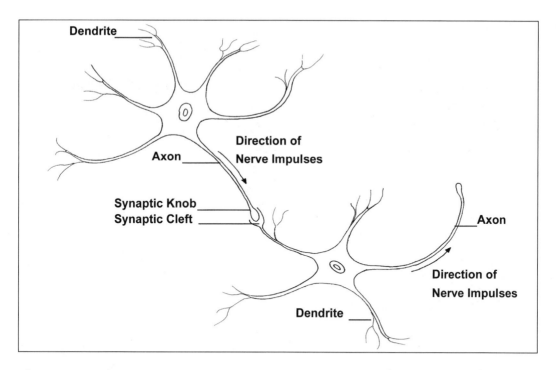

Figure 3-1   Neurons

Between each of the membrane layers are spaces. The space between the dura mater and the inner surface of the bony covering is the **epidural space**. The space between the dura mater and the arachnoid membrane is the **subdural space** and the space between the arachnoid membrane and the pia mater is the **subarachnoid space**.

The central nervous system is also protected and cushioned by **cerebrospinal fluid** (*CSF*), which is formed by specialized capillaries called the *choroids plexus* in inner chambers within the brain called **ventricles.** The cerebrospinal fluid bathes the brain and spinal cord, circulating from the ventricles into the subarachnoid space (see Figure 3-2). From the subarachnoid space it flows to the back of the brain, down around the spinal cord, and then back to the brain, where it is reabsorbed into the blood through the arachnoid membrane. The amounts of cerebrospinal fluid produced and absorbed are equally balanced, so that under normal conditions, the amount of cerebrospinal fluid within the central nervous system remains constant.

Another protective device is the *blood–brain barrier*, a structural arrangement of capillaries that selectively determine which substances can move from the blood into the brain. While substances such as oxygen and glucose are necessary to brain survival and consequently move freely across the blood–brain barrier, other potential harmful substances, such as toxins, are prevented from crossing into the brain.

The central nervous system is composed of white matter and gray matter. **White matter** makes up the inner part of the brain and the outer portion of the spinal cord and consists of myelinated covered axons that conduct nerve impulses. It is called white matter because of its whitish appearance due to the myelin covering. **Gray matter** makes up the thin outer layer of the brain and the inner

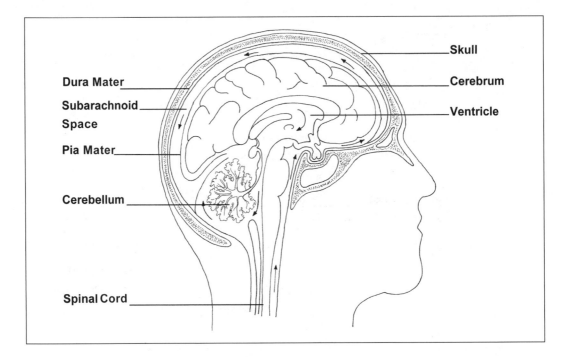

Figure labels:
Dura Mater
Subarachnoid Space
Pia Mater
Cerebellum
Spinal Cord
Skull
Cerebrum
Ventricle

Figure 3-2   Circulation of the cerebrospinal fluid

portion of the spinal cord. Small segments of gray matter are also embedded deep within certain parts of the white matter of the brain. Gray matter consists of groups of neuron cell bodies. It is called gray matter because of its grayish appearance. Gray matter of the brain receives, sorts, and processes nerve messages, while gray matter of the spinal cord serves as a center for reflex action (automatic response to stimuli).

The Brain

The brain is directly connected to the spinal cord and serves as the primary center for the integration, coordination, initiation, and interpretation of most nerve messages. It regulates and monitors many unconscious body functions, such as heart rate and respiration, and coordinates most voluntary movements. In addition, it is the site of higher cognitive processes such as learning, generating and relaying thoughts, reasoning, judgment, memory, consciousness, and emotion. The brain also has a sensory function, which is responsible for vision, hearing, touch, taste, and smell. Language function, including the ability to communicate and to comprehend, is also controlled by the brain. Finally, the brain controls basic behavior patterns and the display of general personality traits, which are characteristic of how each individual responds to stimuli.

The brain is protected by bony covering of the skull (**cranium** or *cranial bones*). The largest part of the brain, the **cerebrum**, is covered with a thin outer layer of gray matter called the **cortex,** which contains billions of nerve cells. The cortex has three specialized areas, which serve three major areas of function:

- The **motor cortex** coordinates voluntary movements of the body.
- The **sensory cortex** is responsible for the recognition or perception of sensory stimuli, such as touch, pain, smell, taste, vision, and hearing.

- The *associational cortex* is involved in cognitive functions such as memory, reasoning, abstract thinking, and consciousness.

The cerebrum is divided into two halves, called the *right hemisphere* and the *left hemisphere*. These two hemispheres communicate with each other. Dividing the hemispheres and connecting specific areas of the two hemispheres are bundles of nerve fibers called the *corpus callosum*. Each hemisphere has centers for receiving information and for initiating responses. The left hemisphere mostly receives information from and sends information to the right side of the body, whereas the right hemisphere mostly receives information from and sends information to the left side of the body.

Deep within the cerebral hemispheres are groups of gray matter called **basal ganglia**, which are part of the *extrapyramidal system*. ("Extrapyramidal" denotes nerve fiber tracts that lie outside the pyramidal tract, a relatively compact group of nerve fibers that originate from cells in the outer layer of the brain.) Extrapyramidal function is concerned with postural adjustment and gross voluntary and automatic muscular movements. The basal ganglia help to maintain tone in muscles in the trunk and extremities, enabling individuals to maintain balance and posture and to engage in movements such as walking. The basal ganglia also play a role in enabling individuals to react swiftly, appropriately, and automatically to stimuli that demand an immediate response, such as after tripping, enabling the individual to adjust movement to avoid a fall.

Each hemisphere of the cerebrum is divided into lobes that contain areas related to specific functions (see Figure 3-3). The **frontal lobe** is located in the front of each hemisphere and contains motor areas that initiate voluntary movement and skilled movements, such as those, involved in handwriting. Other areas in the frontal lobe control higher intellectual functions such as foresight, analytical thinking, and judgment. The **parietal lobe** is located in the middle of each hemisphere and is primarily the sensory area, integrating and interpreting sensation such as touch, pressure, pain, and temperature. Some memory functions are also located in the parietal lobe, especially those responsible for storage of sensory memory. The **temporal lobe** is located under the frontal and parietal lobes and is primarily responsible for the interpretation of and distinction between auditory stimuli. The **occipital lobe** is located at the back or posterior portion of each hemisphere. It is the primary area for reception and interpretation of visual stimuli.

Several parts of the cerebrum are involved in language function, which consists of the process of receiving, interpreting, and integrating visual and auditory stimuli as well as the ability to express thoughts in a coordinated way so that others can comprehend them. Language function is located in the left hemisphere of the cerebrum in most individuals, whether they are right- or left-handed. An area located over the temporal and parietal lobes, called **Wernicke's area**, is the major area responsible for *receptive function* (speech understanding), or the ability to integrate visual and auditory information so as to understand communication received. An area located in front of the temporal lobe and in the frontal cortex, called **Broca's area**, is responsible for speaking ability and is closely associated with motor areas that control the muscles needed for articulation. This area contributes to *expressive function* (speech formation), or the ability to integrate and coordinate words so that the meaning can be comprehended.

A structure known as the *thalamus* lies within the center of the brain. The thalamus acts as a relay station that sorts, interprets, and directs sensory information. Below the thalamus is the *hypothalamus,* which coordinates neural and endocrine activities. It helps

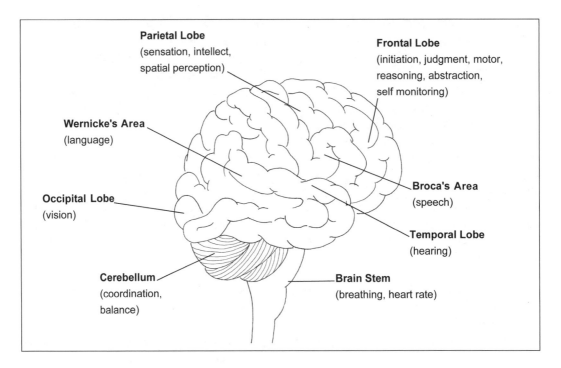

Figure 3-3   Areas of brain function

regulate the body's internal environment and behaviors that are important to survival, such as eating, drinking, and reproduction. Below the hypothalamus is the *pituitary gland*, an endocrine gland that will be discussed in more detail in a later chapter.

The *limbic system* is a group of structures consisting of both gray and white matter that surround the thalamus. The limbic system plays a role in expression of instincts, drives, and emotions and as the formation of memories. A band of gray matter called the *hippocampus* is involved in learning and long-term memory, helping to determine where important and relevant aspects of facts will be stored.

Beneath the occipital lobe of the cerebrum is a structure called the *cerebellum*. The cerebellum is primarily responsible for the coordination and integration of voluntary movement and for the maintenance of equilibrium, posture, and balance of the body. The cerebellum also regulates and coordinates fine movements of the extremities, which are initiated by the frontal lobe.

The **brain stem**, located beneath the cerebellum at the base of the brain just above the spinal cord, acts as a relay station, transmitting nerve impulses between the spinal cord and the brain. It is the primary center of involuntary functions. Control of vital organ functions, such as regulation of heartbeat or respiration, occurs in the brain stem. Areas in the brain stem also regulate the diameter of blood vessels, contributing to the control of blood pressure. Reflex actions, such as coughing and swallowing, are controlled in the brain stem as well. Finally, the brain stem contains scattered groups of cells, called the **reticular formation,** which are involved in the initiation and maintenance of wakefulness and alertness.

The brain requires both oxygen and nourishment in the form of *glucose* in order to function and to survive. Oxygen and glucose are transported to the brain by blood carried by four major arteries: two *carotid arteries* and two *vertebral arteries*. The vertebral arteries join to form the *basilar artery*. The carotid and basilar arteries then connect at the base of the brain to form the *circle of Willis,* from which *cerebral arteries* branch out to carry blood to the rest of the brain.

Brain Damage

The brain, like any other tissue, needs oxygen to function. Anything that interferes with the brain's ability to get oxygen or causes damage to the brain directly will impact its ability to function effectively. The manifestations of brain damage depend on the following factors:

- The cause of the damage
- The area of the brain damaged
- The extent of the damage

Generally, brain damage is classified as one of two types:

- Nontraumatic brain damage
- Traumatic brain injury

Nontraumatic brain damage refers to conditions in which the brain has sustained damage due to conditions unrelated to traumatic injury. It occurs at the cellular level in the brain, affecting its physical structure, metabolic activity, or the ability of brain cells to function (Pah-Lavan, 2006). Nontraumatic brain damage can be caused by interference with oxygen reaching the brain (such as with choking, carbon monoxide poisoning, or infection) or by problems within the brain itself (such as stroke or structural problems within the brain or blood vessels in the brain).

Specifically, *nontraumatic brain damage* is caused by conditions that cause restriction or interference with blood and oxygen reaching parts of the brain. When a part of the brain receives no oxygen (**anoxia**) or too little oxygen (**hypoxia**), the tissue can die. Examples of conditions that can cause acquired brain damage are stroke, congenital malformations [such as arteriovenous malformations (AVMs), in which blood vessels are abnormal at birth], **aneurysms** (in which a weakened area in an artery located in the brain balloons out and can rupture), infections or inflammations of the brain or surrounding membranes (such as **meningitis** or **encephalitis**), or other conditions that deprive the brain of oxygen such as strangulation, near-drowning, and inhalation of noxious gases.

Traumatic brain injury (TBI) (described in greater detail later in this chapter) is caused by an outside force that causes brain damage, such as a blow to the head or a gunshot. Owing to the nature of the injury and resulting impact on the brain, the damage with a TBI may be more diffuse than damage experienced in some acquired brain injuries. Although some of the same manifestations and sequelae may be present, nontraumatic and traumatic brain damage are categorized differently than brain damage that is associated with genetic or congenital conditions or degenerative disease.

■ NONTRAUMATIC BRAIN DAMAGE

Infections of the Central Nervous System

Any infection of the brain or the membranes that surround the brain and spinal cord can cause serious neurological effects, some of which may be permanent.

Meningitis

Meningitis refers to an inflammation of the **meninges** (membranes surrounding the brain and spinal cord). It can be caused by bacteria, viruses, or other organisms. Many types of meningitis exist, and the specific name given to the meningitis infection is frequently related to its cause or location. For instance, *cerebral meningitis* refers to meningitis of the brain, whereas *cerebrospinal meningitis* refers to meningitis of both the brain and the spinal cord. *Meningococcal meningitis* (commonly known as *spinal meningitis*) is caused by bacteria that settle in the lining of the throat and are spread easily through respiratory secretions. These organisms are relatively common. Normally, the lining of the throat is sufficient to act as a barrier to the bacteria; however, when the barrier is insufficient, the infecting organisms invade the bloodstream and reach the meninges, causing them to become inflamed. The organisms also gain access to the cerebrospinal fluid and begin to multiply.

The hallmark of meningitis is its rapid onset. Diagnosis is made by a *lumbar puncture* (spinal tap), in which a needle is inserted between the vertebrae and into the subarachnoid space. Cerebrospinal fluid is aspirated and examined microscopically for organisms.

Individuals with meningitis are usually acutely ill, initially with fever and flu-like symptoms. Within a short period of time they develop severe headache, neck rigidity, and visual discomfort when exposed to bright lights (*photophobia*). If the cause is bacterial in origin, prompt treatment with antibiotics reduces the chance of progression of the condition. The use of medication and prompt treatment have greatly reduced the number of fatalities from meningitis; however, if it occurs in individuals whose physical state is weakened or if diagnosis and treatment are delayed, it can still be fatal. Although most individuals with meningitis recover completely, some may have residual neurological deficits such as deafness, paralysis, or cognitive difficulties.

Immunization against *Haemophilus influenzae group B* (Hib) has greatly reduced the incidence of meningitis caused by this organism, which was formerly the most common type of meningitis in infancy. A vaccine against meningococcal disease is also available.

Encephalitis

Encephalitis is an inflammation of the brain due to direct invasion of an organism. It may be caused by an endemic virus, such as the West Nile virus, a mosquito-borne virus (Marfin & Gubler, 2001; Huhn, Sejvar, Montgomery, & Dworkin, 2003), or it may occur secondary to another infection, such as measles or chickenpox. Some individuals with encephalitis may experience severe headache, stiff neck, and coma. There is no adequate treatment for encephalitis, except for maintaining comfort

and preventing complications. The symptoms can subside in a few weeks, leaving no permanent damage; however, the condition can also be life-threatening. Some individuals develop irreversible neurological changes as a result of encephalitis.

Although encephalitis (or meningitis) and resulting deficits can occur in any age group, children and older adults are often the most susceptible to more severe manifestations of the disease. Individuals with compromised immune systems such as those with HIV or AIDS, individuals with cancer, or those who have received organ transplants are also at greater risk.

Stroke

Stroke, also known as **cerebral vascular accident (CVA),** is an acquired brain injury in which there is a sudden alteration in brain function resulting in weakness or paralysis in a body part as well as other neurological deficits due to decreased blood flow to a part of the brain. Stroke is usually the culmination of a progressive disease that has occurred over the course of many years. Heart disease or *ischemic vascular disease* (arteriosclerosis), **hypertension** (high blood pressure), and diabetes are often associated with stroke (Greenberg, 2006). Other risk factors include obesity, high cholesterol levels, physical inactivity, and alcohol and/or drug abuse, especially cocaine and amphetamine abuse (Gebel, 2007; Zivin, 2004).

Strokes may be caused by one of two events:

- Rupture of a blood vessel (*hemorrhagic stroke*)
- Occlusion of a blood vessel that diminishes blood flow (*ischemic stro**ke**).

Hemorrhagic Stroke

Hemorrhagic stroke occurs because of rupture of a blood vessel, causing hemorrhage. Death of brain tissue occurs in this instance not only because a certain area of the brain has been deprived of oxygen, but also because the escaped blood compresses brain tissue against the skull causing further damage.

A common cause of cerebral hemorrhage is **hypertension** (high blood pressure). When blood vessels are weakened because of disease such as arteriosclerosis or diabetes, or because of congenital weakness as with **aneurysm**, increased pressure may cause the blood vessel to burst. Blood vessels may rupture directly in the brain (*intracerebral hemorrhage*), causing a buildup of pressure and subsequent damage to the brain. Often when aneurysms burst, blood flows into the **subarachnoid space**, the space that is filled with cerebrospinal fluid. As blood fills the subarachnoid space, **acute hydrocephalus** (sudden buildup of fluid in the brain) may occur, impeding the normal flow and absorption of cerebral spinal fluid (Ellegala & Day, 2005), which in turn causes additional buildup of pressure in the brain. Additional risk factors for subarachnoid hemorrhage, in addition to hypertension, are cigarette smoking, cocaine use, and heavy alcohol use (Suarez, Tarr, & Selman, 2006).

Ischemic Stroke

Ischemic stroke is caused by diminished blood flow to the brain. A common cause of ischemic stroke is blocking of a cerebral artery by a clot (**thrombus**) that has formed inside the artery, a condition referred to as cerebral thrombosis. Formation of the thrombus blocks blood flow to an area of the brain. Because brain tissue needs oxygen contained in blood to survive, tissue, that cannot obtain needed oxygen because of the blockage dies within a short period of time. This tissue death is called an **infarct**. The amount of damage depends on the size of the area of the brain that has been deprived of blood supply.

Another cause of ischemic stroke is **embolism**. In this case, a clot, or other substance from another part of the body, forms and breaks off, traveling through the blood to the brain and lodging in one of the cerebral arteries. When the clot occludes blood flow to a part of the brain, surrounding brain tissue dies. Individuals who have a mechanical prosthetic valve in the heart to counteract atrial fibrillation (see Chapter 13) are at higher risk for ischemic stroke, as are individuals with *carotid stenosis* (narrowing of the carotid artery due to atherosclerosis) (Wirkowski, 2007).

At times, temporary blocking of the cerebral arteries causes slight, temporary neurological deficits. These "ministrokes" are referred to as **transient ischemic attacks (TIAs).** Although neurological deficits experienced from TIAs are usually temporary, their occurrence forewarns of the possibility of a larger stroke unless treatment controls the underlying condition.

Functional Consequences of Stroke

The amount and degree of function lost as the result of stroke depend on the following factors:

- The side of the brain affected
- The specific area of the brain that has been damaged
- The amount of damage that has occurred

Often after a stroke produces the initial damage to an area of the brain, surrounding brain tissue becomes **edematous** (swells) and inflamed, causing additional damage (Brown & Morgenstern, 2005). Although death of brain tissue causes permanent damage, areas of the brain that have experienced only swelling may recover, and function in these areas may be restored. Consequently, individuals experiencing stroke may not know the extent of their permanent functional limitations until months after the stroke has occurred.

Cognitive, language, and motor skills are often affected by stroke. Some individuals may also experience seizures after stroke. Other manifestations of stroke may include the following consequences:

- Weakness or paralysis in an extremity or one side of the body (**hemiplegia**)
- Loss of coordination (**ataxia**)
- Loss of sensation in half of the body (*hemiparesis*)

- Visual defects
- Loss of perception of visual depth and distance
- Auditory or other sensations (**agnosia**)
- Inability to organize and sequence specific muscle movements (**apraxia**)
- Difficulty with speech (**aphasia**)
- Cognitive losses
- Bowel or bladder dysfunction (Sandin, 2007)

Extensive physical rehabilitation as well as other therapies is often required for months to years after stroke. One of the functional consequences of stroke that may lead to the need for extensive physical rehabilitation is the inability to walk or to use an upper extremity due to spasticity or paralysis. Another functional consequence of stroke is aphasia, which also requires extensive therapy. Approximately 20% of individuals have difficulty with expression and comprehension of language after stroke (Dobkin, 2005).

Left-Sided versus Right-Sided Brain Damage

Although manifestations of brain damage vary with individuals, outward signs and symptoms of stroke are frequently related to which side of the brain has been damaged.

Left-Sided Brain Damage

The most visible sign of left-sided brain damage, regardless of the underlying cause, is right-sided motor and sensory paralysis. For individuals who are right-handed, everyday tasks such as feeding oneself, dressing, writing, or a number of other activities may be significantly affected.

For most people, regardless of whether they are right- or left -handed, the language center, which processes verbal symbols, is located in the left side of the brain. Consequently, individuals with left-sided damage will most likely have problems with verbal and/or written communication (aphasia). Although individuals

with left-sided brain damage may be able to understand more than they can speak or write, they often have difficulty understanding verbal and/or written communication as well. Even though individuals may have difficulty with speech and language, their ability to learn and communicate should not be underestimated. By the same token, individuals' ability to understand speech should not be overestimated. Usually individuals with this type of communication difficulty will be able to understand short, concise statements better than they can understand long, complicated sentences.

In general, besides having problems with language, individuals with left-sided brain damage tend to be slow, hesitant, anxious, and disorganized when presented with new or unfamiliar situations. Reassurance and frequent reinforcement for tasks performed correctly help reduce anxiety and enhance the individuals' ability to perform.

Right-Sided Brain Damage

The most visible sign of right-sided brain damage is left-sided motor and sensory paralysis. Often right-sided brain damage is accompanied by some degree of visual perception loss or loss of visual motor integration that affects spatial/perceptual function. Functional consequences of spatial/perceptual difficulty can be manifested in several ways. Individuals may experience loss of depth perception or lack of awareness of stimuli on the left side of the body, causing difficulty with navigation within the environment. For instance, individuals may miss the table with a glass when putting it down or bump into a doorway when attempting to go through it. Individuals with right-sided brain damage may also have difficulty processing visual cues. Consequently, an uncluttered, simple, and structured environment can help to prevent distraction and may enhance the individual's ability to perform certain tasks. Spatial/perceptual manifestations of right-sided brain damage may also affect the individual's ability to read. For instance, they may have an inability to move down the page without skipping lines.

Problems with memory may also be present with right-sided brain damage such that individuals are unable to recognize familiar people or places. In other instances, memory consequence is manifested as disorientation in familiar environments, so that individuals may require specific instructions about how to get from place to place. In other instances, memory difficulty may result in individuals forgetting where they have placed personal items and then concluding that someone else must have taken the items.

Because language function is often not affected with right-sided brain damage, the abilities of individuals with right-sided brain damage may be overestimated by others as well as by the individuals themselves. Individuals may be disinhibited and unaware of these consequences, and they may overestimate their own abilities to perform tasks, acting quickly and impulsively. As a result of diminished self-awareness, they tend to set unrealistic goals and appear insensitive to the needs of others. In other instances, individuals may have difficulty decoding nonverbal cues from others and, as a result, be oblivious to others, reactions or feelings.

Management of Stroke

After stabilization in the early phases of stroke, the major focus of treatment is restoration of function and reduction of limitations (Diller & Moroz, 2005). Most natural motor and functional recovery occurs in the first three months after stroke (Bjorkdahl, Nilsson, Grimby, & Sunnerhagen, 2006; Dobkin, 2005), although additional progress can be made through continuing therapy. *Physical therapy* and *occupational therapy* are often provided during the post-acute phase. In the early stages of therapy, focus is on helping individuals increase strength and prevent deformity, such as **contractures** (permanent contraction of a muscle that causes deformity of a joint), which can further limit function. As recovery progresses, goals such as achieving independent walking or walking with an assistive device, such as a cane or walker, and performing transfers such as from bed to chair become primary goals. When the hand and arm are affected, management is directed to helping individuals achieve self-care tasks such as feeding, bathing, and toileting. Individuals who experience aphasia may also receive *speech therapy*. Because the types and severity of aphasia vary widely, treatment is based on individual needs. The goal of treatment and rehabilitation is to help the individual reestablish, as much as possible, his or her independence, and to return to preexisting roles and relationships (Koch, Egbert, Coeling, & Ayers 2005).

Psychosocial Issues in Stroke

Many of the same psychosocial issues that present after a stroke are the same as those experienced in other types of brain injury (see the discussion of psychosocial issues in brain injury later in this chapter). Not only is stroke associated with many physical and neurobehavioral impairments, but it has many long-term psychological and social consequences as well (Jones, 2006). Depression is common after stroke (Chemerinski, Robinson, & Kosier, 2001). Stroke results in loss of functional independence, which in turn alters the individual's capacity for social role functioning. Stroke can alter the individual's perception of competency, identity, self-concept, and self-esteem (Vickery, 2006). In some instances the individual may not accurately perceive the functional consequences of the stroke, which may interfere with effective rehabilitation efforts (Powell, Johnston, & Johnston, 2007).

The psychosocial, physical, and economic consequences of stroke can be a major challenge to the family as well as to the individual (Sandin, 2007; Palmer, Glass, Palmer, Loo, & Wegener, 2004). Stroke can create a psychosocial crisis for the family not only because of the functional consequences experienced by the individual, but also because of the resulting increased caregiving responsibilities that family members must assume, often with little training or support (Palmer & Glass, 2003). After stroke, individuals are often discharged from acute care facilities much earlier today than they were in the past, so that much of the rehabilitation that had previously taken place in the hospital prior to discharge is now being conducted on an outpatient basis. Families are often unprepared for the complexity of interventions needed, the economic consequences, and their own role in contributing to effective rehabilitation outcomes for the individual after stroke (Palmer, Glass, Palmer, Loo, & Wegener, 2004).

Stroke rehabilitation must focus not only on recovery of muscle strength, range of motion, or mobility, but also on rebuilding individuals' identity, roles, and relationships (Palmer & Glass, 2003). Depending on the extent of brain damage experienced with stroke, individuals often require extensive and ongoing rehabilitation. The functional consequences of stroke are far-reaching.

■ CEREBRAL PALSY

Damage to the brain before, during, or shortly following birth may result in a condition known as **cerebral palsy**. Cerebral palsy is not a disease, but rather a complex of symptoms covering a wide number of neurological consequences that interfere with motor function and daily activities (Ostensjo, Carlberg, & Vollestad, 2004). Because it occurs prior to the age of 18, it is considered a *developmental disability*.

Cerebral palsy is characterized by chronic disorders of movement or posture. It may be accompanied by seizure disorders, sensory impairment, and cognitive limitation (Nelson, 2003). No two people with cerebral palsy are alike. Cerebral palsy is not progressive, communicable, or inherited. The condition is also not curable, because once damage to the brain

is sustained, damage is permanent. Nevertheless, different therapies and training programs can help individuals manage their symptoms and increase their functional capacity. Consequently, management is designed to enhance individuals' abilities, rather than to reverse the condition.

Causes of Cerebral Palsy

The causes of cerebral palsy vary widely:

- Birth injury in which the infant experiences direct damage to the brain, such as from ruptured blood vessels or compression of the brain
- Exposure of the mother to toxic chemicals or infectious disease during pregnancy
- Other causes, such as Rh or A-B-O blood type incompatibility between parents of the infant
- Lack of oxygen to the brain of the fetus before birth or shortly after birth resulting from conditions such as umbilical cord strangulation, prolonged labor (which stresses the fetus), or premature separation of the placenta from the uterus

Manifestations of Cerebral Palsy

The word "cerebral" refers to the brain. The word "palsy" refers to movement or posture. One characteristic of cerebral palsy is the inability to totally control and coordinate movement. The type of cerebral palsy and symptoms experienced depend on the location and the extent of the damage to the brain. Some individuals have minor, barely detectable symptoms; whereas other individuals have severe functional consequences.

Depending on the type of cerebral palsy, individuals may experience a number of symptoms affecting movement. One symptom may be **spasticity**, in which abnormality of muscle tone results in muscle stiffness and exaggerated muscle contraction. Spasticity interferes with dexterity and the ability to perform various muscle movements. Some individuals with cerebral palsy experience **ataxia** (disorder in the accuracy of muscle movement), which affects balance and coordination of gait. Still others have **dyskinesia** (unwanted, involuntary muscle movements), which interferes with the ability to conduct purposeful movements or causes movement when none is desired. Some individuals have a combination of spasticity, ataxia, or dyskinesia. In rare instances, **atonia**—in which there is lack of muscle tone and muscles are flaccid—may be present.

Abnormal movements may include any of the following:

- Purposeless, jerky, or abrupt movements (**chorea**) especially of the upper extremities
- Slow, continuous writhing movements (**athetosis**)
- A combination of chorea and athetosis (**choreoathetosis**)

Although cerebral palsy primarily affects muscle control, the brain is responsible for many other activities as well. Consequently, additional manifestations of cerebral palsy may include visual or hearing impairments, perceptual disorders, seizures, communication difficulties, intellectual disability, learning difficulties, or behavioral disorders, depending on the parts of the brain affected (Odding, Roebroeck, & Stam, 2006).

Classification of Cerebral Palsy

Clinically, cerebral palsy is classified according to the type of movement manifestations, their location, their degree, and the tone of muscles at rest. Clinical types of cerebral palsy based on classification of movement involved are as follows:

- *Spastic cerebral palsy*, in which individuals experience high muscle tone (**hypertonia**) so that muscles and joints are tight and stiff, limiting movements in areas of the body that are affected. Individuals often experience an increase in hypertonia with activity and interference with residual motor function.

- *Ataxic cerebral palsy*, in which individuals have difficulty with balance and coordination.
- *Athetoid cerebral palsy*, in which individuals exhibit uncoordinated, jerky, or twisting movements in affected body parts, particularly in fingers and wrists.
- *Mixed type cerebral palsy*, in which individuals experience manifestations of more than one clinical type of cerebral palsy.

Cerebral palsy can also be classified according to the location of the manifestations:

- **Hemiplegia** indicates that manifestations are found on only one side of the body, such as an arm and a leg on the right side.
- **Quadriplegia** indicates that manifestations affect all four extremities.
- **Diplegia** indicates that all extremities are affected, but lower extremities are more severely affected.
- Other classifications, such as **monoplegia**, in which only one limb is involved, and **triplegia**, in which three limbs are involved, are rare.

Another way of classifying cerebral palsy is by degree:

- *Mild cerebral palsy* describes manifestations that affect only fine motor movement.
- *Moderate cerebral palsy* describes manifestations that affect general muscle movement, fine motor movement, and clarity of speech so that activities of daily living and communication may be affected, but the individual is still able to function.
- *Severe cerebral palsy* describes manifestations that significantly affect the ability to walk, use the hands, or communicate so that the individual's ability to function in activities of daily living or communicate is extensively compromised.

Lastly, cerebral palsy may be classified according to muscle tone at rest:

- **Isotonic,** in which muscle tone is normal
- **Hypertonic,** in which there is increased muscle tone
- **Hypotonic,** in which there is decreased muscle tone

Management of Cerebral Palsy

Management of cerebral palsy is directed toward providing functional supports to individuals based on specific symptoms exhibited so that functional capacity can be enhanced and additional functional limitations prevented. Although cerebral palsy itself is not progressive, altered tone or activity of muscles may cause conditions that, in turn, result in additional limitations and consequences such as **contractures** (loss of range of motion or fixation of a joint) or **scoliosis** (lateral curvature of the spine). Consequently, in addition to helping individuals reach their maximum functional capacity, management of cerebral palsy is directed toward prevention of detrimental conditions that could impede function.

All aspects of management of symptoms of cerebral palsy should be directed toward giving individuals the opportunity to control and manage their own situation as much as possible. Major goals of management often include maintenance of range of motion of joints, so as to prevent contractures and other deformities, and increasing muscle control and coordination, so as to help individuals counteract abnormal postures. In addition, environmental modifications that help individuals perform activities of self-care, mobility, and social function are also important to help individuals achieve optimal functioning (Ostensjo, Carlberg, & Vollestad, 2005).

Interventions begin at an early age and include a number of services depending on specific needs and symptoms of the individual. *Physical therapy* may be instituted to increase and enhance motor skill and balance. *Occupational therapy* may be utilized to help individuals learn how to manage activities of daily living as well as other daily functions. *Orthotics* in the form of prescribed braces or splints may be used to help prevent or correct deformity. Braces can help individuals improve both functional mobility and appearance; the type of brace selected depends on the type of physical manifestation experienced.

Medical interventions may also be involved in the management of cerebral palsy. In some instances, medications may be prescribed to promote muscle relaxation when excessive muscle spasticity or excessive muscle tone is present. Anticonvulsant medications may be prescribed if individuals also have a seizure disorder associated with cerebral palsy. *Orthopedic surgery* may be needed to correct joint deformities or to lengthen muscles or tendons so as to decrease muscle spasm, thereby increasing functional capacity.

The best management of complications is through prevention. Contractures can be prevented through regular passive exercise or surgical intervention to lengthen already contracted muscles. Bowel and bladder incontinence can be managed through training programs that aim to help individuals establish dietary control and a regular evacuation schedule, as well as programs to increase awareness of sensory stimuli that indicate a need for evacuation. Individuals may decrease dental problems though training on oral hygiene and regular dental care. A specific program of weight-bearing and muscle activity as well as diet adequate in calcium can help to prevent osteoporosis. Training that helps individuals increase posture control and the use of bracing and splinting can decrease development of degenerative joint disease and scoliosis. Training to help individuals develop improved breathing patterns, coughing, and lung expansion can decrease the chances of aspiration, and consequently, respiratory infection.

Although cerebral palsy is not a progressive, degenerative condition, individuals with cerebral palsy have increasing functional impairment throughout life (Ando & Ueda, 2000).

For example, 35% of the adults in one study reported reduced walking ability, and 9% had stopped walking completely (Andersson & Mattsson, 2001). To maintain walking ability, individuals need to exercise regularly and have changes in walking ability monitored (Andersson, Asztalos, & Mattsson, 2006).

Due to their enhanced energy expenditure, fatigue may be an issue for individuals with cerebral palsy. Adequate rest at night and establishment of rest periods throughout the day can decrease fatigue. Evaluation of individuals' total energy output and adjustment of tasks and schedule to fit individual needs can help preserve energy and prevent excessive fatigue.

Complications of Cerebral Palsy

Due to the manifestations of cerebral palsy, a variety of complications that are secondary to the condition itself can alter the individual's function or well-being (Sandstrom, 2007). For example, contractures can limit both passive and active joint movement and interfere with self-care, walking, and sitting. Some individuals with cerebral palsy also experience bowel and bladder incontinence because they cannot attend or respond to sensory stimulus indicating the need to urinate or defecate. Other individuals may experience dental problems, which are exacerbated by an inability to brush the teeth adequately. Because of insufficient muscle activity, some individuals may be more prone to osteoporosis, which in turn can cause pain and increase susceptibility to fractures. Poorly aligned joints may predispose individuals to degenerative joint disease, resulting in pain and increased immobility. If individuals have poorly supported sitting posture, scoliosis (lateral curvature of the spine) may occur, compromising both breathing and functioning of internal organs. In cases in which coughing and swallowing abilities are insufficient, aspiration of food or fluids may place individuals at risk of development of respiratory infections or pneumonia.

Although not necessarily a complication, fatigue secondary to manifestations of cerebral palsy may interfere with individuals' ability to function efficiently. Because individuals with cerebral palsy may experience difficulty with motor control and coordination, more energy may need to be expended to carry out even routine motor activities. Involuntary movement or spasticity may also increase the amount of energy expended. As a result, individuals with cerebral palsy may become more easily fatigued.

Psychosocial Issues in Cerebral Palsy

Chronic illness or disability in childhood has implications for the psychosocial well-being of both the individual and his or her family (Barlow & Ellard, 2006). Positive peer interactions in childhood are associated with a number of developmental benefits, but individuals with a congenital condition may not have the same opportunities for developing positive relationships and may consequently be at increased risk for social difficulties (Cunningham, Thomas, & Warschausky, 2007).

Although data regarding psychosocial adjustment of adults with cerebral palsy are limited, cerebral palsy as a developmental disability poses many of the same problems as other developmental disabilities. Misunderstanding of the condition by parents, teachers, or others with whom individuals with cerebral palsy come in contact can perpetuate a sick and dependency status rather than a sense of empowerment. How individuals with cerebral palsy were treated in childhood can influence their self-perception and functioning in adulthood. In particular, childhood conditions can influence body image and prevent affected individuals from becoming involved in social relationships (Cho, 2004).

With any type of developmental disability, there is the risk of overprotectiveness from parents and others, which can impede the individual's emotional development by restricting access to experiences that are vital to the development of adequate coping strategies. As a result, children may learn, at an early age, to use maladaptive behavior to achieve goals. If this behavior continues into adulthood, it may impede the individual's ability to integrate effectively into the larger social milieu. When children have been kept overly dependent on parents, have been given little responsibility for home chores, have not been confronted with typical consequences of behavior, or have not learned acceptable means of expressing emotions, their lack of experience and mature social development can serve as a handicapping factor in adulthood.

In other instances, children who have been the focus of a wide variety of services and activities from an early age may continue these expectations into adulthood, demonstrating a sense of egocentricity, which in turn may limit positive social interactions and lead to further social isolation. If these behaviors persist into adulthood, they may become more of an impediment to social integration than any manifestations of the condition itself. In some individuals, brain damage associated with cerebral palsy may also create behavior deficits, which can interfere with development and maintenance of social relationships.

Activities and Participation

As adolescents, opportunities to participate in social activities, information related to sexuality, and opportunities to engage in sexual exploration and relationships may have been limited for individuals with cerebral palsy. Although there may be specific physical limitations and barriers associated with sexual activity, the largest barrier to establishing social and sexual relationships may be related to lack of information or resources (Wiegerink, Roebroeck, Donkervoort, Stam, & Cohen-Kettenis,

2006). In addition, adolescents with cerebral palsy may have a distorted body image and lowered self-concept, which may negatively affect their social competence, dating, and sexual behavior. Although individuals with cerebral palsy experience normal desires as both adolescents and as adults, they may lack the skills necessary to fulfill those needs. In addition to barriers of inadequate information, skill, or opportunity for appropriate sexual expression, individuals with cerebral palsy may experience physical barriers because of their condition that make sexual expression more difficult.

Communication issues for individuals with cerebral palsy may include hearing or auditory comprehension problems, visual disorders, or speech deficits. Individuals with communication problems as the result of cerebral palsy may have grown up in an environment in which family, friends, and others became accustomed to their adaptive communication methods. In adulthood, however, when relationships change and higher standards of performance are expected, communication may become increasingly difficult. For instance, those unfamiliar with the individual or with cerebral palsy itself may misinterpret problems with hearing or unintelligible speech as lack of cognitive ability. In other instances, because the individual may be difficult to understand, acquaintances may begin to avoid interactions with the individual so that he or she becomes socially isolated. Depending on the severity and type of cerebral palsy, decreased mobility, problems with eating, or problems with personal hygiene may further restrict the individual's social interactions.

Although the life expectancy for individuals with a variety of health conditions has, in the past, been less than the life expectancy for the general population, awareness of the importance of preventing complications and advances in medical care have expanded the number of adults with cerebral palsy living into older age. Older individuals with cerebral palsy experience many of the same issues as older adults without cerebral palsy, but recent studies have shown that older adults with cerebral palsy experience more loneliness than other adults in the older age category (Balandin, Berg, & Waller, 2006). In some instances, increasing levels of dependency due to the aging process and possible relocation due to a change in the individual's ability or a caregiver's inability to continue giving care may contribute to loneliness if the separation necessitates separation from family or friends. Encouraging individuals to develop leisure and recreational activities can facilitate social networking and provide opportunities for developing new friendships, although frequent contact alone does not necessarily protect one from loneliness (Balandin, Berg, & Waller, 2006). Although there may be a tendency to provide individuals with cerebral palsy the opportunity for social involvement through specialized disability services or organizations, involvement in community-integrated activities can facilitate social communication as a way to prevent loneliness, provide for development of friendships, and enhance the individual's sense of personal control (Ballin & Balandin, 2005).

Vocational Issues in Cerebral Palsy

Cerebral palsy is not a progressive condition, and progressive deterioration does not occur as a direct result of the cerebral palsy itself. Cerebral palsy is, however, a life-long condition. Consequently, follow-up throughout the individual's life may be necessary. As individuals age with their condition, additional limitations may occur. For instance, fatigue is a consideration for individuals with cerebral palsy regardless of their age. As individuals become older, however, their endurance for the same activities once performed over time may be decreased.

Long-term goals for persons with cerebral palsy are appropriate and desirable. The degree to which individuals are able to achieve their goals in a specified occupation will depend on their physical, psychosocial, and language abilities, as well as their motivation and social support networks. Specific skills and abilities may be enhanced with compensatory measures and/or with practice. Given that functional limitations associated with cerebral palsy are individualized, specific vocational limitations will depend on the symptoms that each individual experiences. In some instances, verbal communication is severely impaired; in other cases, it may be totally unaffected. Some individuals may have limited mobility or ambulation problems, whereas others may have significant difficulty with mobility or ambulation. While some individuals will be ambulatory, others may require use of a wheelchair. In some instances, individuals may have difficulty concentrating or remembering; in other instances, individuals' cognitive abilities are unaffected.

Because most jobs require some degree of social skill, when individuals have difficulty in this area, social skills training may be of benefit (Salkever, 2000). Matching the work setting to the individual's specific needs, interests, and abilities is important for anyone with disability; however, in the case of cerebral palsy, attention to these factors may be even more important to increase the potential for vocational success.

■ SEIZURE DISORDERS AND EPILEPSY

Seizures (temporary loss of control over certain body functions) may be caused by *extrinsic* (systemic) factors or *intrinsic* (brain) factors (St. Louis & Granner, 2007). Seizures can occur as a result of temporary dysfunction of the brain brought on by extrinsic factors in which permanent changes in brain function do not exist. Provoked seizures due to extrinsic factors may be caused by severe alcohol intoxication or withdrawal; abuse of drugs such as amphetamines or cocaine; prescription drugs, such as psychotropic drugs or pain medications; or insulin shock or diabetic coma (see Chapter 11). Provoked seizures may also be caused by acute conditions such as **meningitis** (infection of the covering of the central nervous system), **encephalitis** (inflammation of the brain), or **hypoxia** (too little oxygen to the brain). Each of these extrinsic factors can cause temporary brain dysfunction resulting in the symptom of a seizure. If the underlying cause of brain dysfunction is reversible so that no permanent alteration of brain function exists and seizures do not recur, individuals are not considered to have epilepsy.

Epilepsy is a chronic condition of the nervous system in which there are recurrent, unprovoked seizures. Epilepsy is not a disease, but rather a symptom of an underlying neurological condition in which neurons in the brain create abnormal electrical discharges that cause seizures. There is no single cause of epilepsy. It can affect anyone at any age. It can be caused by a number of conditions, such as head injury or stroke, in which a function of the brain has been affected. Sometimes, however, no clear-cut cause can be identified. In this case, epilepsy is considered to be **idiopathic**.

Although the essential feature of epilepsy is recurrent seizures, not all seizures are due to epilepsy. The term "epilepsy" is reserved for individuals with recurring seizures due to a chronic abnormality of the brain that results in seizures.

Classification of Seizures

Individuals with epilepsy can exhibit a variety of seizures, with symptoms ranging from muscle spasms or confusion to total loss of consciousness. Seizures can be mild or severe, can occur frequently or rarely, and can change their pattern of occurrence over time. Depending on the type, seizures usually last only seconds to minutes. Between seizures, most individuals are able to function normally.

Seizures are classified according to the part of the brain that demonstrates abnormal electrical activity and the type of seizure experienced. The International League Against Epilepsy (ILAE) has defined different seizure types and established descriptions of epilepsy syndromes (St. Louis & Granner, 2007). Classification of seizures in epilepsy is important so that appropriate management can be determined.

Seizures in epilepsy are classified as *generalized*, in which nerve cells discharge abnormally throughout the brain, or *partial*, in which abnormal nerve cell discharge is limited to one specific part of the brain. Table 3-2 summarizes the common types of seizures, and a brief description of generalized and partial seizures follows.

Generalized Tonic–Clonic Seizures (Grand Mal)

An abnormal discharge of nerve cells throughout the brain results in a **generalized tonic-clonic seizure**, sometimes called a grand mal seizure. Some individuals experience an **aura**

Table 3-2   Common types of Seizures Associated with Epilepsy
Generalized Seizures   1. Tonic–clonic (grand mal)   2. Absence (petit mal)   **Partial Seizures**   1. Simple partial (focal)   2. Complex partial (psychomotor)

(warning sign) immediately before the seizure begins. Auras can consist of things such as seeing a flash of light, having an unusual taste in the mouth, or having other unusual sensations. As the seizure develops, individuals lose consciousness and fall down, entering a **tonic** state in which there is generalized body rigidity. Muscles then enter a **clonic** state such that the whole body undergoes rapid, jerky movements. The teeth are clenched tightly together, and control of the bladder or the bowel may be lost. The seizure generally lasts less than a few minutes. When it ends, consciousness is gradually regained, but individuals may experience confusion, difficulty in speaking, and headache. Although post-seizure symptoms usually disappear within several hours, the fatigue experienced may be overwhelming, often necessitating an extended period of rest or sleep.

Although a tonic–clonic seizure may be frightening to those who witness it, individuals experiencing the seizure are usually in no imminent danger unless there are hard, sharp, or hot hazards within the immediate environment. No attempt should be made to move individuals experiencing a seizure except as necessary to protect them from such hazards. To avoid injury, there should be no attempt to restrain individuals during a tonic–clonic seizure, to pry open clenched teeth, or to place hard objects in the individual's mouth. Individuals should be placed on their side during a seizure so that secretions can drain from the mouth and do not compromise the airway.

Absence Seizures (Petit Mal)

Like tonic–clonic seizures, **absence seizures** are classified as generalized seizures because nerve cells discharge throughout the brain. Children most commonly experience this type of seizure. Absence seizures are characterized by brief blank spells or staring spells and a loss of awareness of the surroundings. The seizure generally lasts for only seconds. The individual does not fall, and there are usually no out-ward motor manifestations of absence seizures, although abnormal blinking or slight twitching may occur occasionally. Because of the limited visible symptoms of the seizure, those around the individual may misinterpret absence seizure as daydreaming or inattentiveness.

When children experience frequent absence seizures, their school performance may be disrupted. Because there may be no significant signs that are easily observed during the seizure, the seizure disorder may not be diagnosed and the poor school performance may be erroneously attributed to other causes. Recognition of symptoms and appropriate diagnosis are crucial to enable children to achieve their maximum potential. Absence seizures may disappear spontaneously with age, although some individuals who have had absence seizures later go on to develop tonic-clonic seizures.

Partial Seizures

When nerve cells discharge in an isolated part of the brain, partial seizures occur. One type of partial seizure is a **focal seizure**, in which there is no loss of consciousness and symptoms are very localized, depending on the part of the brain affected. One type of focal seizure, a **Jacksonian (simple-partial) seizure**, begins with convulsive symptoms in one part of the body, such as a hand or foot. The convulsive muscle movement then progresses in an orderly manner up the extremity. Jacksonian seizures can remain limited to one part of the body or can go on to develop into full-blown tonic–clonic seizures.

Other types of partial seizures may have more complex symptoms. **Complex-partial (psychomotor) seizures** are characterized by a loss of awareness of the surroundings. Individuals may pace, wander aimlessly, make purposeless movements, and utter unintelligible sounds. The seizure may last as long as 20 minutes, with mental confusion persisting for a few minutes after the seizure is over. Observers may misinterpret symptoms of complex-partial seizures, often attributing the symptoms to alcohol, drug abuse, or mental illness.

Status Epilepticus

Status epilepticus is a term used to describe seizures that are prolonged or that come in rapid succession without full recovery of consciousness between seizures. This condition is a medical emergency that can be life-threatening. Consequently, status epilepticus requires immediate medical attention and treatment (Pedley, 2004; Lowenstein & Alldredge, 1998).

Diagnosis of Epilepsy

Individuals having a seizure for the first time usually undergo medical evaluation by a neurologist to determine whether the seizure is a symptom of acute medical or neurological illness that can be treated and resolved, or a symptom of a chronic neurological problem that will require ongoing treatment for control. Extensive physical examination and blood tests are usually part of initial screening as well as a detailed history of precipitating factors that appeared to trigger the seizure.

When individuals have more than one seizure, or when other symptoms or history indicate that epilepsy may be the cause of seizure activity, a more extensive medical evaluation is conducted. A primary diagnostic tool for evaluating individuals after seizures is **electroencephalography (EEG),** a noninvasive procedure in which the electrical activity of the brain is recorded on a graph. **Magnetic resonance imaging (MRI),** a noninvasive procedure that produces rapid detailed pictures of body structures, may also be used to identify structural anomalies in the brain that are related to seizures.

Management of Epilepsy

Treatment of epilepsy depends on the cause of the seizure activity and the types of seizures experienced. Generally individuals who have had only a single seizure are not considered to have epilepsy. Although they may be thoroughly evaluated in an attempt to determine the cause of the seizure, they usually are simply monitored and not given medication (Willmore, 1998). If seizures are caused by a tumor, scar tissue, or another abnormality that can be corrected, surgical intervention to remove or repair the abnormality may be indicated. In some instances when seizures are not controlled by medication and are severely disabling, surgery may be directed toward resection of the part of the brain responsible for the seizure activity (St. Louis & Granner, 2007). In most cases, however, the standard treatment of epilepsy is the regular use of one or more anticonvulsant or antiepileptic medications.

Although medications do not cure epilepsy, they can effectively control seizures and enable many individuals to carry on full and productive lives. Successful control of seizures, however, requires the individual's strict, long-term compliance with medication instructions. Medications used to manage epilepsy are also not without side effects. Toxic effects are common during long-term management with anticonvulsant medications. Depending on the medication, side effects may include gum overgrowth, nausea, dizziness, clumsiness, visual difficulty, or fatigue.

Once medication for management of seizures has begun, it is generally maintained for at least two years, regardless of whether the individual has remained seizure free (Browne & Holmes, 2001). If there have been no recurrent seizures after this time, the physician may consider withdrawing the medication. Individuals who have had no additional seizures after beginning the medication or who have experienced side effects may be tempted to alter or discontinue their medication. The consequences of this course of action could be dangerous or even life-threatening. Consequently, individuals should never attempt to alter or discontinue their medication without consulting their physician.

Medication is prescribed based on which type of seizure the individual experiences and whether he or she has experienced more than one type of seizure. The general goal of intervention with medication is to maximize control of seizures without causing toxic side effects, such as liver damage or bone marrow suppression. The physician periodically monitors levels of the medication in the blood. Based on the medication's concentration in the blood and its effectiveness in controlling seizure activity, the physician may subsequently alter medication dosages. Measurement of blood levels of an anticonvulsant also helps the physician monitor the individual's compliance with the medication regimen and identify any toxic effects of the medication.

In some cases, even when individuals are compliant with taking anticonvulsant medications, seizures remain uncontrolled. Many of these individuals experience several seizures per month or, at times, several seizures per day, despite following a strict treatment regimen. When seizures are severely disabling and cannot be controlled by medication, surgery may be recommended to manage epilepsy. Under these circumstances, surgery may involve removing a portion of the brain structure, resecting a portion of the brain, or disconnecting the affected portion from the rest of the brain. The surgery itself may leave residual effects. The amount of disability experienced, if any, after this type of surgery depends on the individual circumstances. In fact, some individuals may still need anticonvulsant medications even after surgery.

Alcohol can lower a person's seizure threshold and, therefore, precipitate seizures. Alcohol and antiepileptic medications may also interact and cause untoward effects. Consequently, individuals with epilepsy should consult their physician about alcohol use.

Individuals with epilepsy should be helped to identify factors that may trigger a seizure. They should avoid activity that would be hazardous if a seizure should occur, such as swimming alone or operating heavy equipment. A medical identification bracelet should be worn by individuals with epilepsy at all times.

The general prognosis for individuals with epilepsy depends on the type of seizure, the underlying cause, the administration of appropriate treatment, and the individual's willingness and ability to follow the prescribed management regimen. If their condition is accurately diagnosed and appropriately managed, most individuals with epilepsy can live active, productive lives. Prompt detection and early medical intervention can greatly improve the ability to control seizures and enhance the general quality of life for the individual with epilepsy.

Psychosocial Issues in Epilepsy

Individuals with epilepsy may face many psychological and psychosocial challenges. They must learn to deal with uncertainty related to whether and when another seizure will occur. No matter how well-controlled seizures are, individuals live with the possibility—even if remote—that another seizure will occur. The time, place, and social circumstances under which a seizure may occur are unknown. If individuals experience a seizure in public, they risk feelings of embarrassment and onlookers' potential misperception of the seizure. Individuals may feel they have no control over their lives and behavior. At times, even when seizures are adequately controlled, anxiety over the possibility of having a seizure or other psychosocial consequences may be the most disabling factor associated with the condition. As a result, individuals may have difficulty establishing interpersonal relationships, building self-esteem, and obtaining or maintaining employment.

Activities and Participation

Family is crucial to the adjustment of an individual with a condition that has associated disability. Depending on the point at which the diagnosis of epilepsy is made and the reaction of the individual's family to it, both adjustment and emotional development of the individual can be affected. When epilepsy is diagnosed in childhood, parental feelings of fear, anxiety, guilt, overprotectiveness, or mourning can influence not only the child's ability to accept his or her condition and associated manifestations, but also the child's self-concept and social adjustment. Overly protective parents may foster dependency in their child. Children in turn, may learn to use their condition as an excuse for inactivity or avoidance of responsibility. As teenagers, concerns related to whether they will drive a car, participate in sports, or engage in dating may cause additional stress and lessening of self-esteem.

Diagnosis of epilepsy in adulthood can also disrupt interpersonal and family relationships. Individuals' social identity may be threatened, such that they go to great lengths to conceal their condition to avoid potential rejection. Partners of individuals with epilepsy may be fearful of observing a seizure or may be concerned that the disorder is hereditary. Due to anxiety and misinformation, they may be unwilling to learn more about the condition or to provide the support that the individual with epilepsy needs.

Sexual activity, in most cases, need not be affected by epilepsy (Frazer & Gumnit, 1990). Although some medications used to treat seizures may have some effect on libido, most do not. Psychological issues of low self-esteem or poorly developed social skills may produce greater limitations. Individuals may be reluctant to form intimate relationships because of the fear of having a seizure. Counseling may be necessary to help individuals overcome fear so that appropriate intimate relationships can be established.

When a person is between seizures, epilepsy is an invisible disability. Unless individuals are having a seizure, there are no outward signs of disability. Although considerable effort has been devoted to educate the public about the condition, misinformation and lack of acceptance still exist and epilepsy continues to carry a stigma for many individuals. In some cultures, historical misconceptions about epilepsy have linked it to demonic possession and insanity. In other instances, people with epilepsy were not permitted to participate in various events because of their diagnosis. Attitudes have changed for the better in recent years thanks to public education programs, improved placement of individuals with epilepsy into the world of work, and increased ability to control seizures. Nevertheless, individuals with epilepsy may still experience unjust restrictions, denying them access to participation in routine activities. The stigma and shame associated with epilepsy may cause individuals or their family to deny or minimalize the condition. Individuals may try to pass as someone without a disability because of anticipated rejection due to real or perceived public attitudes.

In the past, individuals with epilepsy were restricted from driving motor vehicles because of concerns for both public safety and their own personal safety. Although today most states permit individuals with epilepsy to obtain driver's licenses, the length of time they must be seizure free in order to obtain the license varies from state to state. State laws do not always take into account individual differences, instead making blanket rules that apply to all individuals with epilepsy regardless of their personal circumstances. The ability to operate a motor vehicle has a direct impact on the individual's independence and social well-being. Specifically, inability to drive can limit social interaction, educational experiences, and employment opportunities. In most instances, individuals with epilepsy can drive without significant risk of accident due to seizure if seizures are controlled with medication.

Alcohol consumption is frequently a part of social occasions. Individuals with epilepsy should always consult their physician about alcohol consumption, especially in regard to taking alcohol when they are also taking anticonvulsant medication. However, each individual situation must be considered in terms of the person's specific needs.

Sports activities are another important means of socializing as well as helping individuals build self-confidence and self-esteem. In some situations, restrictions on participation in various activities are placed on individuals with epilepsy even though no basis for limiting activity exists. Although some individuals may have seizures precipitated by fatigue or other sports-related circumstances, others may experience a reduction in the incidence of seizures with exercise. Consequently, the individual's specific circumstances should be considered rather than issuing blanket restrictions; each case should be considered individually. Restrictions may be necessary for specific activities that present a hazard should a potential seizure, which involves loss of consciousness, take place. For instance, individuals with epilepsy should not swim alone. Likewise, activities such as flying an airplane, rock climbing, or other activities in which a seizure could cause severe and possibly fatal consequences should be avoided. In most instances, applying common sense enables individuals to participate in activities while avoiding potential hazards.

Even when seizures are relatively well controlled, individuals may still fear having the "occasional" seizure and the physical and social consequences the seizure may bring. In addition to the embarrassment of having a seizure in public, individuals may fear injury. Injury during seizure while performing routine tasks, such as setting clothes on fire from gas stoves or falling in the bathtub, can occur. Consequently, individuals may need help in establishing common-sense safety precautions for activities of daily living. Family, friends, and co-workers should also be informed about appropriate measures to take if a seizure occurs.

Despite control of seizures, individuals may still feel the weight of restrictions of freedoms, activities, and events, which others take for granted. For instance, in most states individuals are required to report that they have epilepsy when applying for a driver's license. Individuals may be required to obtain a written statement from the physician to verify that they can return to regular activities after a seizure occurs. If flickering lights precipitate seizures, individuals may need to avoid certain theaters, bars, or other places that use strobe lights for decoration or effect. Taking medication regularly as prescribed, obtaining proper rest, and reduction of stress are other self-management issues that individuals with epilepsy must consider. In addition, the social stigma associated with epilepsy—whether real or perceived—can cause stress and influence social function. The uncertainty associated with the condition, as well as restrictions, potential social isolation, and difficulty with employment, may require adjustment and coping skills for the individual to achieve his or her full potential.

Vocational Issues in Epilepsy

Most individuals with epilepsy have the same range of IQ as the general population, unless other conditions that affect intellectual function are involved. Even so, individuals with epilepsy are likely to experience both unemployment and underemployment (Bishop, 2004; Fisher, 2000). Many problems in the workplace related to individuals' ability to obtain or maintain employment continue to be inspired by misperceptions and stigma rather than physical limitations. Although some individuals with epilepsy, especially when epilepsy is associated with head trauma, may have neuropsychological limitations that can impact on employment, many do not. Consequently, special considerations for individuals in the workplace should reflect their individual situation rather than any general pattern of limitation.

Epilepsy is a chronic condition, meaning it requires a continuous relationship with the medical community. Medication is, of course, a major part of management and necessitates close medical supervision. Multiple medications may be needed to control seizures, and the medications themselves may have associated side effects. Individuals must be diligent in taking mediation because missed doses may precipitate a seizure. When individuals are in denial of their condition, the denial may be manifested as poor compliance with medication, which in turn causes poor seizure control and may, consequently, affect the person's employment potential.

Because of the chance of unpredictable loss of consciousness, which may place individuals with epilepsy or others at risk of injury, some occupations—such as airplane pilot or interstate truck driver—may be unrealistic for the individual to pursue. Understanding how seizures affect job function is critical. It is important to assess the types and numbers of seizures individuals have, the degree to which seizures are controlled with medication, and individual's level of compliance in following the management regimen. Determination of situational patterns for seizures (such as a regular time when seizures occur) or factors that precipitate seizures (such as fatigue, stress, or flickering lights) is key to help individuals avoid or alter situations in which seizures may occur. If fatigue tends to precipitate a seizure, care should be taken so that the individual does not become overly fatigued. Likewise, if seizures are related to the individual's sleep pattern, he or she may be unable to work on a rotating shift. It is also helpful to know whether individuals experience an aura prior to the seizure and, therefore, would be able to remove themselves from dangerous situations prior to the seizure's onset. Individuals who experience seizures should probably not work alone in an isolated environment, especially if the environment imposes some threat of danger if a seizure should occur.

Individuals may question whether they should disclose that they have a seizure condition. Job seekers may choose to disclose their condition to an employer after they have outlined their qualifications and skills for the job, or they may want to establish credibility in the workplace before disclosing that they have a seizure condition (Fraser & Miller, 2005). If, when, and how an individual discloses his or her condition is dependent on the individual variables and the particular situation.

Employers who fear risk of lawsuits arising from workplace injuries may be overly conservative with restrictions for employees with epilepsy. Nevertheless, many jobs once thought to be inappropriate for individuals with epilepsy may not be contraindicated if proper safety equipment is used. In addition, many states have specific regulations protecting employers from excessive liability if injury occurs even though adequate safety precautions were maintained. Work potential can be maximized with continued education of employers, adequate safety precautions, and consideration of individual needs.

■ TRAUMATIC BRAIN INJURY

Brain damage associated with trauma are among the most common types of traumatic injury (Lemke, 2007) and are a major source of disability (Dixon, Layton, & Shaw, 2005). *Traumatic brain injury (TBI)* is broadly defined as an injury to the brain from external forces, such as vehicular accidents, falls, violence, or sports or recreational injury, or penetration of the skull by a foreign object (NIH Consensus Development Panel on Rehabilitation of Persons with Traumatic Brain Injury, 1999). It is not degenerative, is not the result of a disease, and is not congenital in origin. Damage to the brain can occur from a blow to the head in which the skull remains intact, but the force of the blow causes the brain to move within the skull resulting in injury (**closed head injury**). Damage can also occur from penetration of the skull (**open head injury**) by a foreign object causing injury to the brain directly, or from damage occurring when the skull itself is fractured from a blow to the head and bone fragments cause injury.

TBI can result in any combination of cognitive impairment, emotional and/or behavioral change, or physical manifestations and affects every aspect of an individual's life, often resulting in significant disability (Coetzer, 2007). The changes associated with a traumatic brain injury can limit an individual's ability to maintain or attain employment, engage in leisure activities, or carry on social relationships (Anson & Ponsford, 2006). The wide range of functional consequences associated with TBI and the resulting impact on the individual's daily life present unique challenges in rehabilitation.

Types of Traumatic Brain Injuries

Generally, two types of traumatic brain injuries are distinguished:

- Open or penetrating head injury
- Closed head injury

Open (penetrating) injuries refer to injuries in which the skull is fractured (such as with a blow to the head in which the skull is broken) or penetrated (such as with a gunshot wound). The functional consequences experienced with open or penetrating injury may be more localized and are usually related to the specific area of the brain affected. Sometimes, the functional consequences in an open head injury may be more extensive if additional damage is sustained. For example, in addition to the trauma to the brain itself, bone fragments from the injury may lacerate and injure the

brain, blood vessels, or meninges (the lining surrounding the brain).

In a *closed head injury* (such as a blow to the head or violent shaking of the head, such as in shaken baby syndrome), the skull is not fractured. Nevertheless, the brain is damaged because the head has been hit with sufficient force such that the brain slams against the other side of the skull or twists within the skull, causing tearing or shearing of blood vessels or nerve fibers throughout the brain (**diffuse axonal injury**). Injury is caused to the brain from both the external force and the movement of the brain within the skull. The initial impact to the brain is called the **coup**; the impact of the brain to the opposite side of the skull is called the **contre coup**. The functional consequences associated with a closed head injury depend on where and how much shearing occurred in the brain and may be more diffuse because of the more extensive damage to the brain itself.

Additional injury may occur as an indirect result of **edema** (swelling) of the brain, hemorrhage, or the formation of a **hematoma** (a sac filled with blood) within the skull as a direct result of the injury itself. Bleeding within the cranial vault is referred to as **intracranial hemorrhage**. Because the brain is confined within the skull, there is no space available for expansion if swelling or bleeding should occur. As a result, swelling or bleeding will compress the brain, increasing intracranial pressure and interfering with brain function. Unless recognized and treated promptly, these events can cause additional permanent brain damage or death.

Bleeding and blood clots (hematomas) compress the brain, increasing intracranial pressure. An **epidural hematoma** is bleeding that occurs in the space between the outer membrane of the brain (the **dura mater**) and the skull. Although bleeding generally occurs rapidly, it may not be recognized immediately after an injury. Individuals who have been injured may carry on a lucid conversation, only to slip into drowsiness and unconsciousness hours later. Epidural hematomas carry a high mortality rate because they may not be immediately recognized and consequently not immediately treated (Vitaz, 2007).

A **subdural hematoma** is a hemorrhage that occurs in the space beneath the dura mater. Although symptoms may be apparent immediately, they may also appear more gradually, becoming evident days or even weeks after the injury. In both instances, immediate action is essential to stop the bleeding and to relieve the intracranial pressure before permanent damage to the brain occurs.

Measuring the Severity of Traumatic Brain Injury

A variety of instruments are available to measure the level of severity for a TBI. These instruments are utilized as predictors of discharge disposition and as indicators of the type of rehabilitation services needed in early stages of management of TBI after hospitalization (Wagner, Hammond, Grigsby, & Norton, 2000).

Brain injuries are classified as mild, moderate, or severe. One basis of classification is the length of time the individual is unconscious after the injury and the depth of his or her unconsciousness or coma. The length of unconsciousness is also used as a predictor of prognostic outcome. Generally, the longer the period of unconsciousness, the more severe the injury to the brain and the greater subsequent residual effects (Hodge, 2004).

An instrument called the **Glasgow Coma Scale** (Jennett, Snoek, Bond, & Brooks, 1981) has become widely accepted as a classification system for rating the seriousness of brain injury. This scale is used to assess the level of consciousness along a continuum ranging from alert to coma. Scores are assigned according to the level of response in each of three areas: eye opening, motor response,

and verbal response (Table 3-3). The range of scores that may be obtained on the scale is from 3 to 15. The lower the score, the deeper the level of unconsciousness and generally the greater the functional consequences. The Glasgow Coma Scale provides a means whereby individuals' level of consciousness can be assessed systematically. An initial assessment provides a baseline from which changes in neurological status can be measured. The Glasgow Coma Scale is typically used in the early post-injury period in the emergency and the critical care unit.

Another scale used to measure level of brain injury is the **Rancho Los Amigos Cognitive Scale** (Hagan, Malkmus, & Durham, 1972). This scale basically describes levels of arousal and cognitive functioning (Table 3-4). It measures increasing levels of consciousness, so it often is used to give a gross indication of stages of recovery after brain injury. The range of the scale is from 1 to 7, with higher scores indicating higher functional level. In the treatment and rehabilitation phase after injury, individuals may remain at one level of unconsciousness or coma for an extended period of time or may move from one level of consciousness to the next. The Ranchos Los Amigos Scale, as a measure of cognitive function, is typically used to assess changes in levels of consciousness during the post-injury period and as a broad indicator of the extent to which independent functioning is possible. In this way a specific treatment can be instituted to promote appropriate behavior as the individual moves through different levels.

The **Disability Rating Scale** (Rappaport, Hall, Hopkins, Belleza, & Cope, 1982) is also used to estimate functional capacity after brain injury. This scale evaluates individuals on eight categories of disability and their ability to function. The highest score possible is 30. The lower the individual scores on the Disability Rating Scale, the better. Functional ability is scored on the following areas:

- Level of arousal, awareness, and responsiveness

Table 3-3   The Glasgow Coma Scale

Category		Score
Eyes open	Never	1
	To pain	2
	To verbal stimuli	3
	Spontaneously	4
Best verbal response	None	1
	Incomprehensible sounds	2
	Inappropriate words	3
	Disoriented and converses	4
	Oriented and converses	5
Best motor response	None	1
	Extension (decerebrate rigidity)	2
	Flexion abnormal (decorticate rigidity)	3
	Flexion withdrawal	4
	Individual localizes pain	5
	Individual obeys	6
		Total 3-15

Source: White and Likavec (1992).

Table 3-4   Los Amigos Scale of Cognitive Functioning

Level I	No response to sounds, light, or touch.
Level II	Generalized response to stimuli, such as responding to a loud noise, but not turning toward the noise. Movement is not consistent and does not appear to have a purpose. When eyes are open, they do not appear to be focusing on anything in particular.
Level III	Localized response. The individual begins to open eyes and look at specific objects. The head turns in the direction of sound. Simple commands are followed, such as "Squeeze my hand."
Level IV	Confusion and agitation. The individual becomes very restless and agitated regardless of the circumstances. Conversation may at times appear to be coherent. The individual may become verbally abusive.
Level V	Confused, with conversation often not making sense. The individual appears confused, although he or she may be able to follow simple instructions. The individual seems less agitated, but may become frustrated
Level VI	Confused, but verbal responses are appropriate. Some memory problems regarding recent events may be present. Capable of most self care activities. Some judgment and problem-solving difficulties, but the individual is often aware of this deficit.
Level VII	Purposeful and appropriate. Independent. Can process new information and problem solve.

- Cognitive skills needed for self-care
- Dependence on others
- Psychosocial adaptability, including flexibility and ability to adapt to different people and situations

Levels of Traumatic Brain Injury

Mild brain injuries account for approximately 70% of all TBIs (Busch & Alpern, 1998) and are characterized by a traumatically induced disruption of brain function, in which there is at least one of the symptoms listed in Table 3-5. Individuals with mild brain injuries have a Glasgow Coma Scale score of 13 or higher and may have few, if any, outer signs of brain injury or no detectable anatomic damage to the brain. As a result, the brain injury itself may be undiagnosed and consequently untreated (Clements, 1997). Individuals with mild brain injury may experience subtle but disruptive symptoms that persist months or even years after the initial injury. This group of symptoms has come to be known as **post-concussion syndrome** and can consist of symptoms such as headache, **vertigo** (dizziness), **tinnitus** (ringing in the ears), sleep disturbance, depression, irritability, reduced attention span, or memory impairment. Because there often are few, if any, objective signs of brain damage with mild brain injury, individuals experienc-

ing these symptoms may have their credibility questioned and they may be labeled as malingerers (Koch, Merz, & Torkelson Lynch, 1995). Cognitive deficits associated with mild brain injury may cause individuals considerable distress and adversely affect both social and occupational functioning.

Moderate brain injury is defined by a Glasgow Coma Scale score of 9 to 12. Individuals with moderate brain injury may have loss of consciousness for a few minutes or several hours. There may be confusion or disorientation, which may last for a few days or several weeks. Individuals with moderate brain injury may experience physical, cognitive, or psychosocial deficits, which last for weeks to months or may be permanent.

Severe brain injury is defined as having a Glasgow Coma Scale score of 8 or less. Individuals with severe brain injury remain in a coma for an extended period of time ranging from days to months. **Coma** is defined as prolonged unconsciousness in which there is little, if any, meaningful response from the individual and the person is unable to be awakened. Individuals are said to be in a "vegetative state" when they react to painful stimuli and may open their eyes in response to stimulation, but have no meaningful response with the environment (Giacino & Zasler, 1995). The more severe the injury, the more serious the permanent conse-

---

Table 3-5   Manifestations of Mild Brain Injury

Individual experiences at least one of the following:

(1) Brief loss of consciousness (30 minutes or less)
(2) Brief period of time after the injury during which the individual feels stunned and disoriented
(3) Loss of memory for events occurring immediately before or after the injury lasting no longer than 24 hours
(4) Temporary neurological deficit
(5) Initial Glasgow Coma Scale score of 13–15.

Source: Berrol, 1992.

quences or deficits experienced. Potential consequences of brain injury vary tremendously depending on the type of injury and the area of brain damaged as well as premorbid factors.

Conditions Associated with Traumatic Brain Injury

Post-traumatic epilepsy is experienced by some individuals after traumatic brain injury. In the early post-injury period, seizures may be related to increased intracranial pressure or other direct results of injury. Seizures occurring later may be due to the formation of scar tissue in the brain and may occur more than a year after the initial injury.

Individuals with traumatic brain injury may also develop *post-traumatic hydrocephalus*, in which there is interference with reabsorption of cerebrospinal fluid. Post-traumatic hydrocephalus can cause increasing neurological or functional deterioration. It may be treated by surgically implanting a shunt in the brain to divert and drain the cerebrospinal fluid. The prognosis for individuals who develop post-traumatic hydrocephalus varies.

Functional Consequences of Brain Damage

Because the brain is responsible for so many functions, damage to the brain, whether *traumatic* or *nontraumatic*, can have a profound impact on all areas of an individual's life. Regardless of whether brain damage is caused from an accident, a blow to the head, stroke, infection of the brain, exposure to toxins, or lack of oxygen, manifestations of brain damage may affect many areas of function. The effects experienced from brain damage depend on which part of the brain was damaged and the extent of the damage incurred. In general, potential consequences of brain damage can be classified into four categories (Groswasser & Stern, 1998):

- Motor control and perception
- Communication effects
- Cognitive changes
- Personality changes and affective response

TBI occurs most frequently in children, young adults, and older adults. Although considerable attention has been given to the functional consequences of brain damage in adulthood, less attention has been paid to the functional consequences experienced by adults who received brain damage in childhood (Brenner, Dise-Lewis, Bartles, O'Brien, Godleski, & Selinger, 2007). Brain injury in the context of the developmental stage when the injury was sustained adds a layer of complexity to the functional implications experienced.

Motor and Perceptual Consequences of Brain Damage

Motor and perceptual consequences of brain damage depend on whether the damage was diffuse or local. Functional impact can affect any of the following areas:

- Movement, coordination, or balance
- Visual–spatial relations
- Perception
- Vision or hearing
- Touch, taste, or smell
- Eating/swallowing
- Endurance
- Bowel or bladder function

In addition, individuals with brain damage may experience seizure disorders and, in some instances, persistent pain.

Movement, Coordination, or Balance

Whether brain damage is nontraumatic (such as stroke) or traumatic (such as from a gunshot) in origin, damage confined to one hemisphere of the brain will result in symptoms related to the extent of damage and the hemisphere affected. Because one side of the brain controls the opposite side of the body, damage to one hemisphere of the brain affects function of the body on the opposite side. Consequently, right cerebral damage can cause paralysis or weakness of the left side of the body (*left hemiplegia*), affecting the left arm and leg, while left cerebral damage can result in paralysis or weakness of the right side of the body (*right hemiplegia*), affecting the right arm and leg. The resulting paralysis or weakness may interfere with the individual's ability to walk so that there may be need for assistive devices such as a cane, a walker, a brace, or, in some instances, a wheelchair.

When individuals experience diffuse axonal injury, such as in closed head injury, changes in movement affecting both sides of the body may be present. Individuals may experience problems with muscle coordination (**ataxia**) affecting balance, causing them to walk with an unsteady gait or to lurch from side to side as they walk. They may also experience other motor changes, including **dyskinesias** (abnormal movements), or **dystonia**, (abnormal muscle tone). Dystonia can consist of too little tone (**flaccidity** or **hypotonicity**), which decreases the ability to move, or too much muscle tone (**spasticity** or *hypertonicity*), which heightens reflexes or exacerbates abnormal movement.

Even when motor function of muscles remains intact and muscle strength, coordination, and sensation are normal, there may be loss of ability to organize and sequence specific muscle movements to perform a task (**apraxia**). Individuals with apraxia are aware of what they want to do and how to do it, but are unable to organize their muscle movements properly to perform the task. Consequently, a number of tasks, from dressing and eating to performing more complex activities such as typing or driving, may be affected.

Visual–Spatial Relations

Visual–spatial deficits cause problems with depth perception and judgment of distance, size, position, rate of movement, form, and the relation of parts to wholes. Visual–spatial changes as a result of brain damage interfere with the ability to interpret visual information accurately. Consequently, there may be difficulty orienting position and navigating movement within the environment, or individuals may demonstrate inaccurate judgment of space or distance or under- or over-estimate the relationship of distance between two objects. As a result, individuals may appear careless or clumsy, frequently bumping into furniture, having difficulty navigating doorways, knocking items off tables or counters, or missing the table when attempting to put a glass down.

Visual–spatial consequences of brain damage can affect other activities of daily living as well. For example, individuals may find it difficult to read because they continually lose their place on the page, or they may have difficulty dressing because they confuse the inside and outside of clothes as well as left and right. Because of difficulty judging distances, individuals with even minor visual–spatial deficits may have difficulty driving a car.

Perception

Perceptual consequences affect the ability to understand or interpret stimuli or objects within the environment. Depending on which part of the brain is damaged, many different perceptual problems may occur. Although some perceptual consequences may improve over time, others will be permanent.

There may be loss of comprehension of sensations (**agnosia**), in which individuals lose the ability to recognize familiar things such as words, faces, or objects. Individuals with localized brain damage (especially to the right side), may experience a condition called **anosognosia** (one-sided or unilateral neglect) in which body parts or objects on one side of the body are ignored. For instance, an individual with anosognosia may shave only one side of the face or put on only one shoe. In some instances, anosognosia is visual, such that there is an inability to perceive objects on either the right or left side of the central field of vision. In these instances, individuals may bump into things on the ignored or neglected side of the body.

Sometimes, signals from all senses on one side of the body are involved such that individuals may not recognize their own arm or leg or are unresponsive to auditory stimuli that originate from the environment on the affected side of the body. Nonresponsiveness to auditory stimuli on the affected side is different from merely losing hearing in one ear. All stimuli on the affected side are ignored, while stimuli on the individual's unaffected side continue to evoke a response.

Vision and Hearing

Visual consequences may be present even though the eye itself is not injured. When part of the brain that receives, perceives, or interprets nerve impulses from the eye has been damaged, visual deficits may still be present. Visual consequences can include total blindness, **diplopia** (double vision), blurred vision, visual field loss such as cuts in the peripheral field of vision (*blind spots*), **hemianopsia** (loss of vision in half the visual field), or color blindness.

As with vision, even though the ear has not been damaged directly, hearing deficits may be present if the area of the brain responsible for receiving, perceiving, or interpreting sound has been damaged (**sensorineural hearing loss**). Individuals may experience ringing in the ears (tinnitus) as well as partial or total loss of hearing.

Touch, Taste, and Smell

Brain damage that involves parts of the brain responsible for sensation can lead to a variety of consequences, such as decreased or absence of feeling in various body parts. These changes may result in numbness (**anesthesia**), the inability to feel pain (**analgesia**), or the inability to sense movement of body parts. Individu-

als may also experience abnormal sensations (**paresthesia**) such as pain, tingling, or burning in various locations in the body.

If the olfactory nerve or corresponding area of the brain has been damaged, the individual may have no sense of smell (**anosmia**). Although loss of sense of smell may not appear to be a significant consequence of brain damage, it does have important functional implications, which can significantly affect the ability to function. Loss of sense of smell can affect the ability to detect hazards such as smoke, gas leaks, or other important warning signs. Lack of sense of smell also has implications for the ability to taste. Inability to taste may affect the individual's will to eat and, consequently, the person's nutritional status and ability to detect spoiled food.

Eating/Swallowing

Swallowing reflexes may be affected so that individuals have difficulty with swallowing (**dysphagia**) and, in some instances, difficulty with chewing. The gag reflex may also be impaired, such that there is increased susceptibility to choking. Because of difficulty with swallowing or performing chewing movements, food may be pocketed in one side of the mouth, increasing the risk of gagging or choking. Inability or difficulty related to swallowing can be dangerous because of the risk of **aspiration** (food or liquid entering the lungs rather than the stomach). When individuals are unable to swallow food because of swallowing difficulty, a special diet consisting of pureed food may be needed or tube feedings may be necessary to prevent aspiration of food into the lungs. In addition, because of difficulty or inability to swallow, saliva may build up in the mouth, causing the individual to drool.

Endurance

After developing brain damage, individuals may experience extreme fatigue when completing both mental and physical tasks, especially when tasks are unfamiliar or require significant concentration. Mental fatigue as a consequence of brain damage appears to be the most prominent type of fatigue, followed by physical fatigue (Ouellet & Morin, 2006). Mental and physical activities that, prior to the injury, were easy for the individual to complete may also be exhausting to complete post-injury. Sleep patterns may also be altered so that quality of sleep is affected, compounding the problem. Fatigue can exacerbate other symptoms related to brain injury and have detrimental effects on daily functioning and well-being (Strober & Arnett, 2005). Tasks may be performed better earlier in the day, as performance levels can deteriorate later in the day owing to fatigue.

Bowel and Bladder Function

In some instances, control of bladder or bowel function may be lost (**incontinence**) after brain damage. At times, problems are caused by the individual's inability to recognize the need to urinate or defecate. In other instances, individuals are unable to urinate at will or to completely empty the bladder when urinating. There may be a need for bladder and/or bowel retraining. Some individuals may need to wear adult incontinence protection garments or utilize a *catheter* (a tube inserted into the bladder to drain urine).

Post-Traumatic Seizures

Seizures may be experienced in the period immediately after the brain damage occurs. Post-TBI seizures can be mild or severe, temporary or permanent. In some instances, seizures occurring in the immediate post-damage phase resolve after swelling of the brain recedes. In many other cases, however, individuals continue to have seizures, a condition called post-traumatic epilepsy.

Communication Consequences

Brain damage can affect all forms of communication, including the ability to speak, comprehend, or convey language through either written or verbal means. **Speech** refers to the physical ability to produce sounds and/or movement of the lips, tongue, or other structures that are used to produce language. **Language** refers to how words, as symbols, are put together to convey and understand concepts. Both the ability to use certain muscles to form words and project speech and the ability to use and understand words (language) are controlled by the brain. When the area of the brain that controls either speech or language is damaged, limitations in either area may occur.

Motor difficulty in structures related to speech may affect the individual's ability to speak. Coordination and accuracy of movement of the muscles, lips, tongue, or other parts of the speech mechanism may be impaired secondary to weakness or paralysis of muscles needed to speak, a condition called **dysarthria**. Impairments may range from speech that is slightly slurred to speech that is unintelligible. Paralysis or weakness of muscles may also cause vocal cord dysfunction, which in turn can affect voice quality.

Other motor problems can cause **articulation disorders** in which there is no significant weakness or incoordination for reflexive action, but rather the inability to position and sequence muscle movements properly. For example, individuals may be able to scrape a food particle off their teeth with their tongue, yet be unable to coordinate the muscles that move the tongue so as to produce a phonetic sound, a condition known as **apraxia of speech.**

Another communication consequence of brain damage may be the inability to comprehend or use language (aphasia). Aphasia can affect either verbal or written communication. It is the result of dysfunction of language centers in the brain, rather than impairment of the musculature involved in producing speech. Although there are a number of types of aphasias, two categories are commonly distinguished:

- Nonfluent (expressive or motor) aphasia
- Fluent (receptive or sensory) aphasia.

Broca's aphasia is a type of nonfluent aphasia characterized by misarticulation, laborious speech, hesitancy, and reduced vocabulary and grammar. Individuals may be able to understand and read simple material; however, as the complexity or length of the message increases, difficulty in completing these tasks becomes more apparent. Although individuals are able to comprehend material, they may have difficulty expressing their thoughts in speech and writing because of difficulty putting words and sentences together logically. Word-finding difficulties (**dysnomia**) are also common. Reading ability may be better than writing ability. Speech may be labored, slow, or difficult to understand, and small connecting words, such as prepositions, may be omitted.

Wernicke's aphasia is a type of fluent aphasia in which there is effortless speech, relatively normal grammatical structure, and increased verbal output, but with reduced information content, so that what the individual says makes little sense. Auditory and reading comprehension is usually poor. Individuals with Wernicke's aphasia are typically unaware of their communication difficulties.

In some instances, individuals may experience **global aphasia**, in which there is severe difficulty communicating because of both the inability to use language (inability to use words and organize them into coherent sentences) and severe difficulty in understanding language, either written or spoken.

Language impairment may differ depending on the area of the brain damaged. Because the center of language function is located in the left cerebral hemisphere for most individuals, communication deficits can occur when damage involves the left side of the brain. By contrast, individuals with right cerebral damage often have intact language function.

Cognitive Consequences

Brain damage can alter a variety of cognitive skills:

- Memory

- Attention and concentration
- Self-awareness
- Problem solving and decision making
- Information processing and concept formation
- Judgment

Memory

Memory encompasses the ability to store and retrieve information. Memory problems affect the individual's ability to recognize and recall people, places, facts, and concepts as well as to problem solve, form goals, organize, and plan. Memory for both new and old information may be affected.

Several types of memory exist:

- *Immediate memory* lasts only seconds or minutes unless converted into short-term memory. An example of immediate memory is remembering a phone number long enough to dial the number but not committing it to memory for later use.
- *Short-term memory* lasts from minutes to hours, but is then lost if not converted to long-term memory. An example of short-term memory may be learning facts for a test but not committing the facts to long-term memory for continued use.
- *Long-term memory* refers to memories that are stored and are able to be retrieved in the future, whether weeks or years ahead.

A variety of memory problems may be experienced after brain damage. Some individuals may be able to remember facts, but unable to remember how to do specific tasks. For instance, an individual may be able to remember names and birth dates of family members, but unable to remember how to operate a washing machine. Some individuals experience **retrograde amnesia** in which they are unable to remember things that occurred prior to the time of brain damage. Individuals with **remote memory impairments** may have forgotten their own personal history, so they do not recognize family members, or remember what type of work they had been engaged in prior to the brain damage occurring.

After experiencing brain damage, individuals can have difficulty remembering or learning new information so that they are unable to acquire new memories or recall recent conversations and events. In some instances individuals make up answers to questions, or make up situations or events (**confabulation**). This behavior results not from faulty memory, but rather from the tendency to juxtapose unrelated memories together. At other times, in conversation, individuals may get stuck on one theme, repeating a question, phrase, or concept again and again (**perseveration**). Perseveration can also pertain to tasks, which the individual repeats over and over, such as continuing to wipe the same spot on a counter until someone intervenes.

Individuals with brain damage may be unable to remember skills that were once very familiar. For instance, they may be unable to complete simple daily tasks, such as dressing, because they are unable to remember the steps involved or because, after completing the first steps of the task, they forget their original goal.

Memory problems can be the most limiting of all of the potential cognitive consequences of brain damage because they may affect the individual's ability to learn, store, and retrieve information. The ability to profit from experience is often limited as well. Consequently, individuals may continue to make the same mistakes over and over because the ability to apply what was learned from past experience is usually diminished. Likewise the ability to generalize from one situation to another may be impaired, such that what is learned in one setting may not be able to be transferred to another. For example, an individual who has learned a skill in a rehabilitation setting may be unable to perform the same skill in his or her own home.

Attention and Concentration

After experiencing brain damage, individuals may find it difficult to focus attention and to concentrate on a specific activity (Chan, 2005). Consequently, they may be unable to follow a train of thought or perform multiple-step instructions. They may have difficulty focusing on one task, they may be easily distracted, or they may unable to "shift gears" from one task to another. Individuals with brain damage may find it difficult to perform multiple tasks at one time, such as writing down messages or notes while talking on the phone, or carrying on a conversation while polishing furniture.

Self-Awareness

One of the consequences frequently associated with brain injury is that individuals have limited awareness of their limitations and the implications of their injury. They may underestimate the severity of their physical, cognitive, and behavioral limitations (Trahan, Pépin, & Hopps, 2006; Sawchyn, Mateer, & Suffield, 2005). They may also have limited ability to recognize or understand any limitations they are experiencing. They may lack insight into the appropriateness of their behavior and be unaware of how certain aspects of their behavior affect other people, remaining oblivious to subtle reactions or emotional cues from others. Because they may be unaware of their deficits, they may be unable to assess the extent of their disability and may, therefore, set unrealistic goals. There may also be inability to monitor and adjust their own actions according to feedback from others. When they do receive feedback, they may discount it because they disagree with others' observations regarding their behavior or performance.

Problem Solving and Decision Making

Planning, organizing, and problem solving may be difficult after brain damage. Individuals may have difficulty sequencing tasks so that even apparently simple tasks become problematic. For example, when preparing a meal, there may not be the realization that food items that take more time to cook should be prepared first. Consequently, when cooking dinner, the individual may fully prepare the mashed potatoes before even starting to make the meatloaf. In other instances, there may be difficulty following steps in order. For instance, when dressing, individuals may put on their slacks before they put on underwear or put their socks on over their shoes.

Individuals may be unable to recognize problems as they occur; if a problem is identified, they may be unable to generate alternative solutions or to select a solution when one is presented. Reasoning and decision making may also be affected. Individuals may consider only immediately apparent information rather than look at the situation as a whole. For example, if they want to visit a friend in another city, they may recognize that they can take a train to get there, but may not be able to consider how they would obtain money for the train fare, how they would obtain a ticket, or how they would get to the train station.

Individuals with brain damage sometimes have difficulty thinking or planning for the future. For instance, they may see no need to go to the grocery store for supplies if they are not currently hungry, or they may use all of their money on a taxi ride to reach a destination without thinking about how they will be able to pay for the ride back.

There may also be a lack of ability to initiate and sustain activity. For example, an individual may be assigned a task of straightening a room, but after several hours still not have begun, or may pick up one or two items from the floor but then discontinue the task before finishing. Performance can also become inconsistent, such that tasks performed well on one day may not be performed well on subsequent days.

Problem solving may be especially difficult for individuals with damage to the left side of the brain. If presented with a new problem,

they may respond slowly and in a cautious, disorganized fashion. Dividing tasks into smaller steps to avoid confusion in performance and providing frequent feedback throughout even simple tasks such as dressing may be helpful in such cases.

Information Processing

Even when hearing and vision are unaffected by brain damage, more time may be needed to synthesize verbal or visual input received. There may be a delayed response to visual or verbal stimuli, so that individuals find it difficult to maintain the pace in a social setting. In some instances, comprehension of input itself may be severely disrupted. Information processing may be disrupted not only in terms of speed, but also in terms of the ability to sequence and categorize information such that there is difficulty understanding concepts. As a result, individuals may experience problems with abstraction and tend to think only in concrete terms, taking cues and stimuli literally. For instance, in money exchange, the phrase "Do you have anything smaller" may be taken quite literally by individuals with brain damage because they are unable to distinguish between "smaller" as referring to denomination and "smaller" as referring to size of the bill.

Judgment

Due to loss of ability to learn from experience, problem solve, self-monitor, or interpret cues from other individuals or the environment, judgment may be affected by brain damage. Individuals may demonstrate rigidity of response, which precludes alternative responses. For instance, because of the inability to recognize and synthesize information and then adjust plans or to plan alternative activities accordingly, an individual who had planned to go swimming may proceed with those plans, even though the weather has become cold and rainy. Lack of judgment can cause individuals to endanger themselves or others if they attempt to perform tasks or engage in situations for which they have limited skills. For example, an individual who has never ridden a motorcycle before may believe that he or she can take a young neighbor for a ride on a busy highway. Individuals may behave impulsively and act quickly without thinking or anticipating the consequences of their behavior.

Personality Changes and Affective Response

Psychosocial effects of brain damage not only pose serious limitations for individuals but can also be the most difficult challenge for family and friends to face. Potential psychosocial effects can consist of the following:

- Personality changes
- Anger or irritability
- Nonconformance to social norms
- Apathy and depression
- Loss of self-esteem

Personality Changes

Personality changes associated with brain damage may be slight or extreme, or even be severely disabling. Individuals who were very meticulous and precise prior to developing brain damage may become careless and sloppy post-damage. Individuals who were once jovial and outgoing may become quiet and withdrawn. In other instances, individuals who, prior to brain damage, had been calm and tolerant may be emotionally explosive post-damage, demonstrating outbursts of anger or episodes of severe anxiety.

Family and friends may not recognize such changes as being a result of brain damage and misinterpret these behaviors as laziness, disinterest, or uncooperativeness, rather than viewing them as a symptom of the condition itself. Social interactions are often affected by these

personality changes, so that individuals are unable to maintain relationships. Once personality changes are recognized as symptoms associated with brain damage, compensatory behaviors can be learned to overcome them.

Anger or Irritability

Aggressive behavior displayed after brain damage may be the result of frustration, or it can be a direct physiologic consequence of the damage to the brain itself. Aggression can be expressed actively or passively, verbally or physically. There may be decreased patience or overreaction to stresses in the environment, or individuals may be more sensitive to environmental stimuli and become distracted or react to stimuli with irritation. Because individuals with brain damage may have low frustration tolerance, aggressive behaviors and emotional outbursts can be common. Individuals may have sudden mood swings, turning from happy to sad or from complacent to volatile with little or no provocation.

Nonconformance to Social Norms

Disinhibition can be a consequence of brain damage, meaning that affected persons may have inadequate social skills to function effectively within the environment. As a result, individuals may make rude or embarrassing remarks to others, exhibit inappropriate sexual behavior in public, or make inappropriate sexual remarks. They may misinterpret gestures of others, such as a hug, as an indication that the individual desires a more passionate encounter. In some instances, individuals with brain damage may have heightened sexual drive and become over-demanding sexually.

Substance abuse is frequently a contributor to accidents that resulted in the original traumatic brain injury. If substance abuse or dependence was a problem prior to injury, it may also contribute to problems post-injury. Given the stress of adjusting to changes associated with brain damage, lack of self-awareness and insight, and inability to recognize cues from the environment, substance abuse may become problematic for some individuals after they experience such an injury. Brain damage can increase sensitivity to the effects of alcohol or drugs, so that use of these substances often contributes to greater impairment of cognitive, psychomotor, and psychosocial skills, making it more difficult for individuals to become integrated into the community or the workplace. In addition, drugs and alcohol may interact with other prescribed medications, causing serious effects. As mentioned earlier, individuals with brain damage are more prone to seizures. Alcohol and drugs can lower the seizure threshold, increasing the risk of seizures for individuals with brain damage. As individuals with brain damage achieve greater levels of independence, the likelihood of substance abuse increases. Ongoing assessment of alcohol and drug use should continue throughout the rehabilitation process.

Apathy and Depression

Depression is a natural reaction to the losses that individuals experience with many disabilities. Individuals with brain damage, for example, can experience a number of losses related to cognitive, motor, sensory, social, and vocational functions. At times, it may be difficult to discern the extent to which depression is the direct consequence of physiologic damage to the brain versus a personal reaction to losses associated with the condition itself. As individuals become increasingly aware of the losses, restrictions, and alterations in lifestyle that may follow brain damage, they may go through a grieving process, which leads to depression. As a consequence, they may become increasingly withdrawn and have difficulty in taking the initiative to interact socially with others.

Loss of Self-Esteem

After experiencing brain damage, some individuals have no memory of what they were like prior to the injury. Others may develop an increasing awareness of their condition and its implications, or an awareness that they are unable to perform tasks they performed previously. They may recognize role changes they are experiencing and sense that their status has changed within family, social, and work settings. Loss of status may diminish individuals' self-image so that they become preoccupied with feelings of worthlessness and grief because they are unable to assume their former roles.

Management of Brain Damage

Comprehensive, individualized interdisciplinary management and rehabilitation provided by a diverse team of professionals is necessary to achieve both short-term goals and global outcomes for individuals with brain damage. Interventions are directed toward preventive, restorative, and compensatory strategies. The course of recovery and rehabilitation of individuals with brain damage is variable, but is almost always lengthy, ranging from months to years. The rate of recovery may vary over time.

Physicians involved in the care of individuals with brain damage usually include a primary physician such as an internist or family physician, as well as specialists such as a neurologist, a neurosurgeon, and a physiatrist. Other health professionals involved in the individual's care, treatment, and rehabilitation may include a variety of health professionals such as nurses, respiratory therapists, physical therapists, dietitians or nutrition specialists, speech/language pathologists, audiologists, pharmacists, occupational therapists, recreational therapists, clinical or counseling psychologists, neuropsychologists, cognitive retrainers, social workers, and rehabilitation counselors.

Initial Treatment of Brain Damage

The initial treatment for individuals experiencing brain damage, whether from traumatic or nontraumatic causes, is intended to stabilize the condition and enhance the recovery process by preventing complications.

Damage to the brain can cause increased muscle tone, paralysis, or weakness. If these changes are left untreated, permanent deformities such as **contractures** (deformity and immobility of a joint due to permanent contraction of a muscle) can occur, which could interfere with the individual's future function. In the initial stages after brain damage, individuals are kept immobile, predisposing them to complications such as pneumonia, pressure sores, urinary tract infections, and blood clots. Should these complications arise, the potential for recovery could be compromised. Consequently, in the initial stages of treatment, special attention is given to maintaining nutritional status and preventing complications.

With traumatic brain damage, there is often at least one other major organ system injury as well. These injuries may include spinal cord injury, musculoskeletal injury, or injury to internal organs. Treatment of any complicating associated injury is necessary to prevent deterioration, which could jeopardize recovery, rehabilitation, and—in some instances—survival. In the case of nontraumatic damage, direct treatment of any underlying conditions (such as infection in the case of meningitis or hypertension or diabetes in the case of stroke) is also important to stabilize the condition and prevent further damage from occurring.

Neurosurgical procedures are sometimes indicated in the immediate-treatment phase of brain damage. Careful observation is essential to detect early signs of increased intracranial pressure due to swelling of the brain or intracranial bleeding, which, unless relieved, could cause additional damage or death. Treatment of increased intracranial pressure can be surgical or nonsurgical. Surgical intervention may involve placement of a *shunt* that allows excess cerebrospinal fluid to drain into the general body circulation. If individuals with traumatic brain damage have an open skull fracture, surgery may be necessary to remove fragments of bone or other foreign materials and to repair the skull. If increased intracranial pressure is caused by a blood clot (e.g., a subdural or epidural hematoma) or hemorrhage, two small holes may be placed into the skull (*burr holes*) and the blood clot removed or bleeding controlled. In some instances, individuals may undergo a **craniotomy**, a surgical procedure in which the skull is surgically opened and the clot or foreign object removed or bleeding controlled through the surgical incision.

Nonsurgical interventions for increased intracranial pressure consist of giving medications to remove fluid and decrease swelling of the brain or to prevent further clot formation.

If the individual has an aneurysm or malformed arteries or veins, surgery to remove the aneurysm or correct the malformation may be performed.

Post-Acute Treatment and Rehabilitation of Brain Damage

After the condition has stabilized, appropriate post-acute management requires early and active intervention by the interdisciplinary team. In the early phases after brain damage, *physical therapy* may focus on activities to prevent joint and muscular complications. *Physical therapists* work with individuals early after the initial phase of brain damage to provide range-of-motion exercise to extremities, thereby preventing deformity, and later in the recovery period to assist with ambulation. Later physical therapy may be directed toward helping individuals improve balance, muscle control, ambulation, and other physical movements. Individuals who experience hemiplegia (paralysis on one side of the body) may need special instruction in ambulation techniques (*gait training*). Depending on the extent of permanent damage to the brain, individuals may use assistive devices to perform a variety of functions and activities. Braces or splints may be necessary to help individuals increase their functional capacity and become independent. Individuals with paralysis of an arm may be taught to use special tools such as a plate guard to keep food from sliding off the plate, or special eating utensils or other tools designed to help in daily living activities. If there is paralysis of an upper extremity, the weight of the paralyzed arm can cause separation of the arm from the shoulder joint (**subluxation**). To prevent separation from occurring, individuals with this condition may wear a sling to support the arm.

Individuals with brain damage may need assistance to increase their awareness or orientation to time, place, and person. *Occupational therapy* can help individuals with brain damage integrate available sensory information so that they can use it as a basis for motor activity and increase their ability to perform activities of daily living. Helping individuals learn skills and use assistive devices that would help them with activities of daily living, such as skills related to personal hygiene, dressing, or eating, may also be a focus of therapy.

Speech and language therapies may focus on the mechanical difficulties of speech, the formation and execution of language, or the development of alternative communication systems. *Speech and language therapists* may help individuals with both verbal and nonverbal communication. Focus may be on speech or language acquisition, or on conversational skills training. The speech therapist can also help individuals with brain damage develop social skills that relate to communication so that they learn techniques to enhance communication and ways to structure the environment to maximize their communication

effectiveness. In some instances, alternative methods of communication, such as writing or using a picture board, may be used.

If individuals have impaired swallowing capabilities, *speech pathologists* may be involved in helping individuals learn how to swallow again. In some instances, speech pathologists may also be involved in cognitive remediation.

Clinical or counseling psychologists may conduct psychotherapy or counseling with the individual with brain damage and family members to facilitate the adjustment process. *Neuropsychologists* (psychologists who specialize in neurological testing and assessing brain function) may be involved in neurological assessment, conducting comprehensive neuropsychological evaluations. Some neuropsychologists may also be involved in cognitive retraining or remediation in which individuals with brain damage learn ways to compensate for areas of cognitive function with which they may have difficulty.

Often cognitive changes—rather than physical changes—hamper effective daily functioning for individuals with brain injury. In these instances, **cognitive remediation** strategies designed to ameliorate sensory/perceptual, language-related, and problem-solving deficits may be a major focus of the rehabilitation effort. The goal of therapy is to return individuals with brain injury to as much independent functioning as possible in as many areas as possible. Cognitive strengths and weaknesses are identified through observation and *neuropsychological assessment*. How cognitive abilities and limitations in areas such as memory, organizational ability, reasoning, or judgment affect the individual's ability to function in the environment is evaluated, and cognitive strategies are devised to help the person compensate for or remediate those shortcomings as needed. Individuals are then helped to transfer these strategies from the clinical setting to their own environment. In some instances, depending on the individual's life circumstances and the extent of his or her brain damage, long-term supportive care may be needed.

Most individuals who have experienced brain damage should abstain from alcohol and all drugs that have not been medically prescribed. The use of alcohol and other substances can increase potential for seizures after brain damage. In addition, taking alcohol or drugs in combination with prescribed medications can have dangerous effects. Furthermore, alcohol and other substances may accentuate any residual deficits from brain damage, increasing the chances of additional accident or injury as well as impairing individuals' ability to function to their optimal capacity.

Several approaches are utilized for individuals with brain damage after they are medically stable to help them reach their full functional capacity—namely, *home-based programs, outpatient rehabilitation programs, community reentry programs, day treatment, residential community reentry* or *transitional living programs,* or *neurobehavioral programs.* These programs offer therapies designed to improve individuals' functioning or assist them in developing social behaviors. Some programs provide care and supervision for individuals who require some assistance in meeting basic needs, as in a supported living program or independent living center.

Functional Implications of Brain Damage

Psychosocial Issues in Brain Damage

Emotional adjustment after brain injury appears to be influenced by a number of factors (Anson & Ponsford, 2006). The range of emotional reactions experienced by individuals after brain damage can be immense, including symptoms varying from depression to mood swings to psychosis (Busch & Alpern, 1998). Just as physical, cognitive, and emotional changes associated with brain injury can

cause stress, anxiety, and depression, so stress, anxiety, and depression can influence physical, cognitive, and emotional symptoms (Kit, Mateer, & Graves, 2007). How individuals view the brain damage in terms of its cause and the extent to which they blame themselves or others for the injury can influence both their emotional reactions and their subjective well-being (Hart, Hanks, Bogner, Millis, & Esselman, 2007).

Although the extent of personality changes and other psychological symptoms will vary from individual to individual, it is safe to assume that, whether damage is mild or severe, some psychological symptoms will be experienced. Symptoms may differ at different phases of recovery. Individuals in the early stages of recovery may deny the extent of their limitations. Later they may experience feelings of frustration because of difficulty with memory or because they are unable to carry out tasks that they were once able to perform. Feelings of anger, grief, anxiety, or helplessness may also occur, or there may be feelings of worthlessness or guilt.

Because of the damage sustained, some individuals may no longer be able to comprehend the world around them or respond to it in the same way they did before the injury. They may show loss of emotional control in the form of emotional liability, in which they suddenly switch from laughing to crying, or from crying to laughing, when there is no apparent cause. Sometimes emotional liability is expressed as prolonged crying that, rather than being caused by depression or sadness, is instead a direct result of damage to the brain itself. If emotional lability exists, the family may need support and guidance in dealing with the individual's outbursts. The emotional reaction can often be diverted if the individual's attention can be directed to another activity.

Individuals with brain damage may demonstrate impulsivity with regard to money, sex, drugs, or interactions with others in general. In some instances, they may demonstrate verbal outbursts of aggression or outbursts of physical violence. They may also lack sensitivity to the impact of their behavior on others. If individuals are aware of their unusual behavior, they may become self-conscious and anxious, avoiding contact with others or becoming over-cautious and hypervigilant.

Personality traits that were present prior to brain damage may become exaggerated after the damage has occurred, or a dramatic personality change may occur such that an individual who was quiet and passive prior to brain damage becomes boisterous and aggressive after the injury. A person who was once self-directed and took initiative may, in turn, become apathetic and be unable to complete tasks independently. Although many of these personality changes may be the direct result of the injury itself, others may be associated with adjustment to the injury (Rush, Malec, Brown, & Moessner, 2006).

Counseling and psychotherapy are important parts of total rehabilitation in the case of most disabling conditions and can be used to treat depression, reduce denial, increase self-esteem, or help individuals form realistic goals. In the case of individuals with brain damage, however, additional challenges may be present if the individual has lost the capacity for insight or is unable to participate in abstract reasoning. Counseling may be directed toward providing emotional support for both the individual and the family and toward helping all involved adjust and relate to one another in the context of the changes brought about by the individual's brain damage.

In the case of traumatic brain injury, substance abuse is often a contributor to the original accident that caused the injury. After the injury has occurred, individuals may maintain the same pattern of substance abuse behavior they followed prior to the injury. Conse-

quently, substance abuse evaluation should be conducted routinely and treatment instituted as needed. For some individuals, substance abuse may be a maladaptive means of coping with the stress and depression they experience following brain damage. In either case, the effects of alcohol or other drugs will further impair already impaired function and have the potential to interact with other medications that the individual may be taking. In addition, substance abuse may precipitate a seizure, which the individual is already more prone to experience. Abstinence is, therefore, the best policy for individuals with traumatic brain injury.

Some individuals may believe that substance use has been a significant part of their social relationships. In these instances, individuals with brain damage may need to identify other circumstances under which to engage in social activity and should be encouraged to participate in social and recreational activities that do not involve alcohol or other drugs.

Life Activities

The complexity of brain damage has far-reaching consequences, including impacts on general activities of daily living. After their discharge from acute care facilities, many individuals fail to receive adequate services presumed to be critical to maintain activities of daily living and to prevent secondary complications (Pickelsimer, Selassie, Sample, Heinemann, Gu, & Veldheer, 2007). The degree to which home modifications or assistance in independent living is needed will depend on the physical, cognitive, and perceptual limitations that the individual experiences. Although the goal of rehabilitation is to assist the individual in achieving as much independence in as many areas as possible, safety can also be an issue because of issues of problem solving, judgment, and impulse control associated with brain damage.

Depending on which physical limitations individuals experience as the result of their brain damage, accommodations, modifications, and assistive devices in the home may be necessary. For example, if the individual experiences paralysis of an upper extremity, items kept in cabinets and cupboards should be moved for ease of reach, and special adaptive devices may be needed for eating or to assist in dressing. In the case of limitations in lower extremities, bathroom modifications such as a raised toilet seat, grab bars, and bench in the shower or tub may be needed, or doorways may need to be modified to accommodate a wheelchair. In other instances, adaptive devices such as a leg brace may be needed.

The capability of individuals to operate a motor vehicle post brain damage depends not only on their physical capability, but also on any cognitive and emotional limitations that could cause harm to either the individual or the general public. Driving is a complex task, requiring organizational ability, problem solving, decision-making ability, reflex actions, visual–motor skills, coordination, and physical manipulation. Limitations in any of these areas could affect individuals' ability to drive. If a seizure disorder is present, the problem is compounded. Comprehensive assessment may be needed to evaluate the individual's capability to drive. Unfortunately, because facilities or professionals qualified to provide this type of assessment may be limited except in urban areas, such evaluation may not be available to all who need it (Handler & Boland Patterson, 1995).

In some instances, eating behavior is affected by brain damage, such that monitoring of eating habits, weight gain or loss, and nutrition may be needed. In some cases, individuals may refuse to eat; in other instances, they may experience a constant urge to eat without feeling full. Specific strategies to assure adequate nutrition and stabilization of weight may need to be implemented. For instance, individuals may need to follow a regular schedule so that they take meals at the same time each day. If the person has problems with eating or swallowing, or if tube feedings are necessary, privacy should be provided for these activities.

Memory problems can interfere with individuals' ability to perform what might seem even small tasks of daily living following injury. Encouraging individuals to keep a notepad on which to list scheduled events, appointments, and important information can help them remember specific events. Keeping notes that have been strategically placed in the home or at work can help individuals remember specific tasks that might otherwise be overlooked, such as turning off the lights or closing the door.

Brain damage can cause a myriad of consequences that affect an individual's sexuality as well. Brain damage will, almost inevitably, cause cognitive, psychological, and sometimes physical changes that in some way affect the sexuality of the individual who has sustained the damage (Dombrowski, Petrick, & Strauss, 2000). Sensory–motor changes can cause erectile dysfunction in males, or motor changes leading to spasticity or ataxia may affect sexual behavior. Cognitive changes that inhibit or regulate emotional responses can result in disinhibition, impaired judgment, or other cognitive factors that regulate impulse control and can also impact sexual activity. Psychological factors such as depression or decreased self-esteem can decrease sex drive. Anxiety or emotional reactions of the individual's sexual partner may also adversely affect sexual function and drive.

A primary issue related to sexual activity may be social isolation and limited social contacts for individuals with brain damage. Individuals may have lost friends and contacts, or may not have had a sexual partner at the time of the injury. When opportunities to increase social interaction do occur, individuals with brain damage may, in their desire to be accepted, be overly anxious to be accepted, become vulnerable, and be taken advantage of. Individuals with brain damage who do not have a sexual partner may need to learn acceptable outlets through which they can express sexual needs.

Some individuals with brain damage may experience disinhibition, impairment in judgment, or inability to control sexual impulses. In these instances, the individual may engage in socially inappropriate behaviors such as inappropriate sexual advances or responses or masturbation in public. Individuals may need help in learning to interpret social and environmental cues and in learning more socially appropriate ways of expressing sexual need.

Individuals or family members may be reluctant to bring up sexual problems, or in some instances the individual with brain damage may be unaware that a problem exists. Talking openly about sexuality and assessing specific sexuality issues in the context of their specific values enable individuals to discuss specific concerns and to identify ways to adapt to changes in sexuality. In addition, identification of specific sexuality issues can lessen the effects of any problems that do arise (Hibbard Buffington, 1996).

Participation

Role changes as a result of brain injury affect not only the individual but also his or her family. Because of changes in the individual's temperament, behavior, and personality, there is often a disruption in family cohesion and feelings of entrapment experienced by family members (Degeneffe & Lynch, 2006). Depending on the extent of their role change, individuals may feel a diminishment of social status, social isolation, and consequently loss of self-esteem. Often more troublesome for family and friends are not the physical ramifications and residuals of the injury, but rather the behavioral and personality changes that

are a direct result of brain damage. Such personality changes may also put a strain on family relationships.

After they experience a brain injury, social relationships for individuals are often drastically altered. No relationship is more significantly modified than that of the family. Brain damage dramatically and permanently affects not only the individual experiencing it, but the whole family system. Severe brain damage produces prolonged stress in the family. Not only must the family cope with profound physical, cognitive, and emotional changes in the individual, but the stress of caregiving and financial burden can also be extreme. Because brain damage—whether traumatic or nontraumatic—occurs suddenly, neither the family nor the individual has the opportunity to prepare for its emotional and economic impact. Normal family development is disrupted, and any prior family stress may be exacerbated.

The family also significantly influences how the individual reacts to the damage and its residual effects. Depending on the circumstances of the injury, family members may place blame on the individual or on others, may be angry, or may express other negative emotions, which can have a negative impact on the individual and his or her rehabilitation potential. Family members may misinterpret personality changes or specific behaviors of the individual as deliberate or spiteful, coming from deep-seated anger toward the family, or they may assume the individual could control behavior if he or she wanted to. Individual family members may feel trapped and resent the caregiving role they must now assume, reminding the individual with brain damage of his or her dependence or belittling the individual. In other instances, family may enforce dependence. Glad to have the individual home again, rather than fostering independence and achievement of fullest functional potential, the family may instead encourage the person's dependence.

Family structure may be altered because the individual's condition may necessitate alterations in roles and functions of individual family members. In many cases, individuals who were once self-sufficient and living independently may, post injury, need support and care from a spouse or other family member. Depending on the severity of the brain damage, the personality and coping ability of the caregiver, and the previous relationship between the individual and his or her family, the situation can breed resentment and stress, which in turn can negatively affect rehabilitation potential. Even when a spouse or other family members willingly assume caregiving duties and do not consider their new responsibility to be a burden, most still undergo tremendous emotional turmoil as they adjust to changes in the individual with brain damage. The primary caregiver may neglect his or her own physical and emotional needs, as well as the needs of other family members. In some instances, the behavior of the individual with brain damage may make even simple social interactions embarrassing, so that the family eventually feels it is easier to stay within their home environment. As a result, they may become increasingly socially isolated.

Marital relationships can also begin to deteriorate. If significant marital strain was present prior to the brain damage, post-damage stress will merely be increased and consequently increase the strain. Determining pre-morbid family function can be helpful in identifying problems and working toward solutions.

Support, counseling, and education of the family about the nature of the condition, ways to cope with the individual's behavior, and identification of resources can be of considerable help in restoring a family's equilibrium. Family members should be given the opportunity to work through their feelings and be assured that their feelings are natural. Emphasis should be placed on maintaining the well-being of self and others in the family unit as well as attending to the needs of the individual with brain damage. Overall, the individual and family should be assisted in attaining realistic expectations and directed to pursuing reasonable goals.

Vocational Issues of Brain Damage

Unemployment rates for individuals with brain injury are high and often become higher over time (Schonbrun, Kampfe, & Sales, 2007). Return to work for individuals with brain damage has a multifactorial perspective. Because of the wide variation of manifestations related to brain damage, no one model can be applied to all individuals. The disparate changes that may occur as a result of brain damage present challenges not encountered with many other disabilities. The degree to which individuals with brain damage are able to maintain employment depends on the extent of the damage and any associated functional limitations as well as their prior background, age at the time the brain damage occurred, preinjury education, occupation, and work history (Wagner, Hammond, Sasser, & Wiercisiewski, 2002; Keyser-Marcus et al., 2002; Kreutzer et al., 2003). Personal motivation and support from family are also important factors in determining the individual's rehabilitation potential. Owing to the fact that behavioral and cognitive disabilities in TBI are often less visible and, therefore, less easy to categorize, services to address these needs may not be obtained, further impeding the individual's ability to return to work (Hart et al., 2006).

Factors that seem most closely related to the ability to return to work and to maintain employment after brain damage include the severity of damage experienced, the individual's age, preinjury behavior problems, and work history prior to brain damage. (Devitt, Colantonio, Dawson, Teare, Ratcliff, & Chase, 2006; Wagner, Hammond, Sasser, Wiercisiewski, & Norton, 2000; Felmingham, Baguley, &

Crooks, 2001). As the severity of brain damage increases, the rate of successful return to work decreases. Persons with greater manifestations and associated limitations have been shown to require more extended time and more extensive rehabilitation services before placement (Malec, Buffington, Moessner, & Degiorgio, 2000). Although the majority of individuals with mild brain damage may be able to return to work, individuals with moderate and severe brain damage have poorer outcomes (Fabiano & Daugherty, 1998). Even when job placement is accomplished, for individuals with moderate to severe manifestations, job retention may be difficult.

The type of occupation individuals were in prior to their injury also appears to influence the return to work outcome, with the highest rates of return to work being found among persons with higher decision-making jobs (Orr, Walker, Marwitz, & Kreutzer, 2003). Likewise, age also appears to be a significant determinant of return to work. Generally, the older the individual is at the time of injury, the less likely he or she is to return to work (Rothweiler, Temkin, & Dikmen, 1998).

Lastly, work history prior to brain damage appears to be related to ability to return to work post damage. Those individuals with a poor work history prior to experiencing brain damage are more likely to have more problems returning to work after brain damage has occurred (Rubin & Roessler, 2001).

Cognitive deficits and psychosocial difficulties may have more profound implications for an individual's ability to return to work than do any physical limitations. Individuals who retain average to above-average intellectual abilities and interpersonal skills after brain damage occurs are often better able to compensate for other limitations and maintain or gain employment. For others, however, levels of interpersonal functioning and cognitive self-awareness are often limited. Brain damage may result in drastic changes in personality

and personal ability as well as impaired self-awareness, which is also a frequent contributor to employment problems. Individuals who experience emotional liability may have more difficulty in reentering the workplace and in dealing with co-workers.

Memory impairment may be a debilitating effect of brain damage. Individuals with memory problems may forget what they have learned and may benefit from experience to only a limited extent. Helping individuals find alternative ways to perform tasks and develop strategies to reduce, organize, and retrieve information can reduce disabling effects of memory impairment. Given that individuals may have difficulty organizing their day, implementing structured routines, using written notes or lists, or audiotaped reminders may help improve performance. Usually the use of notes or lists will be most effective if information is kept simple, with no extraneous details. Too much information may cause the individual to become overwhelmed and confused.

Individuals with brain damage may not be aware of their deficits and may overestimate their abilities. Judgment may also be affected. Poor self-awareness or inaccurate self-perception can, in turn, contribute to employment problems. Individuals may be unable to recognize job errors and may consistently rate their performance more highly than their employer does. As a result, they may realize only a limited benefit from feedback.

The ability to communicate verbally or in writing or to comprehend words and concepts influences all aspects of job selection, training, and performance. Special considerations need to be given when limitations in ability to communicate are present. Visual–perceptual skills are integral to many jobs, both skilled and unskilled. The ability to perceive details, and to scan, match, or accurately perceive patterns may affect a number of daily life activities, including reading, driving, and general ability to navigate the environment.

Motor skills limitations affecting finger dexterity, eye–hand coordination, or eye–foot coordination may also be present in case of brain damage. When these limitations exist, work involving precision or operation of certain tools or equipment may be difficult. Individuals who have experienced paralysis of one of the upper extremities may be limited in their ability to lift, carry, or pull or push. If one of the lower extremities has been affected, individuals may require assistive devices such as a cane, walker, braces, or a wheelchair. Consequently, ambulation may be restricted to short distances. Ambulation on uneven surfaces should be avoided and, if a wheelchair is used, environmental modifications may be required. Reduced speed of performance of various tasks, physical stamina, and endurance should also be taken into account. Often individuals may be able to perform a task well if they are allowed to take their time, rather than feeling pressured to rush. Competitive environments in which speed is a priority may not be the best choices for individuals with brain damage and may actually contribute to decreased quality of work.

Brain damage is not a progressive condition, and, unless accompanying chronic illness produces additional symptoms or increases the chance of another stroke occurring, the individual's overall life expectancy is not affected by such injury. Brain damage is, however, a lifelong disability. Just as rehabilitation needs of individuals vary depending on the age at which the damage occurred, so will rehabilitation needs change over the individual's lifetime. Consequently, ongoing monitoring and contact with individuals may be necessary to help them maintain their maximum potential in the workplace.

In some instances, supported employment or job coaching may be appropriate. In other instances, performance-based feedback or prompts may be sufficient to help the individual maintain employment. Returning to gainful employment represents a series of complex challenges because of the number, complexity, and interaction of problems possible, all of which may contribute to difficulty in maintaining long-term employment. Monitoring performance and maintaining communication with the employer can contribute to job retention. Helping individuals learn compensatory strategies, providing appropriate workplace accommodations, and educating employers about the nature of brain damage and its consequences can greatly increase the chances of successful job placement.

■ OTHER CONDITIONS INVOLVING THE BRAIN

Central Sleep Apnea

Sleep apnea is one of the most widespread chronic disorders affecting adults. Among working adults, the prevalence of sleep-disordered breathing is estimated to be 25% among men and 9% among women (Weaver, 2001). Sleep apnea is characterized by frequent episodes of **apnea** (cessation of breathing) during sleep (Gottlieb, 2002) and daytime sleepiness. The latter problem can contribute to increased incidence of traffic accidents (Yamamoto, Akashiba, Kosaka, Ito, & Horie, 2000). Lack of sleep also causes stress, such that affected people become irritable, undergo changes in personality, or have difficulty with memory, leading to social and family disruption (Findley, Smith, Hooper, Dineen, & Suratt, 2000). It can also lead to more serious health consequences because of the increased risk of **hypertension** (high blood pressure) and heart disease associated with sleep apnea (Nieto et al., 2000; Shahar et al., 2001; Roux, D'Ambrosio, & Mohsenin, 2000) and, in some instances to death (Drazen, 2002; Veale et al., 2000).

There are two types of sleep apnea. The most common type, *obstructive sleep apnea*, is discussed in Chapter 14. The second type of sleep apnea, *central sleep apnea*, occurs when the brain fails to send appropriate messages to muscles needed for breathing to initiate respiration. It can be caused by stroke or by infections affecting the brain stem; it can also be caused by neuromuscular diseases that involve respiratory muscles.

Narcolepsy

Narcolepsy is a complex neurological sleep disorder involving the central nervous system that is linked to a disruption of the sleep control mechanism (Siegel, 2000). It is characterized by episodes of excessive sleepiness and uncontrollable sleep that occurs during the day (Stansberry, 2001). It can occur at any time, and during any activity, such as while engaging in conversation, while driving, while eating, or even when reading (Siegel, 2000).

Diagnosis is usually based on a persistent history of excessive daytime sleepiness not due to other causes; this diagnosis is confirmed through tests conducted at a sleep-disorders clinic. Treatment usually consists of planned short nap periods during the day and, in some instances, prescription of medications—namely, central nervous system stimulants.

The physical, psychosocial, and vocational implications of narcolepsy can be devastating. Individuals who are not adequately diagnosed and treated have a high risk of motor vehicle accidents and may have difficulty reaching their full potential either in school or in employment (Siegel, 2000). Even with treatment, symptoms of narcolepsy may not be adequately managed. Fear of embarrassment, which may result from the unpredictability of narcolepsy attacks, can cause individuals to limit their social interactions. Safety concerns regarding operation of potentially dangerous equipment may be an issue if the individual's symptoms are not adequately controlled. Employers, teachers, and others coming in contact with the individual should be educated to understand the individual's condition

so that if an attack does occur, symptoms will not be misinterpreted.

Diagnostic Procedures Used for Conditions of the Nervous System

Skull Roentgenography

Roentgenograms (radiographic studies or x-rays) of the skull provide visualization of the bones making up the skull as well as structures such as the sinuses. They are helpful for identifying fractures or other abnormalities of surrounding structures. X-ray films are usually taken by a radiology technician. The films are then read and interpreted by a **radiologist** (a physician who specializes in radiology).

Computed Tomography

A noninvasive radiographic technique, **computed tomography** (**CT scan**) applies computer technology and digital imaging techniques to x-ray studies and produces images of the body. Unlike conventional x-rays, computed tomography produces images of cross sections of the body, showing one "slice" of the structure being studied at a time, in sequence. On regular x-ray films, bone (e.g., the skull) can block the view of parts lying behind it (e.g., the brain). By contrast, computed tomography scans show both the bone and the underlying tissue and can detect abnormalities that cannot be visualized on plain x-rays.

A scan of the head by computed tomography can detect tumors and blood clots inside the brain. It can also reveal an enlargement of the ventricles of the brain due to inadequate drainage of cerebrospinal fluid (**hydrocephalus**) as well as other types of abnormalities in the brain and skull. In addition, a CT scan can be used to identify tumors or other sources of pressure on the spinal cord.

Individuals who are undergoing a scan by computed tomography are placed within a large cylinder that contains an x-ray tube and a receptor mounted opposite of each other.

Usually a special substance (contrast medium) is administered to the individual intravenously to highlight certain structures and make the results more readable. The tube is then rotated around the individual. X-rays are sent from the tube to the receptor, which measures the amount of radiation that each body tissue or organ absorbs during each rotation. A computer converts this information to a visual image on a screen. Images are monitored on a video screen and later photographed for more careful study by the radiologist, who has been specially trained in the field of radiology and reads and interprets the results from the radiological testing.

Magnetic Resonance Imaging

Magnetic resonance imaging (**MRI**) is a noninvasive procedure that may be used to obtain detailed information about body organs, especially soft tissue. It is used in disorders of the brain to aid in diagnosis or evaluation of conditions such as brain tumor, aneurysm, or malformation of blood vessels in the brain, stroke, multiple sclerosis, hydrocephalus, or abscess. This imaging technology may also be useful in determining the extent of traumatic brain injury.

During the MRI, the individual is placed in a narrow cylinder. When in the cylinder, a strong magnetic field causes positively charged biological substances in the body (*protons*) to become aligned in a certain direction. During the MRI, the individual's body is bombarded with radiowaves, which stimulate the protons to change their alignment. When the radiowaves are discontinued, the protons return to their normal positions. The changes are recorded electronically, and a computer translates the degree of change into highly detailed images, which helps the physician distinguish between normal and abnormal body tissues.

Although the procedure is relatively safe, MRI may be contraindicated for some individuals. Due to the confining nature of the cylinder used for the test, individuals with claustrophobia, individuals who are confused or agitated, or individuals with severe intellectual disability may be unable to be tested. Likewise, individuals who are extremely obese may not fit inside the cylinder. Open MRI machines, which do not require individuals to be placed into a confining cylinder, are available at some medical facilities. Because of the use of magnetic force in conducting the MRI, the test is contraindicated for individuals with cardiac pacemakers, metal implants, or other metal fragments, such as shrapnel, because of potential injury.

Brain Scan

Brain scan (also called brain nuclear scan) is not used as frequently as it once was owing to the advent of the CT scan and MRI (described earlier). This technique uses *radionuclides (radioisotopes)* to identify changes in brain tissue, including tumors, *infarction* (death of tissue), or infection, or blockage of blood vessels in the brain. A small amount of the radioactive material is injected intravenously and localizes in abnormal areas of the brain. A small camera records the concentration of radioactive material that has accumulated in various parts of the brain. These data are then transcribed by a computer to form images on film. The scan is usually performed by a radiologist or nuclear medicine technician.

A refinement of nuclear scanning is *SPECT (single photon emission computed tomography)*. This test uses computer methods similar to that of CT scan (described earlier), with a scanning camera that rotates around the body recording images of the collection of radionuclides in areas of abnormality of the body. SPECT scans are used to examine blood flow to the brain.

The radiation hazard in nuclear scanning is very slight, because the dosage of the radionuclide is very small and the duration of the exposure is brief. In many instances, nuclear scanning can provide useful information so that more dangerous, invasive tests can be avoided.

Positron Emission Transaxial Tomography

To study the biochemical or metabolic activities in cells of body tissue, **positron emission transaxial tomography** (**PET scan**) may be used. Individuals are injected with or inhale a biochemical substance tagged with a radionuclide. When the particles from the radionuclide combine with particles normally found in the cells of certain tissues, they emit special rays of radioactive particles (gamma rays) that a scanner can detect. The scanner then translates these emissions into color-coded images.

PET scans are able to assess chemical activities in body tissue, especially related to blood flow and metabolism. Consequently, information from the PET scan not only shows the structure of an area of the body, but also provides information about how body tissues function. In the brain, this type of scan can be used to evaluate tumors or the effects of disorders that may alter cerebral metabolism, such as Parkinson's disease, multiple sclerosis, or epilepsy.

Cerebral Angiography

Abnormalities of circulation in the brain can be visualized radiographically through **cerebral angiography**. Because blood vessels cannot be readily observed on regular x-rays, a contrast dye must be injected to make vessels visible on x-ray films. Cerebral angiography is considered an invasive procedure because a catheter is inserted into an artery and radiopaque dye is injected into the person. A series of x-ray films are then taken. The test enables physicians to study blood flow and to identify blockages that may be interfering with blood flow to certain parts of the brain.

Lumbar Puncture

When a laboratory analysis of an individual's cerebrospinal fluid is needed, a **lumbar punc-** **ture** (also called cerebrospinal fluid analysis or spinal tap) is done. To remove the fluid, a physician inserts a needle into the subarachnoid space of the spinal column at the lumbar area. The test may be done to determine whether there is blockage of the flow of spinal fluid, to detect bleeding, to detect infection such as encephalitis or meningitis, or to identify other central nervous system disorders. Although a lumbar puncture is often performed for diagnostic purposes, it can be done for therapeutic reasons, such as to reduce increased CSF pressure or to instill medications. It is often performed in an outpatient setting under local anesthesia.

Electroencephalography

A graphic recording of electrical activity of the brain (brain waves) can be obtained through electroencephalography (EEG). This procedure is helpful in identifying tumors, seizure disorders, and other types of brain dysfunctions, such as drug intoxication, and in determining brain function after brain injury. It may also be used to evaluate sleep disorders.

EEG is a noninvasive procedure in which electrodes are placed on various areas of the scalp and connected to a machine that records brain waves graphically. It may be performed by a physician or by a specially trained technician. The test is usually evaluated by a **neurologist** (a physician who is trained to diagnose and treat conditions of the nervous system).

Neuropsychological Tests

Neuropsychological tests are procedures that are used to assess major functional areas of the brain and to describe the impact of brain dysfunction on many areas of an individual's life, including the emotional, social, educational, and vocational spheres, to name a few. The tests are performed by a *clinical neuropsychologist*, an individual with advanced graduate training in the field of neuropsychology. Information gained from these tests may be used for diagnosis, monitoring changes, or treatment planning. In addition to assessing cognitive processes, most neuropsychological tests assess perceptual and motor skills. These tests can be used to assess memory, abstract reasoning, problem solving, spatial abilities, and emotional and personality consequences of brain damage or dysfunction.

Examples of commonly used neuropsychological tests are the *Wechsler Intelligence Scales, the Wechsler Memory Scales, Halstead–Reitan Neuropsychological Test Battery,* and *Luria Nebraska Neuropsychological Battery.*

Psychosocial Activities and Participation Issues Linked to Nervous System Conditions Involving the Brain

Conditions that involve the brain have widespread effects. Individuals can experience consequences affecting not only cognitive function, but also physical and emotional function. Physical consequences of brain injury can have manifestations that interfere with the ability to communicate, the ability to perform routine self-care, and other activities related to work and daily living.

The consequences of conditions affecting the brain have implications for both the individual and his or her family. Self-care or activities of daily living are often altered so that help from family members or others becomes necessary. Family members may become overly protective, shielding individuals from responsibility. They may exclude the individual from family problems or decision making or limit the individual's inclusion in family activities. In some instances, families may be reluctant to express their own feelings of frustration or helplessness, leading to stress and disruption in family functioning.

Although adjustment to any chronic condition or disability can be difficult, manifestations of conditions affecting the brain may offer particular challenges. To compound the issue, it is sometimes difficult to determine the degree to which behavioral and affective changes associated with brain conditions are physiologic and the degree to which they are situationally induced. Significant role changes may be necessary because of the manifestations of the condition. Individuals may need to adopt compensatory mechanisms or strategies to be implemented in a variety of social interactions, learn alternative methods of performing routine tasks, or learn how to use assistive devices to maximize performance. Consequently, psychological adaptation becomes a multifaceted endeavor.

Fatigue is often associated with conditions affecting the brain. It may be necessary for individuals with such conditions to space out activities or to arrange for frequent rest periods during the day. Activities that were once able to be completed in a short amount of time may need to be divided into a series of smaller tasks carried out over time.

Sexual function may also be affected. Personality changes may alter relationships with significant others so that sexual relationships change as well. In some instances, conditions affecting the brain cause emotional changes that interfere with judgment, insight, or ability to control sexual expression. In other instances, physical consequences, such as paralysis or spasticity, may make sexual activity more difficult.

Difficulties with social interaction may be associated with conditions affecting the brain that can alter social performance, cause social anxiety, and produce low self-esteem. Individuals may experience frustration and less self-assurance in the struggle to cope with social demands. Decreased capacity for social perceptiveness, distractibility, an absence of social initiation, or behavioral problems such as disinhibition or impulsivity may significantly affect individuals' ability to interact effectively in social or work settings. Social skills training or continuing supervision or prompting in the social setting can help individuals to become more fully integrated into social situations.

Not all manifestations of conditions affecting the brain are visible. Fatigue, visual or perceptual problems, or a predisposition to seizures may create a conflict in expectations when others do not understand the reason behind certain behaviors or when behaviors are misinterpreted as laziness, clumsiness, or unwillingness to participate in various activities. When conditions involve emotional liability or problems with memory, attention, or judgment, individuals may be perceived as rude, insensitive, or irresponsible, rather than having these characteristics be recognized as manifestations of the condition itself. Individuals who experience gait disturbance or slurring of speech as a manifestation of the condition may be thought by others to be intoxicated rather than to be affected by the condition.

Some conditions affecting the brain, such as epilepsy, are still associated with many myths and misconceptions and, as a result, may be accompanied by social stigma. Erroneous beliefs about the cause or meaning of seizures, or fear of knowing what to do if a seizure occurs, can cause disruption in social relationships, as others avoid social contact with the individual. Social contact may also be interrupted when conditions affecting the brain lead to altered speech, because others may be uncomfortable in their attempts to understand what the individual is trying to communicate.

Vocational Issues in Conditions Involving the Brain

Implications for vocational function for individuals with conditions involving the brain vary widely, depending on the extent and location of the brain area affected and the resulting manifestations. In many conditions affecting the brain, such as traumatic brain injury, there is no progression of the condition and, therefore, capabilities and function remain stable.

Conditions of the brain affect a number of functions, all of which should be assessed. Not only should cognitive functions, such as memory, problem-solving ability, and spatial and temporal orientation, be assessed, but motor abilities, such as coordination, balance, speed of performance, and muscle dexterity, should also be addressed.

Job stress may lead to fatigue—a manifestation that may already be a consequence of the condition. In conditions such as epilepsy, stress may precipitate symptoms. When individuals experience poor motor speed or decreased processing ability as a result of their condition, they may feel rushed or stressed when trying to perform tasks, and, as a result, their productivity and the quality of their work may be affected.

When communication skills are affected, alternative means of communicating in the workplace or job modifications may be needed. In many instances, even though individuals' communication may be difficult to understand, patience and practice will enable co-workers to establish basic patterns of communication that make interchange in the workplace possible.

For many conditions, specific characteristics of the condition as well as workplace conditions may need to be evaluated. For example, for individuals with epilepsy, it is important to assess the degree to which seizures are controlled and to identify whether any stimuli in the work environment might precipitate seizures. Transportation to and from work may also need to be considered. Although regulations vary from state to state, individuals with epilepsy may have to demonstrate that they have been seizure free or that medication has adequately controlled their seizures over a number of months or years before they are permitted to drive a motor vehicle. Individuals with physical or motor manifestations of a condition affecting the brain may need other structural modifications in the work environment or specific assistive devices to assist them in the workplace.

Other factors that may enhance or diminish individuals' ability to reach their full vocational capacity may be the availability of transportation, the attitudes of others, and realistic expectations about their level of performance. Expectations that are too high or too low may not match individuals' abilities and result in a less-than-satisfactory vocational experience. Considering each individual's abilities and needs, as with all other disabilities, is a key to vocational success.

CASE STUDIES: CONDITIONS

INVOLVING THE BRAIN

Case I

Ms. A. is a 29-year-old veterinary technician who received a brain injury when she slipped and fell on ice, hitting her head on the pavement. When evaluated at the trauma unit at the hospital, her Glasgow Coma Scale score was 7. After her condition stabilized, Ms. A. was referred for post-acute treatment and rehabilitation. Residuals experienced as consequences to her injury are post-traumatic seizures, information processing, and short-term memory difficulty.

1. What level of brain injury did Ms. A. experience based on the Glasgow Coma Scale score?
2. What types of other health professionals might you expect Ms. A. to have encountered during her post-acute rehabilitation, and what type of information may be important to have when considering Ms. A.'s ability to return to work?
3. What particular information would you want to assess related to Ms. A.'s seizures?
4. Which specific accommodations would you expect Ms. A. to need because of her injury?

Case II

Mr. D., a 20-year-old college student, experienced damage to the right side of his brain due to a ruptured congenital aneurysm. The aneurysm was surgically repaired.

1. What potential residual effects might you expect with right-sided brain damage?
2. Although you will obviously need additional information about the manifestations of brain damage Mr. D. experienced, how would you expect the damage to affect his ability to return to school?
3. Which specific services or accommodations might Mr. D. need in the event that he returns to school?

■ REFERENCES

Andersson, C., Asztalos, L., & Mattsson, E. & 2006). Six-minute walk test in adults with cerebral palsy: A study of reliability. *Clinical Rehabilitation, 20,* 488–495.

Anderson, C., & Mattsson, E., (2001). Adults with cerebral palsy: A survey describing problems, needs, and resources, with special emphasis on locomotion, *Developmental Medicine and Child Neurology, 43*(2), 76–82.

Ando, N., & Ueda, S. (2000). Functional deterioration in adults with cerebral palsy. *Clinical Rehabilitation, 14,* 3000–3006.

Anson, K., & Ponsford, J. (2006). Coping and emotional adjustment following traumatic brain injury. *Journal of Head Trauma Rehabilitation, 21*(3), 248–259.

Balandin, S., Berg, N., & Waller, A. (2006). Assessing the loneliness of older people with cerebral palsy. *Disability and Rehabilitation, 28*(8), 469–479.

Ballin, L., & Balandin, S. (2005). Community participation: Experiences of three older people with cerebral palsy. *AGOSCI News,* 15–18.

Barlow, J. H., & Ellard, D. R. (2006). The psychosocial well-being of children with chronic disease, their parents and siblings: An overview of the research evidence base. *Child Care, Health and Development, 32*(1), 19–31.

Berrol, S. (1992). Terminology of post-concussion syndrome. *Physical Medicine and Rehabilitation: State of the art reviews, 6,* 1–19.

Bishop, M. (2004). Determinants of employment status among a community-based sample of people with epilepsy: Implications for rehabilitation interventions. *Rehabilitation Counseling Bulletin, 47*(2), 112–120,122.

Bjorkdahl, A., Nilsson, A. L., Grimby, G., & Sunnerhagen, K. S. (2006). Does a short period of rehabilitation in the home setting facilitate functioning after stroke? A randomized controlled trial. *Clinical Rehabilitation, 20,* 1038–1049.

Brenner, L. A., Dise-Lewis, J. E., Bartles, S. K., O'Brien, S. E., Godleski, M., & Selinger, M. (2007). The long-term impact and rehabilitation of pediatric traumatic brain injury: A 50 year follow-up case study. *Journal of Head Trauma Rehabilitation, 22*(1), 56–64.

Browne, T. R., & Holmes, G. L. (2001). Epilepsy. *New England Journal of Medicine, 344*(15), 1145–1151.

Brown, D. L., & Morgenstern, L. B. (2005). Stopping the bleeding in intracerebral hemorrhage. *New England Journal of Medicine, 352*(8), 828–830.

Busch, C. R., & Alpern, H. P. (1998). Depression after mild traumatic brain injury: A review of current research. *Neuropsychology Review, 8*(2), 95–108.

Chan, R. C. K. (2005). Sustained attention in patients with mild traumatic brain injury. *Clinical Rehabilitation, 19,* 188–193.

Chemerinski, E., Robinson, R. G., & Kosier, J. T. (2001). Improved recovery in activities of daily living associated with remission of post-stroke depression. *Stroke, 32,* 113–117.

Cho, S. R. (2004). Characteristics of psychosexual functioning in adults with cerebral palsy. *Clinical Rehabilitation, 18,* 423–429.

Clements, A. D. (1997). Mild traumatic brain injury in persons with multiple trauma: The problem of delayed diagnosis. *Journal of Rehabilitation, 63,* 3–5.

Coetzer, R. (2007). Psychotherapy following traumatic brain injury: Integrating theory and practice. *Journal of Head Trauma Rehabilitation, 22*(1), 39–47.

Cunningham, S. D., Thomas, P. D., & Warschausky, S. (2007). Gender differences in peer relations of children with neurodevelopmental conditions. *Rehabilitation Psychology, 52*(3), 331–337.

Degeneffe, C. E., & Lynch, R. T. (2006). Correlates of depression in adult siblings of persons with traumatic brain injury. *Rehabilitation Counseling Bulletin, 49*(3), 130–142.

Devitt, R., Colantonio, A., Dawson, D., Teare, G., Ratcliff, G., & Chase, S. (2006). Prediction of long-term occupational performance outcomes for adults after moderate to severe traumatic brain injury. *Disability and Rehabilitation, 28*(9), 547–559.

Dixon, T. M., Layton, B. S., & Shaw, R. M. (2005). Traumatic brain injury. In H. H. Zaretsky, E. F. Richter III, & M. G. Eisenberg (Eds)., *Medical aspects of disability* (3rd ed., pp. 119–149). New York: Springer.

Dobkin, B. H. (2005). Rehabilitation after stroke. *New England Journal of Medicine, 352*(16), 1677–1684.

Dombrowski, L. K., Petrick, J. D., & Strauss, D. (2000). Rehabilitation treatment of sexuality issues due to acquired brain injury. *Rehabilitation Psychology, 45*(3), 299–309.

Drazen, J. M. (2002), Sleep apnea syndrome. *New England Journal of Medicine, 346*(6), 390.

Ellegala, D. B., & Day, A. L. (2005). Ruptured cerebral aneurysms. *New England Journal of Medicine, 352*(2), 121–124.

Fabiano, R. J., & Daugherty, J. (1998). Rehabilitation considerations following mild traumatic brain injury. *Journal of Rehabilitation, 64*(14), 9–11.

Felmingham, K. L., Baguley, I. J., & Crooks, J. (2001). A comparison of acute and postdischarge predictors of employment 2 years after traumatic brain injury. *Archives of Physical Medicine Rehabilitation, 82*(4), 435–439.

Findley, L., Smith. E., Hooper, J., Dineer, M., Suratt, P. M. (2000). Treatment with nasal CPAP decreases automobile accidents in patients with sleep apnea. *American Journal of Respiratory and Critical Care Medicine, 161*(3 part 1), 857–859.

Fisher, R. S. (2000). Epilepsy from the patient's perspective: Review of results of a community-based survey. *Epilepsy and Behavior, I* (suppl 1), S9–S14.

Fraser, R. T., & Miller, J. W., (2005). Epilepsy. In H. H. Zaretsky, E. F. Richter III, & M. Eisenberg (Eds.), *Medical aspects of disability* (pp 268–288). New York: Springer.

Frazer, C., & Gumnit, R. J. (1990). Sexuality and the person with epilepsy. In Gumnit, R. J. (Ed.), *Living well with epilepsy* (pp. 105–108). New York: Demos.

Gebel, J. M. (2007). Intracerebral hemorrhage. In R. E. Rakel & E. T. Bope (Eds.), *Conn's current therapy* (pp. 1036–1039). Philadelphia: W. B. Saunders.

Giacino, J., & Zasler, N. (1995). Outcome after severe traumatic brain injury: Coma, the vegetative state, and the minimally responsive state. *Journal of Head Trauma Rehabilitation, 10,* 40–56.

Gottlieb, D. J., (2002). Cardiac pacing—A novel therapy for sleep apnea? *New England Journal of Medicine, 346*(6), 444–445.

Greenberg, S. M. (2006). Small vessels, big problems. *New England Journal of Medicine, 354*(14), 1451–1453.

Groswasser, Z., & Stern, M. J. (1998). A psychodynamic model of behavior after acute central nervous system damage. *Journal of Head Trauma Rehabilitation, 13*(1), 69–79.

Hagan, C., Malkmus, D., & Durham, P. (1972). *Rancho Los Amigos scale.* Rancho Los Amigos Hospital.

Handler, B. S., & Boland Patterson, J. (1995). Driving after brain injury. *Journal of Rehabilitation, 61,* 43–49.

Hart, T., Dijkers, M., Fraser, R., Cicerone, K., Bogner, J. A., Whyte, J. et al. (2006). Vocational services for traumatic brain injury: Treatment definition and diversity within model systems of care. *Journal of Head Trauma Rehabilitation, 21*(6), 467–482.

Hart, T., Hanks, R., Bogner, J. A., Millis, S., & Esselman, P. (2007). Blame attribution in intentional and unintentional traumatic brain injury: Longitudinal changes and impact on subjective well-being. *Rehabilitation Psychology, 52*(2), 152–161.

Hibbard Buffington, A. L. (1996). Sexuality issues among survivors of traumatic brain injuries. *Journal of Applied Rehabilitation Counseling, 27*(1), 45–48.

Hodge, C. J. (2004). Head injury. In L. Goldman & D. Ausiello (Eds.), *Cecil textbook of medicine* (22nd ed., pp. 2241–2243). Philadelphia: W. B. Saunders.

Huhn, G. D., Sejvar, J. J., Montgomer, S. P., & Dworkin, M. S. (2003). West Nile virus in the United States: An update on an emerging infectious disease. *American Family Physician, 68*(4): 653–660.

Jennet, B., Snoek, J., Bond, M. R., & Brooks, N. (1981). Disability after severe head injury: Observations on the use of the Glasgow outcome scale. *Journal of Neurology and Neurosurgical Psychiatry, 44,* 285–293.

Jones, F. (2006). Strategies to enhance chronic disease self-management: How can we apply this to stroke? *Disability and Rehabilitation, 28*(13–14), 841–847.

Keyser-Marcus, L. A., Bricout, J. C., Wehman, P., Campbell, L. R., Cifu, D. X., Englander, J. et al. (2002). Acute predictors of return to employment after traumatic brain injury: A longitudinal follow-up. *Archives of Physical Medicine Rehabilitation, 83*(5), 635–641.

Kit, K. A., Mateer, C. A., & Graves, R. E. (2007). The influence of memory beliefs in individuals with traumatic brain injury. *Rehabilitation Psychology, 52*(1), 25–32.

Koch, L., Egbert, N., Coeling, H., & Ayers, D. (2005). Returning to work after the onset of illness: Experiences of right hemisphere stroke survivors. *Rehabilitation Counseling Bulletin, 48*(4), 209–218.

Koch, L., Merz, M. A., & Torkelson Lynch, R. (1995). Screening for mild traumatic brain injury: A guide for rehabilitation counselors. *Journal of Rehabilitation,* October/November/December, 50–56.

Kreutzer, J. S., Marwitz, J. H.,Walker, W., Sander, A., Sherer, M., Bogner, J., et al. (2003). Moderating factors in return to work and job stability after traumatic brain injury. *Journal of Head Trauma Rehabilitation, 18*(2), 128–138.

Lemke, D. M., (2007) Sympathetic storming after severe traumatic brain injury. *Critical Care Nurse, 27*(1), 30–37.

Lowenstein, D. H., & Alldredge, B. K. (1998). Status epilepticus. *New England Journal of Medicine, 338,* 970-976

Malec, J. F., Buffington, A .L., Moessner, A. M., & Degiorgio, L. (2000) A medical/vocational case coordination system for persons with brain injury: An evaluation of employment outcomes. *Archives of Physical Medicine Rehabilitation, 81*(8), 1007–1015.

Marfin, A. A., & Gubler, D. J. (2001). West Nile encephalitis: An emerging disease in the United States. *Clinical Infectious Disease, 33*(10), 1713–1719.

Nelson, K. B. (2003). Can we prevent cerebral palsy? *New England Journal of Medicine, 349*(18), 1765-1769.

Nieto, F. J., Young, T. B., Lind, B. K., Shahar, E., Samet, J. M., Redline, S., et al (2000) Association of sleep-disorder breathing, sleep apnea, and hypertension in a large community based study. *Journal of the American Medical Association, 283*(14), 1829–1836.

NIH Consensus Development Panel on Rehabilitation of Persons with Traumatic Brain Injury. (1999). Rehabilitation of persons with traumatic brain injury. *Journal of the American Medical Association, 282*(10), 974–983.

Odding, E., Roebroeck, M. E., & Stam, H. J. (2006). The epidemiology of cerebral palsy: Incidence, impairments and risk factors. *Disability and Rehabilitation, 28*(4), 183–191.

Ostensjo, S., Carlberg, E. B., & Vollestad, N. K. (2005). The use and impact of assistive devices and other environmental modifications on everyday activities and care in young children with cerebral palsy. *Disability and Rehabilitation, 27*(14), 849–861.

Orr, M. R., Walker, W. C., Marwitz, J. H., & Kreutzer, J. (2003). Occupational categories and return to work after traumatic brain injury. *Archives of Physical Medicine Rehabilitation, 84*(9), E5.

Quellet, M. C., & Morin, C. M. (2006). Fatigue following traumatic brain injury: Frequency, characteristics, and associated factors. *Rehabilitation Psychology, 51*(2), 140–149.

Pah-Lavan, Z. (2006). Traumatic brain injury: The cloud of unknowing. *Journal of Community Nursing, 20*(12), 4–12.

Palmer, S., & Glass, T. A. (2003). Family function and stroke recovery: A review. *Rehabilitation Psychology, 48*(4), 255–265.

Palmer, S., Glass, T. A., Palmer, J. B., Loo, S., & Wegener, S. T. (2004). Crisis intervention with individuals and their families following stroke: A model for psychosocial service during inpatient rehabilitation. *Rehabilitation Psychology, 49*(4), 338–343.

Pedley, T. A. (2004). The epilepsies. In L. Goldman & D. Ausiello (Eds.), *Cecil textbook of medicine* (22nd ed., pp. 2257–2268). Philadelphia: W. B. Saunders.

Pickelsimer, E. E., Selassie, A. W., Sample, P. L., Heinemann, A. W., Gu, J. K., & Veldheer, L. C. (2007). Unmet service needs of persons with traumatic brain injury. *Journal of Head Trauma Rehabilitation, 22*(1), 1–13.

Powell, R., Johnston, M., & Johnston, D. W. (2007). Assessing walking limitations in stroke survivors: Are self-reports and proxy-reports interchangeable? *Rehabilitation Psychology, 52*(2), 177–183.

Rappaport, M., Hall, K. M., Hopkins, K., Belleza, T., & Cope, D. N. (1982). Disability rating scale for severe head trauma: Coma to community. *Archives of Physical Medicine and Rehabilitation, 63,* 118–123.

Rothweiler, B., Temkin, N. R., & Dikmen, S. S. (1998). Aging effect on psychosocial outcome in traumatic brain injury. *Archives of Physical Medicine and Rehabilitation, 79*(8), 881–887.

Roux, F., D'Ambrose, C. & Mohsenin, V. (2000). Sleep-related breathing disorders and cardiovascular disease. *American Journal of Medicine, 108*(5), 396–402.

Rubin, S. E., & Roessler, R. T. (2001). *Foundations of the vocational rehabilitation process* (5th ed.). Austin, TX: Pro-ed.

Rush, B. K., Malec, J. F., Brown, A. W., & Moessner, A. M. (2006). Personality and functional outcome following traumatic brain injury. *Rehabilitation Psychology, 51*(3), 257–264.

Salkever, D. S. (2000). Activity status, life satisfaction, and perceived productivity for young adults with developmental disabilities. *Journal of Rehabilitation, 66*(3), 4–13.

Sandin, K. J. (2007). Rehabilitation of the stroke patient. In R. E. Rakel & E. T. Bope (Eds.)., *Conn's current therapy* (pp. 1042–1046). Philadelphia: W. B. Saunders.

Sandstrom, K. (2007). The lived body—experiences from adults with cerebral palsy. *Clinical Rehabilitation, 21,* 432–441.

Sawchyn, J. M., Mateer, C. A., & Suffield, J. B. (2005). Awareness, emotional adjustment, and injury severity in postacute brain injury. *Journal of Head Trauma Rehabilitation, 20*(4), 301–314.

Shahar, E., Whitney, C. W., Redline, S., Lee, E. T., Newman, A. B., Javier Nieto, F., et al. (2001). Sleep-disordered breathing and cardiovascular disease: Cross sectional results of the Sleep Heart Health Study. *American Journal of Respiratory Critical Care Medicine, 163*(1), 19–25.

Siegel, J. M., (2000) Narcolepsy, *Scientific American, 282*(1) 76–81.

St. Louis, E. K., & Granner, M. A. (2007). Seizures and epilepsy in adolescents and adults. In R. E. Rakel & E. T. Bope (Eds.), *Conn's current therapy* (pp. 1046–1055). Philadelphia: W. B. Saunders.

Stansberry, T. T. (2001) Narcolepsy: Unveiling a mystery. *American Journal of Nursing, 101*(8), 50–53.

Strober, L. B., & Arnett, P. A. (2005). An examination of four models predicting fatigue in multiple sclerosis. *Archives of Clinical Neuropsychology, 20,* 631–646.

Suarez, J. I., Tarr, R. W., & Selman, W. R. (2006). Aneurysmal subarachnoid hemorrhage. *New England Journal of Medicine, 354*(4), 387–396.

Trahan, E., Pépin, M., & Hopps, S. (2006). Impaired awareness of deficits and treatment adherence among people with traumatic brain injury or spinal cord injury. *Journal of Head Trauma Rehabilitation, 21*(3), 226–235.

Veale, D., Chailleux, E., Hoorelbeke-Ramon, A., Reybet-Degas, O., Humeau-Chapuis, M. P., Alluin-Aiquoy, F., et al. (2000). Mortality of sleep apnoea patients treated by continuous positive airway pressure registered in the ANTADIR observatory, *European Respiratory Journal, 15*(2) 326–331.

Vickery, C. D. (2006). Assessment and correlates of self-esteem following stroke using a pictorial measure. *Clinical Rehabilitation, 20,* 1075–1084.

Vitaz, T. W. (2007). Management of head injuries. In R. E. Rakel & E. T. Bope (Eds.)., *Conn's current therapy* (pp. 1117–1122). Philadelphia: W. B. Saunders.

Wagner, A. K., Hammond, F. M., Grigsby, J. H., & Norton, H. J. (2000). The value of trauma scores: Predicting discharge after traumatic brain injury. *American Journal of Physical Medicine Rehabilitation, 79*(3), 235–242.

Wagner, A. K., Hammond, F. M., Sasser, H. C., & Wiercisiewski, D. (2002). Return to productive activity after traumatic brain injury: Relationship with measures of disability, handicap, and community integration. *Archives of Physical Medicine Rehabilitation, 83*(1), 107–114.

Wagner, A. K., Hammond, F. M., Sasser, H. C., Wiercisiewski, D., & Norton, H. J. (2000). Use of injury severity variables in determining disability and community integration after traumatic brain injury. *Journal of Trauma, 49*(3), 411–419.

Weaver, E. M. (2001). Obstructive sleep apnea syndrome: When to suspect, how to help. *Consultant, 41*(3), 397–398; 400-403; 408-409.

White, R. J., & Likavec, M. J. (1992). The diagnosis and initial management of head injury. *New England Journal of Medicine, 327*(21), 1507–1510.

Wiegerink, D. J., Roebroeck, M. E., Donkervoort, M., Stam, H. J., & Cohen-Kettenis, P. T. (2006). Social and sexual relationships of adolescents and young adults with cerebral palsy: A review. *Clinical Rehabilitation, 20,* 1023–1031.

Willmore, L. J. (1998) Epilepsy emergencies: The first seizure and status epilepticus. *Neurology, 51* (suppl 4), S34–S38.

Yamamoto, H., Akashiba, T., Kosaka, N., Ito, D. & Horie, T. (2000) Long-term effects of nasal continuous positive airway pressure on daytime sleepiness, mood and traffic accidents in patients with obstructive sleep apnoea. *Respiratory Medicine, 94*(1), 87–90.

Wirkowski, E. (2007). Ischemic cerebrovascular disease. In R. E. Rakel & E. T. Bope (Eds.), *Conn's current therapy* (pp. 1039–1042). Philadelphia: W. B. Saunders.

Zivin, J. A. (2004). Approaches to cerebrovascular disease. In L. Goldmman & D. Ausiello (Eds.), *Cecil textbook of medicine* (22nd ed., pp. 2280–2287). Philadelphia: W. B. Saunders.

Chapter 4

Conditions of the Nervous System
Part II. Spinal Cord, Peripheral Nervous System, and Neuromuscular Conditions

■ **STRUCTURE AND FUNCTION OF THE SPINAL CORD AND PERIPHERAL NERVOUS SYSTEM**

The Spinal Cord

The spinal cord is part of the central nervous system (see Chapter 3) and extends from the brain stem to the lower part of the back. Bony coverings called *vertebrae* surround the spinal cord and protect it. This bony covering, as a whole, forms the vertebral column. The *vertebral column* consists of 7 *cervical vertebrae*, located in the neck area; 12 *thoracic vertebrae*, located in the upper and middle back; and 5 *lumbar vertebrae*, located in the lower back. The *sacrum*, located below the lumbar vertebrae, consists of fused (joined) bone. At the tip of the sacrum is the *coccyx*, or tailbone (see Figure 4-1).

The spinal cord conducts impulses to and from the brain. The outer white matter of the spinal cord, which consists of bundles or tracts of myelinated fibers of sensory (afferent) and motor (efferent) neurons, conveys electrical impulses up and down the spinal cord between the **peripheral nervous system** (those nerves lying outside the central nervous system) and the brain. In most instances, sensory information traveling up the right side of the spinal cord crosses over to the left side of the brain, so the left hemisphere of the brain

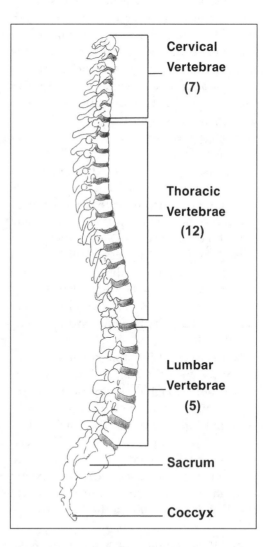

Figure 4-1 The spine

would, for example, interpret pain in the right hand. Conversely, motor impulses originating in the left brain cross to the right side of the spinal cord and initiate a response to the right side of the body. Because of this crossover effect, damage on one side of the brain typically causes symptoms on the opposite side of the body.

The inner gray matter of the spinal cord, which is composed of cell bodies and unmyelinated neurons, acts as a coordinating center for reflex and other activities, such as voluntary movements and control of internal functions. A reflex center in the gray matter of the spinal cord is where sensory and motor neurons connect; this part of the spinal cord serves as a center for spinal reflexes. A **reflex** can be defined as an automatic response to a given stimulus. Spinal reflexes control not only muscle reflexes, but also the reflexes of internal organs.

The gray matter within the spinal cord resembles the letter "H." The projections of the H are named according to the direction to which they project. The *posterior horns* extend toward the back, and the *anterior horns* project toward the front. Cerebrospinal fluid, which nourishes and protects the spinal cord, fills both the *central canal*, located within the center of the gray matter, and the subarachnoid space surrounding the outer portion of the spinal cord.

Motor (*efferent*) impulses originate in the motor cortex of the brain, extend down the spinal cord through *descending tracts*, and exit through motor spinal nerve roots that extend through openings between the vertebrae that surround the spinal cord. Sensory (*afferent*) impulses from the body enter the spinal cord through spinal nerve roots that also extend through openings between vertebrae and then travel up *ascending tracts* in the spinal cord to the brain.

Spinal nerve roots are named for the vertebral level from which they exit. For example,

the nerve roots that leave the spinal cord at the *cervical* level are labeled C1 through C8, and the nerve roots that leave at the **thoracic** level are labeled T1 through T12 (see Figure 4-2). The *sensory* (afferent) nerve fibers from outside the central nervous system carry body sensations into the *sensory nerve roots* (posterior roots) at the back of the spinal cord, where they are then carried up the spinal cord to the brain. *Motor* (efferent) impulses travel from the brain down the spinal cord and exit from *motor nerve roots* (anterior roots) at the front of the spinal cord. Motor nerve fibers then carry impulses to the voluntary muscles of the body.

Many types of neurons work together to transmit impulses through the spinal cord. Sensory impulses entering the spinal cord at the lumbar region are relayed vertically to the brain through a number of connecting sensory neurons. Motor impulses from the brain to the peripheral nerves, however, are conducted through two separate categories of motor neurons. *Upper motor neurons* originate in the brain and are contained entirely within the central nervous system. *Lower motor neurons*, although originating in the central nervous system, have fibers extending to the peripheral nerves in voluntary muscles. Alteration of function of either upper or lower motor neurons can generally affect the voluntary muscles. The location of the alteration of function determines the nature of the manifestations.

The Peripheral Nervous System

A nerve is a bundle of fibers outside the central nervous system that transmits information between the central nervous system and various parts of the body. The peripheral nervous system consists of all nerves that extend from the brain and spinal cord. To function effectively, the peripheral nerves must be connected to the central nervous system. Some peripheral nerves connect directly to the brain (*cranial nerves*); others connect directly to the

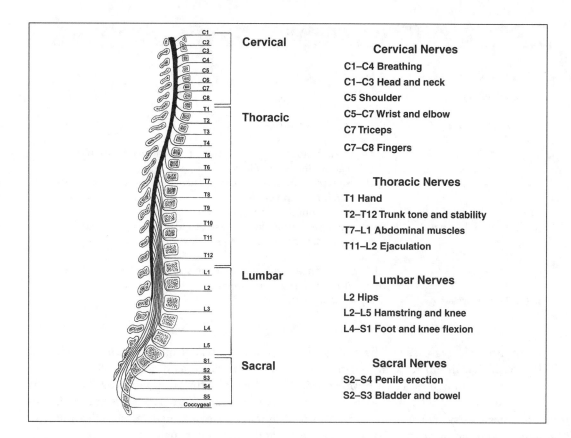

Figure 4-2   Spinal nerves

spinal cord (*spinal nerves*). Cranial and spinal nerves are essential links between the rest of the body and the central nervous system.

The 12 pairs of peripheral nerves that connect and transmit messages directly to the brain are called **cranial nerves**. Some cranial nerves contain only sensory fibers, whereas others contain both sensory and motor fibers. Cranial nerves mediate many aspects of sensation and muscular activity in and around the head and neck. Cranial nerves and their related functions are described in Table 4-1.

The 31 pairs of peripheral nerves that connect and transmit messages directly to the spinal cord are called **spinal nerves.** Each nerve divides and then subdivides into a number of branches. Nerves at each level travel to specific parts of the body, conveying information

between those areas and the central nervous system. Spinal nerves and their related functions are described in Figure 4-2.

Nerves control both voluntary and involuntary functions in the body. Nerves that control voluntary functions (such as movement of the muscles in the extremities) are called **somatic nerves.** Nerves that are concerned with the control of involuntary functions are part of a subcategory of the peripheral nervous system called the **autonomic nervous system**.

The autonomic nervous system integrates the work of vital organs, such as the heart and lungs. Its primary function is to coordinate the activity of internal organs so that they can make adaptive responses to changing external situations, thereby maintaining internal equilibrium. Nerve fibers monitor the activi-

Table 4-1   Cranial Nerves and Related Functions

Cranial Nerve	Area of Function
I. Olfactory	Smell
II. Optic	Vision
III. Oculomotor	Movement of eye muscles
IV. Trochlear	Eyelids
V. Trigeminal	Sensation in head, face, and teeth, motor activity of chewing
VI. Abducens	Pupil dilation, focusing of lens
VII. Facial	Taste, sensation of external ear, control of salivary glands, tears, muscles in facial expression
VIII. Vestibulocochlear	Sensation of sound, balance, orientation of head
IX. Glossopharyngeal	Swallowing, sensation of pain, taste, touch from tongue and throat
X. Vagus	Heartbeat, digestion, speech, swallowing, respiratory function, gland functions
XI. Accessory	Movement of head and shoulders, muscles of pharynx and larynx in throat, production of voice sounds
XII. Hypoglossal	Tongue movement, speech, swallowing

ties of internal organs as well as changes in the external environment. When changes are necessary to maintain internal **homeostasis** (equilibrium) or to protect the body, the autonomic nervous system stimulates an immediate, involuntary response. For example, in response to a speck of dust in the eye, tears are produced. In response to a fearful situation, the heart beats faster.

The autonomic nervous system is divided into two subsystems:

- The sympathetic nervous system
- The parasympathetic nervous system

These two systems work both together and in opposition to control internal organs and regulate their function. Hormones and emotions can affect both systems.

The sympathetic nervous system becomes active during stress and emergencies. It prepares the body for action, deepening respirations, making the heart beat faster, dilating the pupils, stimulating production of stress hormones, and increasing blood supply to the large muscles of the body.

In contrast, the parasympathetic nervous system dominates when the body is a rest. It activates mechanisms that focus on body conservation, such as decreasing the heart rate and constricting the pupils of the eye. The parasympathetic nervous system is also an important component of sexual arousal in both males and females.

■ SPINAL CORD INJURIES

Spinal cord dysfunction can result from a number of causes:

- Accidents causing direct injury to the spinal cord (such as motor vehicle accidents, sports injuries, or acts of violence, such as gunshot wounds)
- Compression of the spinal cord (such as a herniated disk or spinal tumors)
- Infectious conditions (such as polio or tetanus)
- Degenerative disorders (such as multiple sclerosis)
- Congenital disorders (such as spina bifida)

Most spinal cord dysfunction is due to injuries from motor vehicle accidents, with the second highest cause being falls (Hodge,

2004). Ultimately, spinal cord dysfunction results in some combination of sensory, motor, or reflex deficit (Johnson, Mowrey, & Bergman, 2008). When the spinal cord is injured, transmission of impulses between the brain and other parts of the body below the level of injury is interrupted. Consequently, some degree of motor, sensory, or reflex function below the injury is affected. There may be numbness, complete paralysis, or exaggerated, absent, or diminished reflexes below the level of the injury. The extent of the functional consequence or loss depends on which part of the spinal cord is injured and whether the cord is bruised, compressed, or severed. For instance, in some cases, swelling, bleeding, or a tumor may compress the cord without severing it. In these instances, removal of the source of compression may restore function, if the spinal cord has not been permanently damaged. When the spinal cord is severed, however, transmission of nerve impulses may be permanently lost or impaired.

Total severance of the spinal cord results in *complete spinal cord injury*, so that there is no nerve function below the level of the injury and no voluntary motor or sensory function exists below that level. When severance is not complete, the injury is called an *incomplete spinal cord injury* meaning that the individual has some motor or sensory function below the level of the injury. In these instances, one portion of the spinal cord may be nonfunctional, while another portion maintains some function; or certain nerve tracts may still be functioning, but in an abnormal way. The term **paraparesis** refers to partial paralysis and indicates that some function remains below the level of the injury. Sometimes even when the spinal cord is not completely severed, all motor and sensory function below the level of the injury may be lost if the remaining nerves are destroyed owing to lack of blood supply, degeneration, or compression. In general, the higher the level of the spinal cord injury, the greater the functional consequences.

Manifestations of Spinal Cord Injury

Symptoms of spinal cord injury specifically reflect the level of the injury and the function of the neurons involved (see Figure 4-2). If spinal nerves are unable to transmit messages between the central nervous system and the peripheral nervous system, function below the level of injury will be disrupted. The degree of functional loss depends on the degree to which the spinal cord is injured. For example, if the afferent nerve roots in the ascending tracts (*sensory tracts*) were injured, it would be expected that some degree of sensory loss below the level of injury would exist. If the efferent nerve roots in the descending tracts (*motor tracts*) were injured, some degree of motor loss below the level of injury would be expected. When both sensory and motor tracts are injured, as with complete severance of the spinal cord, both motor and sensory loss occurs below that level.

Ambulation is affected to some degree regardless of the level of injury, with the exception of injury at the sacral level (S2–S4) in which ambulation may return to normal. Individuals with spinal cord injuries above T12 usually require a wheelchair for ambulation. At lower levels of injury, ambulation for short distances may be possible with braces or crutches.

Most individuals lose voluntary control of bladder and bowel function after spinal cord injury. In case of *neurogenic bladder* (a condition in which bladder muscles are paralyzed and the individual is unable to empty the bladder voluntarily), a number of bladder evacuation devices may be used: external collection devices, such as condom/Texas catheters; indwelling catheters inserted into the bladder through the urinary meatus; indwelling catheters inserted through a surgical opening created on the lower abdomen above the bladder (*suprapubic*). These devices are used in conjunction with external drainage systems such as a leg bag. Bladder incontinence pads may also be used. When feasible, intermittent catheterization may be used several times a day. In lower-level injuries, such as at the lumbar level, bladder evacuation may be accomplished by applying external pressure to the lower abdomen.

Neurogenic bowel is the term used to describe paralysis of the lower rectal and anal muscles such that the individual is unable to control bowel evacuation. Loss of voluntary bowel function is frequently one of the most distressing factors for individuals with spinal cord injury, altering their body image (Coggrave, Burrows, & Durand, 2006). Consequently, an effective bowel management program is important to individuals' overall rehabilitation. A bowel management program is required to empty the lower bowel and to establish a consistent routine so that involuntary bowel evacuation can be avoided (Johnson, Mowrey, & Bergman, 2008). Bowel management may be accomplished through use of suppositories, digital stimulation or manual evacuation of stool, or small-volume enema, in addition to consumption of a diet with high fiber content, avoidance of gas-producing foods, and adequate hydration.

Spinal Cord Injuries at the Cervical Level (C1 through C8)

Diving accidents, motor vehicle accidents, or a blow to the head with a heavy object may cause fractures of the cervical vertebrae. An injury to the spinal cord at the cervical level (C1 through C8) results in **quadriplegia** (paralysis of both upper and lower extremities). Injuries at C1 or C2 are often fatal because the functioning of all muscles, including the muscles of respiration, is lost. Individuals who survive these injuries require ventilatory support to breathe and are totally dependent on others for self-care. Individuals with injuries at C3 or C4 also have compromised ventilatory capacity and require special respiratory equipment; in addition, they will be dependent on others for self-care. However, at this level of injury, wheelchair ambula-

tion may be possible through use of a mouth stick, which individuals can employ to manipulate an electric wheelchair. Most individuals with spinal cord injuries at C4 or above must have an attendant for personal care, dressing, and transfers.

With an injury at the C5 level, some gross movement of the upper extremities is possible, such as bending the arm at the elbow. Individuals may be able to hold a light object between the thumb and finger, or they may be able to maneuver small objects with the assistance of hand splints. Assistance will still be required for most activities, but individuals may be capable of transfer on their own with the assistance of special equipment. Total independent living is probably not feasible, although independent electric wheelchair ambulation may be possible.

Individuals with injury at C6 also have gross motor movement of upper extremities and may be able to retain some independence in self-care, such as feeding and dressing with the aid of special orthotic equipment. Propelling a wheelchair manually may be possible, with a modified hand rim, although many individuals continue to operate a motorized chair. With the use of hand splints, individuals may also be able to write. Independent transfer from bed to chair or to a car may also be possible, as is driving with the use of special adaptative devices.

Individuals with C7 injuries are capable of straightening their arm and are able to sit up in bed, dress themselves, and transfer. Thus almost total independence with some adaptations in the environment may be achieved. Fine motor movements of the hands are impaired, but writing may be possible with the use of a special device that can be strapped to the hand. Driving is possible with hand controls.

With C8 injuries, individuals have some sensation in their hands and may become totally independent with a modified environment and some adaptative devices.

Spinal Cord Injuries at the Thoracic Level (T1 through T12)

Spinal cord injuries occurring at T1 or below result in **paraplegia** (paralysis of the lower extremities). Upper extremities for the most part are unimpaired, with the exception of T1 injuries, in which there may be slight weakness and some loss of flexibility in the hands. Individuals with an injury between T1 and T3 may need a brace or other support to maintain posture in an upright position; even though the upper extremities are functional, in these persons, the muscles of the trunk are paralyzed. In most cases, individuals with injuries at T1 through T12 are able to attain total independence in self-care, wheelchair ambulation, and transfer. Individuals with injuries at T7 to T12 may be able to walk with the use of long leg braces. Nevertheless, because of the strenuous nature of the activity, ambulation may be possible for only short distances.

Spinal Cord Injuries at the Lumbar Level (L1 through L5)

Many of the muscles of mobility are intact with L1 through L5 injuries. All upper body muscles and many of the leg muscles are functional. Ambulation with braces and/or use of a cane or crutches may be possible, especially for short distances. Individuals are able to gain total independence in care, although hand controls may be necessary for operating a motor vehicle. Although bowel and bladder function are still impaired, reflex emptying of bowel and bladder may be possible.

Spinal Cord Injuries at the Sacral Level (S1 through S4)

Ambulation is usually possible with little or no equipment. Bowel and bladder function may still be impaired to some degree.

Initial Management of Spinal Cord Injury

The initial treatment of spinal cord injuries focuses on preventing further injury, stabilizing individuals' physical condition, and, in some instances, performing surgery to realign the spinal column or achieve decompression of the spinal cord. Many individuals with spinal cord injuries—especially those who received the injury as the result of an accident—will have other injuries such as fractures, injuries to internal organs, or brain injuries that further complicate their care.

Individuals with injuries to the cervical spine are usually placed in skeletal traction to immobilize the spine. In some instances, individuals may have cervical orthoses, such as a *halo brace* (see Figure 4-3). With this device, metal pins are inserted into the skull and attached to a metal "halo" that surrounds the head. The "halo" is attached with two metal rods to a "vest" worn on the torso of the individual. The halo brace is used to allow mobility while keeping the head and neck in proper position. Traction is rarely used to stabilize and immobilize thoracic or lumbar fractures because there is no effective way to provide it.

After their condition has been stabilized and any acute medical needs met, individuals are usually transferred to a rehabilitation unit, where they learn skills or learn to use adaptive devices that will help them to achieve the maximum level of independence. A wide variety of health professionals are usually involved in this phase of rehabilitation. Health professionals involved may include *physiatrists, physical therapists, rehabilitation nurses, occupational therapists, orthotists, psychologists, social workers, and rehabilitation counselors.*

Physical therapy begins as soon as possible to prevent deformities such as *contractures* (permanent contraction of a muscle such that a joint becomes fixed or immobile) or footdrop, as well as to build strength. An immediate treatment goal is to have individuals with either paraplegia (involvement of lower extremities) or quadriplegia (involvement of all four extremities) placed into an upright position as soon as possible to prevent complications such as respiratory

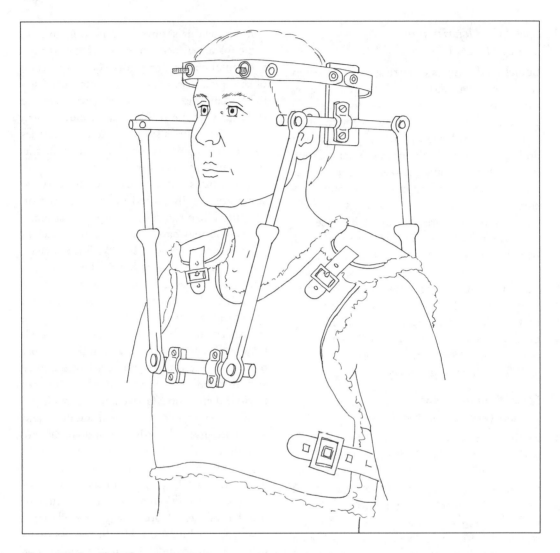

Figure 4-3   Halo brace

problems from occurring. The use of a *tilt board* or *circular bed* is used to accomplish this goal. Individuals are strapped securely to the tilt board or circular bed while in a prone position; the board is then gradually raised or the circular bed rotated until the individual is upright.

As an individual's condition stabilizes, treatment is directed toward teaching self-care. Most individuals with spinal cord injury become mobile with the use of a wheelchair. Many types of wheelchairs with a variety of options, including detachable armrests and footrests, removable back panel, lapboard, and carryall bag, are available. Power-operated wheelchairs are available for individuals who have little or no use of their upper extremities. These battery-operated chairs can be controlled with a switch adapted to the particular individual's ability. Because of the size of these wheelchairs, they are heavy and, therefore, more difficult to transport.

As part of rehabilitation, individuals are taught a variety of self-care skills, including dressing, hygiene, and grooming. It may be necessary to install specific adaptive devices, such as grab bars and a raised toilet seat, in the home. Because most spinal cord injuries affect bladder and bowel function, instructions in catheter care and bowel retraining are usually necessary.

Potential Complications Associated with Spinal Cord Injury

In addition to altered functional capacity, individuals with spinal cord injury are confronted with a number of short-term and long-term issues that require ongoing medical attention (Bloemen-Vrenchen, deWitte, & Post, 2005). Individuals with spinal cord injury are at risk of developing additional health problems that could result in a secondary condition and, consequently, more functional limitations. Development of complications can hamper individuals' ability to work as well as interfere with their social relationships. Some complications associated with spinal cord injury can also be fatal.

The risk of developing complications is related to the level of injury. In general, the higher the level of injury, the greater the risk of developing secondary disabling conditions. It is, therefore, imperative that individuals with spinal cord injuries, family members, and professionals working with them be aware of this risk and the prevention strategies to lessen the risk. When complications do arise, it is crucial that they be treated immediately.

Altered Symptoms of Illness

Because of the lack of sensation that accompanies most spinal cord injuries as well as the interruption to nerve pathways, symptoms of various conditions unrelated to the spinal cord injury itself may not be recognized and, as a result, may not receive prompt treatment. For example, because pain is not felt, appendicitis may not be discovered until the appendix ruptures.

In some instances, symptoms may be expressed differently in individuals with spinal cord injury than in individuals without spinal cord injury. For example, individuals without spinal cord injury may experience severe flank pain in response to a kidney infection, whereas individuals with spinal cord injury may experience an abrupt increase in spasticity with the same infection. As a result, the symptom may not be recognized as being related to kidney infection and, consequently, the kidney infection may not be immediately diagnosed and treated. Individuals with spinal cord injuries, caregivers, and professionals should be made aware of alterations in the presentation of symptoms and should be alerted to report or investigate new symptoms or accentuated old symptoms as soon as they are noted.

Pressure Sores (Decubitus Ulcers)

One of the most common complications associated with spinal cord injury is pressure sores, also called *decubitus ulcers* (Catz, Zifroni, & Philo, 2005). People with spinal cord injuries are at increased risk of developing pressure sores, which result from lack of blood supply to a body pressure point, such as the buttocks, sacrum, heel, or back. Pressure sores develop when continuous pressure is exerted to a body part over time (Woolsey & McGarry, 1991; Pires & Adkins, 1996). Pressure on a body part interferes with blood supply, eventually resulting in breakdown and ulceration of the skin. Because individuals with spinal cord injury are often immobile, areas of pressure on certain bony prominences are more likely to develop. As individuals with spinal cord injury usually have no sensation below the level of injury, they are unable to feel pressure, and because of the paralysis, they are unable to easily shift their weight to relieve the pressure. Inadequate skin care, irritation, and nutritional deficiency can further contribute to the development of pressure sores.

Pressure sores may appear to be small on the surface, but the depth of the ulcer may be more extensive. Untreated pressure sores can progress from redness to breakdown of the skin, infection, and eventually death (**necrosis**) of skin tissue, which could extend through the tissue all the way to the bone. Pressure sores are not only debilitating but can be potentially life-threatening (Catz, Zifroni, & Philo, 2005).

Individuals with spinal cord injury must be aware of the risk of pressure sores and the importance of self-monitoring of skin. Education about the importance of decreasing the amount of pressure on bony prominences by regularly changing position, good nutrition, and good skin care is an important part of the rehabilitation process. A number of prescribed wheelchair cushions are available that can help distribute pressure to prevent skin breakdown and extend endurance in a wheelchair. In addition to having the correct cushion prescribed, individuals with spinal cord injury should be helped to learn how to position the cushion properly.

Urinary Tract and Bowel Complications

Individuals with spinal cord injuries are especially prone to urinary tract infections because of the abnormal emptying of their bladder. The bladder may not empty often enough or may not empty completely, leaving urine in the bladder that then acts as a reservoir for infection. Because individuals with spinal cord injury are generally unable to control their bladder, they may need to have a catheter inserted into the bladder to drain urine and prevent incontinence. The bladder and its contents normally contain no pathologic organisms, but there is always the potential for the introduction of infectious organisms when a catheter is inserted into the bladder. For individuals with spinal cord injury, urinary tract infections can be a serious, debilitating, and, at times, life-threatening problem. Untreated urinary tract infection can lead to **pyelonephritis** (infection of the kidney; see Chapter 15) and in severe cases, **septicemia** (infection in the blood).

After paralysis, due to the individual's inactivity, the amount of calcium in the blood increases. As a consequence, the risk of developing kidney stones (*renal calculi*) increased. A stone may form in the kidney itself or may lodge in the *ureters* (tubes leading from the kidney to the bladder) so that it obstructs urine flow, causing urine to back up into the kidneys (**urinary reflux**) and eventually damaging to the kidney itself.

Education of individuals with spinal cord injuries about the urinary tract, risk of its infection, and ways to decrease the risk of infection or stone formation is crucial in preventing secondary urinary tract complications. In addition, individuals with spinal cord injuries should be made aware of the importance of self-monitoring and promptly reporting symptoms so that prompt diagnosis and treatment may be instituted.

Secondary conditions related to bowel elimination may also be problematic. Incontinence of fecal material may not only contribute to skin breakdown and urinary tract infection, but also result in social isolation if individuals become concerned about the probability that incontinence will occur. Other problems may relate to *impaction* (fecal matter that becomes hardened and is unable to be evacuated) or *paralytic ileus* (a condition in which the intestine ceases to function). Individuals can decrease their risk for developing these conditions by establishing a pattern of regular elimination, monitoring their diet and fluid intake, and learning specific techniques to enhance optimal bowel function.

Contractures

Contractures (loss of range of motion, or fixed deformity of a joint) may occur in paralyzed limbs if the joints are not moved through their regular range of motion. Contractures of the upper extremities in individuals with quadriplegia can interfere with the use of assistive devices. If individuals with paraplegia or quadriplegia develop contractures of the hip or knee, it may be difficult to assume adequate positioning in a wheelchair. Regular movement of joints through the full range of motions via passive exercise conducted by another person or through use of special equipment can prevent contractures from occurring. In addition, proper wheelchair seating and correct positioning of joints can help reduce the risk of contractures.

Spasticity

Spasticity refers to exaggerated involuntary movement of paralyzed muscles. It can restrict activities of daily living, cause pain and fatigue, disturb sleep, contribute to the development of contractures, and affect individuals' self-image (Adams & Hicks, 2005). Although spasticity may be absent immediately after injury, it can occur subsequently long after individuals leave the rehabilitation facility.

Because communication between the peripheral nervous system and the brain is interrupted by spinal cord injury, signals received by the peripheral nerves are "short-circuited." Rather than traveling to the brain to be interpreted and appropriately adapted, the signal instead returns from the spinal cord directly to the muscle. The resulting muscle contractures can sometimes be violent and can occur with even slight stimulation. Spasticity can be debilitating, not only because it is disruptive and can potentially cause embarrassment to the individual, but also because in some instances it can be so strong that it causes individuals to fall from their wheelchairs. Spasticity can also contribute to formation of contractures. Although in some instances spasticity can be useful to help individuals perform certain functions, such as shifting position or standing, more often it is a source of discomfort.

When spasticity is a cause of concern for the individual, a physical rehabilitation program using a variety of modalities may help diminish its frequency. In other instances, antispasticity medications may be used to reduce spasticity, although side effects of sedation, and generalized weakness, may make this treatment less desirable (Adams & Hicks, 2005). When oral medications are not effective, medications may be administered through a surgically implanted pump with a reservoir that delivers medication (baclofen) directly into the cerebrospinal fluid (Kita & Goodkin, 2000). In other instances, medications that block nerves may be injected so that nerve conduction is disrupted, hence relaxing muscles (Jozefczyk, 2002). Botulinum toxin—a neurotoxin— may also be injected into a muscle to temporarily inhibit spasms (Burchiel & Hsu, 2001). In severe cases, when other treatments are ineffective in controlling spasticity, individuals may resort to surgery, such as *tenotomy*, the release of a tendon from a severely spastic muscle); tendon lengthening, to reduce pull on spastic muscles; or tendon transfer, in which the tendon attachment to the bone is moved closer to the muscle to relieve spasticity (Adams & Hicks, 2005; Jozefczyk, 2002).

Osteoporosis

Bone is a dynamic substance that is characterized by continual deposition and reabsorption of calcium. The combined stress of weight bearing and muscle pull that occurs with activity helps bones maintain their calcium content. Conversely, inactivity can contribute to softening and weakening of bones (**osteoporosis**). Individuals with spinal cord injuries have an increased rate of calcium removal from the bone and, therefore, are more susceptible to fractures, which could be caused by either falls or simple activities such as wheelchair transfer (Chen, Lai, Chan, Huang, Tsai, & Chen, 2005). Calcium, which is excreted through the urinary system, can also contribute to urinary tract stones, as noted earlier. In some instances, calcium is deposited in soft tissues so that the function of a joint or muscle is disrupted.

Adequate diet, passive and strength-building exercises, and electrical stimulation to the muscles are all techniques that can be used to help reduce the risk of developing osteoporosis. In addition, proper training in safety procedures when operating a wheelchair and transferring can help prevent occurrence of falls and potentially broken bones if osteoporosis is present.

Cardiovascular Complications

In the initial stages after a spinal cord injury, individuals are susceptible to **thrombophlebitis** (formation of blood clots in the legs) or *pulmonary embolism* (a blood clot that travels to the lungs), a potentially life-threatening disorder. As the individual's condition stabilizes, this complication becomes less of a threat. In the initial period after injury, individuals may also experience *orthostatic hypotension*, a condition in which the blood pressure becomes significantly lower when the individual is moved from a flat position to an upright position (Claydon, Steeves, & Krassioukov, 2006).

Although these complications become less likely after the first month, individuals with spinal cord injuries continue to be more prone to developing respiratory disorders, especially conditions such as pneumonia, which can be both debilitating and life-threatening. Individuals with high cervical or high thoracic injuries, because of their weakened chest muscles, have a more difficulty in expanding the lungs and clearing respiratory secretions. Consequently, they are more susceptible to infection of the lungs.

Individuals with spinal cord injury also have a more sedentary lifestyle, which can affect the cardiovascular system. Because of this increased susceptibility to cardiovascular conditions, individuals with spinal cord injuries should refrain from smoking or use of tobacco products as well as excessive alcohol consumption. Good nutrition, an exercise program, and weight control are also important measures for prevention of cardiovascular disease. Individuals with spinal cord injuries, because of their increased risk of developing cardiovascular conditions, should engage in regular medical examinations and comprehensive healthcare programs that accommodate the needs of individuals with spinal cord injury.

Autonomic Dysreflexia

Autonomic dysreflexia is an abnormal reflex condition characterized by a sudden rise in blood pressure, profuse sweating, and headache as the result of excessive neural discharge from the autonomic nervous system. It may be triggered by events as simple as overdistention of the bowel or bladder, pressure sores, or constipation (Jennings, 2007). Unless the individual receives immediate treatment to decrease the blood pressure, there is risk of stroke. Autonomic dysreflexia commonly occurs in individuals who have experienced an injury to the upper spinal cord. Identifying and avoiding situations or conditions that trigger autonomic dysreflexia are important in the prevention of this condition.

Pneumonia and Other Respiratory Problems

Pneumonia and other respiratory complications are common in individuals with spinal cord injuries, especially those with quadriplegia (Johnson, Mowery, & Bergman, 2008). Individuals with higher-level injuries may have difficulty deep-breathing and removing secretions, contributing to an increased risk of respiratory complications. Individuals with spinal cord injuries should avoid exposure to persons with respiratory infections as much as possible, as well as avoid smoking and air pollution.

Other Neurological Complications

Diaphoresis (profuse sweating) and **paresthesia** (abnormal painful sensations below the level of injury) are other potential sequelae of spinal cord injury. About one-third of individuals with spinal cord injury report experiencing chronic pain (Jensen, Hoffman, & Cardenas, 2005).

Sexual Dysfunction

Nerves to the genital region are almost always affected to some degree by spinal cord injury (Ducharme, 2006). This does not mean, however, that other aspects of sexuality—such as sexual attraction to others, sexual desire, and the need to express oneself as a sexual being—are changed. Many men and women remain sexually active after spinal cord injury, although modifications of sexual behavior and function typically need to be made.

Genital function is controlled by the parasympathetic and sympathetic nervous systems as well as by motor nerves; the amount of function retained after spinal cord injury depends on the level of injury as well as on whether the injury is complete or incomplete. The higher the level of injury, the more significantly genital function will be affected. Most individuals with a spinal cord injury—both males and females—will have little sensation directly in the genital area. Because mobility is affected in spinal cord injury, individuals will also need to use an alternative technique for sexual performance.

Many males, regardless of the level of spinal cord injury, continue to have reflex erections. Also, in many instances, erection can be produced through manual stimulation. The ability to produce an erection through psychological arousal is absent in most men with spinal cord injuries; although individuals with lower spinal cord injuries may have a weakened sexual response due to psychological stimuli. Some individuals have used techniques such as penile implants to achieve intercourse.

Ejaculation is absent for most men with spinal cord injury; if it does occur, individuals may experience retrograde ejaculation, such that semen is deposited into the bladder rather than externally (Ducharme, 2006). As a result, fertility in males is significantly affected, especially in males with complete severance of the spinal cord. Techniques such as *electro-ejaculation*, in which ejaculation is stimulated through electrical means, have been used to obtain sperm for artificial insemination.

Females with spinal cord injuries are still able to engage in sexual intercourse, although the lubrication produced by psychological arousal is usually absent. Menses typically are absent the first months after injury; with the return of menstruation occurring within six months after injury. In most instances female fertility is unaltered by spinal cord injury. Consequently, women who do not wish to become pregnant need to use some form of contraception. When women with spinal cord injuries become pregnant, they are able to carry the pregnancy to term, although because of altered sensation, it may be more difficult for them to determine when labor begins.

Psychological Issues in Spinal Cord Injury

Spinal cord injury interrupts and alters not only physical functioning, but also psychosocial functioning. Post-traumatic stress disorder (PTSD) as well as other psychological consequences has been linked to spinal cord injury (Chung, Preveza, Papandreou, & Prevezas, 2006; Lude, Kennedy, Evans, Lude, & Beedie, 2005). Individuals with spinal cord injury, in addition to experiencing changes in movement and sensation, decreased mobility and independence, changes in bowel and bladder functioning, and changes in sexual functioning, experience altered self-concept and, in many instances, loss of self-esteem. Frustrated goals, loss of self-regard, or loss of illusion of omnipotence and control can result in internalized anger, anxiety, and guilt. To a great degree, how individuals adjust will be related to how they conceptualize losses they experience as a result of the injury, their individual coping style, and the amount and type of social support available.

Although depression is common after spinal cord injury, it is not universal and is not necessary for adjustment to occur (Cushman & Dijkers, 1991). Some individuals are more likely to exhibit depressive symptoms after spinal cord injury than others. Individuals who had difficulty coping with stress or who had a history of substance abuse or relationship problems prior to the injury tend to demonstrate increased difficulty adjusting after injury, whereas those who have greater personal resources and demonstrated optimal adjustment prior to injury are more likely to display adequate adjustment post injury (Elliot & Frank, 1996).

Lack of social support is strongly associated with depressive symptoms after spinal cord injury (Rinala, Young, Hart, Clearman, & Fuhrer, 1992). Outward displays of depressive symptoms may result in avoidance by others, creating social isolation, which in turn causes the individual with spinal cord injury to be more depressed. In general, individuals who demonstrate grater internal locus of control (Livneh, 2000) and a sense that the world is manageable and meaningful (Lustig, 2005) also demonstrate less psychosocial distress and better adaptation.

Activities and Participation in Spinal Cord Injury

Spinal cord injury affects the injured individual as well as the network of others around him or her (Rothrock, 2006). Given the changes in physical needs that result from spinal cord injury, in order to function effectively in personal, social, or occupational spheres, individuals must make modifications to their daily routines to accommodate the injury's physical ramifications. For example, extra time may be needed for daily activities related to personal hygiene. Individuals may need to conform daily routines to a structured bowel and bladder program. Transportation or moving from one place to another may require extra time and planning. Awareness of the demands

involved in routine self-care enables individuals to establish and adjust daily routines in order to enhance their ability to participate in social and occupational activities.

Individuals with spinal cord injuries continue to be sexual beings. Sexual adjustment is an integral and necessary part of total psychological adjustment. Changes in sexual functioning as a result of spinal cord injury may be a source of extreme frustration for adults. Individuals who experience spinal cord injury in adolescence or pre-teen years may have added challenges with acceptance, self-worth, and self-esteem. Discussion of sexual needs and reassurance that sexual expression is still possible in their life are important parts of rehabilitation. Elimination of physical barriers and provision of appropriate accommodations are also important aspects of enabling individuals with spinal cord injuries to express their sexuality. Depending on the extent of the functional consequences of the injury regarding use of upper extremities, personal assistance may be required to engage in sexual activities, meaning more than two people may be involved in the process (Sakellariu, 2006). This type of accommodation, just as other accommodations, should be handled with delicacy and sensitivity.

Sexuality is not based solely on physical performance, but also is connected to emotional intimacy (Sakellariou, 2006). Individuals should be provided with opportunities to obtain accurate and complete information about sexual activity in conjunction with spinal cord injury, and information should be provided in the context of their personal values.

Not only must individuals with spinal cord injuries incorporate new behaviors and mobility techniques to function, but they must continually adapt to their changing environment as well. Although spinal cord injury causes radical changes in mobility and independence, most individuals are able to return to their community, and many can return to their own homes with environmental modifications. The degree of successful reentry into the community depends to a great degree on the individual's social support, access to adequate housing and transportation, and availability of quality attendant care if needed.

In some instances, establishment of new relationships and reestablishment or maintenance of old ones may be difficult. Relationships may need to be reexamined and redefined. Significant others may experience many of the same reactions as those experienced by the individual with the spinal cord injury. Losses experienced by family members may also parallel those of the injured individual. Sudden incapacity of a family member or significant other owing to spinal cord injury may result in shock, denial, anger, or depression in other family members. Perceived avoidability of the cause of spinal cord injury, or blaming the individual or others for the injury, may contribute to hostility, pessimism, anxiety, and higher levels of social distress. Family relationships may be strained if family caregivers experience stress related to financial strains, or the need to help the individual with activities of daily living and self-care. Family members and significant others may need the same degree of help and support as the individual with spinal cord injury so that they can cope with the condition and, in turn, offer support to the individual. Role obligations may need to be shifted, negotiated, and shared.

The focus of many rehabilitation programs in spinal cord injury is on helping individuals attain optimal function related to self-care activities or employment, with minimum attention being given to recreational activities, which could enable individuals to become active in a larger social sphere. Lack of structured peer recreation activities and peer support can lead to social isolation and impede individuals' feeling of living effectively with their condition (McAweeney, Forchheimer, & Tate, 1996). After spinal cord injury, the level of participation in social and recreational activities will depend on the attitude and interests of the individual, the number of recreational opportunities and resources available, and access to appropriate adaptative devices and adequate sources for equipment repair. Adaptive devices that enable individuals with spinal cord injuries to participate in many sports and other recreational activities are available, although other considerations—such as adequate transportation, quality attendant care if needed, and other environmental restrictions—must also be considered.

The trend toward increased access to public buildings, businesses, and services is enabling individuals with spinal cord injuries to participate more fully in a broader range of community activities as well as exploring and pursuing a number of social roles. Unfortunately, many architectural and attitudinal barriers still exist. Consequently, to live most effectively with their condition, individuals with spinal cord injuries must also learn self-efficacy and the role of self-advocate (Suzuki, Krahn, McCarthy, & Adams, 2007).

Vocational Implications of Spinal Cord Injury

Employment rates for individuals with spinal cord injury vary widely, from approximately 16 to 69% (Meade, Armstrong, Barrett, Ellenbogen, & Jackson, 2006; Chan & Man, 2005). Employment for an individual with spinal cord injury, just as with other disabilities, depends on the person's psychosocial characteristics as well as the physical, social, economic, and political environment (Meade, Barrett, Ellenbogen, & Jackson, 2006).

Unless affected individuals have an associated brain injury, they should experience no cognitive deficits from the spinal cord injury. The level of injury determines, to a great extent, the amount and kind of activity in which individuals are able to engage and the assistive device or special accommodations needed. Individuals with very low spinal cord injuries (sacral or lumbar level) may be able to walk short distances with the assistance of braces and crutches, whereas individuals with injuries at higher levels, such as at the thoracic level, will probably require a wheelchair for mobility and individuals with cervical injuries may require a powered wheelchair. When the injury is at the cervical area, individuals will have limited ability to use the upper extremities; at higher levels of injury, they will be unable to use the upper extremity at all. Consequently, special adaptive equipment will be required to work a telephone, computer, or other equipment that requires hand use.

Environmental barriers such as steps, table heights, and width of doorways will need to be considered in the work environment. Given that many individuals with spinal cord injuries also have difficulty with temperature regulation, the work environment should be climate controlled.

Pre-injury education, vocational interests and skills, and congruence with level of functional capacity after injury are important considerations in vocational placement. Age and the presence of financial disincentives are other factors that may influence an individual's employment status.

Spinal cord injury is a lifetime condition. Consequently, periodic check-ups should be instituted to identify individuals who are experiencing difficulty in the workplace or who encounter new barriers to access so that appropriate accommodations can be instituted (Roessler, 2001).

■ SPINA BIFIDA

Spina bifida is one of several congenital conditions collectively known as *neural tube defects*. These defects involve incomplete development of the brain, spinal cord, and/or coverings of these structures. Other neural tube defects include *anencephaly* in which infants are born with underdeveloped brains and incomplete skulls, and *encephalocele*, in which infants are born with a hole in the skull through which brain tissue protrudes. In most cases, infants with either of the latter conditions do not survive or, if they do, they experience severe mental retardation.

Spina bifida, however, does not involve the brain, but rather involves the spinal column. In this condition, one or more vertebrae are left open so that the spinal cord is exposed.

Types of Spina Bifida

Three types of spina bifida are distinguished (See Figure 4-4):

- **Spina bifida occulta** refers to an opening in one or more vertebrae of the spinal column. The mildest form of spina bifida, it does not involve any damage to the spinal cord. Many individuals with this form of spina bifida may be unaware that their condition even exists.
- **Meningocele** refers to a more serious type of spina bifida. In this form of the condition, the **meninges** (the protective covering around the spinal cord) protrude through the opening in the spinal column. The protruding part, called a meningocele, contains only the meninges, not portions of the spinal cord. In some cases, surgery can correct this problem so there is little or no damage to the nerves of the spinal cord. In other instances, individuals with meningocele may have residual effects resulting from spinal cord damage.
- **Myelomeningocele,** the most common and most severe form of spina bifida, is a condition in which nerves of the spinal cord as well as the meninges protrude through the opening of the vertebrae to the outer part of the body. Because there is no protective covering of the skin, spinal fluid may leak from the protrusion

and the risk of infection is great. When this defect occurs, it usually results in **paraplegia** (paralysis of the lower extremities) as well as poor bladder and bowel control. Although surgery is usually performed immediately to correct the defect, symptoms of paralysis of lower extremities usually persist.

Manifestations of Spina Bifida

Manifestations of spina bifida depend on the type, the part of the spinal cord affected, and the severity of the condition. The severity can range from mild, in which there are few if any symptoms, to severe, in which there is muscle paralysis, loss of sensation, and loss of bowel and bladder control. Many children with the severe type of spina bifida also experience **hydrocephalus**, a condition in which fluid builds up in the brain. In these cases surgical implantation of a shunt is necessary so that the fluid can be drained to prevent excessive pressure to the brain. If hydrocephalus is not corrected, mental retardation can result.

Because spina bifida is congenital, more severe forms of the condition may impinge on normal motor development. Depending on the social, economic, and psychological circumstances of the individual and the resources available to him or her, cognitive development could also be affected. Although the condition itself is not progressive, problems associated with the condition itself may increase over time. For example, in more severe cases when paralysis is present, uneven posture compounded by vertebral abnormalities may lead to **scoliosis** (lateral S-shaped curvature of the spine). Scoliosis can lead to respiratory problems; impede effective functioning of other internal organs, and decrease endurance. Paralysis and associated bowel and bladder problems can also predispose individuals to develop decubitus ulcers (pressure sores). In addition, bowel and bladder problems increase the potential for chronic urinary tract infections.

Adult males with more severe forms of spina bifida may have difficulties maintaining an erection and may have difficulties with

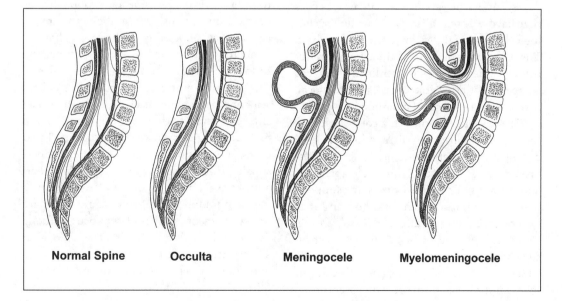

Normal Spine   **Occulta**   **Meningocele**   **Myelomeningocele**

Figure 4-4   Types of spina bifida

fertility. Conversely, females may be capable of engaging in sexual relations and have normal fertility, although sensation to the genital area may be absent.

Management of Spina Bifida

Given that the presence of spina bifida is obvious at birth, and in more severe forms, treatment is usually instigated within 24 hours of birth. Intervention depends on the extent of neurologic problems present, the level of the lesions, and the existence of any complications, such as hydrocephalus or infection. Early surgical interventions available have significantly increased the survival rate for people with spina bifida as well as their quality of life. In addition, greater awareness of the potential for complications as a result of spina bifida has led to increased early treatment of symptoms of complications as soon as they occur as well as implementation of active measures to prevent complications from occurring.

Psychosocial Issues in Spina Bifida

Spina bifida, as a congenital condition, produces important variances in life experiences that have a potential impact on the psychological and social development of the child. The degree to which the child achieves maturity and independence in later life is shaped to a large extent by the biological, psychological, and social experiences of childhood.

When a child is born with a congenital condition, common parental reactions include denial, guilt, anxiety, rejection, anger, or overprotectiveness. If, during this vulnerable time, parents are not provided necessary support, parent–infant attachment and bonding may be altered, leading to disorders of parenting. Child-rearing style has a profound effect on the child's personality development. Parents who do not establish norms and expectations for a child's behavior may create psychosocial

manifestations that have a greater impact than the physical consequences associated with the congenital condition. In addition, a secondary consequence—social isolation—may result from the amount of time needed for medical care and hospitalization. Early intervention, active steps to promote socialization, and family counseling may help to overcome many of these problems.

A normal part of development is gradual separation of parent and child emotionally. When this does not occur because of overprotectiveness or overinvolvement of parents, the child may experience prolonged dependence and the inability to take control, which in turn adversely affects his or her normal development and delays or impedes the ability of the child to form his or her own identity. As a result, the individual may develop emotional dependence and remain in the home of the parents past maturity, rather than establishing an independent living environment.

Children with spina bifida and resulting physical limitations may not be provided with the same opportunities to test their physical and intellectual capabilities as are provided to individuals of the same age group without physical limitations. Doubt about the child's capabilities, or setting expectations that are either too high or too low, can also contribute to low self-esteem and increased dependence. At times, in an attempt to boost the child's self-concept, parents, teachers, and others may shower a child with attention, emphasizing or humoring unrealistic expectations. In so doing, it is possible to foster an egocentric personality that may be more of a handicap than any physical limitation the child experiences.

During adolescence, when a normal part of development consists of the focus on body image and quest for identity, the child with spina bifida may experience anxiety over appearance, acceptance by peers, and sexuality. Difficulties with interpersonal relationships may arise from having had only limited experience in learning and practicing social skills. Helping the individual develop appropriate social skills throughout his or her development can assist the person with spina bifida to form relationships during adolescence and adulthood.

Sexual education is important regardless of the disability or the age of its occurrence. In the case of congenital conditions, issues of sexuality may be ignored as the individual reaches adolescence. As a result, individuals may have limited opportunities to explore or express their sexual desires.

Anticipatory guidance provided to parents from the time they were first told their child's diagnosis can be extremely helpful in preventing many of the problems that can negatively affect the child's psychosocial development and can help the child gain full affective and personality growth and maturity. As the child goes through each stage of development, new needs and new demands inevitably arise. Social encounters outside the home should be encouraged, as well as participation in sports, camping, and other adaptive recreational events designed to promote physical independence and social maturity.

Vocational Issues in Spina Bifida

Unless the individual has associated intellectual limitations because of other complications associated with spina bifida, his or her intellectual ability should not be altered by this condition. Limitations associated with spina bifida depend on the severity of the condition. Those individuals with paraplegia have the same functional limitations as individuals with paraplegia from other causes. The vocational success and ability to function in society are determined primarily by the emotional and personality development achieved throughout childhood. An individual's personal develop-

ment and social environment may make a significant contribution to the degree to which they achieve their goals (Andrén & Grimby, 2004).

■ POLIOMYELITIS AND POST-POLIO SYNDROME

Poliomyelitis (or simply *polio*) is an acute infectious viral disease that was prevalent in the United States in the first half of the twentieth century. Although the condition has been largely eradicated in industrialized nations, it is still prevalent in many developing countries (Pallansch & Sandhu, 2006). The virus enters the body when contaminated water or food is ingested or when hands that have been contaminated with the virus touch the mouth.

Poliomyelitis targets the nerve cells that control muscles. The brain stem, spinal cord, and neuromuscular system may be affected (Salcido, 2000). The nerve cells or motor neurons damaged by the poliovirus are located in the anterior horn of the spinal cord and extend to the muscles. As neurons are affected, muscle cells lose the ability to contract, resulting in paralysis. If motor cells are able to overcome the virus, paralysis may be temporary. If, however, motor cells are unable to overcome the virus, they die, resulting in permanent paralysis or, in some instances, ongoing weakness of affected muscles. The extent of paralysis is unpredictable. Although the disease primarily affects children, devastating epidemics of polio that spread across North America and Europe from the 1930s to the mid-1950s severely disabled adults as well.

In 1955, Dr. Jonas Salk developed the inactivated poliovirus vaccine (IPV). Its introduction was followed in 1960 by the development of a live, attenuated oral poliovirus vaccine (OPV) by Dr. Albert Sabin. When the vaccines became available, widespread immunization against polio was begun, nearly abolishing polio in the United States and other countries in which immunization programs are widely available. Although poliomyelitis has been nearly eradicated in the industrialized world with the advent of active immunization programs, the residuals of the condition experienced by those who had contacted the disease prior to immunization persist. In addition, small outbreaks continue to occur in developing countries and small numbers of cases continue to appear in the industrialized world as well.

Manifestations of Poliomyelitis

Individuals in the initial stages of polio are acutely ill. Early symptoms are usually nonspecific, such as gastrointestinal or upper respiratory symptoms accompanied by fever. Symptoms later progress to headache, stiff neck, and muscle pains. Affected muscles become paralyzed or weakened. In some individuals, only a small group of muscles are affected; in others, paralysis is widespread and may include the whole body. Extremity involvement is often asymmetrical, such that one extremity may have major paralysis while the opposite limb has only slight weakness or is not affected at all. Although muscles are paralyzed, functions of sensation, bowel, bladder, and sexual response are left intact.

When an extremity is affected by polio in childhood, during a time of continued growth, the rate of growth of the affected extremity is delayed, resulting in a smaller extremity when full growth is reached. The legs are most frequently affected; however, sometimes all four extremities are affected, sometimes only one extremity is affected, or sometimes paralysis extends to only the lateral half of the body (**hemiplegia**), with one arm and one leg being affected. This type of polio is called *paralytic polio*. When the poliovirus affects the brain stem, muscles that control breathing and swallowing are also affected; this is called *bulbar polio*. When respiration is affected, individuals

require mechanical respiratory support such as the "iron lung."

Functional limitations resulting from polio depend on the nerves affected and the degree of damage. Individuals with lower extremities affected have difficulty with ambulation and may require a wheelchair, cane, or braces. When upper extremities are involved, self-care skills may also be affected. Having trunk muscles affected may also create a muscle imbalance leading to scoliosis (lateral curvature of the spine), which can interfere with breathing and functioning of internal organs.

After the initial acute episode of poliomyelitis, some degree of function may return; however, some of the residuals are permanent. The degree of residual manifestations depends on the extent of the permanent damage to nerves.

Manifestations of Post-Polio Syndrome

Poliomyelitis itself is not a progressive condition. Consequently, many individuals who contracted the disease 30 or more years ago adapted to residual paralysis, muscle weakness, or other symptoms and have gone on to live productive lives with little medical intervention needed. In the 1980s, however, individuals who had previously been diagnosed as having poliomyelitis began to seek medical advice because of new symptoms that ranged in severity from mild to severely debilitating (Gordon & Feldman, 2002). At first, individuals reporting symptoms were not taken seriously. Many were classified as having "emotional disturbances" or symptoms were merely attributed to "aging." As more and more individuals who had had polio sought help for new symptoms, however, their symptoms were taken more seriously and the term *post-polio syndrome* was coined to describe this phenomenon.

Post-polio syndrome is a noncontiguous neurological disorder that produces a variety of symptoms in individuals who had recovered from poliomyelitis many years earlier. Common symptoms of post-polio syndrome appearing 30 to 40 years after the acute bout of poliomyelitis include the following:

- Abnormal muscle fatigue and generalized fatigue
- New muscle weakness in muscles not previously affected
- Muscle pain (**myalgia**) and/or joint pain
- Respiratory difficulty

The cause of post-polio syndrome is unknown (Burk & Agre, 2000). It appears that most of the motor neurons originally damaged in the initial bout of polio are involved in post-polio syndrome and that most individuals who had polio are at risk to develop the syndrome. Individuals who initially had experienced severe polio seem to be at greatest risk for developing post-polio syndrome; however, other individuals who were less severely affected initially also can experience a decline in function. Those who had been able to walk without use of assistive devices may require them because of post-polio symptoms. Those who had used assistive devices for ambulation may find it necessary to begin to use a wheelchair.

Post-polio syndrome is progressive, meaning that deterioration will continue. Despite increasing decline, however, individuals will not experience the level of functional manifestations they experienced when polio was in its acute state. With appropriate exercise, strength and function can be improved and deterioration slowed, if not halted.

Diagnosis of Polio and Post-Polio Syndrome

The diagnosis of poliomyelitis in its acute state is based primarily on the medical history of the individual and on the symptoms. A spinal tap or fecal sample can be used to confirm the diagnosis. The diagnosis of post-polio syndrome is, at times, more difficult.

One step in diagnosis of post-polio syndrome is to identify or eliminate other conditions that may be responsible for the symptoms. Symptoms of post-polio syndrome may be difficult to distinguish from symptoms associated with other degenerative disorders of muscles and joints, such as osteoarthritis or osteoporosis. General medical evaluation, routine laboratory tests, *electromyographic* studies (a graphic record of the contraction of a muscle as the result of electrical stimulation), and *nerve conduction* studies may help to identify and exclude other diseases. Magnetic resonance imaging may be used to exclude other conditions of the spine that could cause similar symptoms (Burk & Agre, 2000).

Management of Post-Polio Syndrome

No specific intervention is available to alter the course of post-polio syndrome. Individuals with symptoms of increasing muscle weakness, fatigue, and pain should first have a thorough physical examination by a physician to rule out other potential causes of symptoms. Interventions are largely directed toward managing symptoms experienced with post-polio syndrome and assisting individuals to maintain their functional status and independence as long as possible. Good health practices, including proper nutrition and adequate rest, are important to maintain optimal function.

Generalized fatigue is treated with lifestyle changes consisting of energy conservation measures. Physical activities should be paced to prevent excessive fatigue. Individuals may require frequent rest periods throughout the day. Use of additional assistive devices, such as using a wheelchair rather than crutches, may help to conserve energy.

Increasing muscle strength through nonfatiguing exercise may be used to treat mild to moderate weakness. Exercises that are tolerable and that do not contribute to more weakness and fatigue may be prescribed. Physical therapists generally instruct individuals about proper exercise protocols so that overuse and excessive fatigue can be avoided. Individuals are typically instructed to exercise for short intervals, resting between bouts of exercise, and to exercise only every other day to prevent excessive muscle fatigue.

Individuals with respiratory difficulty may require noninvasive positive-pressure ventilation at night. Because individuals with post-polio syndrome are more susceptible to infectious diseases, pneumonia and influenza vaccines are usually recommended. Tobacco use should be avoided.

The use of braces to decrease mechanical stress on the joints may be used to minimize muscle and joint pain. Changes in orthotics or in the mode of ambulation may be required. Moving from braces or crutches for ambulation to a wheelchair can also reduce stress on joints. If the individual with post-polio syndrome is overweight, weight reduction may be recommended to reduce fatigue and stress on the muscles and joints. For individuals whose respiratory muscles were also affected by the initial infection, weight control can help to prevent respiratory difficulty as well.

Psychosocial Issues in Post-Polio Syndrome

Given that poliomyelitis is not a progressive disease, many individuals believed their recovery to be permanent and have adapted and adjusted to the functional limitations and residual effects associated with the condition, going on to lead full and productive lives. Individuals with residual manifestations from polio have worked for years to minimize their limitations and maximize their assets. New, unexpected symptoms associated with post-polio syndrome threaten function and independence and can be psychologically devastating.

The symptoms of this new "secondary disability" can be both frightening and frustrating for the individual, who again must adjust and adapt to continuing functional consequences, potential use of new assistive devices, and alteration of lifestyle. After regaining function previously through much physical and emotional effort, being forced to deal again with new symptoms, which are much like the initial symptoms, can be discouraging. Individuals may reject new assistive devices because they are symbols of loss of physical ability that the individuals feel they earned through great effort.

Vocational Issues in Post-Polio Syndrome

Many individuals with poliomyelitis have achieved gainful employment and lived productive lives with residuals of polio. The onset of symptoms related to post-polio syndrome, however, may make a number of alterations necessary in the work setting. In some instances, depending on performance requirements, the individual may be unable to perform all of the job duties. Thus alteration of job duties or retraining for other job duties may be necessary.

Even when remaining in the current job is possible, individuals may experience increased fatigue, or altered stamina and strength, so that frequent rest periods may be needed; some persons may also need a more sedentary job structure. The ability to lift, reach, walk, or climb may be altered owing to increased muscle weakness and fatigue, making such job restructuring necessary.

Symptoms of post-polio syndrome—whether pain, weakness, or fatigue—may necessitate use of additional assistive devices. Individuals who once ambulated without assistive devices may require a cane, crutches, or braces. Individuals who once used crutches or braces may require a wheelchair for ambulation. Adaptation in the workplace for accommodation of assistive devices may be needed. If, owing to increased symptoms, the individual's current mode of transportation is no longer accessible, transportation to and from work may become a barrier to employment. In addition, because of increased manifestations that diminish physical capabilities or stamina, individuals may require additional time to get ready for work.

In some instances, the onset of new symptoms and increasing limitations may result in depression, which can interfere with the individual's ability to work effectively. Supportive counseling may be necessary to enable the individual to cope with increasing manifestations of the post-polio syndrome.

■ NEUROMUSCULAR CONDITIONS

Parkinson's Disease

Parkinsonism

Parkinsonism is a general term used to describe a syndrome characterized by the following symptoms:

- Tremor at rest
- Slowness of movement (**bradykinesia**)
- Rigidity
- Postural instability (Jankovic, 2004)

Individuals who exhibit these symptoms are said to have Parkinson syndrome. A number of conditions in addition to Parkinson's disease can cause these symptoms, including infections, drugs, toxins, endocrine disorders, Huntington's disease (discussed later in this chapter), and Alzheimer's disease.

Parkinson's disease is a slowly progressive disorder of the central nervous system that leads to progressive loss of motor function. Although its cause remains unknown, evidence suggests that both genetic and environmental factors may play a role (Janson, Leone, & Freese, 2002; Nussbaum, & Ellis, 2003). Parkinson's disease involves extensive degenerative changes in the basal ganglia (gray matter embedded in the white matter of the brain, which has a role in complex movements) and the loss of or decreases in levels of *dopamine* (a neurotransmitter) in the basal ganglia. Most of the disabling symptoms associated with Parkinson's disease are due predominantly to drastic reductions of levels of dopamine in the brain. Although Parkinson's disease occurs most commonly after the age of 50 (Litvan, 1998), greater awareness and improved methods of detection have increased the number of diagnosed cases of Parkinson's disease among younger individuals.

Secondary parkinsonism is a term used to describe a parkinsonian syndrome in which individuals experience Parkinson's disease-like symptoms, but symptoms are due to other causes. Secondary parkinsonism can be associated with the ingestion of certain drugs (prescription or illicit) or exposure to toxic substances, such as carbon monoxide or other chemicals. Secondary parkinsonism gained attention in the early 1980s when the "designer drug" MPTP, which mimicked the action of heroin, entered the street market. A number of young adults, after taking the drug, suddenly developed permanent signs and symptoms of severe Parkinson's disease. Some medications used to treat mental illness may also produce parkinsonian-like side effects if not closely monitored.

A variety of other conditions mimic Parkinson's disease, causing similar symptoms (i.e., parkinsonism). These symptoms should be distinguished from true Parkinson's disease.

Manifestations of Parkinson's Disease

The four most common symptoms of Parkinson's disease are tremor, muscle rigidity, bradykinesia (slowness of movement), and postural instability (Janson et al., 2002).

In early stages of the condition, individuals may exhibit extreme slowness in initiating or maintaining movements (bradykinesia). Individuals who have Parkinson's disease may walk with small, shuffling steps (*shuffling gait*) and may have difficulty in rising from a chair or bed. They may also find it difficult to initiate or to stop voluntary movements. While walking, for example, they may experience *gait hesitation* when they suddenly "freeze," taking seconds to regain motion; in other instances, they may continue five or six more steps beyond where they want to stop. Bradykinesia can interfere with activities such as shaving, buttoning clothes, or cutting food, all of which take longer and become more difficult to perform as the disease progresses. Because Parkinson's disease affects both the central and autonomic nervous systems, some individuals may also experience urinary or bowel problems.

Individuals with Parkinson's disease are sometimes said to have a poverty of spontaneous movement. They may blink less frequently and develop a mask-like, expressionless face. They may develop difficulty swallowing (**dysphagia**), which results in saliva accumulation and drooling. Because the individual is unable to swallow quickly, the rate of swallowing food decreases and eating becomes slower and more deliberate as the condition progresses. As food collects in the mouth and in the back of the throat, individuals may be prone to coughing and choking episodes.

Motor changes related to Parkinson's disease may cause speech changes related to in- coordination and reduced movement of those muscles that control breathing, voice, pronunciation, and rate of speaking. Volume of speech may be decreased (*hypophonia*), and there may be no verbal inflections. Individuals' ability to write may also be affected. Reduction in amplitude of movement may affect an individual's ability to write so that handwriting gradually becomes smaller and smaller (**micrographia**) until it is no longer legible.

Tremor of a limb, usually most noticeable in one hand, is the most frequent early symptom of Parkinson's disease. The tremor intensifies when the hand rests in the lap (*resting tremor*) and diminishes with voluntary movement. The tremor is not present during sleep, however.

The posture of individuals with Parkinson's disease becomes stooped, and their arms fail to swing with their stride when they are walking. The loss of postural reflexes makes it difficult for these individuals to maintain an upright position if they are suddenly bumped, increasing the risk of falls. To keep from falling, individuals may inadvertently quicken their steps as if to "catch up" with their own center of gravity. Muscle tone is increased, creating muscle rigidity, which also interferes with movement and causes severe immobility. Because greater effort is necessary to engage in voluntary movement, fatigue is also increased.

Mental and behavioral changes do not always occur as a result of Parkinson's disease, but both cognitive changes, and changes in emotions and behavior can be part of the symptoms. Dementia can also occur in some individuals later in the course of the condition. Risk factors for dementia associated with Parkinson's disease include advanced age, longer duration of the condition, and later age of onset for the disease (Leegwater-Kim & Waters, 2007). Apathy, passivity, depression, and loss of initiative may be noted. Some studies indicate that depression is present in a large number of individuals with Parkinson's disease and can have a more dramatic effect on quality of life than symptoms of the condition or side effects of treatment (Phillips, 1999). As the individual becomes aware of his or her decreasing cognitive abilities, depression related to losses may result. The degree to which depression reflects physiological changes and the degree to which they reflect a reaction to the disease itself, however, are not known.

There is no cure for Parkinson's disease. This condition is characterized by progressive debilitation, although the progression occurs slowly over years. Intervention, usually in the form of medication, physical therapy, and exercise, along with maintenance of general health, can reduce the effects of the symptoms so that the affected individual may remain active longer.

Diagnosis of Parkinson's Disease

There is no single test that can be used to diagnose Parkinson's disease. Individuals with initial symptoms are usually referred to a neurologist (a physician who specializes in the evaluation and treatment of nervous system disorders) for evaluation. Physicians usually base their diagnosis on the presence of tremor, stiffness, and slow movement. Because many other conditions may have similar symptoms in early stages of development, and because initially symptoms may be attributed to aging, misdiagnosis occurs frequently (Aminoff, Burns, & Silverstein, 1997).

Management of Parkinson's Disease

Currently, there is no cure for Parkinson's disease. As noted earlier, intervention includes both nonpharmacologic and pharmacologic approaches. Nonpharmacologic approaches include regular exercise, physical therapy, speech therapy, and psychosocial support (Leegwater-Kim & Waters, 2007). Exercise and activity are especially important for individuals with Parkinson's disease because of the tendency of the muscles to be stiff and rigid. Muscles can **atrophy** (become smaller, or shrink) without the stimulation that exercise provides, decreasing the individual's capacity for self-care. Individuals are usually encouraged to engage in a daily exercise routine, such as walking a prescribed distance, doing simple calisthenics, or performing active range-of-motion exercises. Other interventions are directed toward preventing complications. Individualized physical therapy focusing on joint mobility, correction and prevention of postural abnormalities of trunk and limbs, and maintenance of normal gait is important to help individuals maintain function as long as possible. Passive stretching of extremities, muscle massage, resistive exercises and training are techniques used by physical therapists to achieve this goal.

The administration of a medication called *levodopa* (L-dopa) can decrease the symptoms of Parkinson's disease. Levodopa works by helping to increase the level of the neurotransmitter dopamine in the brain. At first, small amounts are usually prescribed; the dosage is then gradually increased. Although helpful, levodopa can have serious side effects and limited long-term efficacy (Janson, Leone, & Freese, 2003; Jankovic, 1999). Some individuals may experience side effects, such as nausea or abnormal involuntary movements called **dyskinesia**. These effects are generally related to the dosage of the medication, occurring more frequently with higher dosages. In some individuals, levodopa causes mental confusion or decreases alertness.

Neurosurgical intervention as a treatment for Parkinson's disease continues to be explored. The *deep brain stimulation (DBS)* technique has been used with some success at specialized clinics in Europe and North America. This procedure involves implanting an electrode into a target area of the brain. The electrode is then tunneled under the skin to an external stimulator, which can be switched on or off by the person with Parkinson's disease (Phillips, 1999). Another surgical procedure, *pallidotomy*, consists of identifying and destroying a part of the basal ganglia that secretes substances that are believed to destroy portions of the basal ganglia (Leegwater-Kim & Waters, 2007). Surgical procedures appear to be most helpful for those individuals whose symptoms are not satisfactorily controlled with medication.

Parkinson's disease is a chronic, lifelong condition characterized by progressive deterioration. Because of its gradual onset and slow progression however, with appropriate assistive devices and other therapies most individuals have many years after diagnosis during which they can remain productive and functional.

Psychosocial Issues in Parkinson's Disease

Parkinson's disease has a profound impact on the affected individual's life, but it can also have a profound effect on the individual's family. Parkinson's disease is a visible neurological disorder. Not only is it difficult for the individual to move, but there is also stooped posture, flexed arms with lack of swinging of the arms when walking, and often tremor of an extremity. One aspect of the movement disorder is lack of facial expression and of spontaneous movements when talking. Because of the inability to use these sources of body language, individuals have reduced capability for nonverbal communication. They may also experience speech disturbances as a result of motor difficulties, so both verbal and nonverbal communication may be difficult. Acquaintances or strangers as well as family members may attribute lack of expression to disinterest, dementia, or low intellectual ability (Lyons, Tickle-Degnen, Henry, & Cohn, 2004). Individuals may become stressed or frustrated by the attitudes of others and consequently begin to withdraw from or be reluctant to participate in social interactions.

Anxiety may occur from the time of initial diagnosis and may continue as symptoms progress. In addition, many people with Parkinson's disease experience depression, which can have a more significant impact on quality of life and life satisfaction than many of the physical symptoms (Gage & Storey, 2004; Dural, Atay, Akbostanci, & Kucukdeveci, 2003). For individuals who had prided themselves on their efficiency, communication, or manual skills, deterioration of these skills can be particularly stressful. Stress can make symptoms of Parkinson's disease worse, further contributing to the individual's social isolation. Because Parkinson's disease is progressively debilitating, the individual and his or her family must continually readjust to increasing loss of functional capacity, which can in turn contribute to anxiety and depression. If mental deterioration, confusion, or personality changes occur, family members may have increased difficulty coping with these changes. In some instances, individuals with Parkinson's disease may demonstrate decreased initiative and impaired judgment,

which can be another source of stress for the family. As the individual becomes more dependent on others for self-care, the social support system may become further eroded.

Information about sexual function in Parkinson's disease is scarce, although sexual problems are frequently present in neurological disorders. Depression is considered a contributor to sexual problems in the general population. Consequently, given that individuals with Parkinson's disease frequently experience depression, it stands to reason that some sexual problems may exist. Medications taken to treat symptoms of Parkinson's disease may also contribute to sexual dysfunction. Furthermore, factors common to many types of chronic illnesses can cause lack of interest in sexual activities. As time needed for activities of daily living (such as dressing, eating, and personal hygiene) and for treatment requirements increases, interest in and energy for sexual activity may decline.

Activities of daily living such as dressing or bathing can be very tiring and time-consuming for persons with Parkinson's disease. Individuals should allow enough time so they don't feel rushed. Given that balance is sometimes a problem, special safety precautions, such as grab bars, or a tub bench or shower chair should be used when bathing. Clearing the environment of potential hazards that could cause the individual to fall can prevent complications that could result from the fall. Use of walking aids, such as crutches or a walker, may also help individuals prevent falls.

Vocational Issues in Parkinson's disease

Whether persons with Parkinson's disease can continue working is an individual decision that is based on the specific circumstances. In most instances, work that is more sedentary and that does not require significant verbal communication may be continued longer than work that requires more strenuous activity. Because affected individuals have difficulty with balance and gait, jobs that require considerable walking, stooping, or bending should be avoided. Transportation to and from work may be the largest obstacle to maintaining employment.

Highly stressful occupations should be avoided because increased stress tends to increase the severity of symptoms that the individual experiences. For some individuals, work becomes increasingly difficult and the effort to continue working may produce a tremendous strain. For these individuals, not working may bring a sense of relief from the physical and mental stress of attempting to continue carrying out various tasks and responsibilities. For others, the inability to work may have a detrimental effect. In most cases, individuals will be able to continue working if the work is not extremely demanding physically or does not require manual dexterity. Scheduling frequent rest periods and restructuring the workload may help to increase the total amount of work that can be done during the workday. Because stiffness and muscle rigidity are common symptoms of the condition, working in a cold environment should be avoided because of the increase in muscle stiffness that could be experienced.

Huntington's Disease (Huntington's Chorea)

Huntington's disease is a progressive, genetic condition of the central nervous system in which neurons in the basal ganglia of the brain degenerate. It is characterized by disorders of movement, cognition, and/or behavior (Leng, Woodward, Stokes, Swan, Wareing, & Baker, 2003). Most individuals develop symptoms between the ages of 30 and 50 years of age. The condition advances slowly and progressively. Although the rate of deterioration varies from person to person, as does the rate at which symptoms appear, Huntington's disease leads to severe functional conseqeunces and death after 15 to 20 years (Zinzi et al., 2007; Cattaneo, Rigamonti, & Zuccato, 2002).

Manifestations of Huntington's Disease

Huntington's disease is characterized by three types of symptoms:

- Cognitive deficits
- Motor consequences
- Behavioral changes

Cognitive changes usually occur in the early stages, with the individual at first becoming increasingly absent-minded and having difficulty with concentration. As the condition progresses, mental deterioration (**dementia**) occurs.

Early signs of motor consequences involve movements of the fingers that give the impression that the individual is fidgeting. As the condition progresses, movement and coordination continue to deteriorate, with bradykinesia (slowness of movement) and rigidity interfering with the individual's ability to walk. Jerky, involuntary movements (**chorea**) are present as well. Motor difficulty also affects the individual's ability to speak and to swallow.

The individual also experiences personality change. Behavioral changes associated with the condition range from delusions to impulse-control problems.

Diagnosis of Huntington's Disease

Diagnosis is usually based on the individual's symptoms and family history. In most instances, extensive neurological testing is not necessary. Evaluation is usually done by a *neurologist* (a physician who evaluates and treats neurological disorders).

Management of Huntington's Disease

There is no intervention known to slow the progression of or cure Huntington's disease. Interventions are usually directed toward preventing complications and treating symptoms.

Physical therapy is a major component of the management program for individuals with Huntington's disease. It can assist the individual in improving or stabilizing motor ability, prevent contractures, or adapt the environment to promote safety as well as maximum independence. Occupational therapists may help individuals improve coordination abilities and activities of daily living skills. Speech therapists may help individuals maximize their speech capability and their ability to swallow. In some instances, cognitive retraining and memory training may be useful. Training in ways to avoid exposure to upper respiratory infections as well as other communicable diseases is also advised.

It is sometimes difficult to distinguish which behavioral symptoms are related to the condition itself and which are related to the individual's anxiety about having the condition. Psychotropic medications may be used to help alleviate or control behavioral symptoms regardless of their cause. Medication may be prescribed for anxiety or depression, irritability, or mood swings. In some instances, psychotropic medication may be used to control some of the involuntary, jerky movements individuals may be experiencing.

A major portion of management is directed toward assisting individuals and their family in managing self-care as the condition progresses. Individual counseling, family counseling, and genetic counseling of family members may be important interventions.

Psychosocial Issues in Huntington's Disease

Individuals and their families must cope with continued losses, both physical and mental, as the condition progresses as well as with the knowledge that Huntington's disease is a progressive condition in which continued deterioration can be expected. For individuals with Huntington's disease, their condition-related cognitive and behavioral changes may make it more difficult for them to cope. Both affected individuals and family members may feel helpless and hopeless. As a result, they may be reluctant to participate in activities

designed to maintain or improve their current level of function.

Faulty judgment and impulsivity related to behavioral changes may sometimes result in unsafe situations for individuals with Huntington's disease. Individuals who are in denial about their condition and their limitations may also expose themselves to situations that could result in unsafe practices or injury.

As the condition progresses, individuals become less able to care for themselves and, therefore, more dependent on others. As communication becomes more difficult, social interactions also become more challenging and, increasing social isolation may result. Personality changes that may produce violent or hostile behaviors further stress support systems.

Because Huntington's disease has a genetic component, family members may be under additional stress given the possibility that they may themselves be at risk for developing Huntington's disease. Counseling, education, and support can help to reduce the stress that family members may be experiencing.

Vocational Issues in Huntington's Disease

Huntington's disease is a progressive, degenerative disease. However, in the early stages before mental deterioration and physical incapacitation are present, short-term training may be appropriate. As the condition progresses and individuals have increasing difficulty with memory, communication skills, and physical ability, sheltered employment may be the most feasible alternative.

Amyotrophic Lateral Sclerosis

Amyotrophic lateral sclerosis (ALS), also sometimes referred to as Lou Gehrig's disease in memory of the baseball player who died of ALS in 1941, is a progressive, degenerative condition in which there is destruction of motor neurons (nerve cells that convey impulses to initiate muscular contraction) in the brain, spinal cord, and peripheral nervous system (Orrell, 2007). Damaged portions of the nerve tracts are replaced by scar tissue or plaques.

The cause of ALS is unknown, although current medical theory suggests a multifactorial etiology, which may include genetic, viral, autoimmune, and neurotoxic factors (Roland & Schneider, 2001; Walling, 1999.). Individuals are usually affected in middle or later life, with males being affected more frequently than females.

Manifestations of ALS

Symptoms of ALS depend on the area of the nervous system affected and may involve both upper and lower extremities. There are two primary forms of ALS: the spinal form and the bulbar form.

The spinal form of ALS is characterized by muscular weakness, muscle **atrophy** (decrease in size), spasticity, and hyperactive reflexes. Individuals may first complain of tripping, stumbling or awkwardness when walking or running. Others may complain of difficulty with simple activities such as buttoning a shirt, or picking up small objects. In the bulbar form, individuals may first notice difficulty with breathing, slurring of speech or lowered volume when speaking, or difficulty with swallowing.

As the condition progresses, symptoms become worse, spreading to other parts of the body. Eventually, whether the individual first experienced the bulbar or spinal form of ALS, he or she develops all the symptoms. Individuals become increasingly weak and immobile. Progressive paralysis leads to increasing loss of function, until individuals are completely dependent on others for help with all activities of daily living. Excessive production of saliva and difficulty in swallowing can cause drooling. Some individuals may also experience muscle pain as a result of spasticity of muscles. Individuals may develop respiratory muscle weakness leading to breathing problems, and in later stages of the condition affected persons may require ventilatory assistance to breathe. Cognitive function, sensation, vision, hearing, and bowel and bladder function are usually not affected.

Diagnosis of ALS

There is no reliable laboratory test to detect the presence of ALS. Diagnosis of ALS is usually based on the symptoms the individual exhibits and their progression, the individual's medical history, and the process of ruling out other causes for the symptoms.

Management of ALS

There is no cure for ALS, and no effective treatment for it is currently available. Management goals are generally directed toward helping individuals and families cope with manifestations of the condition, assisting individuals with ALS to remain independent as long as possible, promoting comfort, and preventing complications. Management of symptoms focuses on maintaining muscle function, relieving discomfort, and forestalling complications such as respiratory infections and decubitus ulcers. Medications to reduce spasticity may be used, although they can also increase muscle weakness and cause sedation. Physical therapy may be helpful to maintain function and to reduce painful symptoms brought on by muscle spasm.

Occupational therapists can provide support and help individuals to adapt their environments so as to maximize function. Individuals with speech difficulties may utilize speech therapists to help them learn techniques to communicate. Speech pathologists may be required to help individuals who have difficulty with swallowing. If individuals have breathing difficulty, respiratory therapists may be consulted to help individuals learn techniques to assist with respiratory management.

Psychosocial Issues in ALS

The social, economic, and psychological implications of ALS are substantial. It is common for individuals with ALS to experience fear, anxiety, and depression, especially as the condition progresses and the individual experiences rapid deterioration of physical function. Because of the loss of mobility and increased dependency, feelings of helplessness and powerlessness are also common. Some individuals may experience discouragement and become angry as their physical limitations increase. They may experience grief with each subsequent loss of function. There may also be loss of social relationships, leading to social isolation.

Changes in physical appearance and physical ability may cause individuals to question their self-worth. They may feel guilty because of their increased dependence on others and may express concern and frustration over the burden they feel is being placed on family members.

Family members are also affected. Modifications of roles of family members are often required. Because individuals with ALS need substantial help with most activities of daily living, family members most often find themselves in a care-giving role even in the early stages of the disease. Expenditures for medical care and equipment can be sizable. If the individual with ALS is also the major breadwinner, financial issues may become a major concern. Family members may quit work to assume the caregiving role, which further contributes to financial distress. Family members may also have feelings of powerlessness, anger, or anxiety about the future. They may vacillate between resentment and guilt.

Despite the significant manifestations of their condition, individuals with ALS retain their cognitive and intellectual ability and still have needs for recreation, entertainment, and companionship. Utilization of special techniques and equipment, especially those that enhance individuals' functional capacity and independence in self-care, can help them exert personal control over their life and thus maintain self-esteem. Given that communication is usually significantly affected, equipment, to facilitate communication, such as voice amplifiers, or techniques such as eye blinking if the individual's condition has progressed such that he or she can communicate no other way, is a means to help the individual maintain meaningful relationships.

Vocational Issues in ALS

As ALS progresses, the degree of physical limitation increases, with activity becoming increasingly more difficult. This condition generally progresses fairly rapidly over a course of three to five years, although some individuals survive for as long as ten years. Many individuals live productive lives after their diagnosis is made, continuing to work despite advanced symptoms. As new interventions emerge that may retard progression of ALS and prolong survival, the ability to maintain competitive employment also increases (Norquist, Fitzpatrick, & Jenkinson, 2004). The degree to which individuals are able to continue working depends on the requirements of the job and the way in which symptoms affect the individual's ability to perform. Older age, female gender, short time from symptom onset to diagnosis, and disease severity are key prognostic factors (del Aquila, Longstreth, McGuire, Koepsell, & van Belle 2003).

Physical demands of work should be light and sedentary for persons with ALS. Even if the individual is still ambulatory, a wheelchair-accessible work environment should be considered, as the person will require a wheelchair for ambulation as the condition progresses. Transfer may become more difficult in later stages of his or her condition. Because communication can be a problem, occupations in which the ability to speak makes up an important part of the job should be avoided.

■ CONDITIONS OF THE PERIPHERAL NERVOUS SYSTEM

Guillain–Barré Syndrome

Guillain–Barré syndrome is an inflammatory condition of the peripheral nerves (nerves lying outside the central nervous system). The exact cause of Guillain–Barré syndrome is unknown, but it appears to be an immune-mediated condition, often following infection that appears to sensitize the immune system to antigens (see Chapter 10) that are shared between the infecting organism and the peripheral nerves (Griffin, 2004).

Manifestations of Guillain–Barré Syndrome

The severity of Guillain–Barré syndrome varies greatly. Some individuals may have only mild muscle weakness, whereas others may become totally paralyzed and develop complications such as inability to breath, abnormal blood pressure or heartbeat, or other life-threatening conditions. An acute and progressive condition, it is characterized by muscular weakness that usually begins in the lower extremities and spreads upward (ascending paralysis). Paralysis of both upper and lower extremities can occur, and chest and facial muscles can be affected. Breathing can be affected so that ventilatory support is needed. The amount of paralysis varies: Some individuals experience only mild footdrop, while others develop complete paralysis (Blank-Reid, Kaplan, & Santora, 2008). Abnormal sensations, such as numbness, tingling, or sense of something crawling under the skin in the feet, hands, or face, may also be present. Individuals may also experience muscle aches or back pain as early symptoms.

Symptoms develop rapidly, over hours to days or sometimes over a few weeks.

Generally, symptoms reach their maximum intensity within three to eight weeks. For the most part, symptoms are reversible and recovery occurs after progression of the symptoms ceases. Although most individuals recover completely, the rate of recovery is variable and can take as long as to two years (Forsberg, Press, Einarsson, de Pedro-Cuesta, & Holmqvist, 2005). Permanent disability or even death can result in some instances. Some individuals, even though they appear to have recovered, may develop fatigue with sustained activity. Poor endurance with regard to walking or other activities of daily living can be an ongoing problem.

Diagnosis of Guillain–Barré Syndrome

Diagnosis is usually based on symptoms and physical examination.

Electromyography may be used to differentiate symptoms from other causes of generalized weakness.

Management of Guillain–Barré Syndrome

Due to the potential for rapid deterioration, individuals with Guillain–Barré require hospitalization for observation. Because respiratory muscles can be affected, respiratory failure can be a potentially life-threatening condition that may require ventilatory assistance. Other early treatments may consist of *plasmapheresis* (exchange of the individual's plasma for albumin) or intravenous infusion of *human immunoglobulin,* both of which may shorten the time to recovery (Griffin, 2004).

Other interventions are primarily symptomatic and used to prevent additional complications. General physical rehabilitation is started early, usually under the guidance of a physiatrist, (a physician who specializes in rehabilitation and physical medicine). Physical therapists are usually involved in the early stages of the condition to help individuals prevent muscle atrophy (shrinkage), contractures, or pressure sores. Occupational therapists help individuals learn how to strengthen muscles, use energy conservation techniques, and perform activities of daily living. If speech or swallowing is affected, a speech therapist may be needed to help individuals improve speech patterns or facilitate swallowing.

Prognosis and recovery vary with age and severity of the condition (Griffin, 2004).

Psychosocial Issues in Guillain–Barré Syndrome

The initial stages of this syndrome can be extremely frightening. Individuals who were healthy suddenly find themselves paralyzed and unable to care for themselves. If respiration is affected and individuals are placed on mechanical ventilation. The inability to breathe in itself is frightening. In addition, individuals on a respirator are unable to communicate, further adding to their apprehension and feelings of helplessness.

Even though most individuals regain function, the unpredictability of the condition and progression of symptoms lead to fear, frustration, and concern for the future. Depending on the individual's situation and the extent of time needed to recover, financial concerns, fear of permanent limitations, and loss of dependence can be extremely stressful and can have long-standing psychological effects even after the individual has reached maximum recovery.

Vocational Issues in Guillain–Barre Syndrome

Because individuals with Guillain-Barré syndrome have, in many instances, been incapacitated for a lengthy period of time, most will require an extensive period of rehabilitation. This intervention may include driver retraining, learning to pace activities, and, in some instances, reemployment training. Individuals may, after a certain amount of activity, continue to experience muscle aches or other sensations that interfere with normal activity. Initially individuals may consider returning to work on a part-time basis and anticipate

the need for periodic rest periods during the day. In the case of individuals who require wheelchair use for a period of time after hospital discharge, architectural barriers at their employment site should be considered.

Myasthenia Gravis

Myasthenia Gravis is a neuromuscular condition characterized by weakness and fatigability of the muscles. It is an autoimmune condition in which symptoms are caused by a decrease in a neurotransmitter, *acetylcholine,* at the point at which nerves initiate contraction of a muscle (Robinson & Kothari, 2007). Eyelids, muscles of the throat, and often muscles of the extremities are affected. A common symptom is *ptosis* (drooping) of the eyelid. Speech, chewing, and swallowing may also be affected.

Diagnosis is usually based on symptoms and physical examination. Intervention with medications in most instances enables individuals to live productive lives with no significant limitations.

Muscular Dystrophy

Muscular dystrophy refers to a group of hereditary conditions that are characterized by progressive muscle weakness, muscle wasting, contractures of the joints, and deformity. Some forms of the condition are rapidly progressive.

Manifestations lead to difficulties with ambulation, mobility, and (often) arm function. If facial muscles or muscles of the gastrointestinal tract are affected, feeding and speech difficulties may also be present. In some forms of muscular dystrophy, mental retardation may be present.

There is no specific interventions for muscular dystrophy. Nevertheless, physical therapy is essential to help individuals prevent contractures of the joint and maintain muscle strength and maximum functional capacity.

■ OTHER CONDITIONS OF THE NERVOUS SYSTEM

Multiple Sclerosis

Multiple sclerosis is a multifaceted, progressive condition of the central nervous system with a myriad of physical, psychological, social, vocational, and economic consequences (Khan, McPhail, Brand, Turner-Stokes, & Kilpatrick, 2006). Numerous studies indicate that multiple sclerosis is caused by a complex set of factors including genetic predisposition and largely unknown environmental factors (Peltonen, 2007). It is one of the most common disabling neurological diseases in young adults (Renoux et al., 2007; Noseworthy, Lucchinetti, Rodrigues, & Weinshenker, 2000; McDonald, 2000; Confavreux, Vukusic, Moreau, & Adeline, 2000). Most experts now believe that multiple sclerosis is an autoimmune condition in which the body's immune system attacks segments of **myelin**, the protective sheath that surrounds and insulates message-carrying nerve fibers (*axons*) in the brain and spinal cord (Werkerle & Hohlfeld, 2003; McDonald, 2000; Dyment, Cader, Willar, Riseh, Sadovnick, & Ebers, 2002). The term "multiple sclerosis" comes from the multiple areas of scarring (**sclerosis**) that occur when myelin surrounding nerve fibers in the brain and spinal cord is destroyed. Scar tissue replaces areas of myelin that have been destroyed and interferes with the transmission of nerve impulses, causing neurological deficits.

What triggers the autoimmune response causing the body to attack myelin is unknown. Genetic predisposition and geographic factors appear to have some role in determining susceptibility to multiple sclerosis. Individuals with northern European heritage as well as individuals living in more temperate climates appear to be more susceptible. (Lutton, Winston, & Rodman, 2004). There is speculation that genetic factors alone do not increase susceptibility, but rather the interaction of genetic predisposition with environmental factors or exposure to a virus that predisposes individuals to develop the condition (Dyment et al., 2002). Multiple sclerosis most often affects young adults between the ages of 20 and 40, with about 70% of cases being women (Renoux et al., 2007; Rudick, 2004; Johnson & Baringer, 2001).

Manifestations of Multiple Sclerosis

The course and manifestations of multiple sclerosis are variable. Both manifestations and the extent of the consequences experienced with multiple sclerosis vary from individual to individual, being largely dependent on the location and extent of destruction of myelin. Manifestations are diverse and unpredictable, appearing in varying combinations and patterns. Consequently, not all persons with a diagnosis of multiple sclerosis experience the same manifestations or progression of the condition.

Types of multiple sclerosis can be divided into several categories, based on the progression of the condition:

- Relapsing–remitting: fluctuating course of relapses with associated neurologic deficits, followed by periods of relative quiet
- Secondary progressive: cessation of fluctuations with slow deterioration
- Secondary progressive with relapses: fluctuation with relapses and deterioration between relapses
- Primary progressive: deterioration from beginning
- Progressive relapsing: progressive with relapses (Schapiro, 2007)

The most common initial manifestations of multiple sclerosis are dizziness; sensory disturbances, including numbness, weakness, and spasticity, especially of the lower extremities; unsteadiness; visual problems; or poor bowel and bladder control. Weakness and fatigue frequently accompany other manifestations. Symptoms fluctuate, becoming worse at times (**exacerbation**) and better at other times (**remission**) (Antel, & Bar-Or, 2003). The condition often progresses over time with manifestations becoming irreversible (Ransohoff, 2007).

Changes in motor, sensory, intellectual, or emotional function may be associated with multiple sclerosis, depending on the part of the central nervous system affected.

Not only do manifestations vary greatly from person to person, but they can also vary from time to time in the same person. Because of the variability and fluctuation of manifestations, diagnosis of multiple sclerosis is often a challenge. Before being diagnosed with this condition, many individuals have gone from one health provider to another with a host of vague complaints and clinical manifestations, which the health professional may attribute to fatigue, stress, or even laziness and withdrawal. Often, the condition is not recognized or diagnosed immediately, because the manifestations have resolved by the time the individual sees a physician. Prior to having the condition diagnosed, individuals may experience considerable anxiety, self-doubt, and depression owing to the continuing vague manifestations, which cannot be explained.

As manifestations become more pronounced, permanent consequences in a variety of areas becomes more apparent. Manifestations may include paresthesia (a sensation of numbness or tingling in some part of the body); weakness of an extremity; visual disturbances, such as **diplopia** (double vision) and dimness of vision; and **vertigo** (dizziness or false sensation of circular movement). Individuals with multiple sclerosis may develop difficulty with coordination and balance (**ataxia**), a manifestations that may be misinterpreted

by the casual observer as indicative of intoxication. There may be a partial or complete paralysis of any part of the body or spasticity of muscles, especially in the lower extremities. A particular tremor of the hands may be present; it is called an *intention tremor* because it occurs only when the individual tries to engage in a purposeful activity, such as reaching for a glass.

Speech may be slurred, or there may be scanning speech, in which the individual enunciates slowly with frequent hesitations at the beginning of a word or syllable. Individuals with multiple sclerosis may also have difficulty in swallowing (**dysphagia**), which can contribute to choking.

Multiple sclerosis may also affect the genitourinary tract, causing **incontinence** (loss of control of the bladder or bowel). Some individuals may experience **urinary retention** (the inability to empty the bladder of urine). Sexual function can also be affected. Men may experience erectile dysfunction, and women may experience decrease in sexual desire, lubrication problems, or inorgasmia (McCabe, McDonald, Deeks, Vowels, Cobain, 1996). Women with multiple sclerosis are, however, able to become pregnant and carry pregnancy to term. There is no evidence that pregnancy causes an increase in symptoms or exacerbations of the condition (Hansell, 1995).

Some individuals experience cognitive changes as a result of multiple sclerosis (Shevil & Finlayson, 2006), although intellectual function often remains intact. Some individuals, however, may experience difficulties performing tasks that require conceptualization, memory, or new learning, as well as difficulty with tasks that require either rapid or precise motor responses. Some individuals may have difficulty with abstract reasoning and problem solving. Depression is common, although the degree to which it is a reaction to the disease and the degree to which it is a manifestation of neurological dysfunction is not known. Other individuals, rather than experiencing depression, experience an inappropriate euphoria.

Management of Multiple Sclerosis

Diagnosis of multiple sclerosis is based on manifestations, the results of a full neurological examination, and as tests such as magnetic resonance imaging (MRI). There is no a cure for multiple sclerosis, and deterioration that has taken place cannot be reversed. Intervention is usually directed toward controlling individual symptoms, preventing exacerbations and complications, and maintaining function. Intervention may improve manifestations somewhat or help to prevent or delay future exacerbations of symptoms. At the same time, treatments can have risks that must be carefully weighed by each individual against the potential benefit for functional capacity or delay of decline.

A variety of medications, such as interferons, can calm the immune system thereby decreasing relapses, increasing time between relapses, and minimizing damage to the nervous system (Schapiro, 2007). Other medications are used to "fool" the immune system by mimicking myelin and blocking cells before they can attack the myelin. Medications that suppress the immune system *(immunosuppressant)* have also been used to decrease damage during relapses (Rudick, 2004). All of these medications, in addition to being expensive, can cause serious side effects and exaggerate symptoms such as depression. Some medications have the potential to impair memory and learning. Consequently, the type of medication prescribed varies with the individual. Other medications may be used to treat specific manifestations, such as medications for bladder management, control of spasticity, or emotional manifestations.

Although some individuals with multiple sclerosis never experience urinary problems, for those who do, **anticholinergic medications,** which inhibit the effects of the para-sympathetic nervous system, are sometimes helpful in relieving bladder manifestations such as frequency and urgency. Conversely, *cholinergic medications,* which stimulate the effects of the parasympathetic nervous system, may be helpful in relieving urinary retention. When urinary problems are present, individuals may be referred to a urologist (a physician who specializes in evaluation and treatment of the genitourinary tract). Bladder training may be helpful in reducing and managing bladder control problems. Use of a catheter or sanitary pads may also decrease embarrassment associated with possible leakage of urine. Other ways of managing bladder control focus on monitoring the times of day when fluids are ingested and ensuring ready availability of restrooms to minimize the chance of accidents. If the individual has problems with urinary retention, he or she may be taught to insert a catheter into the bladder to drain accumulated urine.

Most persons with multiple sclerosis experience spasticity. Some degree of *muscle relaxants* or *antispasmodics* may be prescribed for muscle spasm or spasticity, unfortunately, at doses high enough to control spasticity, weakness may be exacerbated.

Steroids are sometimes prescribed, especially in acute phases of exacerbations to suppress the manifestations, although they do not affect the progression of the disease. Because of the potential harmful effects of steroids taken over extended periods of time, they are usually prescribed only on a temporary basis to decrease exacerbations and not as an ongoing therapy.

Individuals who experience depression or anxiety may have *antianxiety agents* or *antidepressants* prescribed. Given that suicide rates are relatively high among individuals with multiple sclerosis (Livneh & Antonak, 1997), psychiatric consultation may also be indicated.

In general, individuals with multiple sclerosis should remain as active as they can without developing excessive fatigue. Physical therapy may be prescribed to help individuals with problems of mobility or to train them in the use of assistive devices, such as walkers, if needed. Specific exercises that help to decrease calcium loss from bones, strengthen weak muscles, and maintain muscle strength and joint mobility may be prescribed as well. Physical therapy that includes massage and passive range-of-motion exercises may also be beneficial. Individuals with multiple sclerosis who experience speech problems may be referred to a speech therapist or may use assistive devices, such as a communication board and voice amplifier.

For many individuals with multiple sclerosis, exposure to heat can have a temporary adverse effect on manifestations. Environments in which body temperature is increased, such as during hot or humid weather, illness with fever, or even a hot bath, can make these individuals feel worse, although heat does not necessarily cause a worsening of the condition itself. Individuals should, therefore, avoid hot and humid environments.

Because there is no cure for multiple sclerosis, it is a lifelong condition. This disease is usually not fatal, and most individuals with this condition can expect to live a normal life span, albeit with varying degrees of consequences. There is no formula for estimating the general outcome for all individuals. Manifestations often fluctuate with periods of remission (when manifestations get better) and periods of exacerbation (when manifestations get worse). Although the manifestations may partly resolve when the disease is in remission, exacerbations can leave permanent residual defects.

The condition and deterioration of function show no established pattern. The general prognosis for individuals with multiple sclerosis is unpredictable, with varying rates of progression and varying rates of disability. For some individuals (about 20%), the condition remains relatively stable with only mild manifestations, such as slight weakness, unsteadiness, or vision problems and no long-term disability. The majority of individuals (about 65%) develop a relapsing-remitting form of the condition, in which there are continuing exacerbations when manifestations become worse, along with periods of complete or partial remission in which there is no significant overall disability or restriction of general activity. Many of these individuals retain mobility 20 or more years after diagnosis, with limited disability (Schapiro, Scheinberg, Weiner, & Wolinsky, 1997). Some individuals experience a chronic progressive course of the condition, characterized by slow progression with no remissions and gradually increasing limitations. Still others experience rapid progression of the condition with total disability.

Psychosocial Issues in Multiple Sclerosis

Most individuals with multiple sclerosis are young adults who have lived through formative years of childhood and adolescence as relatively healthy individuals and are at a stage of their life in which they are beginning to assume many social and economic responsibilities, such as engaging in a career, establishing intimate personal relationships, and perhaps starting a family. When the diagnosis of multiple sclerosis has been established, the limitations and unpredictability of the condition can severely alter the individual's self-concept. Restrictions on abilities, activities, and social relationships call for significant initial psychosocial adjustment and alteration of self-concept as well as continual readjustment as exacerbations and remissions occur and as new disabling features of the condition emerge. Consequently, the long-term experience of living with multiple sclerosis through young adulthood, middle age, and older adulthood requires not just initial acceptance of the condition, but continued flexibility and adjustment as the condition changes.

The ambiguity of multiple sclerosis and the erratic nature of the symptoms produces significant stress (McNulty, Livneh, & Wilson, 2004). When the diagnosis of multiple sclerosis is finally established, individuals may react in a number of ways. Some who have been newly diagnosed may be unwilling to accept the diagnosis and continue to search for someone who will provide an alternative diagnosis. In other cases, individuals who have searched for years for an explanation for their vague and elusive neurological manifestations may feel a sense of relief at finally being given a diagnosis to explain what they have been experiencing Others may react with shock and disbelief, still others may demonstrate fear and anxiety. As with other chronic conditions, the individual's reaction to the diagnosis of multiple sclerosis depends on a number of person-specific factors.

As the diagnosis and implications of multiple sclerosis are accepted, individuals may attempt to gain some control over the disease and its symptoms. Although individuals may adapt to the realization that multiple sclerosis is a lifelong condition, its unpredictability is still a source of stress. Despite planning, unforeseen exacerbations may occur, interfering with plans and activities without warning. Exacerbations can renew a sense of vulnerability, undermining optimism or enthusiasm for long-range planning, and causing anxiety about the future.

Activities and Participation in Multiple Sclerosis

As multiple sclerosis progresses, the ability to perform a number of activities of daily living becomes reduced. Limitations in performance of daily activities can have a major impact on personal independence, quality of life, social roles, and family relationships (Mansson & Lexell, 2004). Although individuals may be able to continue to carry on a number of personal activities of daily living, such as toileting, grooming, dressing, and ambulation, there may be increasing need for assistance to carry out more complex tasks such as housekeeping, cooking, shopping, and transportation. Increasing loss of function by the individual may necessitate additional caregiving roles for family members.

Multiple sclerosis affects not only the individual, but also the family. Because many individuals are diagnosed with multiple sclerosis during young adulthood, the implications of this condition for the family, especially children, can be profound. Social support can be a strong predictor of the family's ability to cope and function effectively (Coles, Pakenham, & Leech, 2007) and the individual's perception of quality of life (Motl, McAuley, & Snook, 2007). Individuals with multiple sclerosis may experience a number of qualitative changes in social networks and personal relationships (Williams et al., 2004). Due to worsening mobility or function, they may experience a decrease in social interaction or a deterioration in social relationships (Fong, Finlayson, & Peacock, 2006). Even when individuals have mild cases of multiple sclerosis, manifestations of the condition can be stressful. In mild cases, individuals may have few visible symptoms or may experience only vague symptoms of weakness or fatigue. Family, friends, or colleagues, who are unable to observe visible signs of disability, may not understand why the individual cannot keep pace with others or continue to perform tasks in the same time frame as they were once able to do. The individual may be accused of being lazy or attempting to get out of an activity when, in fact, his or her level of energy is reduced due to the condition. As a result, individuals may attempt to push themselves beyond their capability or beyond what is in their own best interest with regard to management of their disease.

Bladder problems resulting from multiple sclerosis may cause embarrassment, causing an individual to withdraw from social and work activities. A variety of steps can be taken to minimize the social limitations that such problems may present, as described previously.

Although alcohol is not contraindicated for most people with multiple sclerosis, if balance problems are experienced as a result of the condition, alcohol will compound the problem. Likewise, alcohol can be dangerous when taken in combination with some medications. Consequently, individuals with multiple sclerosis should always consult their physician before deciding whether alcohol may be consumed on social occasions. Because of the wide variation in the course of progression of multiple sclerosis and associated functional limitations, a comprehensive evaluation of the individual's environment must be performed to ensure that adequate modifications and compensations are made to allow maximal function. Increasing the functional capabilities of the affected person has the potential to reduce the social and psychological impacts of multiple sclerosis.

Vocational Issues in Multiple Sclerosis

Many individuals with multiple sclerosis experience problems with unemployment and underemployment (Bishop, Tschopp, & Mulvihill, 2000). Multiple sclerosis is usually diagnosed during the peak years of employment, and it can significantly affect individuals' ability to remain in the workplace (Pompeii, Moon, & McCrory, 2005). Educational attainment, manifestation severity, and presence of cognitive limitations appear to be significant predictors for employment status for many individuals with multiple sclerosis (Roessler, Rumrill, & Fitzgerald, 2004). The course of the condition varies greatly among different persons; however, consequently, each individual's vocational potential must be considered separately. Individuals with mild manifestations, those with slowly progressive multiple

sclerosis, or those who have extended periods of remission are capable of being gainfully employed for many years. Others, who have more serious manifestations of the condition can, with appropriate accommodations and assistive devices, often remain employed despite exacerbations or progression of the condition.

Functional abilities related to mobility, communication, vision, and cognitive function are common areas that need to be addressed. Specific accommodations and needs for each person with multiple sclerosis must be evaluated individually. For example, those individuals who experience manifestations requiring use of a wheelchair will need wheelchair accommodations. Individuals with communication difficulties, such as slurred speech, may need other types of accommodations or considerations regarding job placement. Individuals with balance problems may need to avoid situations in which falling could be hazardous or may need a walking aid, such as a cane or crutches, which could be helpful in preventing a catastrophic fall. If vision is affected, specific accommodations related to visual needs may be warranted. If cognitive function is affected, individuals may benefit from cognitive retraining or memory enhancement programs (Roessler, Fitzgerald, Rumrill, & Koch, 2001).

Both emotional stress and physical stress can cause a temporary worsening of manifestations for individuals with multiple sclerosis. The degree of emotional stress the individual experiences on the job, as well as the level of physical activity required, should be considered. Excessive fatigue, particularly to the point of overexhaustion, should be avoided. Although individuals do not need to curtail their physical activity, they should avoid pushing themselves to exhaustion. Individuals may minimize the effects of fatigue on their job productivity by learning to self-pace so that more strenuous activities are planned when energy levels are higher, such as at the beginning of the day. Individuals should learn to moderate their pace and find activity levels conducive to optimizing their energy. Frequent rest periods may be needed throughout the day. It may be important for individuals to break tasks into smaller steps, resting at intervals in between steps. Adapting work hours to individual needs, involving individuals in more sedentary work, or using energy-saving technology may be advisable to increase work capacity.

Because heat also affects symptoms, individuals with this disease should avoid hot and humid environments. They should avoid prolonged exposure to the sun and during hot days stay in an air-conditioned environment as much as possible.

Individuals with multiple sclerosis have increased susceptibility to complications from infectious disease. For this reason, they should avoid environments in which there is significant exposure to people with colds, flu, or other infectious diseases.

Although there are limitations associated with the condition, many people with multiple sclerosis are able to continue to work with only minor adjustments. Even so, discrimination in the workplace continues to be a barrier for some individuals with multiple sclerosis (Roessler, Neath, McMahon, & Rumrill, 2007; Rumrill, Roessler, McMahon, & Fitzgerald, 2005). Loss of time at work during exacerbations should be expected; however, generally these episodes are not excessive. Provision of assistive devices, new equipment, ready access to restrooms, or job restructuring can enhance the individual's ability to continue work. Specifically, environmental factors, accommodations that allow for more sedentary work, flexibility in schedule, and use of technology

can all be instrumental in helping individuals with multiple sclerosis maintain employment (Rumrill, Roessler, Vierstra, Hennessey, & Staples, 2004).

Lyme Disease

Lyme disease is a multisystem inflammatory condition that affects the nervous system as well as joints and muscles. It is the result of an infection caused by a type of organism called a *spirochete* and is transmitted by the bite of an infected tick. In the early stages, this disease is characterized by a reddened area around the site of the tick bite. Lyme disease is rarely, if ever, fatal and is not contagious. Although most people, if treated early, have no permanent effects from this condition, some individuals can go on to develop other consequences affecting the central nervous system, including gait spasticity, facial palsy, memory loss or mild confusion, joint pain, or meningitis (Hayes & Piesman, 2003).

Diagnosis is usually based on manifestations and blood tests. Early treatment with antibiotics can significantly improve outcomes and prevent the chronic effects.

Bell's Palsy

Sudden partial or complete paralysis of one side of the face is characteristic of *Bell's palsy* (Salinas, 2002). Affected individuals may experience a sagging eyebrow, inability to close the eye, and drooping of one side of the mouth. Bell's palsy occurs when a nerve running from the brain to the face becomes inflamed. As the inflammation progresses, the nerve swells, becomes compressed, and is no longer able to transmit signals; consequently, paralysis results. A growing body of evidence links reactivation of herpes viruses with the development of a large number of cases of Bell's palsy (Gilbert, 2002).

Although most individuals recover from Bell's palsy within a month, during the acute phase, if individuals are unable to close the eye, the eye may need to be protected with an eye patch or artificial tears may need to be used. Individuals may also have anti-inflammatory steroids prescribed soon after the symptoms appear.

■ DIAGNOSTIC PROCEDURES IN CONDITIONS OF THE SPINAL CORD, NEUROMUSCULAR SYSTEM, AND PERIPHERAL NERVOUS SYSTEM

In addition to the diagnostic procedures discussed in Chapter 3, x-ray and electromyography may be used in diagnosis of neuromuscular conditions or conditions involving the peripheral nerves.

Spine Roentgenography (X-Ray)

X-ray films of the spine are called *spinal x-rays* and are used to identify fractures or other abnormalities of the vertebrae, including evaluation of spaces between vertebral disks of the spinal column. X-ray films are usually taken by a radiology technician. The films are then read and interpreted by a radiologist (a physician who specializes in radiology).

Electromyography and Nerve Conduction Velocity

Electromyography (EMG) is a procedure used to evaluate the electrical activity of certain muscles and is helpful in the diagnosis of some muscle diseases. It maybe performed by a physician, a physical therapist, or a specially trained technician. A small needle that is attached to an electrode is inserted into the muscle being examined, and the electrical activity of the selected muscle is recorded both at rest and during exercise.

Nerve conduction studies are often performed in conjunction with EMG and are helpful in diagnosing conditions affecting peripheral nerves. For the nerve conduction portion of the procedure, a stimulating electrode that delivers a mild electrical charge is placed on the skin over a nerve. An electrode placed over a muscle records the activity of the nerve distally at the nerve–muscle junction.

Electromyography makes it possible to identify defects in the transmission of impulses from nerves to muscles. It may be used in the diagnosis of a number of neuromuscular disorders and peripheral nerve injuries.

■ PSYCHOSOCIAL ISSUES IN CONDITIONS OF THE SPINAL CORD, PERIPHERAL NERVOUS SYSTEM, AND NEUROMUSCULAR SYSTEM

While conditions such as spinal cord injury remain relatively stable after injury, conditions such as multiple sclerosis, Parkinson's disease, and peripheral nerve disease may be progressive, so that functional capacity continues to change. Management of spinal cord injury after rehabilitation is directed at prevention of complications. When conditions are progressively debilitating, however, as are multiple sclerosis or Parkinson's disease, individuals must continually readjust, as additional functional capacity is lost. Uncertainty about how quickly the condition may progress and how functional capacity may be affected can be a source of continuing anxiety.

The rate of progression and the degree of decline in functional capacity in many conditions are often unpredictable. Uncertainty about whether effects on functional capacity will be minimal or whether they will progress to severe limitation can produce significant anxiety and stress. When individuals experience continued functional loss, they may actively grieve each time additional loss of function is experienced. Additional loss of functional capacity may involve changes in self-concept and body image changes as individuals adjust to new levels of functional ability.

Spinal cord injury, especially when due to trauma, provides no time for gradual adjustment. Individuals who had been previously active suddenly face the prospect of adjusting to loss of functional capacity and alteration in physical appearance. Reactions may range from hostility or anger to withdrawal. Depending on the circumstances of the injury, individuals may experience remorse or self-recrimination for failure to prevent the injury from occurring. If the injury was the result of actions of a third party, such as in the case of a motor vehicle accident or gunshot wound, individuals may feel chronic anger toward the offender or may turn their anger inward with resultant depression. In some instances, the quest for retribution becomes a negative force, eroding the individual's life as he or she continually seeks some sort of justice.

Individuals with spinal cord injuries and some individuals with neuromuscular conditions use a variety of assistive devices, such as wheelchairs, to achieve increased functional capacity. Although wheelchair use can provide mobility and an added sense of freedom and independence, some individuals may have a negative emotional reaction to use of a wheelchair, viewing it instead as a symbol of the inability.

By their very nature, manifestations of many neurological conditions necessitate assistance in care and function. Individuals may harbor resentment over the dependency imposed by the condition. Individuals who, for instance, experience paralysis (as in a spinal cord injury) may feel an increased sense of vulnerability, fearing that escape from a dangerous situation or defending themselves against threats would be difficult or impossible. Individuals' reactions may vary from overdependence to overcompensation, in which persons take unnecessary risks to test or prove their independence and strength.

When there is significant loss of ability to care for basic physical needs, such as feeding, personal hygiene, and bowel and bladder care, acceptance and adjustment to a condition may

be affected. Relying on others to assist with basic needs requires reconstituting views of privacy and self-reliance. Loss of bladder and bowel control may be an especially difficult area of adjustment. Not only are such activities private and mishaps a potential source of embarrassment, but both may also be associated with shame and humiliation experienced in early childhood, when control of these most basic bodily functions is a central issue of development.

Most individuals learn to be self-reliant, despite the fact that their ability to care for their basic physical needs is decreased. Individuals who have experienced a change in functional capacity as a result of an accident may turn their experience into a positive force directed toward broader social issues, such as seat belts in automobiles, helmets for motorcyclists, or laws against drunk driving. Other individuals may use their experience to create greater public awareness of the needs of individuals with disabilities and to educate others about disability issues. Just as neurological conditions have a spectrum of functional consequences, so the adjustment and adaptation of the people experiencing them are highly individualized, such that no two persons with the same condition will have a reaction that is quite the same.

■ ACTIVITIES AND PARTICIPATION IN CONDITIONS OF THE SPINAL CORD, PERIPHERAL NERVOUS SYSTEM, AND NEUROMUSCULAR SYSTEM

The effects of conditions affecting the spinal cord, peripheral nervous system, and neuromuscular system on an individual's lifestyle are varied and complex. Activities of daily living are often altered; meaning that help from family members or others becomes necessary. Subsequent loss of privacy for most intimate details of daily life, such as bathing or other aspects of self-care, may be part of the general condition. Even when individuals are able to manage their own personal care, the additional time required to carry out most activities must be taken into account.

Alteration of living space, including special adaptations within the environment such as widening doorways for wheelchairs, lowering countertops in kitchens, raising toilet seats, and adding ramps and railings, may be necessary. Although not all conditions require the use of a wheelchair, most require some consideration of environmental factors. For example, individuals with multiple sclerosis may be especially sensitive to hot, humid conditions, and they may need to remain in a cool environment with decreased humidity. Individuals with balance or coordination problems may need to avoid uneven terrain or other situations in which they may fall or be thrown off balance.

Alterations in daily schedules and routines may be necessary to allow additional time for dressing, bathing, and other self-care needs. If wheelchairs are utilized, the accessibility of the environment determines the ease of movement from place to place. Wheelchairs can provide more freedom of movement for those with paralysis, for those who have difficulty in walking because of problems with coordination, or for those who fatigue easily and use a wheelchair to conserve energy. Freedom of movement is limited, however, if there are stairs but no elevator, bathrooms that are too small to accommodate a wheelchair, or public transportation that is not equipped with lifts or mechanisms for transporting individuals in wheelchairs.

Individuals with conditions affecting the spinal cord or neuromuscular system can usually drive, even with paralysis, if the vehicle is equipped with special controls. If manifestations of the condition include cognitive or perceptual consequences, however, driving may not be possible.

When fatigue exacerbates manifestations of a condition, as in multiple sclerosis, or when fatigue is part of the manifestations, as in post-polio syndrome, it may be necessary to space out activities or to arrange for frequent rest periods during the day. It is sometimes helpful to divide activities that were once completed in a short amount of time into a series of subtasks, allowing rest periods in between each step.

Sexual activity may also be affected. Generally, physiologic responses require an intact nervous system. Sexual function may be most disrupted by conditions involving the spinal cord. Although women with a spinal cord injury are still capable of intercourse, sensory loss in the genitals is common in both men and women with such conditions. Men may still experience reflex erections but are usually incapable of psychologically stimulated erections. Reproductive function may also be a concern after spinal cord injury. Women with such an injury generally remain fertile and are capable of conceiving and delivering a child. Men with spinal cord injury may be infertile, however, because of inability to ejaculate, retrograde ejaculation, or decreased sperm formation.

Of course, sexuality is more than just genital acts of sex. Some form of sexual expression is possible for almost all individuals who experience disability as a result of their condition. When sexual function is affected by spinal cord injury or, in some instances, by multiple sclerosis, individuals may need to learn new forms of sexual expression to meet their needs. Although loss or alteration of sexual function is initially a severe blow to self-esteem and sense of attractiveness, individuals can express sexual feelings and needs through a variety of alternative means. Individuals who have had sexual function physically affected can still develop long-term intimate relationships that include love, respect, and mutually satisfying expression of sexual feelings.

Many factors associated with conditions of the nervous system can affect social function. The financial impact of many conditions, for example, can be devastating. The costs of medical care, rehabilitation, assistive devices, and environmental restructuring can be significant. Financial adjustments that must be made have a significant effect on the individual's general lifestyle. Assistance by various social agencies can help reduce this financial burden as well as reduce stress caused by financial concerns.

A supportive environment, including family, plays an instrumental role in individuals' response to their condition. Assistive devices, such as a wheelchair, present visible cues to others that alert them to levels of physical capacity. In some instances, such as in multiple sclerosis when there are no readily apparent outward manifestations or assistive devices to provide cues, others in the environment may be unaware that limitations of function or activity exist. Misinterpretation or misperception of the individuals' functional ability can negatively affect social interaction and, in turn, influence personal adjustment.

Although some functional limitations associated with neurological conditions are visible, such as the mobility restrictions indicated by use of a wheelchair, others are not so readily recognizable. For example, fatigue experienced in post-polio syndrome, visual or perceptual problems experienced because of multiple sclerosis, or difficulty with bladder control as in spinal bifida may create a conflict of expectations when others do not understand the reason behind certain behaviors. Fatigue associated with multiple sclerosis may be interpreted by others as laziness or attempts to avoid work if they are unaware that fatigue is a consequence of the condition. Individuals with spinal bifida who need ready access to a restroom may be viewed as having a neurotic preoccupation with the location of restroom facilities. Gait disturbance or slurred speech associated with multiple sclerosis may be viewed by others as a sign of intoxication rather than as part of the individual's condition.

In some cases, manifestations of the condition may be more troublesome to the individual exhibiting the manifestation than to those around the affected person. Individuals may fear becoming a burden on family members and consequently withdraw from close personal interactions, while family members, willing and anxious to provide help and support, are hurt at what they view as the individual's rejection of their attempts to help. In other instances, individuals may assume that others would not want to interact with them because of their condition, when actually they are greatly admired by others because of their ability to cope.

Wheelchair use may also affect social function. Despite legal mandates for accessibility, not all social events or situations are accessible to individuals using a wheelchair. Consequently, they may either avoid the activity or need to make special arrangements to attend an event or participate in an activity. Although most public places have made provisions for accessibility, some means of accessibility are more desirable than others. For example, a multilevel historic site may be accessible to individuals in wheelchairs only through a back entrance or freight elevator. To reach a stage for presentation, individuals may need to be "pushed" up a ramp rather than negotiate the ramp themselves. In addition, different angles of eye contact can have both emotional, and physical implications for individuals in wheelchairs who must continually look upward at their peers. This can relate an impression of differing social stature, both in individuals using the wheelchair and in those with whom they engage in conversation.

■ VOCATIONAL ISSUES IN CONDITIONS OF THE SPINAL CORD, PERIPHERAL NERVOUS SYSTEM, AND NEUROMUSCULAR SYSTEM

Progressive conditions or conditions characterized by remissions and exacerbations, such as multiple sclerosis, require ongoing evaluation of functional capacity. Although functional capacity in spinal cord injury is relatively stable, changing conditions or complications such as pressure sores or contractures may also change functional ability.

Stress and its impact are also factors to be considered. For instance, stress in the workplace for individuals with multiple sclerosis may add to fatigue that is already a consequence of the condition itself. In other instances, such as in Parkinson's disease, stress may precipitate manifestations or make manifestations worse.

Manifestations of the condition must be matched with specific needs and conditions in the workplace environment. For instance, if communication skills are affected, such as in multiple sclerosis or Parkinson's disease, specific devices, techniques, or alternative means of communication may be needed. Hot, humid environments should be avoided by individuals with multiple sclerosis. Individuals with high thoracic spinal cord injuries or cervical injuries also often experience difficulty with heat regulation and consequently should avoid extremes of temperature. In addition, because of the loss of sensation in the extremities with conditions such as spinal cord injury, situations in which there is a possibility of burns or frostbite should be avoided. Individuals with spinal cord injuries, multiple sclerosis, or Parkinson's disease may be especially susceptible to upper respiratory problems. Consequently, exposure to pollutants or exposure to others with respiratory infections should be avoided.

Accessibility of the workplace should be evaluated for individuals who use wheelchairs or other assistive devices in which environmental factors could interfere with mobility. Availability of elevators as opposed to stairs, desk or workbench height, width of doorways, and size of bathrooms are all important environmental considerations. Factors such as availability of transportation, and additional time required for getting ready for work also

need to be considered. In all instances, a realistic appreciation of the individual's strengths and abilities is crucial. Each person and his or her specific needs, abilities, and interests should be considered individually.

CASE STUDIES: SPINAL CORD, PERIPHERAL NERVOUS SYSTEM, AND NEUROMUSCULAR CONDITIONS

Case 1

John, an 18-year-old high school senior, experienced a spinal cord injury (C6) during a high school football game. John had begun work with his father, the owner of a construction company, during the summer and had hoped, after graduating from high school, to go to a technical school to learn more about construction. After graduating, from this school, he had planned to join his father in the construction business.

1. Which types of limitations would you expect John to experience given his level of injury?
2. Which types of adaptive devices will John most likely need to achieve his greatest level of independence?
3. Which types of alternative career choices might John have, given his interests?
4. Which lifestyle issues may need to be considered?
5. How does John's family status influence his rehabilitation goals?
6. Which specific issues would you address when working with John to establish his rehabilitation plan?

Case 2

Mrs. R. is a 50-year-old woman who experienced polio as a child. Residual consequences of polio consisted of weakness in both extremities. Today she ambulates using canes and braces. Mrs. R. works as a legal secretary in a small metropolitan city. As part of her job, she frequently accompanies her employer to various meetings at different locations in the city, as well as to court. Recently she has begun experiencing increasing weakness in her lower legs, and shoulder pain. After consulting her physician, Mrs. R. was told she is experiencing post-polio syndrome.

1. Which issues specific to Mrs. R.'s age should be considered in working with her to develop a rehabilitation plan?
2. Which specific issues regarding post-polio syndrome should be considered?
3. Are there accommodations that Mrs. R. would need in her job to enable her to maintain her optimum level of independence?
4. Will manifestations of her post-polio syndrome prevent Mrs. R. from continuing employment? Which issues would you discuss?

■ REFERENCES

Adams, M. M., & Hicks, A. L., (2005). Spasticity after spinal cord injury, *Spinal Cord, 43,* 577–586.

Aminoff, M. J., Burns, R. S., & Silverstein, P. M. (1997). Update on Parkinson's disease. *Patient Care, 31*(10), 12–14; 16; 19–20, 23–25.

Andrén E., & Grimby, G. (2004). Dependence in daily activities and life satisfaction in adult subjects with cerebral palsy or spina bifida: A follow-up study. *Disability and Rehabilitation, 26*(9), 528–536.

Antel, J. P., & Bar-Or, A. (2003). Do myelin-directed antibodies predict multiple sclerosis? *New England Journal of Medicine, 349*(2), 107–109.

Bishop, M., Tschopp, M. K., & Mulvihill, M. (2000). Multiple sclerosis and epilepsy: Vocational aspects and the best rehabilitation practices. *Journal of Rehabilitation, 66*(2), 50–55.

Blank-Reid, C., Kaplan, L. J., & Santora, T. A. (2008). Neuroscience critical care management. In E. Barker (Ed.), *Neuroscience nursing.* (pp. 278–304) St. Louis; Mosby

Bloemen-Vrencken, J. H. deWitte, L. P. & Post, M. W. M. (2005). Follow-up for persons with spinal cord injury living in the community: A systematic review of interventions and their evaluation. *Spinal Cord, 43,* 462–475.

Burchiel, K. J., & Hsu, F. P. (2001). Pain and spasticity after spinal cord injury: Mechanisms and treatment. *Spine, 26,* S146–S160.

Burk, J. & Agre, J. C. (2000). Characteristics and management of post polio syndrome. *Journal of the American Medical Association, 284*(4), 412–413.

Cattaneo, E., Rigamonti, D., & Zuccato, C. (2002). The enigma of Huntington's disease. *Scientific American, 287,* 93–97.

Catz, A., Zifroni, A., & Philo, O. (2005). Economic assessment of pressure sore prevention using a computerized mattress system in patients with spinal cord injury. *Disability and Rehabilitation, 27*(21), 1315–1319.

Chan, S. K. K., & Man, D. W. K. (2005). Barriers to returning to work for people with spinal cord injuries: A focus group study. *Work, 25,* 325–332.

Chen, S. C., Lai, C. H., Chan, W. P., Huang, M. H., Tsai, H. W., & Chen, J. J. J. (2005). Increases in bone mineral density after functional electrical stimulation cycling exercises in spinal cord injured patients. *Disability and Rehabilitation, 27*(22), 1337–1341.

Chung, M. C., Preveza, E., Papandreou, K., & Prevezas, N. (2006). Spinal cord injury, post-traumatic stress, and locus of control among the elderly: A comparison with young and middle-aged patients. *Psychiatry, 69*(1), 69–80.

Claydon, V. E., Steeves, J. D., & Krassioukov, A. (2006). Orthostatic hypotension following spinal cord injury: Understanding clinical pathophysiology. *Spinal Cord, 44,* 341–351.

Coggrave, M., Burrows, D., & Durand, M. A. (2006). Progressive protocol in the bowel management of spinal cord injuries. *British Journal of Nursing, 15*(20), 1108–1113.

Coles, A. R., Pakenham, K. I., & Leech, C. (2007). Evaluation of an intensive psychosocial intervention for children of parents with multiple sclerosis. *Rehabilitation Psychology, 52*(2), 133–142.

Confavreux, C., Vukusic, S., Moreau, T., & Adeleire, P. (2000). Relapses and progression of disability in multiple sclerosis. *New England Journal of Medicine, 343*(20), 1430–1437.

Cushman, L. A., and Dijkers, M. (1991). Depressed mood during rehabilitation of persons with spinal injury. *Journal of Rehabilitation, 57,* 35–38.

del Aquila, M. A., Longstreth, W. T. Jr., McGuire, V., Koepsell, T. D. & van Belle, G. (2003). Prognosis in amyotrophic lateral sclerosis: A population-based study, *Neurology, 60*(5), 813–819.

Ducharme, S. (2006). Medical and psychosocial aspects of infertility for men with spinal cord injury and their partners. *Sex Disability, 24,* 73–75.

Dural, A., Atay, M. B., Akbostanci, C., & Kucukdeveci, A. (2003). Impairment, disability, and life satisfaction in Parkinson's disease. *Disability and Rehabilitation, 25*(7), 318–323.

Elliot, T. R., & Frank, R. G. (1996) Depression following spinal cord injury. *Archives of Physical Medicine and Rehabilitation, 77,* 816–823.

Fong, T., Finlayson, M., & Peacock, N. (2006). The social experience of aging with a chronic illness: Perspectives of older adults with multiple sclerosis. *Disability and Rehabilitation, 28*(11), 695–705.

Forsberg, A., Press, R., Einarsson, U., de Pedro-Cuesta, J., & Holmqvist, L. W., (2005). Disability and health-related quality of life in Guillain–Barré syndrome during the first two years after onset: A prospective study. *Clinical Rehabilitation, 19,* 900–909.

Gage, H., & Storey, L. (2004). Rehabilitation for Parkinson's disease: A systematic review of available evidence. *Clinical Rehabilitation, 18,* 463–482.

Gilbert, S. C. (2002) Bell's palsy and herpes viruses. *Herpes, 9*(3), 70–73.

Gordon P. A., & Feldman, (2002). Post-polio syndrome: Issues and strategies for rehabilitation counselors. *Journal of Rehabilitation. 68*(2), 28–32.

Griffin, J. W. (2004). Peripheral Neuropathies. In, L. Goldman & D. Ausiello (Eds.). *Cecil Textbook of Medicine* (22nd ed., pp. 2379–2387). Philadelphia: W. B. Saunders.

Hansell, R. (1995) The role of the general medical practitioner in the management of MS. *MS Management, 2*(2), 19–23.

Hayes, E. B., & Piesman, J. (2003). How can we prevent Lyme disease? *New England Journal of Medicine, 348*(24), 2923–2429.

Jankovic, J. (2004). Parkinsonism. In L. Goldman & D. Ausiello (Eds.), *Cecil Textbook of medicine* (22nd ed., pp. 2306–2310). Philadelphia: W. B. Saunders.

Janson, C., Leone, P., & Freese, A. (2002). Parkinson's disease: Part 1. Molecular pathology, *Science and Medicine, 9,* 328–338.

Jennings, W. (2007). Expert opinion—Frequently asked questions (FAQs): Changing urinary catheters in people with spinal cord injury, residing in the community. *Australian and New Zealand Continence Journal, 13*(2), 46–49.

Jensen, M. P., Hoffman, A. J., & Cardenas, D. D. (2005). Chronic pain in individuals with spinal cord injury: A survey and longitudinal study. *Spinal Cord, 43,* 704–712.

Janson, C., Leone, P., & Freese, A. (2003). Parkinson's disease: Part II. Cellular basis of medical treatment. *Science Medicine, 9*(1), 24–35.

Johnson, K. P., & Baaringer, J. R. (2001, April 15). Current therapy of multiple sclerosis. *Hospital Practice,* pp. 21–29.

Johnson, K., Mowrey, K., & Bergman, M. J. (2008). Neurotrauma: Spinal cord injury. In E. Barker (Ed.), *Neuroscience nursing: A spectrum of care* (3rd ed., pp. 368–402. Mosby: St. Louis).

Jozefczyk, P. B. (2002). The management of focal spasticity. *Clinical Neuropharmacology, 25,* 158–173.

Khan, F., McPhail, T., Brand, C., Turner-Stokes, L., & Kilpatrick, T. (2006). Multiple sclerosis: Disability profile and quality of life in an Australian community cohort. *International Journal of Rehabilitation Research, 29*(2), 87–96.

Kita, M., & Goodkin, D. E. (2000). Drugs used to treat spasticity. *Drugs, 59,* 487–495.

Leegwater-Kim, J., & Waters, C. (2007). Parkinsonism. In R. E. Rakel & E. T. Bope (Eds.)., *Conn's current therapy* (pp. 1100–1106). Philadelphia: W. B. Saunders.

Leng, T. R., Woodward, M. J., & Stokes, M. J., Swan, A. V., Wareing, L. A., Baker, R. (2003). Effects of multisensory stimulation in people with Huntington's disease: A randomized controlled pilot study. *Clinical Rehabilitation, 17,* 30–41.

Litvan, I. (1998). Parkinsonian features: When are they Parkinson disease? *Journal of the American Medical Association, 280(19),* 1654–1658.

Livneh, H. (2000). Psychosocial adaptation to spinal cord injury: The role of coping strategies. *Journal of Applied Rehabilitation Counseling, 1*(2), 3–10.

Lude, P., Kennedy, P., Evans, M., Lude, Y., & Beedie, A. (2005). Post traumatic distress symptoms following spinal cord injury: A comprative review of European samples. *Spinal Cord, 43,* 102–108.

Lustig, D. C. (2005). The adjustment process for individuals with spinal cord injury: The effect of perceived premorbid sense of coherence. *Rehabilitation Counseling Bulletin, 48*(3), 146–156.

Lutton, J. D., Winston, R., & Redman, T. C. (2004). Multiple sclerosis: Etiological mechanisms and future directions. *Experimental Biology and Medicine, 229*(1), 12–20.

Lyons, K. D., Tickle-Degnen, L., Henry, A., & Cohn, E. (2004). Impressions of personality in Parkinson's disease: Can rehabilitation practitioners see beyond the symptoms? *Rehabilitation Psychology, 49*(4), 328–333.

Mansson, E., & Lexell, J., (2004). Performance of activities of daily living in multiple sclerosis. *Disability and Rehabilitation, 26*(10), 576–585.

McAweeney, J. G., Forchheimer, M., Tate, D. G. (1996). Identifying the unmet independent living needs of persons with spinal cord injury. *Journal of Rehabilitation, 63*(3), 29–33.

McCabe, M. P., McDonald, E., Deeks, A., Vowels, L. M., & Cobain, M. J., (1996). The impact of multiple sclerosis on sexuality and relationships. *Journal of Sex Research, 33*(3), 241–252.

McDonald, W. I. (2000). Relapse remission, & progression in multiple sclerosis. *New England Journal of Medicine, 343*(20), 1486–1487.

McNulty, K., Livneh, H., & Wilson, L. M. (2004). Perceived uncertainty, spiritual well-being, and psychosocial adaptation in individuals with multiple sclerosis. *Rehabilitation Psychology, 49*(2), 91–99.

Meade, M. A., Armstrong, A. J., Barrett, K., Ellenbogen, P. S., & Jackson, M. N. (2006). Vocational rehabilitation services for individuals with spinal cord injury. *Journal of Vocational Rehabilitation, 25,* 3–11.

Meade, M. A., Barrett, K., Ellenbogen, P. S., & Jackson, M. N. (2006). Work intensity and variations in health and personal characteristics of individuals with spinal cord injury (SCI). *Journal of Vocational Rehabilitation, 27,* 13–19.

Motl, R. W., McAuley, E., & Snook, E. M. (2007). Physical activity and quality of life in multiple sclerosis: Possible roles of social support, self-efficacy, and functional limitations. *Rehabilitation Psychology, 52*(2), 143–151.

Norquist, J. M., Fitzpatrick, R., & Jenkinson, C. (2004). Health-related quality of life in amyotrophic lateral sclerosis: Determining a meaningful deterioration. *Quality of Life Research, 13,* 1409–1414.

Noseworthy, J. H., Lucchinetti, C., Rodriguez, M., & Weinshenker, B. G., (2000). Multiple Sclerosis. *New England Journal of Medicine, 343,* 938–952.

Nussbaum, R. L., & Ellis, C. E. (2003). Alzheimer's disease and Parkinson's disease. *New England Journal of Medicine, 348*(14), 1356–1364.

Orrell, R. W. (2007). Understanding the causes of amyotrophic lateral sclerosis. *New England Journal of Medicine, 357*(8), 822–823.

Pallansch, M. A., & Sandhu, H. S. (2006). The eradication of polio: Progress and challenges. *New England Journal of Medicine, 355*(24), 2508–2511.

Peltonen, L. (2007). Old suspects found guilty: The first genome profile of multiple sclerosis. *New England Journal of Medicine, 357*(9), 927–929.

Phillips, P., (1999). Keeping depression at bay helps patients with Parkinson disease. *Journal of the American Medical Association, 282*(12), 118–119.

Pires, M., & Adkins, R. (1996). Pressure ulcers and spinal cord injury: Scope of the problem. *Topics: Spinal Cord Injury Rehabilitation, 2*(1), 1–8.

Pompeii, L. A., Moon, S. D., & McCrory, D. C. (2005). Measures of physical and cognitive function and work status among individuals with multiple sclerosis: A review of the literature. *Journal of Occupational Rehabilitation, 15*(1), 69–84.

Ransohoff, R. M. (2007). Natalizumab for multiple sclerosis. *New England Journal of Medicine, 356*(25), 2622–2628.

Renoux, C., Vukusic, S., Mikaeloff, Y., Edan, G., Clanet, M., Dubois, B., et al. (2007). Natural history of multiple sclerosis with childhood onset. *New England Journal of Medicine, 356*(25), 2603–2613.

Rinala, D., Young, J., Hart, K., Clearman, R., & Fuhrer, M. (1992). Social support and the well-being of persons with spinal cord injury living in the community. *Rehabilitation Psychology, 37,* 155–163.

Robinson, J., & Kothari, M. J. (2007). Myasthenia gravis and related disorders. In R. E. Rakel & E. T. Bope (Eds.), *Conn's Currrent Therapy* (pp. 1086–1094). Philadelphia: W. B. Saunders.

Roessler, R. T. (2001). Job retention services for employees with spinal cord injuries: A critical need in vocational rehabilitation. *Journal of Applied Rehabilitation Counseling, 32*(1), 3–8.

Roessler, R. T., Fitzgerald, S. M., Rumrill, P. D., Koen, L. C. (2001). Determinants of employment status among people with multiple sclerosis. *Rehabilitation Counseling Bullentin, 45*(1), 31–39.

Roessler, R. T., Neath, J., McMahon, B. T., & Rumrill, P. D. (2007). Workplace discrimination outcomes and their predictive factors for adults with multiple sclerosis. *Rehabilitation Counseling Bulletin, 50*(3), 139–152.

Roessler, R.T., Rumrill, P.D., & Fitzgerald, S.M. (2004). Predictors of employment status for people with multiple sclerosis. *Rehabilitation Counseling Bulletin, 47*(2), 96–103.

Rothrock, J. (2006). Spinal cord injury and vocational rehabilitation. *Journal of Vocational Rehabilitation, 25,* 1–2.

Roland, L. P., & Schneider, N. A. (2001). Amyotrophic lateral sclerosis. *New England Journal of Medicine, 344*(22), 1688–1698.

Rudick, R. A. (2004). Multiple sclerosis and demyelinating conditions of the central nervous system. In L. Goldman & D. Ausiello (Eds.), *Cecil textbook of medicine* (22nd ed., pp. 2320–2327). Philadelphia: W. B. Saunders.

Rumrill, P., Roessler, R. T., McMahon, B. T., & Fitzgerald, S. M. (2005). Multiple sclerosis and workplace discrimination: The national EEOC ADA research project. *Journal of Vocational Rehabilitation, 23,* 179–187.

Rumrill, P. P., Roessler, R., Vierstra, C., Hennessey, M., & Staples L. (2004). Workplace barriers and job satisfaction among employed people with multiple sclerosis: An empirical rationale for early intervention. *Journal of Vocational Rehabilitation, 20,* 177–183.

Sakellariou, D. (2006). If not the disability, then what? Barriers to reclaiming sexuality following spinal cord injury. *Sex Disability, 24,* 101–111.

Salcido, R. (2000) Rehabilitation of the post polio patients. *Topics in Geriatric Rehabilitation, 15*(3), 95–97.

Salinas, R. (2002). Bell's palsy. *Clinical Evidence, 7,* 1140–1144.

Schapiro, R. T. (2007). Multiple sclerosis. In R. E. Rakel & E. T. Bope (Eds.), *Conn's Current Therapy* (pp. 1081–1085). Philadelphia: W. B. Saunders.

Schapiro, R. T., Scheinberg, L., Weiner, H. L., & Wolinsky, J. S. (1997, January, 15) Living with MS: The outlook improves *Patient Care,* pp. 87, 88, 91, 92, 97, 102–104, 106–108, 119.

Shevil, E., & Finlayson, M. (2006). Perceptions of persons with multiple sclerosis on cognitive changes and their impact on daily life. *Disability and Rehabilitation, 28*(12), 779–788.

Suzuki, R., Krahn, G. L., McCarthy, M. J., & Adams, E. J. (2007). Understanding health outcomes: Physical secondary conditions in people with spinal cord injury. *Rehabilitation Psychology, 52*(3), 338–350.

Walling, A. D. (1999). Amyotrophic lateral sclerosis: Lou Gehrig's disease. *American Family Physician, 59*(6), 1489–1496.

Werkerle, H. & Hohlfeld, R. (2003). Molecular mimicry in multiple sclerosis. *New England Journal of Medicine, 349*(2), 185–186.

Williams, R. M., Turner, A. P., Hatzakis, M., Chu, S., Rodriquez, A. A., Bowen, J. D., & Haselkorn,

J. K. (2004). Social support among veterans with multiple sclerosis. *Rehabilitation Psychology, 49*(2), 106–113.

Woolsey, R. M. & McGarry, J. D. (1991). The cause, prevention, and treatment of pressure sores. *Neurology Clinics, 9,* 797–808.

Zinzi, P., Salmaso, D., De Grandis, R., Graziani, G., Maceroni, S., Bentivoglio, A. (2007). Effects of an intensive rehabilitation programme on patients with Huntington's disease: A pilot study. *Clinical Rehabilitation, 21,* 603–613.

Chapter 5

Conditions of the Eye and Blindness

■ STRUCTURE AND FUNCTION OF THE EYE

The eyeballs are spherical organs encased in the orbital cavities of the skull. Muscles located on the top, bottom, and side of each eye enable the eye to rotate in different directions. The eyelid serves a protective function. Through frequent blinking, the eyelid helps keep the eye moist, preventing irritation. The *lacrimal glands*, which lie in the upper, outer side of the eye behind the eyelid, secrete tears to keep the eyeball moist and help rid the eye of foreign material.

In front of the eye is a transparent curved structure called the *cornea*, which admits light and protects the inner eye from foreign particles and organisms? Although the cornea contains no blood vessels, it is richly supplied with nerve cells. Connected to the cornea and completely covering the eyeball (except for the part covered by the cornea) is a fibrous membrane called the **sclera**. The sclera forms the white part of the eye and has the primary function of supporting and protecting the eye and maintaining eye shape. Lining the exposed area of the sclera and inner eyelid is a sensitive membrane called the **conjunctiva**. Lying underneath the sclera and also surrounding the eyeball is the choroid coat, which contains most of the blood vessels that nourish the eye. (See Figure 5-1.)

The colored part of the eye is called the *iris*. At the center of the iris is a round opening called the *pupil*, which admits light to the inner part of the eye. The cornea covers both the iris and the pupil. Smooth muscle fibers on either side of the pupil cause it to contract or dilate, thereby automatically regulating the amount of light that enters the eye. In bright light, the pupil contracts to reduce the amount of light admitted. In the dark, the pupil dilates to admit as much light as possible.

Directly behind the iris is a space called the posterior chamber. Contained in the posterior chamber is a structure called the ciliary process, which produces a transparent fluid called the *aqueous humor*. The aqueous humor escapes from the posterior chamber through the pupil into a space lying between the iris and cornea called the anterior chamber, which lies between the iris and the cornea. The aqueous humor then drains from the eye into lymph channels and into the venous system through a sieve-like structure called the *canal of Schlemm* (*trabecular network*), which is located at the junction of the iris and the sclera. The balance between the amount of aqueous humor produced and the amount drained helps to maintain normal **intraocular pressure** (pressure within the eyeball).

The aqueous humor nourishes both the cornea and a structure located directly behind the iris called the **lens**. The lens is a small

141

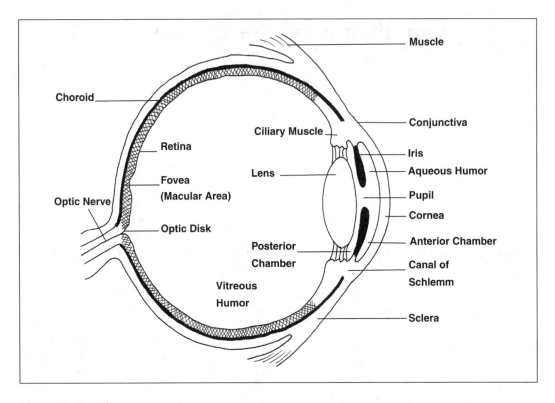

Figure 5–1   The eye

transparent disk enclosed in a transparent capsule. Attachments around the circumference of the lens, called ciliary muscles, automatically contract or expand, changing the shape of the lens from fat to thin (or vice versa) in response to the proximity or distance of an object being visualized. Changing shape of the lens permits the eye to focus for near or far vision, a process called **accommodation**. To focus on objects in the distance, the ciliary muscles relax, thereby thinning and flattening the lens. To focus on objects close by, the ciliary muscles contract, so that the lens becomes more rounded.

Behind the lens is a larger cavity known as the vitreous space. This space is filled with a jelly-like, translucent substance called the *vitreous humor*, which helps to maintain the form and shape of the eyeball.

At the very back of the eye is the innermost coat of the eye, the **retina**. The retina contains two layers: (1) a pigmented layer that is fixed to the choroid and (2) an inner layer that contains special light-sensitive cells called *rods* and *cones*.

Rods are involved with detecting light and dark as well as shape and movement; they are primarily necessary for night vision and peripheral vision. Rods contain a derivative of vitamin A, called *rhodopsin*, a highly light-sensitive substance that breaks down rapidly when exposed to light. This chemical process causes a reaction that activates the rods, so that the eye adjusts to varying amounts of light, enabling individuals see in the dark. This process is called **adaptation**.

Cones are involved primarily in daylight and color vision as well as in the perception of sharp visual detail. Most of the cones are located in a spot on the retina called the **macula**. The macula is the area of clearest central vision. The center of the macula, the fovea, contains no rods and is the area where vision is clearest in good light.

The optic nerve enters the back of the eye through an area called the optic disk. This area is sometimes called the blind spot because it does not contain light-sensitive cells. Light rays pass through the cornea, enter the pupil, pass through the lens, and register on the retina. Sensory cells of the retina receive light stimuli and convert them into electrical impulses. These electrical impulses are then transmitted to the optic nerve, which carries them to the occipital lobe of the brain, where they are interpreted.

After exiting the optic disk, the optic nerves from both eyes join together at the base of the brain just in front of the brain stem to form the optic chiasm. At this point, half of the nerve tracts from each eye cross over to the opposite side of the brain. Both eyes receive information from a combination of both visual fields. *Depth perception* requires that the brain receive input from both eyes. The portion of the visual field detected by both eyes which is called the *binocular visual field*, is necessary for depth perception.

■ MEASURING VISION

The two most common types of testing for vision are **visual acuity testing** and *visual field testing* (Barker, 2008). **Visual acuity** is defined as the sharpness of the visual image perceived. Visual acuity tests are used to measure the level of best vision and to measure the need for corrective lenses.

A standard test of visual acuity is the *Snellen test*. The chart used for this test contains a series of letters on nine lines of decreasing size. Lines are identified according to the distance from which they can be read by individuals

with unimpaired vision. For example, individuals with normal visual acuity can read the top line of the chart at 200 feet and the last line at 20 feet. When taking the Snellen test, individuals view the Snellen chart at the equivalent of 20 feet and read the lines on the chart from the largest to the smallest. The results of the test are expressed as a fraction, with the numerator denoting the equivalent distance from the chart at which the individual being tested views the chart (20 feet) and the denominator denoting the distance from the chart at which a person with normal vision would be able to read the same line. Consequently, a visual acuity of 20/100 means that the individual being tested can see at 20 feet what a person with normal visual acuity could see at 100 feet, and would indicate that the individual has a visual impairment. A result of 20/10 would indicate that the individual being tested has better than normal visual acuity, as he or she can see at 20 feet what individuals with normal visual acuity could only see at 10 feet.

Visual field is defined as the size of the area that individuals can see without turning the head or moving the eyes. *Peripheral vision* (side vision) is measured by a curved device called a perimeter. Individuals look into the perimeter, and a test object is systematically moved from outside the peripheral field of vision toward the center until the individual indicates visualization of the object. *Central vision* (vision in the center of the visual field) is tested with the individual looking at a tangent screen, on which a test object is systematically moved across the screen. The individual's ability to see the object at certain points is then mapped, outlining his or her central field of vision.

■ TYPES OF VISUAL CONDITIONS

When any deviation of normal vision exists, individuals are considered to have a **visual impairment**. Visual impairments range from mild to total loss of vision. In general, conditions involving the eye that result in visual impairment can be categorized as followed:

- Refractory errors
- Difficulty with coordination of the eyes
- Opacities of the eye
- Damage to the eye due to injury
- Damage to the eye secondary to other conditions
- Degenerative changes of the eye

Visual impairments may be temporary, reversible, progressive, or permanent. They may involve any of the following components of vision:

- Central field of vision. Individuals are able to see images in the periphery of the visual field but not images in the center.
- Peripheral field of vision. Individuals are able to see images in the center of the field of vision but not in the periphery (*tunnel vision*).
- Night vision. The individual has difficulty seeing at night (*night blindness*).
- Color vision. Individuals have difficulty distinguishing colors, especially red and green. Rarely, individuals have complete lack of color vision with associated low visual acuity (*achromatopsia*).
- Binocular vision. Individuals have difficulty with the coordinated use of both eyes to produce a single image. As a result, individuals may have double vision **(diplopia).**

Severe visual impairment can be defined as the inability to read ordinary newsprint even with the aid of glasses. When deviations of vision are great enough to cause total loss of light perception, the term **blindness** is used. Many individuals, however, have some usable vision so that special aids or devices can enable them to perform most tasks. When ordinary glasses, contact lenses, medical treatment, or surgery is unable to correct sight to the normal range, individuals are said to have low vision or to be partially sighted. (Butler, 1997). The term **legal blindness** is used to describe both those who have total loss of vision and those who have some remaining visual function but who are significantly disabled by visual impairment. In the United States, legal blindness has been defined as follows:

- Visual acuity not exceeding 20/200 or worse in the better eye with correcting lenses
- Central field of vision limited to an angle of 20 degrees or less

■ CONDITIONS OF THE EYE AND BLINDNESS

Refractive Errors

The most frequent cause for diminished visual acuity is refractive error (Fay & Jakobiec, 2004). *Refractive errors* occur when changes in the cornea, aqueous humor, lens, or vitreous humor prevent proper bending of light rays to converge on the retina. . One type of refractive error, **myopia** (nearsightedness), results from elongation of the eyeball so that light rays focus on a point in front of the retina. Individuals with this condition have good visual acuity for close objects but difficulty seeing objects in the distance. The opposite type of refractive error is **hyperopia** (farsightedness), in which the eyeball is shorter than normal so that light rays focus on a point beyond the retina. Individuals with hyperopia have good visual acuity for objects in the distance but have difficulty focusing on things at close range. Another type of refractive error, **astigmatism,** results from irregularity of shape of the cornea or (at times) the lens so that vision is distorted. Myopia, hyperopia, and astigmatism can occur at any age.

Presbyopia is a condition usually associated with aging in which there is gradual loss of accommodation due to loss of elasticity of the lens and weakening of the ciliary muscle. Individuals with presbyopia must hold small objects and printed material farther and farther away to see clearly because the eye can no longer adjust the shape of the lens to allow clear vision of close objects.

Refractory errors are usually remedied with corrective lenses. A surgical procedure, called *radial keratotomy* (discussed later in this chapter), is now often performed to correct myopia. This procedure attempts to correct nearsightedness by altering the shape of the cornea, causing it to flatten.

Incoordination of the Eyes

To achieve good vision, both eyes must work together so that images from each eye can fuse into one single image. When this does not occur, vision may be impeded to some degree. Incoordination of the eyes can be the result of heredity, disease, or damage to the brain.

Nystagmus is a condition in which the eyes move involuntarily even though the gaze is fixed in one direction. The movement may occur in any direction but most often is horizontal. Nystagmus may be congenital, or it may develop later in life as a result of a neurological disease or other condition. Although this condition may cause little visual disturbance and be unapparent to the individual, it may be distracting and noticeable to others who are interacting with the person.

Strabismus is a condition in which the eyes cannot be directed to the same object or in which the eyes are crossed, turning inward. It is classified according to the type and magnitude of misalignment. When present in children, it is recommended that it be corrected early to decrease the risk of **amblyopia** (discussed later) and to maximize the potential for binocular vision (Donahue, 2007). Strabismus may result from unequal ocular muscle tone or from a neurological condition. It can often be corrected by surgery, by corrective lenses, by medications, or by a combination of the three.

Suppression amblyopia (lazy eye) is a condition in which one eye does not develop good vision, usually because of strabismus. It is usually treated at an early age by placing a patch over the eye. The eye usually responds to early intervention and the condition is corrected. If, the condition is not treated early, however, the condition can persist for life.

Opacities of the Eye

Opacities of the Cornea

Any condition, including injuries, inflammation, or disease that causes scarring or clouding of the cornea, can cause permanent partial or total loss of vision. Because of its rich nerve supply, inflammation or injury to the cornea can cause severe pain. Prompt intervention for corneal inflammation can prevent subsequent formation of scar tissue that can interfere with vision. When clouding or scarring of the cornea causes permanent visual loss, *corneal transplant* (discussed later in this chapter) may be performed. When corneal transplant is successful, vision may be restored with few, if any, restrictions.

Cataracts

A **cataract** is a clouding or opacity of the lens of the eye. Although cataracts are a common cause of visual impairment in older adults, they may also be congenital, inherited, the result of ocular trauma or inflammation, or associated with a variety of other conditions, such as diabetes. They can also be drug-induced, such as occurs with use of high levels of certain types of steroids. Individuals with cataracts often describe their vision as looking through a cloudy pane of glass or through a fog.

Although cataracts are generally bilateral, they may form at different rates in each eye. As the lenses become more opaque, vision gradually diminishes. If cataracts are the result of injury, such as from radiation or a foreign object striking the lens, loss of vision occurs more rapidly. Cataracts associated with aging progress more slowly over time.

Because there is no way to return the lens to its normal transparency, treatment of cataracts involves removal of the lens and its replacement with an implant, with glasses, or with both (Sherwood, 2007). An intraocular prosthetic lens is generally inserted into the eye at the time of surgery. Surgery is usually performed on an outpatient basis. Any implanted lens has a fixed focal length so that vision is clear at only one distance. Thus individuals who have undergone cataract surgery may continue to need corrective lenses, such as bifocals.

Injuries to the Eyes

Eye injuries are common and, in many cases, preventable. The most common type of eye injury is an injury to the cornea caused by a foreign body. Although often considered minor, these injuries can become serious if a scratch or abrasion to the cornea becomes infected or causes scarring, which can in turn impede vision. When the cornea becomes so scarred that vision is severely compromised, a surgical procedure, corneal transplant (**Keratoplasty**), may be performed (Nishida et al., 2004). Corneal transplantation may also be performed when the shape of the cornea is distorted. Donor eyes for corneal transplantation come from individuals who have recently died. During the surgical procedure, the opaque area of the cornea of the recipient's eye is replaced with the clear donor cornea, which is sutured into place. Because the cornea has no blood vessels, the healing process is slow. Although a corneal transplant can restore vision, graft rejection or need for a second operation is also possible.

More serious injuries to the eye include chemical burns, corneal laceration, or bleeding into the anterior chamber (*hyphema*) all of which can threaten vision. Chemical agents with an alkaline base (such as cleansing agents, fertilizers, plaster, and refrigerants) can penetrate the eye rapidly, leading to cell disruption and tissue death. Chemical agents with an acidic base cause protein coagulation in the eye so that penetration is not as rapid, but scarring of tissue can still result in visual loss. In both instances, immediate irrigation of the eye can decrease the amount of damage to the eye, although emergency medical treatment should also be sought immediately.

Some injuries involve puncture or laceration of the eye. Common causes are work-related injuries, such as chopping or sawing wood, or chiseling or hammering metal on metal, such that a stray fragment of material causes the laceration. In some instances, the puncture is so small that it may not be detected immediately. Puncture or laceration of the eye warrants immediate medical attention.

Deep penetration or laceration of the eye can cause bleeding into the anterior chamber (hyphema). Blows to the head or the eye can also damage the internal structures of the eye, leading to hemorrhage, retinal damage, or other injury. When bleeding causes increased intraocular pressure, surgical intervention may be needed to relieve the pressure and prevent further damage from occurring.

Any injury to the eye necessitates a consultation with an **ophthalmologist** (a physician who specializes in diseases and treatment of the eye). The degree of visual loss that results from an eye injury is not only a function of the extent and type of injury, but also, frequently, the consequence of the delay or promptness of emergency intervention.

Most eye injuries are preventable. Using appropriate eye protection for work, home, and sports activities that carry a risk of eye injury is one of the major forms of prevention.

Inflammation and Infections of the Eye

Conjunctivitis is an inflammation of the membrane that lines the eye, the conjunctiva. It may be caused by infectious organisms, such as viruses or bacteria, by allergy, or by chemicals. In most instances, conjunctivitis is easily treated, is self-limiting, and has no permanent effects. Conjunctivitis caused by virus is particularly contagious, however (Cho & Goldstein, 2007). Some types of infectious conjunctivitis, such as *gonococcal conjunctivitis* or *trachoma,* can cause ulceration of the cornea and subsequent blindness (Mariotti, 2004).

Uveitis, is an inflammation of the **uveal tract** (iris, ciliary body, choroid). It may be associated with autoimmune disease such as **ankylosing spondylitis** (see Chapter 16) or *inflammatory bowel disease* (see Chapter 12) or by local or systemic infection, such as HIV. Manifestations may include decreased vision and sensitivity to light (*photophobia*). Uveitis is usually treated with topical medication.

Keratitis is an inflammation of the cornea that can be associated with a number of infectious conditions, including herpes simplex (*herpetic keratitis*), and as a complication of HIV disease. Another common cause of keratitis is use of contacts. Microbial keratitis is associated with the use of contact lenses and is usually caused by improper handling of contact-lens equipment and solutions (Bienfang, Kelly, Nicholson, & Nussenblatt, 1990). The risk of infection decreases with proper hand washing and with use of the appropriate technique for cleaning and applying contact lenses.

Glaucoma

Glaucoma comprises a group of conditions that result in visual field loss, and is the leading cause of irreversible blindness (Syed & Bell, 2007). Although glaucoma was once linked only to increased intraocular pressure, it is now recognized that, while increased intraocular pressure is a risk factor, the condition can be caused by a variety of conditions (Syed & Bell, 2007). If glaucoma is left untreated, permanent damage to the optic nerve can result, causing blindness.

Glaucoma can occur either as a primary condition or secondary to other conditions such as diabetes, trauma, infection, prolonged use of medications such as steroids, or developmental ocular abnormalities occurring in childhood. It develops when the amount of aqueous humor produced exceeds the amount being drained from the eye, much like a sink into which water continues to flow even though the drainage pipe is blocked resulting in overaccumulation of water in the sink.

Several types of glaucoma are distinguished, with the broad categories being based on the reason for the problem with the aqueous flow.

Types of Glaucoma

Primary Open-Angle Glaucoma

The most common type of glaucoma, *primary open-angle glaucoma,* occurs when the outflow of aqueous humor from the eye is reduced. Because the outflow no longer equals the inflow, the amount of aqueous humor builds up, and pressure in the eye increases. Open-angle glaucoma generally progresses slowly over many years, producing no symptoms until the optic nerve is sufficiently damaged to reduce visual acuity and visual field. At this point, the damage is irreversible. Vision loss generally begins with the loss of peripheral (side) vision so that individuals can see only straight ahead, as if looking through a tunnel (tunnel vision). Because loss of peripheral vision is often gradual, individuals may be unaware of the problem until advanced stages of the condition. If left untreated, the field of vision continues to narrow until all vision is lost. There is no cure for chronic open-angle glaucoma. However, if the condition is detected early, appropriate medical intervention can control it for many years. Consequently, early detection is important.

Secondary Open-Angle Glaucoma

Secondary open-angle glaucoma is also due to reduced outflow of aqueous humor, in this case, however, the condition is caused by a preexisting or underlying condition such as trauma or steroid use.

Primary Angle-Closure Glaucoma

Primary angle-closure glaucoma develops much more rapidly than primary open-angle glaucoma and is a medical emergency. Manifestations include sudden severe pain, sharply decreased vision, nausea and vomiting, and rapid damage to the optic nerve with associated vision loss. Acute angle-closure glaucoma results from an abrupt blockage and obstruction of the canal of Schlemm so that aqueous humor rapidly accumulates in the anterior chamber of the eye. Although acute closed-angle glaucoma is much less common than chronic open-angle glaucoma, it must be treated immediately to prevent blindness. Initially it may be treated with medications, but surgical intervention is also often necessary.

Secondary Angle-Closure Glaucoma

Secondary angle-closure glaucoma can result from scarring that blocks the flow of the aqueous humor. Conditions such as diabetes, uncontrolled hypertension, and inflammation of the uveal tract because of other conditions can cause blockage of aqueous humor flow. Intervention usually involves surgery (Syed & Bell, 2007).

Management of Glaucoma

Management of glaucoma is directed toward reducing the intraocular pressure by decreasing the amount of aqueous humor produced, or by increasing its outflow. This goal can be accomplished with medication or through surgical creation of a new pathway for drainage.

Medication for the management of glaucoma, whether eyedrops or oral medication, must be used daily for life to control eye pressure and prevent further damage to vision. In any type of glaucoma, early detection and management are critical to prevent irreversible damage to the optic nerve and subsequent

blindness. Regardless of the type of glaucoma, lifetime medical supervision is required. Most people with glaucoma can lead normal, unrestricted lives without blindness if the condition is identified early and the medical regimen is followed as prescribed.

Management of Primary Open-Angle Glaucoma

Primary open-angle glaucoma may be controlled with medication in the form of eyedrops alone to decrease production of aqueous humor or in combination with oral medication that reduces pressure in the eye, thereby halting progression of the disease. Because eyedrops are absorbed into the bloodstream, they may affect other body functions and cause systemic side effects ranging from generalized weakness to central nervous system, cardiovascular, or gastrointestinal symptoms.

Oral medications for the management of glaucoma work by decreasing production of aqueous humor. Like eyedrops, these medications can affect other body functions and cause systemic side effects. Consequently, individuals who use eyedrops or oral medication for management of glaucoma should be under continuing medical supervision—not only to monitor the condition itself, but also to identify any side effects of the intervention.

When intraocular pressure cannot be successfully controlled with medication, individuals with chronic open-angle glaucoma may have surgery, called *trabeculectomy*, to relieve pressure by creating a passageway through which the aqueous humor can drain. Individuals may also need to continue using eyedrops or oral medication after surgery to control pressure; however, in some instances, surgery may eliminate the need for medication.

Management of Angle-Closure Glaucoma

Angle-closure glaucoma results from the forward displacement of the iris, which in turn narrows or obstructs the path for aqueous humor outflow. Eyedrops called *miotics* constrict the pupil, thereby enlarging the drainage passageway and facilitating the outflow of aqueous humor. Because of the emergency nature of angle-closure glaucoma, oral or intravenous medication is given immediately to relieve pressure on the optic nerve temporarily. Once the pressure level has dropped to a safe level, a surgical procedure called **iridotomy** may be performed. Iridotomy involves the removal of a small section of the iris so that the aqueous humor can flow freely from the posterior chamber to the anterior chamber of the eye, preventing further eye damage by relieving built-up pressure. This procedure is often performed with a laser. Iridotomy may sometimes be performed prophylactically in the unaffected eye after an acute attack of glaucoma in the opposite eye.

Surgical procedures also include trabeculectomy, in which an alernative filtration path is created for aqueous drainage. Individuals undergoing trabeculectomy are at increased lifetime risk for serious infection of the eye (Syed & Bell, 2007).

Retinopathy

Any disease or condition that affects the retina is termed a **retinopathy**. Retinopathies are often named for their cause. For example, *arteriosclerotic retinopathy* is produced by changes that occur in blood vessels in the retina because of arteriosclerosis. *Hypertensive retinopathy* results from changes that occur in blood vessels in the retina because of high blood pressure (Wong & Mitchell, 2004). In both instances, treatment of the primary underlying condition can control progress of the retinopathy.

The most common type of retinopathy, and the most common cause of blindness, is *diabetic retinopathy*. Diabetic retinopathy is the result of damage to the retina and is a complication of diabetes mellitus (see Chapter 11). It is an important cause of visual loss that has significant medical, social, and financial consequences (Lamoureux, Hassell, & Keefe, 2004). Usually there are no manifestations in early stages of diabetic retinopathy. Given this fact, regular comprehensive eye examinations by a physician are important in helping to prevent visual loss.

Diabetic retinopathy causes visual loss in several ways. There are two categories of diabetic retinopathy:

- Nonproliferative diabetic retinopathy
- Proliferative diabetic retinopathy

Nonproliferative diabetic retinopathy is caused by changes in blood vessel walls, which allow fluids to leak into retinal tissue. At the same time, small blood vessels in the retina may become occluded, disturbing circulation in the retina so that some retinal tissue receives too little oxygen and dies (**necrosis**).

Proliferative diabetic retinopathy results from extensive areas of closure of the small blood vessels in the retina. As a result, retinal tissues receive too little oxygen (**ischemia**), to which the body responds by stimulating growth of new vessels. These new blood vessels are abnormally fragile and prone to bleeding, causing hemorrhage into the vitreous humor. The degree of vision loss depends on the amount of hemorrhage. Vessels may burst, filling the back of the eye with blood and resulting in significant visual loss. In some instances, scar tissue associated with new vessels can pull on the retina so that it detaches from underlying tissue.

Surgery may be performed to remove hemorrhage (**vitrectomy**), or laser treatment may be performed to stop the bleeding (Ferris, 2004). *Laser photocoagulation* is a procedure in which an intense beam of light from a laser is used to seal leaking blood vessels of the retina. The laser beam passes through the lens of the eye and vitreous fluid without harming the structures. It then is directed to a very precisely defined area to destroy fragile vessels prone to hemorrhage, or diseased areas of the retina in which there may be additional proliferative vessel changes. Laser photocoagulation may help reduce the risk of visual loss, but it does not stop the progression of diabetic retinopathy. Such intervention is usually performed on an outpatient basis.

Retinal Detachment

With a detached retina, the sensory layer of the retina becomes separated from the pigmented (choroid) layer, depriving the sensory layer of its blood supply. A detached retina may result from a sudden blow to the head, a tumor in the choroid layer, retinal degeneration caused by conditions such as arteriosclerosis, or hemorrhage associated with conditions such as diabetic retinopathy.

Manifestations may develop suddenly or slowly over time. Individuals may notice flashes of light or a loss of vision in different areas of the visual field, or they may experience a complete loss of vision in the affected eye. Usually there is no pain. Retinal detachment in one eye may indicate an increased risk of detachment in the other eye. Prompt diagnosis and surgical intervention are essential to prevent permanent vision loss.

A surgical procedure called *scleral buckling* is sometimes used to treat retinal detachment. Scleral buckling mechanically restores contact of the retina with the choroid. The area of the sclera that lies over the retinal defect is depressed with an implant so that the choroid and the retina are pressed together.

Retinitis Pigmentosa

Retinitis pigmentosa is a hereditary, degenerative condition of the retina that causes slowly progressive loss of peripheral vision and, in many cases, blindness (López-Justicia & Córdoba, 2006; Rundquist, 2004). Although progressive restriction of the visual field occurs

as a result of the loss of peripheral vision, the remaining central visual acuity often remains good. Frequently the first manifestation of retinitis pigmentosa is difficulty with night vision (night blindness), which usually begins in late youth or early adulthood. Often, total bilateral loss of vision occurs by age of 50. There is no cure or treatment for this condition, although a number of assistive devices may be utilized to enhance function.

Macular Degeneration

Degenerative changes in the macula—the part of the eye needed for seeing fine detail and central vision—results in a condition known as **macular degeneration**.

Macular degeneration usually occurs after the age of 50, with no apparent cause, although some research has suggested gene mutation may play a role (Johnson & Anderson, 2004). Painless loss of central visual acuity is usually slow, with visual distortion or blurring of vision being the first manifestation. Eventually individuals may develop a blind spot in the center of their field of vision, which gradually increases in size as the condition progresses. Given that warning signs of macular degeneration are absent until central vision is affected, the importance of regular eye examinations cannot be overemphasized.

Macular degeneration does not result in complete blindness, but it does destroy some or all of the sight in the center of the field of vision. Two types of macular degeneration are distinguished: dry form and wet form. Most cases of macular degeneration are *dry form* in which there is atrophy (shrinkage) and thinning of the macula, causing mild to moderate vision loss. The type of macular degeneration called *wet form* is characterized by significant loss of vision due to abnormal blood vessel formation and hemorrhage.

Both types of macular degeneration are characterized by loss of central vision while peripheral vision remains intact. There is no treatment or cure for macular degeneration, but the use of assistive devices may increase visual function. Activities such as reading may become difficult because of distortion of letters or because of parts of words or sentences in the center of the reading material that appear to be missing. Large print with black type and a white background may make reading easier, as may use of assistive devices such as a magnifying glass.

■ DIAGNOSTIC PROCEDURES FOR CONDITIONS OF THE EYE

Comprehensive Eye Examination

Comprehensive eye examinations usually include an external eye exam, which measures eye movements, size of the pupils, and pupils' ability to react to light. They also include testing of visual acuity and visual field as described earlier in this chapter. This part of the exam may be performed by an **optometrist** (a nonphysician who specializes in correcting refractive errors). An **ophthalmologist** (a physician who specializes in evaluation and treatment of conditions of the eye) may conduct tests of visual acuity as well, but also checks ocular movement, function of the optic nerve, and light reflexes of the pupils, and identifies any optic nerve pathology.

As part of the exam, individuals may be asked to view a chart through an instrument called a *refractor*. The physician then shines a light through the refractor onto the retina in order to estimate the eye's ability to focus on distant objects. Also included in a comprehensive eye exam is *tonometry* (described below) and *slit-lamp exam,* which evaluates the eyes' structures, including the cornea and iris, and screens for cataracts. *Retinal examination* to check for retinal disease may be included as well; it requires that the pupil of the eye be dilated and is useful for checking for retinal disease.

Tonometry

Tonometry is used to measure pressure in the eye in an effort to detect glaucoma. An instrument called a *tonometer* is placed directly on the cornea after the cornea has been anesthetized with drops of a local anesthetic. The tonometer measures the amount of pressure within the eye, thus making it possible to detect glaucoma.

Gonioscopy

For *gonioscopy,* a special contact lens that contains a mirror is gently placed on the eye. The ophthalmologist uses the lens like the periscope of a submarine to examine structures inside the eye. This test is especially helpful in detecting glaucoma.

Ophthalmoscopic Examination

A direct *ophthalmoscopic examination* is used to visualize the internal structures of the eye. It is performed with an instrument called an *ophthalmoscope* placed close to the eye. The ophthalmoscope contains a light that shines into the eye and magnifies internal structures so that the physician can note any pathologic changes.

The internal structures of the eye may also be observed with a *slit lamp,* a type of microscope that is placed in front of the eye of the individual being tested. The physician shines a finely focused slit of brilliant light onto the eye to magnify details of the cornea, iris, and lens. A slit amp is especially useful in identifying foreign bodies in the eye, evaluating corneal ulcers, and diagnosing cataracts.

Fluorescein Angiography

The purpose of *fluorescein angiography* is to detect changes in the blood vessels of the retina. A fluorescein dye is either taken orally or injected into the bloodstream. When the dye reaches the blood vessels of the eye, use of special ultraviolet light enables the physician to photograph the vessels for later study. Any swelling or leakage of the vessels of the retina is apparent on the photograph.

■ TREATMENT AND MANAGEMENT OF CONDITIONS OF THE EYE AND BLINDNESS

Eyeglasses and Contact Lenses

Corrective lenses may take the form of either eyeglasses or contact lenses. Because so many different types of eye conditions interfere with visual acuity, corrective lenses must be prescribed individually. They are prescribed by an ophthalmologist (a physician who specializes in the diagnosis and treatment of conditions of the eye, including surgery and prescription of medications and optical corrections) or an optometrist (an individual who does not have a medical degree but is trained to measure refractive errors and perceptual dysfunction of the eye, diagnose visual conditions, and prescribe optical corrections). Optometrists do not prescribe medications or perform surgery. Lenses for glasses are made by opticians, technicians who have been trained to fill optical prescriptions. They grind and construct the lens according to the prescribed specifications.

When visual acuity at several different distances must be corrected, bifocal or trifocal lenses may be prescribed. Individuals with *bifocal lenses* use the lower portion of the lens for near vision and the upper portion for far vision. *Trifocal lenses* have three different divisions: one for near vision, one for intermediate vision, and one for far vision.

Although several types of contact lenses are available, the most common are hard and soft corneal lenses. Hard lenses cover the central area of the cornea and are generally more durable. Soft lenses cover the entire cornea and are generally more fragile. Regardless of the type, contact lenses must be individually prescribed and constructed. They are helpful for counteracting a variety of visual conditions, but they do not correct astigmatism.

Generally, there are no complications associated with wearing eyeglasses. Contact lenses, however, can damage the eye if they are not worn and cared for properly. Not all people can or should wear contact lenses. Overwearing of hard lenses can cause corneal abrasions and associated complications. Individuals who do not use good hygienic practices when inserting the contact lens may develop an infection of the eye, in which case contact lenses should not be worn.

Refractive Surgery

Refractive surgery is an alternative to wearing glasses or contact lenses. Growing numbers of individuals are choosing to have this kind of surgery to correct their vision. **Myopia** (nearsightedness), **hyperopia** (farsightedness), and **astigmatism** (irregularity in the shape of the cornea or lens resulting in distortion of the visual image) are the conditions most commonly corrected with refractive surgery. The changes wrought by such surgery are generally permanent and irreversible (Bower & Stutzman, 2007).

A number of surgical techniques have been developed for refractory conditions since the first surgery, radial keratotomy (RK), was introduced in the late 1970s. RK has largely been replaced now with surgeries that are performed with the *excimer laser*.

- Photorefractive keratectomy (PRK)
- Laser-assisted in situ keratomileusis (LASIK)
- Laser epithelial keratomileusis (LASEK)

Before individuals have surgery, they are required to have a complete eye examination and must be free of cataracts, glaucoma, macular degeneration, or other eye conditions that would require medical intervention. In addition, surgery is contraindicated in the presence of certain medical conditions, such as diabetes, pregnancy, autoimmune conditions, or conditions of the immune system. Although refractive surgery is effective in correcting myopia and hyperopia, there is always the potential for complications (Buckingham, 2000). Individuals should be aware of both the risks and the benefits before undergoing the procedure (Bower & Stutzman, 2007).

Prosthetic Devices and Eye Replacement

When injury or disease necessitates removal of the eyeball, or when there is a congenital absence of the eye (**anophthalmia**), a prosthetic eye may be constructed and worn by the individual. The prosthetic eye, while not contributing to vision, serves a cosmetic purpose and can enhance individual's body image and self-concept.

Visual impairment resulting from conditions in which there is interruption of electrical stimulation somewhere along the visual pathway or to the retina (where photoreceptors are located) has spurred research into the use of electrical stimulation to overcome visual loss. *Optical prostheses*, which emulate the functions of photoreceptors located in the retina, are examples of devices, that have the potential for restoring rudimentary vision (Scarlatis, 2000). Although still in experimental stages, the development of optical prosthetics is an important advance that may make it possible for individuals with retinal damage to have partial vision restored.

Assistive Devices and Low-Vision Aids

Assistive devices and low-vision aids should be part of an overall program to enhance the life of the individual, not just to enhance the individual's visual system. Types of devices used should be based on individual needs as well as willingness and ability to use them. The overall goal with utilization of low-vision aids is to recapture, strengthen, and maintain individu-

als' self-confidence in their ability to realize safe, independent functioning. These devices enhance remaining visual abilities through use of individually prescribed adaptive equipment appropriate to the specific person's lifestyle.

Adaptive equipment for activities of daily living may include both optical devices, such as high-powered lenses and telescopic spectacles, and nonoptical devices, which are readily available and require no special training, such as large-print reading material or large-button telephones. Low-technology devices such as talking watches, raised-dot markings for oven dials, or templates for check signing require little training and may require only simple adaptations. Other devices, such as talking clocks and timers, writing guides, talking books, and audiocassettes, may similarly help to meet the communication needs of individuals with visual impairments.

High-technology devices are more sophisticated electronically and may require specialized training. Examples of high-technology devices include video magnifiers and computer systems. Video magnifiers use closed-circuit television and can magnify a printed page on a television screen for reading. Numerous computer software programs and adaptive devices can be used to enlarge printed materials or to convert print into synthetic speech output. These devices include large-print computer monitors, programs that enlarge print size on the screen, printers that modify font size, synthetic speech software programs with external audio units, and typewriters equipped with synthetic speech output that interfaces with personal computer units. Speech packages allow for adjustments in the rate of speech and the tone of voice to meet the needs of the individual user.

One of the best-known tactile aids is *Braille*. Hard copy Braille uses the familiar raised-dot method, whereas soft-copy Braille is stored on electromagnetic tape and presented as patterns by a set of pins that represent a Braille dot. Individuals place their fingers on display units through which the pins protrude. Another type of product is *refreshable Braille displays*—electronic devices that are used to read information sent from a computer to a monitor. This kind of device produces Braille output on a Braille display.

Another type of tactile aid is an electromechanical vibratory system. A small camera is passed over a line of print, and each printed letter is then displayed as a pattern of vibrations that the individual can feel with the finger.

A number of professionals recommend and provide training in the use of optical, nonoptical, low-technology, and high-technology aids. They include *occupational therapists, low-vision specialists, orientation and mobility* (O&M) *instructors, rehabilitation teachers, and adaptive technology specialists.*

The key to successful use of any assistive or adaptive device is involvement of the individual who will ultimately use the device in selecting it, so that the device meets user requirements, capabilities, and needs. Customization of devices to accommodate special needs of individuals ensures that the device can be integrated into the daily routine, helps individuals view the device positively, and helps them use the device to best enhance their own functional capacity (Lacey & Mac-Namara, 2000).

Orientation and Mobility Training

The goal of orientation and mobility training is to enable individuals with a visual impairment to achieve as much mobility as possible according to their capabilities and desires and to recapture, strengthen, and maintain self-reliance for safe and independent function. Orientation and mobility specialists provide training that helps individuals know where they are in relation to their surroundings and learn how to safely navigate within their environment (Turnbull, Turnbull, Shank, Smith, & Leal, 2002). In particular, O&M specialists help individuals to move independently indoors and outdoors, and in familiar or in unfamiliar environments; they also provide training in the use of public transportation, use of the cane, and use of mobility lights or electronic travel aids. Through individualized training, persons with visual impairments learn to orient themselves to their environment by using compensatory strategies including illumination techniques and use of contrast, magnification, memorization of location, and auditory and tactile feedback. Compensatory strategies may involve such things as listening for the direction of traffic, arm and hand positioning for guidance along walls and railings, and systematic search techniques for dropped or lost objects.

Mobility Aids

Various types of mobility aids, such as sighted guides, guide dogs, canes, and electronic devices, are available to help individuals with visual impairments move about the environment more freely (Cox & Dykes, 2001). Orientation and mobility specialists can help determine the preferred system for individuals.

Guide dogs not only increase the mobility of the individual with a visual impairment, but can also provide protection and companionship. These dogs undergo intensive training before being matched with the individual to whom they are assigned. They are taught how to respond to various commands as well as how to deal with curbs, traffic, and other potential hazards in the environment. The individual and the dog train together for a number of weeks to become an effective team. Not all individuals are able to use a guide dog, and some individuals prefer to use other forms of mobility aids, such as a long cane. In most instances, individuals should be cane proficient before using a guide dog.

The most common mobility aid is the prescription or long cane, which is usually made of aluminum or fiberglass. An O&M specialist prescribes the cane according to the individual's height, length of stride, and comfort. The cane is used by individuals with visual impairments in a systematic way. The person moves the cane rhythmically in an arc in front of the body to ensure a safe space for the next step. Although this provides some protection, it does not account for objects above the waist that are in the individual's path. In an attempt to compensate for this type of obstacle, some canes have tone-emitting radar units that give a differential pitch for the direction and height of obstacles in front of the individual. Some individuals prefer collapsible, folding, or telescopic canes, which are less obtrusive and can be collapsed and slipped into a purse or under a chair when not in use.

Electronic travel aids may also be used. These devices emit light beams or ultrasound waves. When the light beam or ultrasound waves hit an object in the individual's path, the device vibrates or emits a sound.

■ PSYCHOSOCIAL ISSUES IN CONDITIONS OF THE EYE AND BLINDNESS

Special Issues for Individuals Who Are Partially Sighted

Individuals with low vision or who are partially sighted do not quite fit into the category of either the blind or the sighted population. Consequently, they often have special needs that are overlooked. The social community often lacks understanding of the true nature of vision impairment, so that individuals with low vision are ridiculed in public for appear-

ing to see more than would be expected by a person with visual impairment (Vance, 2000). Individuals with partial sight may be viewed as malingerers by family and acquaintances because they can see some things but not others. Even when individuals attempt to function with appropriate assistive devices, they may be suspected of denying their condition by those who expect individuals with visual impairments to be dependent and isolated.

Adjustment to vision loss is not necessarily correlated with the degree of vision remaining. Individuals with partial sight do not have fewer adjustment issues than individuals who are totally blind and, in fact, may have more adaptation difficulties because their partial sight presents an ambiguous situation for others. In addition, individuals with partial sight may exhibit high levels of anxiety because they may be unsure about whether or when they will lose more of their residual vision.

Even when individuals with severe visual impairments function independently for the most part, there may be some activities for which they are more dependent on assistance from others. The greater dependence associated with a severe visual impairment may be a source of conflict and may negatively affect formerly close relationships, especially if others have misperceptions or misunderstanding about the nature of the visual impairment. In other instances, individuals, in an attempt to demonstrate self-reliance and independence, may reject help from family and friends, causing alienation and social isolation. Counseling individuals to understand sighted people's reactions may facilitate social interactions and enhance development of constructive and realistic interactions. At times, individuals with visual impairments may find interactions with others with low vision helpful for their adjustment through shared experiences and problem solving.

Because partially sighted individuals have some remaining sight, they may attempt to "pass" as a sighted person to avoid potential rejection or avoidance by others. They may deny their condition altogether and associate only with sighted persons in an attempt to be accepted by the mainstream of society. They may make excuses for awkward behavior or attempt in other ways to conceal the fact that they have low vision. They may refuse to use low-vision aids, such as a cane, for mobility or reject suitable orientation and mobility training. In extreme cases, they may engage in dangerous activities such as illegal driving. People often view the ability to drive as very important in the maintenance of independence. This perception makes it extremely difficult for individuals who are losing their vision to give up this activity. Furthermore, by its very nature, the gradual loss of vision creates a time period in which the decision to stop driving is particularly difficult. The emphasis on self-care and independence for individuals with partial vision must be tempered with judgment and concern for the welfare of the individual as well as the welfare of others

Psychosocial Issues for Individuals with Blindness or Low Vision

Vision loss often precipitates a sense of fear and reduced personal competence, which may result in isolation and social withdrawal. Visual impairments may be present at birth, or they may develop suddenly or slowly at any time in an individual's life. Often visual loss follows an unpredictable and uncontrollable progression. Adjustment to loss of vision depends on many factors, including the degree of loss and the age at which the individual experiences visual loss (Lifshitz, Hen, & Weisse, 2007).

Persons who have been blind since birth have not, for example, had the opportunity to learn concepts such as distance, depth, propor-

tion, and color. Because of their lack of visual experiences in their environment, such as the observation of tasks or behaviors of others, concepts that sighted individuals often take for granted must be learned by other means. This adaptive learning of tasks then becomes a natural part of their development so that adjustment to visual limitations is incorporated into their self-perception and daily activities as a normal part of growing up.

Individuals who develop loss of vision later in life are able to draw on visual experiences in the environment as a frame of reference for physical concepts, but may find it more difficult to accept blindness than those who have never had vision. Individuals who lose vision later in life are required to make certain modifications of self-perception as a result of their physical changes and subsequent need for restructuring of daily activities. Individuals who are newly blind may experience grief and despair over loss of visual function. They may become dependent, feel insecure in new situations, and perceive a marked loss of autonomy. Some may become reluctant to interact in social situations, because they want to avoid the awkwardness of initial attempts at social interactions. Loss of control over standard methods of initiating conversations (e.g., eye contact and other nonverbal cues), noticeable discomfort or overhelpfulness of sighted persons, and prolonged gaps in conversations may lead newly blind individuals to believe that they are being watched or ignored.

Accommodation to visual loss or blindness is multifaceted. Individuals with a visual loss must adjust their self-concept and personal goals to take into account the realistic limits imposed by vision loss. They must develop adaptive skills and new abilities, and they must draw on personal resources to adjust to their new situation. Individuals who experience traumatic blindness (a condition in which there has been a sudden loss of partial or total vision because of an internal or external event, such as a head injury, direct injury to the eye, or chemical burn) may have to cope not only with the sudden loss of vision, but also with insurance company representatives, attorneys, and other legal and bureaucratic aspects surrounding the circumstance of their condition. In these situations, family members may also react to the situation with responses ranging from anger to revenge to overprotectiveness.

■ ACTIVITIES AND PARTICIPATION IN CONDITIONS OF THE EYE AND BLINDNESS

Vision is crucial for many activities of daily living. Individuals with little or no vision must learn new techniques for carrying out routine activities of self-care and mobility. They must orient themselves to the home environment so that they may move freely from room to room without risk of injury. Family members can contribute to the individual's mobility within the home by never moving furniture within a room without informing the individual and leaving doors either completely open or completely closed after informing the individual of the plan so that he or she does not bump into a partially open door.

At first, tasks such as pouring water into a glass without spilling it, buttering bread, or cutting meat may seem insurmountable for the individual with visual impairment. However, most people with visual impairments learn to prepare their meals and dine independently once they have been oriented to the location of food, tableware, and cooking utensils. Cooking can be learned through techniques such as the systematic placement of cooking equipment and utensils and special labeling on cans, frozen foods, oven dials, and other items.

Through training, individuals with conditions affecting vision are gradually able to assume personal responsibility for self-care. *Rehabilitation teachers* provide in-home train-

ing in skills of daily living. Activities such as bathing, combing the hair, shaving, applying make-up, and dressing in a coordinated fashion can all be performed independently through skills training and systematic organization and labeling of personal items.

Although individuals with moderate to mild visual loss may carry on much of their personal business with low-vision aids, those with severe visual conditions or blindness may need someone else's help to read a bill, a check, an invoice, or a personal letter. Some individuals have difficulty adjusting to this loss of privacy. In other instances, documents or forms must be translated into Braille or read to the individual, perhaps reducing the efficiency of action or response to the document.

Outside the home, individuals with severe visual impairments can learn techniques of mobility in new environments with the use of a cane or guide dog. Through these techniques, individuals with conditions that significantly affect vision or who are blind are able to travel to work or to other destinations of their choice. They can also learn methods of carrying money so as to discriminate between bills as well as ways to discriminate between different coins. Individuals can continue to enjoy leisure activities including many outdoor activities, such as swimming, hiking, and fishing. With special adaptive procedures, even bicycling is possible. A number of sports organizations, such as American Blind Bowlers Association, United States Blind Golfers Association, and Beep Ball Teams have also been formed for individuals who are blind.

Although visual loss does not affect sexual activity directly, loss of vision on self-esteem may impinge on self-esteem. In addition, individuals with severe visual manifestations are unable to see the facial expressions and other nonverbal communication that are an integral part of sexual relationships. Information about relationships that is normally developed through visual modeling may not be available to individuals with conditions that affect vision if they have been without sight since an early age. Consequently, it may be necessary to teach appropriate social behaviors that are generally learned by observation to teenagers or young adults who have a condition in which vision is significantly affected.

Major obstacles to the effective functioning of individuals with visual impairment in social environments include social stereotyping and attitudes of sighted individuals toward individuals with visual impairment. Many sighted individuals view individuals who have severe visual impairments or who are blind as helpless and dependent. Others believe the myth that people who have severe visual impairments or who are blind develop extraordinary powers of hearing and touch to compensate for the loss of vision, rather than recognizing that these individuals simply learn to make more effective use of other senses in their effort to interpret their environment. Negative attitudes or stereotypical views held by friends, employers, and casual acquaintances can have a major impact on individuals with visual impairment (Kef & Bos, 2006). Unfortunately, many people with conditions that affect vision tend to conform to social expectations, thereby limiting their own potential. The ability of individuals with conditions affecting vision to understand and accept that others may be uncomfortable with them because of lack of previous interactions with people with vision loss or because of misinformation provides the basis for formulating proactive strategies for problem solving, perspective taking, and social inferences, which can ultimately result in fuller social integration.

Loss of visual information significantly affects interpersonal communication. Much human communication occurs through nonverbal cues, most of which are perceived visually. The inability of individuals with visual impairment to see the social behavior of others, therefore, affects social interactions.

Much social interaction and communication are mediated by watching nonverbal actions and reactions of others, such as posture, facial expression, or movement. The absence of these visual cues can place individuals with visual impairment at a disadvantage in a social setting, unless all concerned have developed increased awareness and sensitivity to the individual's inability to observe nonverbal cues.

Although attitudes of family members are important factors in adjustment to most disabilities, attitudes appear to have an especially powerful influence on the adjustment of individuals with visual conditions. How families react to individuals with visual loss depends on the particular family's patterns of belief, feelings, and resources. When family members believe that the demands being placed on them exceed their available resources, so that their resources are overtaxed, stress and strain may develop. Conversely, if families are able to meet major needs of their members so that they can pursue realistic goals, they will be better able to cope successfully.

Family attitudes during rehabilitation may determine individuals' motivation to learn and accept major changes in lifestyle. On the other hand, overprotective or overly anxious families who encourage dependency may prevent or impede rehabilitation. On the other hand, families who foster positive attitudes and demonstrate respect and recognition of the individual with visual loss can be a major asset to rehabilitation.

■ VOCATIONAL ISSUES FOR INDIVIDUALS WITH CONDITIONS OF THE EYE OR BLINDNESS

Persons who are blind or who have low vision are underrepresented in the competitive labor market (Crudden & McBroom, 1999). The degree of the vocational impact of a condition that affects vision depends on the nature of the employment, the type and extent of visual loss, and the life stage at which the visual loss occurs. Many individuals with partial vision are able to continue in their field of employment with special adaptive or low-vision aids; others must learn new job skills. When visual loss is progressive, ongoing evaluation and planning for decreasing visual acuity should be part of the rehabilitation plan.

In addition to the signs and symptoms of the specific eye condition, barriers to employment may include deficits in skills or education, lack of work experience, lack of job preparation skills, or lack of motivation or information. Paid reader support may be necessary to gather information about job openings or training opportunities. In other instances, lack of direction or low expectations of family and friends may make it more difficult to continue looking for work or preparing for employment.

In addition to the challenges posed by on-the-job activity, the ability to get to and from work may be a barrier to employment. If individuals are no longer able to drive and no public transportation is available, suitable alternatives for transportation to and from work must be devised. Unreliable transportation can be a major barrier to obtaining and maintaining employment.

For individuals with low vision, level of visual acuity—and, therefore, the individual's ability to resolve visual detail—must be considered in employment in which reading or seeing fine visual detail is required. Accommodations may involve making the image larger through some form of magnification or using an optical device to make the object appear larger. Individuals with low vision may need additional lighting to enhance vision; however, lighting that produces glare can be detrimental to individuals' visual efficiency and comfort. Individuals with visual field deficits may have difficulty with peripheral or central vision. Individuals with peripheral vision problems may have difficulty detecting objects around them. In addition, peripheral field deficiency can interfere with mobility, and with performing near-vision tasks such as reading or writing. Central vision loss affects individuals' straight-ahead vision, with probably concurrent reduction in visual acuity. Consequently, reading and tasks requiring visualization of detail will be affected. The degree of functional consequence depends on the size and location of the loss of vision.

CASE STUDIES

Case 1

Mr. C. is a 28-year-old male with diabetes who completed college with a degree in elementary education. He currently works as an elementary school teacher at an urban school. Early after he began his job, Mr. C. developed increasing difficulty with vision owing to retinopathy. He currently has moderate vision loss. He appears to be quite anxious about his ability to continue to function in his job with his loss of vision.

1. Which factors related to Mr. C.'s condition would you consider when talking with him about his current employment?
2. Which adaptive devices might Mr. C. find helpful at this stage of visual loss?
3. Which factors would you consider when helping Mr. C. plan for the future regarding employment?

Case 2

Ms. L. is a 42-year-old computer programmer who lost her vision as a result of an auto accident. She has total loss of light perception. Ms. L. lives with her husband and teenage son in a small midwestern community. There is no public transportation available. Ms. L. had been commuting by car 25 miles to her place of employment. You have been asked to begin working with Ms. L. on her rehabilitation plan.

1. Which factors and issues would you consider regarding Ms. L.'s condition and her employment?
2. Which specific adaptive devices or other accommodations might Ms. L. require?
3. Which types of services might be helpful to Ms. L. to assist her in reaching her optimal level of independence?

■ REFERENCES

Barker, E. (2008). The adult neurological assessment. In E. Barker (Ed.), *Neuroscience nursing* (3rd ed., pp. 53–129). St. Louis, Mosby.

Bienfang, D. C., Kelly, L. D., Nicholson, D. H., & Nussenblatt, R. B. (1990). Ophthalmology. *New England Journal of Medicine, 325*(14), 956–967.

Bower, K. S., & Stutzman, R. D. (2007). Vision correction procedures. In R. E. Rakel & E. T. Bope (Eds.), *Conn's current therapy* (pp. 213–217). Philadelphia: W. B. Saunders.

Buckingham, B. K. (2000). Refractive eye surgery: Focusing on risks. *Trial, 35*(5), 18–27.

Butler, R. N. (1997). Keeping an eye on vision: New tools to preserve sight and quality of life. *Geriatrics, 52*(9), 48–55.

Cho, S. Y., & Goldstein, M. H. (2007). Conjunctivitis. In R. E. Rakel & E. T. Bope (Eds.), *Conn's current therapy.* (pp. 217–221). Philadelphia: W. B. Saunders.

Cox, P. R., & Dykes, M. K. (2001). Effective classroom adaptations for students with visual impairments. *Teaching Exceptional Children, 33*(6), 68–74.

Crudden, A., & McBroom, L. W. (1999, June). Barriers to employment: A survey of employed persons who are visually impaired. *Journal of Visual Impairment and Blindness,* 341–350.

Donahue, S. P. (2007). Pediatric strabismus. *New England Journal of Medicine, 356*(10), 1040–1047.

Fay, A., & Jakobiec, F. A., (2004). Diseases of the visual system. In L. Goldman & D. Ausiello (Eds.), *Cecil textbook of medicine* (22nd ed., pp. 465–2420). Philadelphia: W. B. Saunders.

Ferris F. L. III. (2004). A new treatment for ocular neovascularization. *New England Journal of Medicine, 351*(27), 2863–2864.

Johnson, L. V., & Anderson, D. H. (2004). Age-related macular degeneration and the extracellular matrix. *New England Journal of Medicine, 351*(4), 320–353.

Kef, S., & Bos, H. (2006). Is love blind? Sexual behavior and psychological adjustment of adolescents with blindness. *Sex and Disability, 24,* 89–100.

Lacey, G., & MacNamara, S. (2000). User involvement in the design and evaluation of a smart mobility aid. *Journal of Rehabilitation Research and Development, 37*(6), 709–723.

Lamoureux, E. L., Hassell, J. B., & Keefe, J. E. (2004). The impact of diabetic retinopathy on participation in daily living. *Archives of Ophthalmology, 122,* 84–88.

Lifshitz, H., Hen, I., & Weisse, I. (2007). Self-concept, adjustment to blindness, and quality of friendship among adolescents with visual impairments. *Journal of Visual Impairment and Blindness, 101*(2), 96–107.

López-Justicia, M. D., & Córdoba, I. (2006). The self-concept of Spanish young adults with retinitis pigmentosa. *Journal of Visual Impairment and Blindness, 100*(6), 366–370.

Mariotti, S. P. (2004). New steps toward eliminating blinding trachoma. *New England Journal of Medicine, 351*(19), 2004–2007.

Nishida, K., Yamato, M., Hayashida, Y., Watanabe, K., Yamamoto, K., Adachi, E., et al. (2004). Corneal reconstruction with tissue-engineered cell sheets composed of autologous oral mucosal epithelium. *New England Journal of Medicine, 351*(12), 1187–1196.

Rundquist, J. (2004). Low vision rehabilitation of retinitis pigmentosa. *Journal of Visual Impairment and Blindness, 98,* 718–724.

Scarlatis, G. (2000). Optical prosthesis: Visions of the future. *Journal of the American Medical Association, 283*(17), 2297.

Sherwood, L. (2007). The peripheral nervous system: Afferent division; special senses. *In Human Physiology*. (pp. 181–231). Belmont, CA: Thomson Brooks/Cole.

Syed, M. F., & Bell, N. P. (2007). Glaucoma. In R. E. Rakel & E. T. Bope (Eds.). *Conn's current therapy* (pp. 222–226). Philadelphia: W. B. Saunders.

Turnbull, A., Turnbull, R., Shank, M., Smith, S., & Leal, D. (2002). *Exceptional lives: Special education in today's schools* (3rd ed.). Upper Saddle River, NJ: Merrill.

Vance, J. C. (2000). A degree of vision. *Lancet, 356*(i9240), 1517–1519.

Wong, T. Y., & Mitchell, P. (2004). Hypertensive retinopathy. *New England Journal of Medicine, 351*(22), 2310–2317.

Chapter 6

Hearing Loss and Deafness

■ STRUCTURE AND FUNCTION OF THE EAR

The ear is made up of two systems, which have two specific functions:

- The *auditory system* is involved with the detection of sound waves and, consequently, with hearing.
- The **vestibular system** is involved with body equilibrium, orientation, and balance.

The ear consists of three divisions: the outer, middle, and inner ear (Figure 6-1).

The Outer Ear

The outer ear includes the *pinna (auricle)* and the *external ear canal* (external auditory meatus). The pinna, the visible portion of the ear, is made up of elastic cartilage covered with skin. The function of the pinna is to collect sound waves and conduct them to the eardrum *(tympanic membrane)*. The external ear canal is a little longer than one inch and extends from the opening of the ear to the eardrum. It contains special glands that produce **cerumen** (earwax), which protects the ear against the entry of foreign material.

The Middle Ear

The tympanic membrane separates the outer ear from the middle ear. The middle ear *(tympanic cavity)* is an air-filled cavity connected to the throat by the *eustachian tube,* which helps equalize air pressure on both sides of the tympanic membrane. Changes of atmospheric pressure, such as occur with change in altitude, necessitate equalization of air pressure in the middle ear. When the ears "pop" during altitude changes, the eustachian tube has allowed air in the middle ear to equalize with the pressure outside the head. When this does not occur, considerable discomfort can result. The eustachian tube, which is normally collapsed in adults, opens with yawning or swallowing, allowing air pressure on both sides of the tympanic membrane to equalize. Another pathway connects the tympanic cavity to the mastoid air cells within the *mastoid process* of the temporal bone.

The middle ear lies between the eardrum and the inner ear. It contains three small movable bones called **ossicles,** which transfer sound vibrations from the eardrum to the inner ear. These small bones—the *malleus,* the *incus,* and the *stapes*—are connected by small ligaments and are attached to the tympanic membrane by the handle of the malleus with the footplate of the stapes connected to a thin membrane called the oval window, which connects to the inner ear. Also connecting the middle ear with the inner ear is an opening called the *round window*.

The Inner Ear

The inner ear (*labyrinth*) is a fluid-filled cavity that lies deep within the temporal bone of the skull. The inner ear is important not only for hearing (as part of the *auditory system*), but also for maintaining body balance and equilibrium (as part of the *vestibular system*). Contained within the inner ear is the *cochlea*, which is part of the auditory system, and the *semicircular canals*, which are part of the vestibular system. The cochlea has a snail-like appearance and contains tiny hair cells within a structure called the *organ of Corti*, the end organ of hearing. Movement of fluid within the inner ear stimulates nerve endings in both the auditory and vestibular systems. Impulses

from both systems are converted into nerve impulses and transmitted from the inner ear to the brain by the *eighth cranial nerve*, sometimes called the *acoustic* or *auditory nerve*. This nerve contains two branches: the *cochlear nerve branch*, which conducts sensory information about sound, and the *vestibular nerve branch*, which conducts impulses regarding body balance and movement.

Mechanism of Hearing

Sound waves enter the external ear and move through the external ear canal, striking the eardrum and causing it to vibrate. The vibration of the eardrum first moves the malleus, which transmits the vibration to the incus; in turn, the incus transmits the vibration to the stapes. The chained movement of the malleus, incus, and stapes conducts sound waves from the eardrum to the oval window, which connects to the inner ear. The stapes' vibration in the oval window activates the fluid in the inner ear, stimulating the tiny hair cells

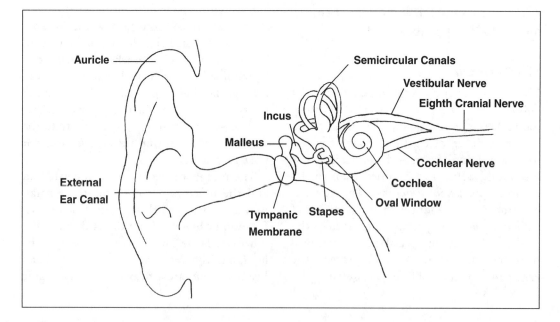

Figure 6-1   The outer, middle, and inner ear

in the organ of Corti. The movement of the hair cells stimulates the nerve endings located around their bases to transmit impulses to the cochlear nerve, which carries the impulses to the auditory center of the brain where they are interpreted as sound.

Equilibrium

The vestibular structures in the ear, concerned with maintaining equilibrium, include the *semicircular canals* and a small rounded chamber at their base called the *vestibule*. The semicircular canals contain the nerve endings through which balance is controlled. Like the organ of Corti, they contain numerous hair cells that project into the fluid of the inner ear. The movement of the head sets this fluid in motion and moves the hair cells, stimulating the nerve endings, which then transmit the impulses to the vestibular nerve. These impulses are carried to the portion of the brain involved with maintaining equilibrium and coordinating movement.

■ HEARING LOSS AND DEAFNESS

Pitch and Intensity of Sound

The sense of hearing is the neural perception of *sound energy* and is based on transmission of external sound to the structures of the outer, middle, and inner ear; the nerves to the brain; and portions of the brain involved in processing acoustic information. Traveling vibrations known as sound waves produces sound. Sound is characterized by both *pitch* (tone) and *intensity* (loudness). Individuals with hearing loss can have diminished hearing with regard to pitch, intensity, or both.

Pitch

Pitch or tone is determined by the frequency of vibrations of sound waves. The faster the vibrations or frequency, the higher the pitch. Frequencies are measured in *hertz (Hz)* or cycles

per second. Hearing loss related to frequency results in a distortion of sound so that individuals may be unable to differentiate between many of the sounds of speech. For example, words with similar sounds, such as "cat" and "rat," may be easily confused. Increasing the volume does not improve the quality of sound or make words clearer if this type of hearing loss exists.

Intensity

Intensity, or loudness of sounds, depends on the *amplitude* of sound waves. The greater the amplitude, the louder the sound. Loudness is measured in *decibels (db)*. Hearing loss related to intensity involves more difficulty in hearing because of reduction in sound volume. With this type of hearing loss, *amplification* of sound may improve hearing.

In instances where individuals have hearing loss related to both frequency and intensity, increasing volume alone will not improve overall hearing.

Definition and Classification of Hearing Loss

Disruption of any part of the hearing system can result in hearing loss. Any degree or type of hearing loss is classified as a hearing impairment. The greater the degree of hearing impairment, the more difficulty individuals have hearing in a number of situations.

Hearing loss may be characterized as follows:

- Partial
- Total
- Temporary
- Permanent
- Mild
- Profound

Hearing loss can affect both the volume and clarity of sound. Some individuals have hearing loss that results in reduced hearing sensitivity; they may be unable to hear soft speech or may have difficulty hearing speech when there is background noise. Other individuals have difficulty with *speech discrimination*; even though volume is adequate, they may be unable to clearly hear certain phonetic elements of speech (for example, consonants such as "x" and "s") because they occur at frequencies where hearing loss is present. Individuals can have both sensitivity loss and discrimination deficit at different degrees.

Hearing loss is classified based on a number of different criteria:

- Cause and location of hearing loss
- Duration of loss or age of onset
- Degree of hearing loss

Cause and Location of Hearing Loss

Cause and location of the loss are classified as one of three types:

- conductive,
- sensori neural, or
- mixed.

Conductive Hearing Loss

Conductive hearing loss occurs when there is damage, obstruction, or malformation in the external or middle ear, which prevents sound waves from reaching the cochlea in the inner ear. In many cases, correction of the underlying problem can restore diminished hearing. Conductive loss may result from the following causes:

- Buildup of earwax in the ear canal
- A foreign object in the ear
- **Otitis media** (infection of the middle ear)
- **Otosclerosis** (hardening of the small bones in the ear that are important for conducting sound)

Conductive hearing loss is a mechanical problem that alters the loudness of sound but does not reduce its clarity because the inner ear, where sound is "processed," is not compromised. Sometimes conductive hearing loss cannot be corrected, so hearing aids may be used to amplify sound and restore normal loudness. Conductive hearing losses are generally of mild to moderate degree. Individuals with mild to moderate conductive hearing loss usually have good success with hearing aids if such devices are necessary.

Sensori neural Hearing Loss

Sensorineural hearing loss results from damage or malformation of the inner ear or the auditory nerve and can lead to total deafness. This type of loss involves damage to the hair cells of the inner ear, which in turn interferes with the reception of nerve impulses. In some cases, the hair cell function of the cochlea is unaffected; rather, the cause of hearing loss is related to the nerve transmission pathway to the brain. With sensorineural loss, hearing is affected not only in terms of loudness, but also pitch or clarity. Individuals may perceive no sound; if sound is perceived, it may be distorted. Sensorineural hearing loss can be caused by a number of factors:

- Hereditary factors
- Genetic (syndrome-related) factors
- Acute infection, such as meningitis or mumps
- *Ototoxic drugs* (drugs that damage nerves of the central nervous system that are associated with hearing)
- Tumors
- Exposure to loud noise

Sensorineural hearing loss may also be due to a disorder of the auditory centers of the brain, such as from head injury or stroke. When this type of hearing loss occurs, the individual is said to have *central deafness*. In this type of deafness, either disruption of the ability of the sound stimulus to reach the hearing centers of the brain is disrupted or the hearing center in the brain incorrectly receives and processes signals.

Sensorineural hearing loss is almost exclusively irreversible. Because it involves damage to the hair cells of the cochlea and/or nerve cell damage, and because the nerve function cannot be restored, associated hearing loss is usually permanent. Although the cause of sensorineural loss should be evaluated medically, individuals with sensorineural hearing loss should also consult with a licensed audiologist for evaluation and potential fitting of hearing aids as well as communication strategies training.

Mixed Hearing Loss

When individuals have mixed hearing loss, there is a combination of conductive hearing loss and sensorineural hearing loss. The conductive component may lend itself to medical intervention, while the sensorineural component remains impervious to intervention. Individuals in some instances may benefit from amplification. The extent of the hearing loss experienced with mixed hearing loss and the success of intervention depend on the degree and type of sensorineural damage.

Duration of Loss or Age of Onset

Another classification of hearing loss is based on when the hearing loss occurred:

- **Prelingual hearing loss** occurs before the individual acquires language, usually before the age of three.
- **Postlingual hearing loss** occurs after verbal language is obtained.
- **Prevocational hearing loss** occurs after an individual acquires language but before entering the workforce, usually before the age of 19.
- **Postvocational hearing loss** refers to hearing loss that has occurred after the individual has started to work.

Degree of Hearing Loss

Hearing loss can also be classified according to the degree of hearing loss:

- *Hard of hearing* refers to individuals with mild to moderate hearing loss. Individuals who are hard of hearing usually have difficulty understanding conversational speech through the ear with or without a hearing aid.
- *Deaf* refers to individuals with severe to profound hearing loss. Deafness is the most severe type of hearing loss. Individuals with severe or profound hearing loss have an extreme inability to understand conversational speech through the ear, precluding their ability to use hearing for communication.

Degree of hearing loss is commonly defined on the basis of the audiogram described later in this chapter.

Causes of Hearing Loss

Hearing loss may be *congenital* (present at birth) or *acquired* (occurs after birth or later in life). In many instances, hearing loss is multifactorial, caused by both genetic and environmental factors (Williams, 2000).

Congenital Hearing Loss

There are three major causes of congenital hearing loss:

- Genetic (syndrome related)
- Prenatal exposure to drugs or toxins
- Prenatal exposure to infections, such as measles (rubella)

Genetic hearing loss may be part of specific genetically linked conditions that involve a variety of other abnormalities, or it may be isolated. Genetically determined deafness may be present at birth or, may appear later in adulthood. The degree, progression, and age of onset of a genetically based hearing loss vary widely, depending on the specific condition or syndrome. In some instances, genetics may not cause deafness per se, but rather predispose individuals to hearing loss induced by noise, drugs, or infection (Steel, 2000).

Maternal exposure to drugs or other substances, or maternal infection such as rubella (measles) during the first trimester of pregnancy, can damage the auditory system of the developing fetus, resulting in congenital hearing loss. Other intrauterine factors that can result in congenital hearing loss include certain endocrine disorders, Rh incompatibility, and difficult deliveries (Baloh, 2004).

Acquired Hearing Loss

There are a number of causes of acquired hearing loss:

- Recurrent ear infections (e.g., otitis media)
- Noise
- Injury
- Viruses
- Degenerative conditions
- Aging
- Ototoxic drugs (drugs that damage the inner ear)
- Tumors (acoustic neuroma)

Recurrent infections of the middle ear, such as otitis media, in early childhood can lead to complications causing conductive hearing loss in young children. Prompt identification and treatment of infections can decrease the probability of hearing loss (Hendley, 2002). It is commonly believed that early intervention when hearing loss is identified in young children can lead to better long-term outcomes, including speech, language, and educational outcomes (Shafer, 2006).

Environmental conditions can also contribute to hearing loss in both children and adults. Noise-induced hearing loss is one of the most common, irreversible, but preventable types of acquired hearing loss worldwide (Nelson, Nelson, Concha-Barrientos, & Fingerhut, 2005). This kind of hearing loss can be caused by a one-time exposure to impulse noise, such as an explosion or gunfire, or it can result from repeated exposure to loud noises over time,

such as a pneumatic hammer, loud music, or noise from heavy equipment. The associated hearing loss may be immediate or hearing may gradually diminish over time.

Avoiding loud noises or wearing ear protectors during exposure to loud noise can drastically reduce the incidence of noise-induced hearing loss. Many industrial sites in which occupational noise presents a hazard now make a concerted effort to inform employees of the necessity of wearing hearing protectors, although compliance with hearing protection policy is often low (Robertson, Kerr, Garcia, & Halterman, 2007). Industries with more intermittent noise, such as construction, also tend to have fewer hearing protection policies in place (Daniell, Swan, McDaniel, Camp, Cohen, & Stebbins, 2006). The degree of permanent damage associated with noise depends on the duration and the intensity of the exposure (Baloh, 2004).

Acquired hearing loss can also result from injuries or other conditions that affect the auditory pathway. Conditions ranging from traumatic brain injury to direct injury to the ear and the acoustic nerve can lead to hearing loss, for example.

Viruses, such as those associated with measles, mumps, and meningitis can produce sensorineural hearing loss (Lerner & Eng, 2005). Stroke that causes damage to part of the auditory system or the area of the brain necessary for interpreting stimuli as sound may also be responsible for hearing loss. Some degenerative diseases, such as multiple sclerosis can be accompanied by loss of hearing. Tumors, such as *acoustic neuroma,* can also compress a portion of the auditory system, causing hearing loss.

Hearing sensitivity declines gradually and progressively with aging (Gordon-Salant, 2005), although the extent to which degeneration of portions of the auditory system is due to the aging process or to cumulative noise trauma throughout life may be difficult to determine. Hearing loss associated with aging is known as **presbycusis.** The most important consequence of aging-related decline in hearing sensitivity is difficulty in understanding speech. Hearing loss, coupled with other perceptual and processing effects of aging, may result in confusion, withdrawal, disorientation, and inappropriate responses, which can lead others to assume erroneously that individuals have a severe cognitive disability (Nichols, 2006).

Drugs or other substances that are harmful to the auditory pathway are called **ototoxic**. Salicylates or certain blood pressure medications taken in high doses can produce transient hearing loss; by contrast, some antibiotics, such as streptomycin and neomycin, can be severely ototoxic, destroying the hair cells of the cochlea (Baloh, 2004).

Manifestations of Hearing Loss

Hearing loss can lead to depression, social isolation, stress, and functional problems such as impaired balance (Nichols, 2006). The type and degree of hearing loss experienced by individuals, regardless of the cause, are varied. Hearing loss usually involves more than a reduction in the loudness of sound. Some hearing losses, for example, also result in a distortion of sound so that words may be heard but are difficult to understand or are garbled. In this case, increasing the loudness is unlikely to enhance individuals's ability to understand what is being said.

Some individuals with hearing loss may develop **recruitment**, a symptom characterized by an abnormally rapid increase in the perception of loudness with small changes in signal energy. Individuals with recruitment have a narrow range between a level of sound loud enough to be understood and a level of sound that causes discomfort or pain. Unexpected sounds may startle individuals with recruitment and distract them from inter-

pretation of the sound's meaning. Therefore, increasing loudness of sound does not correct the hearing problem and can actually cause increased discomfort.

■ CONDITIONS OF THE EAR CONTRIBUTING TO HEARING LOSS

Conditions of the Outer Ear

Conditions of the outer ear can contribute to hearing loss when an obstruction disrupts the mechanical transmission of auditory stimuli decreasing acuity of hearing. Although conditions of the outer ear may not have a major impact on hearing or may be correctable, they may also be disfiguring, leading to cosmetic concerns. Deformities or abnormalities of the outer ear can result from congenital conditions or from trauma. Other conditions of the outer ear that may impede hearing are buildup of earwax, foreign bodies in the ears, or growths (e.g., polyps) that cause obstruction.

For the most part, partial occlusion of the external ear canal has no influence on the efficiency of sound transmission and causes no significant hearing loss. Complete occlusion, however, generally results in a moderate conductive loss. Conditions of the outer ear that cause temporary conductive hearing loss can usually be corrected or alleviated by surgical or mechanical intervention.

Conditions of the Middle Ear

Several conditions of the middle ear may cause temporary or permanent hearing loss.

Perforated Tympanic Membrane

A thickened or perforated tympanic membrane (ruptured eardrum) may or may not impair hearing. Rupture of the eardrum may result from an injury (e.g., a blow to the ear or head, or an explosion), infection, or inflammation.

Otitis Media

Otitis media includes two types of conditions:

- Acute otitis media—inflammation of the middle ear space
- Otitis media with effusion—fluid in the middle ear

Otitis media with effusion can cause conductive hearing losses due to collection of fluid in the middle ear or damage to the tympanic membrane as a result of infection or rupture. Usually, with appropriate intervention, permanent hearing loss will not result.

For the past four decades, concerns about the effects of otitis media with effusion on speech, language, and learning development in young children, led to use of aggressive interventions such as placement of *tympanostomy tubes* to prevent permanent damage. Recent reports have demonstrated little evidence that prompt insertion of tympanostomy tubes improves developmental outcomes in children who have no other conditions confounding development (Berman, 2007; Paradise et al., 2007). Children at risk for speech, language delay, or other developmental issues, such as autism-spectrum disorders, after appropriate testing may still have tympanostomy tube placement recommended (McMurray, 2007).

Mastoididitis

Mastoiditis is an infection of the mastoid cells within the mastoid process located in the temporal bone of the skull. Because of the proximity of the mastoid cells to other important structures in the head, mastoiditis may lead to a number of complications, including paralysis of the facial muscles and infection or abscess of the brain. Mastoiditis is not as prevalent as it once was thanks to the earlier detection of otitis media and intervention with antibiotics. Nevertheless, chronic mastoiditis and associated complications can arise if previous ear infections are left untreated.

Otosclerosis

Otosclerosis is a hardening of the ossicles (incus, stapes, and malleus of the middle ear), which transmit sound impulses to the inner ear. Early symptoms may include trouble hearing on the telephone but not in crowds. The condition appears in part to be hereditary. It causes *conductive hearing loss* because hardening of the ossicles reduces efficiency of the transfer of sound impulses to the inner ear. Otosclerosis produces progressive hearing loss accompanied by **tinnitus** (ringing or noise in the ear). Some individuals may also have vestibular symptoms such as **vertigo** (dizziness) or impaired equilibrium.

Individuals with otosclerosis often hear amplified speech well and without distortions; consequently, they are usually good candidates for hearing aids. Hearing can also often be restored or improved with surgical intervention, although surgery does not fully remedy the loss. When determining if surgery is appropriate, individuals' lifestyle and occupation are considered. Because surgery may affect vestibular function, individuals who require fine balance for employment may find amplification through hearing aids a better choice than surgery. If individuals' hobbies or occupations expose them to large and rapid changes in barometric pressure, or if heavy lifting is required, hearing aids may also be a better choice because of the chance of postoperative complications or vestibular disturbances.

Conditions of the Inner Ear

Many conditions of the inner ear cause permanent hearing loss.

Tinnitus

Tinnitus (ringing or noise in the ears) may or may not be accompanied by hearing loss. It can result from overexposure to loud noise or can be a symptom of a more serious condition, such as tumor, high blood pressure, or head injury. It can also result from side effects or toxic effects of some medications. In some instances, tinnitus may be a separate entity, not associated with a specific condition and with no identifiable cause. The treatment of tinnitus depends on the cause. In some cases, if the cause can be identified and treated, the ringing can be eliminated. In other instances, even though the cause is identified, damage may be permanent and tinnitus cannot be cured.

Most people with tinnitus adjust to its presence and experience no severe residual effects; however, some individuals have difficulty adjusting and experience disabling effects of tinnitus, including sleep disturbances and severe emotional distress (Claussen 2007). Some individuals complain of problems sleeping because of the constant noise and may need background noise, as from a radio, to mask the sound. A number of interventions, including group cognitive therapy, have been used to help people cope with tinnitus. Adjustment to tinnitus does not appear to be related to the severity of the condition, but rather to the coping styles of those affected.

Acute Peripheral Vestibulopathy (Labyrinthitis)

Labyrinthitis (inflammation of the labyrinth of the inner ear) may be acute without resulting in permanent hearing loss. Labyrinthitis may occur as a complication of otitis media, influenza, or upper respiratory infections. Because the inner ear is involved, symptoms of vertigo (dizziness), nausea, and vomiting frequently accompany the condition. Most people gradually improve in one or two weeks, although in some instances manifestations can persist for months (Baloh, 2004).

Benign Paroxysmal Positional Vertigo

Benign paroxysmal positional vertigo (BPPV) is one of the most common causes of vertigo (dizziness) and is related to head movements or changing of position (Hansson & Mansson, 2005; Baloh, 2004). Individuals with BPPV are

at increased risk for falls and may limit their activity for this reason, resulting in decreased independence and quality of life, and subsequent depression (Kovar, Jepson, & Jones, 2006).

This condition results from degenerative debris in the form of free-floating calcium carbonate crystals that enter the semicircular canal (Hansson & Mansson, 2005; Baloh, 2004). Floating of the debris in the fluid causes an illusion of motion, with subsequent vertigo and nausea.

Intervention consists of *particle-repositioning procedures*, often performed by a physical therapist, in which the individual's head is rotated in sequence into different positions, or habituation exercises that reteach the brain so that vertigo does not occur when exposed to stimuli from the debris (Hansson & Mansson, 2005).

Meniere's Disease

Meniere's disease is a chronic condition of the inner ear that encompasses the triad of recurrent severe vertigo, sensorineural hearing loss, and tinnitus (noise or ringing in the ears) (van Cruijsen, Jaspers, van de Wiel, Wit, & Albers, 2006). The cause of Meniere's disease is unknown, but it is believed that the disease results from overabundance of fluid *(endolymph)* in the inner ear, either because of overproduction or underabsorption of fluid (Meyer & Lambert, 2007). It is also thought that disturbances in the fluid dynamics of the endolymph are involved in associated hearing loss. One or both ears may be affected. Exacerbations are episodic, such that the disease is characterized by remissions and relapses. When episodes do occur, they are dramatic, often debilitating individuals during the episode.

During an episode of exacerbation, vertigo usually appears suddenly and is often accompanied by nausea and vomiting. Vertigo associated with Meniere's disease can be severely disabling, lasting from a few minutes to hours (Meyer & Lambert, 2007). Tinnitus may be either intermittent or constant between attacks, becoming worse during an attack. Hearing loss associated with Meniere's disease is variable. Although hearing loss associated with Meniere's disease may at first be transient, it later can become progressive (Thorp & James, 2005). Lower tones may be affected first, but all tones are affected as the condition progresses.

Intervention consists of dietary and lifestyle modifications, including management of dietary sodium to help reduce fluid pressure in the inner ear, and use of diuretic medications to decrease fluid volume by increasing urine production (Meyer & Lambert, 2007; Thorp & James, 2005). Individuals are also asked to decrease their caffeine and alcohol intake and to stop smoking.

A mechanical device (the *Meniett*) has also been found to be helpful for some individuals. Individuals using the Meniett device must first undergo *myringotomy* (discussed later in this chapter) with insertion of a tympanostomy tube. The Meniett delivers low-pressure bursts of air into the external ear canal (Meyer & Lambert, 2007).

Individuals with Meniere's disease who do not respond to other interventions may undergo injection of ototoxic antibiotics into the middle ear to create a partial *labyrinthectomy* (excision of the labyrinth). This procedure can, however cause permanent sensorineural hearing loss (Thorpe & James, 2005). Surgical procedures may include *endolymphatic sac surgery* in which the stent to drain the endolymph fluid is inserted and the endolymphatic sac is decompressed; resection of the vestibular nerve; or labyrinthectomy, in which the semicircular canals are removed, which results in permanent hearing loss (Meyer & Lambert, 2007).

Trauma or Conditions

As discussed earlier in the chapter, hearing loss may result from damage to the inner ear or to the acoustic nerve. Among causes of sensorineural deafness are traumatic head injury or stroke; hypertension and arteriosclerosis, which produce vascular changes in the central nervous system; exposure to high levels of noise, which can damage the hair cells in the inner ear; the ingestion of ototoxic agents (drugs or other chemicals that destroy the hair cells of the inner ear or damage the eighth cranial nerve); and infections, such as meningitis. Growths or tumors inside the head may cause hearing loss by mechanically impinging on the acoustic nerve or by involving it directly. Other neurological conditions, such as multiple sclerosis, may also produce changes in the auditory pathway that contribute to hearing loss.

Presbycusis

Presbycusis, as discussed earlier in the chapter, is caused by degenerative changes in the inner ear, neural pathways, or both; however, the reason that presbycusis occurs is unknown. It has become a catchall term that encompasses many types of auditory deteriorations, but is commonly thought to accompany aging-related structural changes in the ear. Most often presbycusis occurs in both ears equally. Onset is slow, and hearing loss can vary in degree from mild to severe. Ability to hear higher tonal frequencies is usually affected first, but the ability to hear lower frequencies is gradually affected as well. Hearing loss experienced as a result of presbycusis most often is accompanied by word discrimination difficulties, especially if the hearing loss has greatly affected the individuals' perception of the higher-pitched consonants.

Conditions of the Vestibular System

The vestibular system in the ear contributes to sense of balance and equilibrium. Although conditions of the vestibular system can be associated with conditions that affect hearing, such as Meniere's disease, symptoms related to the vestibular system can also exist with other conditions such as stroke or be side effects of certain medications. No matter what their cause, conditions of the vestibular system can cause manifestations that interfere with individuals' functional capacity.

One of the classic manifestations associated with vestibular dysfunction is vertigo. Vertigo is an illusory sense of motion, usually described as a spinning sensation, and often thought of in terms of dizziness. Although vertigo can be associated with many conditions, it is always related to the body's vestibular system.

Episodes of vertigo can last from a few seconds to days. *Vestibular neuronitis* (inflammation of the vestibular nerve), a condition of the inner ear, can cause vertigo that lasts for days or weeks and is extremely disabling during that time. During the episode, individuals become nauseous with vomiting and feel a violent spinning of their surroundings. The cause of vestibular neuronitis is unknown.

Vertigo can also be associated with head injury or other neurological conditions such as brain tumor or multiple sclerosis.

■ DIAGNOSTIC PROCEDURES

Identification of Hearing Loss

Before hearing loss can be evaluated or treated, it must be identified. Individuals with hearing losses may not be aware of the degree of loss, or they may deny that hearing loss exists. An important tool in diagnosis may be simple observation of behaviors that may be indicative of such a hearing loss.

Indications of possible hearing loss in infants and small children include unresponsiveness to sound, delayed development of speech, and behavior problems (e.g., tantrums, inattention, and hyperactivity). School-aged children with undiagnosed hearing loss may have speech impairments, may demonstrate attention disorders, or may demonstrate below-average ability in school.

Adults with undiagnosed hearing loss may be irritable, hostile, or hypersensitive. They may deny their inability to understand or respond appropriately by blaming others for not enunciating distinctly. They often avoid situations in which hearing is more difficult, such as those where large crowds or large groups are present. Individuals with undiagnosed hearing loss may speak excessively loud and may require increased volume to hear the television and radio.

Heightened sensitivity and patience are often necessary when encouraging individuals with suspected hearing loss to obtain evaluation and treatment. Initial resistance to these recommendations is not unusual.

Physical Examination

Physicians may be the first to recognize or be consulted about a potential hearing loss. Although often omitted, screening for hearing loss should be part of every physical exam. Various checklists and questionnaires may be used initially to elicit signs and symptoms associated with hearing loss. During physical examination, physicians may also exam the ear canal for obstruction and visualize the tympanic membrane with an instrument called an *otoscope*. Likewise, rudimentary auditory screening may be performed in the physician's office.

Physicians sometimes use tuning forks in routine physical examinations in their offices as an initial screening method for hearing loss. This method can help differentiate between conductive or sensorineural hearing loss, and problems with both air conduction and bone conduction of sound. It does not quantify the degree of loss, if any exists. The ability to hear by air conduction is tested by placing a vibrating tuning fork in the air near the ear, but out of the individual's sight. Hearing by bone conduction is evaluated by placing a vibrating tuning fork in different positions on the individual's skull, which causes vibration throughout the skull, including the inner ear. The inability to hear the sound in either instance is an indication of hearing loss. Abnormal test results warrant further testing and evaluation. Because of the gross nature of this screening method, it has been widely replaced by other methods.

When problems with hearing are identified, referral for additional testing may be made. For further testing and evaluation, individuals may be referred to an **audiologist**—a person with a master's or doctoral degree in audiology who specializes in the evaluation and rehabilitation of individuals with hearing conditions—for further testing. If testing by the audiologist reveals that medical intervention is necessary, referral is made to an **otolaryngologist** (a physician who specializes in diagnosis and treatment of conditions of the ear and related structures).

Audiometric Testing

Audiometric testing measures the degree of hearing loss with an electronic device called an *audiometer*. An audiologist usually performs the test.

Tests routinely used by audiologists attempt to define three major aspects of hearing:

- Degree of hearing
- Type of hearing loss
- Ability to understand speech under various conditions

A complete audiometric evaluation usually includes *pure-tone air* and *bone conduction testing, speech audiometry,* and *acoustic immittance measurement.* From audiometric results, the type and degree of hearing loss can be determined as well as the degree of speech understanding.

Pure-Tone Audiometry

The accurate measurement of sound is an important component of a hearing test. Changes in sound intensity are measured in decibels and heard as changes in loudness. Changes in sound frequency are measured in Hertz and are heard as changes in pitch. The *audiogram* is a method of recording the softest sounds that individuals can hear. A general guide for describing degrees of hearing loss associated with decibel losses is found in Table 6-1.

The individual's ability to detect sound and pitch in each ear is plotted on the audiogram (see Figure 6-2). A *pure-tone audiogram* is a graph on which an individual's responses to calibrated tones are plotted as *thresholds.* Numbers across the top of the audiogram represent pure-tone frequencies ranging from 125 to 8000 Hz. Along the side of the audiogram are numbers ranging from minus –10 to 110 that represent measurement of decibels.

Table 6-1 Functional Implications of Degrees of Decibel Loss	
26–40 dB	Mild hearing loss. In ideal listening conditions, hearing is minimally affected; there may be difficulty hearing faint, distant speech even in ideal conditions; background noise may interfere with hearing.
41–55 dB	Moderate hearing loss. Hears conversational speech but only at close distances; understanding speech is more difficult with background noses.
56–70 dB	Moderately severe hearing loss. Hears loud conversational speech which is close by. Has difficulty hearing in group situations.
71–90 dB	Severe hearing loss. Conversational speech severely affected. Perception of sound is usually distorted.
Greater than 90 dB	Profound. May hear (or feel from vibrations) only very loud sounds. Hearing is not the primary communication channel.

Source: Moore, D. F., 2001

The audiogram illustrates the degree of hearing loss. The *audometric exam* takes place in a sound chamber to eliminate distracting sounds. An *audiometer* emits sounds (*pure tones*) or words through earphones worn by the individual being tested (*air conduction audiometry*). As the tones are transmitted through the earphones, the individual indicates when sound is first heard. Results of the test are then plotted on the audiogram. The hearing-level scale is constructed so that average normal hearing equals 0 decibels; normal hearing sensitivity ranges from minus 10 to 25 decibels. The higher the number on the decibel scale, the greater the degree of hearing loss. The audiogram tests speech frequencies, which range from 250 to 8000 Hz. The inability to discrim-

inate frequencies within this range may interfere with everyday communication.

Bone Conduction Audiometry

When audiometric testing reveals a hearing loss, the audiologist conducts further testing to determine whether the hearing loss is sensorineural, conductive, or mixed in nature. Tests used for this purpose include bone conduction tests. The procedure for *bone conduction audiometry* consists of placing a vibrator on the individual's mastoid process or on the forehead. Calibrated tones are then transmitted through the vibrator directly into the inner ear, bypassing the external and middle ear systems. The individual's responses to the thresholds are

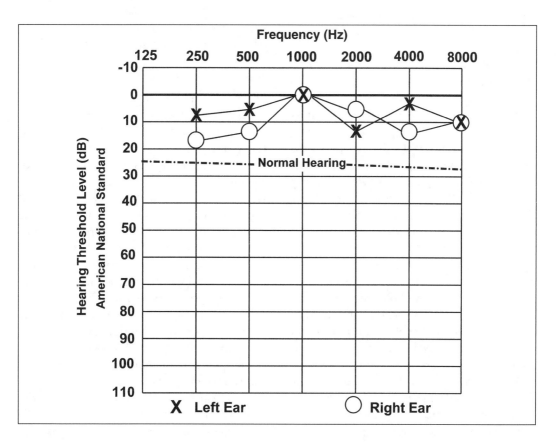

Figure 6-2 Audiogram

plotted on the audiogram and contrasted with the air conduction test results.

To determine the type of hearing loss, thresholds for air and bone conduction are compared. Depending on the differences between the two thresholds, hearing loss is classified as sensorineural, conductive, or mixed.

Speech Audiometry

Although pure-tone audiometry is used to determine individuals' ability to hear specific tones, speech audiometry provides measurements that may indicate more appropriately individuals' ability to understand speech in everyday situations. Two types of speech audiometry measured are the *speech reception threshold (SRT)* and the *speech discrimination threshold*. In both tests, individuals wear headphones and listen to words being transmitted through the headphones without any visual cues.

Tests of speech reception threshold help to identify the lowest intensity, or softest sound level in *decibels*, at which an individual first understands speech. Words with two syllables (such as "baseball," "ice cream," or "cowboy"), taken from a standardized list are presented to the individual through the earphones. The individual then repeats the word, thereby demonstrating his or her acuity for hearing the spoken word. The speech reception threshold should correspond closely to the average pure-tone air conduction threshold and provides a check of the accuracy of the pure-tone measurements. The higher the decibel level required for either threshold, the greater the hearing loss. A speech reception threshold or average pure-tone threshold of 25 decibels, for instance, is considered borderline normal hearing for adults. (Limits for children are reduced to 15 to 20 decibels.) A threshold of 26 to 40 decibels is considered a mild hearing loss.

In addition to measuring how loud speech has to be to be heard, testing involves determining how well individuals understand speech once it is loud enough to hear. Speech discrimination tests (sometimes called *word recognition tests*) help to the provide this information. During the test, words from standardized lists of phonetically balanced one-syllable words are presented to the individual through earphones without visual cues. Words are presented at a supra-threshold level, and the individual must identify and repeat words back to the examiner. The test is scored as the percentage of correctly repeated words. The lower the percentage, the greater the problem in understanding. Individuals with speech discrimination hearing loss may be able to recognize speech but be unable to understand it. The speech discrimination score provides a measure of the ability to understand words at a comfortable volume. It assesses the ability to judge acoustic information and distinguish between similar speech sounds, such as the letters "p" and "b" or the letters "t" and "d."

Acoustic Immittance or Impedance Audiometry

Acoustic immittance measurement includes a battery of tests that evaluate middle ear status. *Tympanometry* is a test of acoustic immittance in which the mobility or flexibility of the tympanic membrane is assessed by measuring how much sound energy is admitted into the ear as air pressure is varied in the external auditory canal. The status of the eardrum is assessed by altering the air pressure in the ear canal and measuring the response of the eardrum to sound transmissions under these varying conditions and different stimuli. As sound energy strikes the eardrum, some is transmitted to the middle and inner ear, but some is reflected back into the ear canal. If the tympanic membrane is stiff, much of the sound energy is reflected back into the external ear canal. The less impedance, the more sound energy admitted to the middle and inner ear. An increased level of resistance is diagnostic of middle ear pathology.

The results of this type of testing are plotted on a graph called a *tympanogram*. The ear's response is plotted on the vertical dimension of the graph, and air pressures are plotted on the horizontal dimension.

Acoustic immittance testing may also be used to measure the *acoustic reflex*—that is, movement of the muscles attached to the malleus and stapes as a response to intense sound. It should occur in both ears in response to a loud sound, even if only one ear is stimulated. Acoustic reflex testing may be helpful in diagnosing conditions or problems that involve the cochlea or auditory nervous system.

Acoustic immittance testing requires no voluntary responses from the individual. Consequently, tympanometry is frequently used to detect or rule out conductive hearing loss in children or in adults who are unable to cooperate fully during pure-tone testing.

Electrocochleography

Electrocochleography is a procedure in which stimulus-related electrical activity generated in the cochlea and auditory nerve is recorded. For the test, the individual reclines, with electrodes being placed in the external auditory canal. Sound stimulus is then delivered through earphones. The test is useful in evaluation of inner ear fluid disorders such as Meniere's syndrome.

Auditory Brain Stem Response

The auditory brain stem response (ABR) records electrical activity generated as sound travels from the auditory nerve through the auditory brain stem pathway. During this test the individual reclines, with electrodes being placed on the mastoid or on the earlobe. A stimulus is then presented through earphones, and electroencephalogram activity is evaluated and the ABR assessed. The ABR is useful in ruling out auditory conditions such as diseases of the cochlea; degenerative or demyelinating diseases of the auditory system, such as multiple sclerosis; and tumors of the auditory system.

Otoacoustic Emissions

Otoacoustic emissions are measured reflections in the outer ear of mechanical activity in the cochlea. Otoacoustic emissions testing enables measurement of hearing in infants, young children, and difficult-to-test persons such as those with dementia or mental retardation. The technology has enhanced the ability to detect hearing loss early in life.

Evaluation of the Vestibular System (Disorders of Balance)

Individuals who experience vertigo (dizziness) or who have problems with balance are frequently tested for inner ear and sensorineural disorders related to vestibular function. These tests are performed either by an audiologist or a physician.

In one test of vestibular nerve function, the *caloric test*, either cold or hot water is introduced into the external auditory canal. The water stimulates the fluids within the inner ear, thus stimulating the vestibular nerve. The introduction of the water into the ear creates a reflex response of the eye called *nystagmus* (involuntary horizontal eye movement). By monitoring the direction of eye movements, the audiologist or physician can determine the origin of the dizziness and identify nerve damage if present. Eye movement may be monitored visually or with *electronystagmography (ENG)*, a procedure in which electrodes are placed near the eye to record eye muscle activity.

■ MANAGEMENT OF HEARING LOSS AND DEAFNESS

Both medical and nonmedical interventions may be used in the management of hearing loss. Medical interventions may involve surgery or medications, whereas nonmedical interventions may include use of hearing aids or other assistive listening devices and special training programs.

Management in most cases involves a variety of professionals. An *otolaryngologist* (a physician who specializes in disorders of the ear and related structures) provides medical evaluation and treatment of hearing loss. *Audiologists,* in addition to conducting evaluations of hearing function, manage the nonmedical treatment of hearing loss, including selecting and fitting amplification devices. The audiologist reviews hearing test results and consults with the individual about his or her listening needs before recommending which style or type of hearing aid would be most beneficial.

Children with hearing loss may also have speech production difficulties because of lack of auditory feedback. *Speech and language pathologists* often work with individuals to help them with particular aspects of speech, language, or both to increase intelligibility.

Auditory training is often helpful for individuals with special problems in communication. Such training may be included in hearing aid orientation and/or special programs on listening for the sounds of speech and other environmental sounds.

Surgical Procedures

Surgical procedures may be performed to eliminate pathologic conditions and to restore or improve hearing.

Myringotomy

When the middle ear is infected, as in otitis media, or when there is a fluid buildup in the middle ear, surgical intervention may be necessary to drain pus or fluid, thereby relieving pressure and preventing rupture of the eardrum (tympanic membrane). A myringotomy is a procedure in which an incision is made into the eardrum for this purpose. Because the procedure is performed under controlled conditions, it seldom leaves enough scar tissue to have a negative effect on hearing.

If fluid has accumulated in the middle ear, the physician may perform a needle aspiration to remove it. Needle aspiration may not remove fluid that has invaded the mastoid air cell system, however, and additional intervention may be necessary if the mastoid system is to be rendered dry. A common procedure performed during myringotomy is the placement of *ventilation* or *pressure-equalizing tubes,* which are placed in the tympanic membrane. The pressure-equalizing tubes act as an artificial eustachian tube, equalizing middle ear pressure. Abnormal eustachian tube function is the most common cause of middle ear problems. The ventilation tubes usually extrude on their own within 3 to 18 months, with complications occurring only rarely. When the ventilation tube is in place and operating properly, conductive hearing loss due to middle ear disease is usually completely eliminated.

Mastoidectomy

Since the advent of antibiotics for treatment of **mastoiditis** (inflammation of the mastoid bone), mastoidectomy is performed less frequently. **Mastoidectomy** is a surgical procedure for removal of infected mastoid air cells, which are located in the mastoid process. Because the mastoid is a portion of the acoustic system of the middle ear, hearing loss could still be present after surgery, depending on the nature of the surgery. Mastoidectomy is frequently completed in conjunction with several of the surgical procedures to treat Meniere's disease (Meyer & Lambert, 2007), as discussed earlier in this chapter.

Tympanoplasty

Surgical procedures involving the middle ear are referred to generally as **tympanoplasty** (repair of the tympanic membrane). **Myringoplasty** is a specific type of tympanoplasty in which the damaged eardrum is repaired. Other types of tympanoplasties may be performed for the surgical repair or reconstruction of the ossicles of the middle ear. Repairing or reconstructing the conductive mechanisms of the middle ear may improve or restore the conductive component of individuals' hearing.

Stapedectomy

The most common surgical treatment for oto-sclerosis is **stapedectomy**, a surgical replacement of an immobile or fixed stapes with prosthesis. The surgery reestablishes a sound pathway between the middle and inner ear; it usually improves hearing but does not totally restore it.

Devices and Aids for Hearing Loss

Cochlear Implant

Approximately 738,000 individuals in the United States have severe to profound hearing loss (Olson, 2006). Increasing numbers of these individuals are using *cochlear implants* to restore partial hearing, including adults with long-term and prelingual hearing loss (Zeng, 2004). In hearing individuals, sound travels from the outer ear to the middle ear, and then to the cochlea, where it is converted into electrical impulses that are transmitted through the auditory nerve to the brain for interpretation. When the hair cells within the cochlea are damaged, however, this conversion process cannot take place. Cochlear implants bypass the hair cells of the inner ear, stimulating the auditory nerve directly.

A cochlear implant is a surgically implanted electronic device that transduces sound signals into electrical signals that stimulate the auditory nerve. It consists of the following components:

- A microphone that picks up sound.
- A speech processor (typically worn behind the ear or, in older models, on a belt) that converts sound into digital impulses according to the individual's degree of hearing loss.
- A headpiece held in place by a magnet attached to the implant that has been surgically placed on the other side of the skin behind the ear.
- The implant, which converts signals into electric currents, sends them through a wire surgically placed into the cochlea, and transmits the impulse to the auditory nerve though electrodes at the end of the wire. The auditory nerve then carries the impulses to the brain, where they are interpreted as sound.

Cochlear implants, which were once used mainly for bilateral deafness and severe hearing loss, are now also prescribed for individuals who are unable to have effective oral communication even with the benefit of a hearing aid (Gates & Miyamoto, 2003). Although these cochlear implants cannot restore total hearing, they can be life-changing for many individuals, so they are able to hear environmental sounds and improve communication (Sherwood, 2007). Cochlear implants can help in speech reading by enabling individuals to distinguish beginnings and endings of words, as well as intonation and rhythm patterns being used. Individuals can typically hear moderate sounds, although they may have difficulty perceiving speech clearly in noisy environments and may have difficulty clearly hearing music. Implants can also have a positive impact in work environments. In addition to experiencing an improvement in verbal communication, individuals with cochlear implants are better able to hear and identify warning signals (Saxon, Holmes, & Spitznagel, 2001).

Although the sound heard with cochlear implants is not like an acoustic signal, individuals with implants become accustomed to hearing via this electrical stimulation. Not all individuals who are deaf are candidates for cochlear implants. For adults, the following criteria should be met before receiving a cochlear implant:

- Severe to profound sensorineural deafness
- Speech recognition at less than 50% with appropriate hearing aid
- Motivated and psychologically suitable for the implant (Zeng, 2004)

The success rate with cochlear implants varies (Olson, 2006). Individuals who have shorter term deafness appear to have greater success with implants than those with long-term hearing loss (Gates & Miyamoto, 2003; Fischetti, 2003). Age does not appear to be relevant to success of cochlear implants, although children who receive a cochlear implant before the age of 5 have been shown to have improved long-term speech perception and production as well as improved oral language and literacy development (Berg, Ip, Hurst, & Herb, 2007; Geers, 2004). Use of a hearing aid in one ear and a cochlear implant in the other ear (referred to as bimodal listening), as well as bilateral cochlear implants, have been shown to improve hearing performance in some persons, especially children (Kirk, Firszt, Hood, & Holt, 2006). In other instances, use of FM systems (discussed later in the chapter) have been found to be useful for some individuals, especially in educational environments in which noise level may interfere with learning of new information (Thibodeau, 2006).

Individuals who receive a cochlear implant should have realistic expectations for their hearing ability after the implantation. Optimal use of the implants requires a commitment to rehabilitation, training, and daily practice. Although the cost of cochlear implants is covered by many insurers, reimbursement for auditory rehabilitation—a key to successful use of implants—may be minimal or non-existent.

Before receiving a cochlear implant, individuals should be well informed about the issues involved and the facts related to implantation (Chute, 2004). Individuals must be carefully screened with an audiological assessment, thorough hearing history and physical examination, and psychosocial assessment. Individuals with prelingual deafness, who have strong ties to the Deaf community, may be unprepared for the social ramifications of cochlear implant. Some individuals in the Deaf culture (as discussed later in the chapter) are strongly opposed to cochlear implants for cultural reasons. Consequently, in some instances, cochlear implants may socially isolate individuals from friends in the Deaf community who reject the idea of implants (Tucker, 1998).

The use of cochlear implants for young children has also raised a number of issues that are still under debate. Improved technological means to test hearing in infants and young children has made early detection of hearing loss or deafness and early intervention possible. Although a number of studies have demonstrated improved cognitive and speech perception outcomes with cochlear implants at a young age (Nicholas & Geers, 2006; Tomblin, Baker, Spencer, Zhang, & Gantz, 2005) others question the social and emotional outcomes of this type of early intervention (Schorr, 2007; Luterman, 2007; Moores, 2005).

Hearing Aids

A hearing aid is any mechanical or electronic device that improves hearing. Prescription of a hearing aid is highly individualized and fitted according to individual need. The advent of digital technology has advanced the quality of hearing aids significantly over the past decade (Edwards, 2007). In the past, hearing aids were mainly designed to amplify sound; today, however, hearing aids are much more complex and combine sound amplification with signal processing for speech, noise reduction, and a number of other functions, including a wireless link with other communication systems (Levitt, 2007). Several types are available:

- Behind-the-ear style, which curves around the back side of the ear
- In-the-ear style, which fits in the ear canal and outer ear bowl
- Canal style, which fits entirely within the ear canal so it is barely visible

All hearing aids, regardless of type or shape, magnify sound and include the following components:

- A microphone to pick up sound
- An amplifier, which makes sound louder

- A receiver, which conveys sound to the ear
- A battery, which provides power for the hearing aid to work

Digital Versus Analog Hearing Aids

Prior to 2000, most hearing aids were analog aids (Fransman & Walker, 2007). *Analog hearing aids* work by increasing volume, but they have little capacity to distinguish pitch (bass sounds versus high-pitched sounds). Because the primary function is to amplify sound, all sounds are amplified indiscriminately. Consequently, although the ability to hear another person talk in a quiet environment is improved, attempting to hear a conversation in a noisy environment is more difficult because all sounds are amplified. Individuals using analog types of aids can control volume; but changing volume repeatedly is cumbersome and not helpful for understanding conversations in noisy environments.

Digital hearing aids change acoustic signals into a discrete series of digital signals so the audiologist can appropriately shape the hearing aid response to the individual's hearing loss. As a result, digital hearing aids can theoretically be programmed for each individual's hearing loss and provide more precision and clarity of sound. Many contain special "noise-reduction circuits" that aid in reducing background noise distraction. Digital hearing aids have become much more affordable in recent years, with technology options ranging from basic digital to premium digital with directional microphones.

Telecoil Circuitry

Some hearing aids have special features called *telecoil circuitry or tone control*. Hearing aids with telecoil circuitry feature have a special switch or push button *(T switch)* located on the hearing aid case, that activates the telecoil. A telecoil is a very small coil of wire that acts as an antenna, picking up electromagnetic energy that is then delivered to the receiver of the hearing aid and converted into sound. Also available is a plug called a boot or shoe, which is designed to fit over the end of a behind-the-ear hearing aid equipped with direct auditory input (DAI). This device enables individuals to be connected to an external sound source, such as a radio signal or microphone. It improves the signal-to-noise ratio, thereby enhancing sound quality. Telecoil circuitry enables individuals to use other assistive listening devices discussed later in this chapter.

Tone control is a feature on conventional analog hearing aids that allows the audiologist to modify frequency sensitivity of the hearing aid amplifier to best respond to the individual's hearing loss. For instance, individuals with hearing loss at higher frequencies have difficulty hearing some higher-pitched tones of speech. Tone control is an attempt to amplify the high frequencies without amplifying the lower frequencies.

Implantable Hearing Aids

Over the last several decades, research has been conducted to develop implantable hearing devices, which would be directly connected to the eardrum or to the small bones in the middle ear (Sichel, Freeman, Eliashar, Fleishman, & Sohmer, 2004). Another type of implantable hearing device is the bone-anchored hearing aid, which is connected to the mastoid bone in the skull with tiny screws. The device then transmits sound waves as vibrations, which through bone conduction, stimulate the cochlea of the ear (Gopen, 2007; Bosman, Snik, Mylanus, & Cremers, 2006; Hodgetts, Scollie, & Swain, 2006). Bone-anchored hearing aids may be used unilaterally or bilaterally (Stenfelt, 2005).

Hearing Aid Prescription

Hearing aid units are dispensed and fitted by audiologists and/or hearing aid dispensers. Hearing aids may be fitted to one or both ears. *Monaural* refers to fitting of a single hearing aid; *binaural* refers to fitting of two hearing aids. Recent trends show binaural fittings are becoming the norm for a variety of reasons, including improved localization skills, safety, and ease of hearing in noisy environments.

Most individuals are given a written contract that provides them with a 30-day trial evaluation period, after which, if they are not satisfied, they can receive a refund for the cost of the hearing aid, less any service charges. Although the hearing aid industry has become more regulated, it is highly recommended that individuals seeking a hearing aid consult with a licensed audiologist who specializes in dispensing of hearing aids. As always, a referral from a friend, family member, or trusted medical professional is the best way to assure the individual is working with a skilled and reputable professional.

Although hearing aids may improve hearing and may be beneficial for many individuals, they do not correct hearing in the way that glasses can improve vision to 20/20 (Desselle & Proctor, 2000). Hearing aids can improve volume but not always clarity of speech. Because analog hearing aids work as amplifiers, they make speech louder but not always clearer. In addition, analog hearing aids amplify not only speech but other sounds in the environment as well, which can interfere with the individual's ability to decipher speech. Individuals with hearing aids may need speech reading to help them fill in gaps in comprehension of speech that persist despite use of the hearing aid. Digital hearing aids have a unique advantage in that they can provide more volume to the soft sounds of speech and less volume to the louder background sounds that can interfere with understanding.

Hearing aids should be carefully prescribed to meet individual needs. For best practice, hearing aids should be dispensed with appropriate verification and orientation regarding proper care and use. Orientation serves a vital role in the success of hearing aid use by helping to establish realistic expectations. Additional audiological rehabilitation training or counseling will help individuals learn ways to enhance communication and minimize communication obstacles.

One potential barrier to effective hearing aid use is the attitude of the individual. Some individuals may resist using hearing aids because they believe society will view them as less capable. Although smaller, less conspicuous hearing aids have improved acceptance, negative attitudes toward hearing aids are one factor that may impede use for many who might benefit from these devices.

Hearing aids are delicate devices that need routine care and maintenance to ensure maximum function. Batteries must be replaced regularly. Individuals using hearing aids must be careful to protect hearing aids from damage to the internal components. Specifically, users should refrain from dropping these devices or, subjecting them to extremes in temperatures, excess moisture, or exposure to other substances, such as hair spray, that could damage the microphone or receiver.

Telephone Devices

Many different types of telephone devices are available to assist with telephone communication. Some of these devices are hearing aid compatible and work in conjunction with the hearing aid telecoil. Such telephones enable the hearing aid user to utilize the telecoil circuitry and thereby receive a more clear signal, without annoying acoustic feedback or squeal. Telecoil circuitry allows the hearing aid user to tap into the electromagnetic signal from the telephone; electromagnetic energy is then transferred to the receiver of the hearing aid and converted into sound. Not all phones in use today are compatible with telecoil, although the Federal Communication Commission (FCC) has made changes in statutes that require all new phones, including cell phones, to be hearing aid compatible.

Some other telephone devices may be used without a hearing aid. *Portable telephone amplifiers* can be slipped over a telephone receiver and may be useful for hard-of-hearing individuals who travel and need a louder signal. Other telephone amplification devices may be wired to the telephone handset so that volume is increased, allowing the user to control the amplification level. Public telephones equipped with amplifier handsets, although not always readily available, are becoming more common. These telephones are usually identified with an access sign.

Telecommunication Display Devices (TDD)

Telecommunication display devices (TDD), also called *teletypewriters (TTY)*, are used to transmit conversations in printed format over regular telephone lines. Individuals on both ends of the line must have compatible devices with which to type their messages and visualize the printed message on a screen or paper. If one individual does not have a TDD, a third-party system may be used or a relay operator may transmit the message to the other individual. Telecommunication relay services allow a person using TDD to communicate with another person using a voice telephone, with the relay operator acting as an interpreter. Special software is also available that allows a personal computer to interact with TDD and provide a synthesized speech signal. In addition, computers are allowing greater access for deaf and hard-of-hearing individuals with e-mail.

Assistive Listening Devices

Assistive listening devices (ALD) include a wide variety of equipment other than hearing aids that can be used by persons with hearing loss. Some devices may be used independently; others supplement hearing aids. As individuals with hearing loss may have more difficulty perceiving high-pitched sounds common in speech or hearing in background noise, assistive listening devices help to improve the signal-to-noise ratio by facilitating listening and reducing background noise and reverberation.

Hard-Wired Systems (Personal Listening Systems)

Hard wired systems are individual devices that amplify speech and minimize outside noise so that speech can be more easily understood. The systems must have a direct connection to the sound source, using either a microphone or a direct plug-in wire, to convey amplified speech signal directly to the receiver (a hearing aid, earphone headset, or neck loop) worn by the individual. When a microphone is used, the speaker talks into the microphone; the sound travels through a cord and then directly reaches the receiver worn by the listener. When a plug-in is used, a wire is plugged into the sound source (such as a television or a radio), and the sound travels through the wire directly to the individual's personal receiver. Using hard-wired systems with television or radio enables individuals with hearing loss to increase the volume on their personal receiver without altering the volume for others in the room.

Hard-wired systems are considered personal listening systems and are more useful in one-to-one communication as opposed to group settings. The systems are small, with the amplifier being contained in a pocket.

Large-Area Systems

Background noise often competes with speech sounds, creating a more challenging listening environment for individuals with hearing loss. Additional reverberation affects sound quality in large groups and brings a more distorted signal to hard-of-hearing individuals. Distance is another factor that has a negative effect for those with hearing loss. A number of devices to enhance hearing in group settings are available. Examples of these *large-area devices* include audio loop systems, FM systems, and infrared systems.

Audio Loop Systems

Audio loop systems are made up of a microphone, an amplifier, and a coil of wire (also called an induction coil) that loops around the seating area. Electricity flows through the coil creating an electromagnetic field that can be picked up by the telecoil of a hearing aid, which is itself activated through a T-switch or push button. The telecoil acts as an antenna and picks up the electromagnetic energy, delivering it to the user's hearing aid. Individuals using the audio loop must sit within or near the loop for it to operate effectively. Audio loop systems can be permanently installed in public meeting rooms, churches, or theaters, or they can be set up on an as needed basis.

FM Systems

FM systems are wireless devices that work much the same way as FM radios. Sound is picked up and transmitted through a frequency-modulated band directly to a receiver worn by the individual with hearing loss. Wireless FM systems have greatly reduced the hardware needed by persons with hearing loss, especially with regard to hearing aid compatibility. FM systems enhance listening in noisy environments by improving the signal-to-noise ratio

Infrared Systems

Infrared systems require installation of an infrared light emitter, which is usually piggybacked onto an existing public address system. Sound is transmitted by invisible, harmless infrared light waves and picked up by a receiver, which can be either a headset for use without a hearing aid or a device intended for use with a hearing aid equipped with a T-switch. These systems are best suited for use in rooms or meeting areas without windows, as sunlight affects the signal.

Captioning Services and Telecaption Adapters

Closed captioning may be used for television or movies in which printed dialog appears on a corner or at the bottom of the screen. Real-time captioning services display the text on a video monitor immediately. All televisions manufactured after July 1993 that are 13 inches or larger must be equipped with closed captioning option. Older models can utilize a decoder that is connected to the television. Captioned feature and educational films are available through a variety of distribution services as well.

Alerting Devices

Hearing enables individuals to respond to sounds such as sirens, the horn of an approaching car, the doorbell, or a baby's cry. Hearing loss can, therefore, hamper individuals' ability to respond to everyday environmental sounds, potentially increasing the risk of accidents and possibly increasing feelings of insecurity. A variety of devices and systems are available commercially to alert individuals with hearing loss to these cues. They may use visual cues, such as flashing lights; auditory cues, such as increased amplification of sound; or *tactile cues*, such as a vibrator. *Certified Hearing Guide Dogs* (International Dogs, Inc.), for example, are trained to react to certain environmental sounds (e.g., a telephone ringing). The dog does not bark but rather makes physical contact with the individual and then runs to the source of the sound.

Speech Reading (Lipreading)

Speech reading is a communication skill in which individuals with hearing loss watch for clues from the lips, tongue, and facial expression of the speaker. Only one-third of the English language is visible on the lips, so individuals who speech read often supplement meaning by observing facial expressions of the speaker and gathering conceptual cues (Myers & Thyer, 1997). Speech reading may also be supplemented with a manual communication system such as *cued speech*.

Speech reading requires good lighting. The speaker must face the individual who is speech reading and must be close enough to enable the individual to see the speaker's lip formation. The speaker should use a natural speaking voice and expression, avoiding distortions of the mouth through movements such as grimacing. Speech reading is more difficult when the speaker speaks very rapidly or enunciates poorly, uses distracting hand movements, or has a beard or a mustache that obstructs view of the lips. Speakers should avoid chewing, turning away from the listener, or moving about while talking. The speaker should get the listener's attention before beginning to speak and clarify statements as necessary.

Considerable concentration is required for most people with hearing loss to grasp the spoken word. It is a complex process that can be very tiring when conversation is extended.

Sign Language

Language is a set of symbols combined in a certain way to convey concepts, ideas, and emotions. There are many ways of transmitting language. *Speech* is the verbal expression of language concepts. *Sign language* is a means of communication in which specific hand configurations symbolize language concepts. Several types of sign language exists, with the two most common being *American Sign Language (ASL)* and *Signed English*.

American Sign Language is a distinct and complete language that contains linguistic components constituting a sophisticated, independent language. It is the native language of Deaf culture. ASL has its own grammar and syntax, idioms, and metaphors. It has no written form. Moreover, it is conceptual in nature, rather than word oriented. Signs of ASL are abstract symbols that are capable of expressing multiple elements simultaneously.

Signed English follows the syntax and linguistic structure of English. Often, people who use Signed English also mouth the words that they sign, a process called *simultaneous communication*.

Cued speech is another system of visual communication. It is phonetically based, using hand shapes to represent speech sounds.

Interpreters

Certified interpreters can provide an important communication link between the deaf or hard-of-hearing individual and the hearing world. Used in both group settings and one-to-one interactions, interpreters are able to translate information so that accurate communication can take place. In situations where it is important for the translation to be precise and accurate, such as professional medical or counseling situations, it is crucial that the interpreter be properly trained and be certified by the *Registry of Interpreters for the Deaf*. In particular situations, such as medical or counseling interactions, it is beneficial to use a professional interpreter with experience in mental health or medical paradigms who can properly assist with complex communication needs. Although family members sometimes serve as interpreters for deaf or hard-of-hearing individuals in more informal situations, in professional situations their use may obscure objective information, so it should be avoided if possible.

The presence of an interpreter can be intrusive and alter the dynamics of the medical or counseling interaction. Use of interpreters means that a third party will be present, reducing the sense of privacy that is normally expected in a number of professional situations. Certified interpreters, however, practice under a stringent code of ethics, which requires that all transactions must be strictly confidential. It takes some adjustment for the employer, counselor, physician, or other person working with the deaf or hard-of-hearing individual to become accustomed to having a third party present in situations that normally take place on a one-to-one basis.

■ PSYCHOSOCIAL ISSUES IN HEARING LOSS AND DEAFNESS

Deafness and Deaf Culture

The needs of people who are deaf or hard of hearing are different from those of individuals with other disabilities. Hearing is vital to verbal communication and to perception of environmental cues; thus all hearing loss interferes with daily function to some degree. The ability of individuals to cope with hearing loss depends on the type and degree of loss, the age of onset, and the extent to which the loss interferes with daily communication and activity.

Hearing loss affects every aspect and activity of an individual's life. It alters speech intelligibility and other basic aspects of hearing such as localization, recognition, or identification of sound.

Severe hearing loss or deafness experienced congenitally or in early childhood also has developmental implications. Hearing loss occurring prior to language development influences individuals' experience and opportunity to gain concepts generally taken for granted in the hearing world. Children learn many concepts from overheard conversations, background information from radio or television, and a multiplicity of other sources. Through this peripheral, daily communication, children learn cultural norms and expectations, generate and shape ideas, and form and enhance values and beliefs. Children who have severe hearing loss or are deaf are not exposed to many elements of communication that would otherwise enrich their language base, help them to formulate concepts, and impart social norms.

Individuals with congenital deafness or with hearing loss acquired before speech development require special programs to help them learn to communicate. Unfortunately, hearing loss in the very young is not always recognized immediately and may be misinterpreted as intellectual deficits, mental retardation, or behavior disorders. Normal development and healthy adjustment of children with hearing loss depend to a large degree on early diagnosis and treatment, early social and cultural influences, and parental attitudes and acceptance.

Diagnosis of deafness in a child often results in parental guilt, overprotection, or rejection. Professional assistance for the family of a newly diagnosed deaf infant may be critical to their acceptance of the child's needs and to their competence in providing a nurturing environment for the child's emotional development.

Individuals who have acquired a hearing loss during adulthood have memories of sound, language, and of previous function. Speech patterns have already been learned and can be maintained through speech and conversation therapy. Individuals who have acquired hearing loss in adulthood may, however, feel uncomfortable and fear that others will reject them if they admit their disability. They may deny that hearing loss exists or may develop strategies to hide hearing loss, such as dominating the conversation to minimize the necessity of understanding anyone else or accusing others of not speaking clearly or mumbling. Some individuals exhibit aggressive behavior as a reaction to their hearing loss; others may withdraw completely from situations in which they have difficulty in hearing. Being unable to understand what is being said, individuals with hearing loss may believe that laughter and talking of others are being directed toward them.

Hearing loss can lead to isolation, loneliness, and frustration, as well as to sensory deprivation. Hearing helps individuals communicate on a daily basis with family and friends, and in social and work settings. At the most basic level, hearing helps individuals keep in touch with the environment. Background sounds, such as the wind in the trees, children playing down the street, or a train whistle in the distance, keep individuals aware of what is happening in the outside world. Hearing also acts as a signal to action. A telephone ringing, a baby crying, the horn of an approaching car, and the sound of footsteps from behind, for example, are all cues for some type of action. Thus, not only must individuals with a loss of hearing alter activities for which hearing is vital, but they also experience a sense of vulnerability because of their inability to hear sounds that once served as cues to action or danger.

A distinction should be made between members of Deaf culture and those who are deaf. Using a capital "D" indicates individuals who describe themselves as a linguistic minority sharing a culture, not a medical condition (Phillips, 1996; Porter, 1999). From the vantage point of Deaf culture, deafness is not a disability, a deficiency, or a handicap, but rather a culture unto itself (Lane, 1995).

Culture influences knowledge, beliefs, attitudes, values, and perceptions. It underlies the meaning given to action and the means by which experiences in the world are organized and understood. One of the key components of culture is language, which is necessary for communication. Language is an important part of every cultural identity and determines to a great extent who talks with whom and what is discussed (Rendon, 1992). For those with hearing loss, there is no common language. Not all

individuals with severe or profound hearing loss use the same language to communicate. Some individuals use Signed English; some use American Sign Language; some rely to a large extent on speech reading to communicate. Especially for individuals who are prelingually deaf who use ASL as their primary language, English may viewed as a foreign language.

American Sign Language is a source of pride for the Deaf community. It is a true language, with its own structure and a syntax that has developed over time and that has no written form (Filer & Filer 2000). Consequently, individuals who use ASL and especially those who are prelingually deaf frequently become part of the larger Deaf culture.

The Deaf community has its own theater, literature, and schools, along with social rules that are different from those of the hearing community (Barnett, 1999). Differences, especially in social norms, patterns, and traditions, can cause misunderstandings and misperceptions by those in the hearing world. Members of the Deaf culture have their own rules for behaviors, such as for getting the attention of individuals with whom they would like to communicate. Stomping a foot or tapping the hand of the individual to get his or her attention may be perfectly acceptable social behavior in the Deaf community, but may be viewed as rude by those in the hearing world. Consequently, individuals in the Deaf community may tend to associate with others in the Deaf community rather than those in the hearing world, may prefer state residential schools for educating the deaf rather than mainstreaming, and may reject efforts to incorporate them into the hearing world. In some instances, pride in the Deaf culture may even preclude procedures such as cochlear implants that could improve ability to hear (Olson, 2006). Individuals in the Deaf community may believe that attempts to correct their hearing imply that they have a medical condition that needs a cure, perpetuating the view of the Deaf as disabled. Some may go as far as to view efforts to cure deafness as an attempt to obliterate Deaf culture (Tucker, 1998).

The Deaf culture does not exist in a vacuum. Individuals may be imbedded in the Deaf culture, but they are also imbued with values, attitudes and behaviors that are part of a larger national culture as well as often part of ethnic minority cultures (Moore, 2001). This fact creates another layer of diversity.

Psychological Issues in Hearing Loss and Deafness

Hearing loss is often associated with isolation because of the very nature of the disability itself. Grief reactions are not uncommon for individuals with acquired hearing loss. These individuals have memories of sounds. Their inability to hear cherished sounds, such as the voices of loved ones, music, or the chirping of birds, may be a difficult loss to accept.

Because hearing loss is an invisible disability, denial is common, especially for those who acquire a hearing loss later in life. They may react with increased sensitivity or irritability when they do not understand words. The increased social pressure to understand may cause anxiety and frustration, and they may avoid activities and interactions that they once enjoyed. Unwillingness to acknowledge hearing loss may result in individuals' refusal to participate in hearing evaluations or reluctance to wear hearing aids.

Individuals with an acquired hearing loss, especially if the onset is sudden, may experience depression. The suddenness of the loss does not permit individuals with the opportunity to adapt gradually as hearing diminishes and, consequently, they are unlikely to have developed signing skills. Depression can also interfere with learning and using new communication skills. Its effects are circular; depression is a barrier to communication, thus intensifying feelings of isolation and making the individual more depressed. Counselors trained in sign language may not be readily available, and the use of an interpreter for counseling sessions may increase individuals' reluctance to participate or to disclose feelings openly.

Any and all of the emotional states experienced by the adult with hearing loss may be experienced by the parents of children who have been identified as hard of hearing or deaf. Just as adults with hearing loss must work through their feelings to achieve a healthy adjustment, so must parents before they can be of optimal assistance to their child.

Individuals who have hearing loss depend heavily on visual channels and on manual means of communication. The development of additional medical conditions that threaten these resources is of increased concern. A visual impairment or a condition that affects the hands, such as rheumatoid arthritis, can seriously hamper an individual's accustomed means of communication if using ASL or Signed English, necessitating additional training in new ways of communicating.

■ ACTIVITIES AND PARTICIPATION WITH HEARING LOSS AND DEAFNESS

Many daily activities involve the sense of hearing. For individuals with hearing loss, even simple transactions—such as purchasing items from a local store, communicating with a repair person, or obtaining directions—requires additional means of communication. In some instances, use of a third party as an interpreter may be a solution; however, individuals who are hard of hearing or deaf may resent the loss of privacy or loss of the sense of independence associated with the use of an interpreter.

Signal dogs trained to alert their deaf owners to environmental sounds or signals are increasing in popularity. Special devices are necessary to make daily environmental sounds, such as a knock on the door, known to individuals with hearing loss. Technology and special aids become, in many instances, a necessity.

Everyday activities with family members may require more effort on the part of all involved. For instance, without awareness and sensitivity of other family members, individuals with hearing loss may be unable to participate actively in family conversations at mealtime or engage in small talk while performing various tasks. They may also find themselves increasingly left out of family decision making and discussions.

Depending on the degree of hearing loss, special activities—such as watching television or attending movies, plays, and concerts—may also be affected. The special devices mentioned previously may help individuals participate more fully in such activities. In addition, decoders that provide captioned programming may be available to enable individuals with hearing loss to enjoy television.

Although hearing loss does not directly affect sexual activity, verbal communication during lovemaking may no longer be possible, which may be viewed by some individuals with hearing loss as an emotional loss. Individuals who are single may have more difficulty meeting potential partners and establishing communication that could lead to a more intimate relationship.

The social environment of individuals with hearing loss is profoundly altered due to the need for alternative means of communication. Individuals who have been deaf since birth or early childhood may integrate well with the Deaf community, where a common language is shared. Those who acquire hearing loss later in life, however, frequently do not join the Deaf community and may feel more isolated, feeling that they fit into neither the Deaf community or the hearing world.

Language plays an important role in regulating social play interactions and is paramount for framing and setting up play activities. Children who are deaf or hard of hearing may have difficulty developing cooperative play with hearing playmates. Promoting socialization between children with hearing loss and hearing peers includes building on the strengths of the children and fostering a shared communication system that encourages social integration. Hearing loss at an early age also has implications for literacy. Individuals who have been deaf from an early age usually have a literacy level of fourth to fifth grade after high school (Barnett, 1999). Low literacy rates may be attributed to lack of consensus on educational methods. Emphasis is often placed on techniques of communication, with less emphasis on content matter. In addition, because English is often a second language to individuals who are deaf, children who are deaf may face the same educational barriers as those experienced by other minority groups whose primary language is not English.

People with acquired hearing loss in adulthood are more likely to maintain social and cultural contacts with the hearing world because they have grown up with the language and culture of the hearing world. Many people, who were deaf from an early age and use ASL as their primary language, however, feel that they are part of the Deaf community, which has established a culture that has its own specific norms and characteristics, along with its own language. Members of this culture tend to view deafness not as a disability, but rather as an alternative culture and associated lifestyle. Individuals who do not speak the language are frequently viewed as outsiders and are not readily integrated into the Deaf culture.

Individuals with hearing loss may limit social contacts to family members and a few close friends, or they may avoid social contacts altogether because of their inability to understand what is being said. Difficulty in understanding verbal communication can cause withdrawal from social situations in an effort to avoid the embarrassment of giving inappropriate responses to questions or statements. Lack of understanding by others can contribute to social isolation. New acquaintances who are unfamiliar with hearing loss or unaware of individuals' inability to hear may perceive them as aloof or even rude because of their failure to respond to a friendly statement that they did not hear.

Individuals with hearing loss may have more difficulty keeping up with conversations in group settings, especially if others in the group are unaware of or insensitive to their needs. Group settings with poor lighting make lip-reading more difficult, and competing sounds, such as the rattling of dishes in a restaurant, may make communication difficult even for individuals with milder hearing loss.

Engaging in conversation requires cooperation from others. Some people may feel uncomfortable or impatient while attempting to communicate with individuals with hearing loss and, consequently, may avoid contact with them. Some may consider deafness to carry a social stigma because of myths and misconceptions about hearing loss. Such attitudes build a barrier to acceptance by others and inclusion in the larger social community. Societal responses can create difficult and stressful situations for individuals with hearing loss, discouraging their further participation in social functions.

A number of support groups directed toward individuals with adult- or late-onset hearing loss are available, including Self Help for Hard of Hearing People (SHHH) and the Association of Late Deafened Adults (ALDA). In addition to offering support to individuals who are hard of hearing or deaf, SHHH and ALDA strive to increase community understanding about the rights and needs of individuals with hearing loss as well as to make social environments more accessible. Many communities also have other types of support groups for people with hearing loss.

Although family members serve as a support group for individuals with hearing loss, their attitudes may also impede individuals' acceptance of their condition and subsequent rehabilitation. Family members may perceive a hearing loss as feigned or may attribute the difficulty to inattention. As a result, they may become angry, ignore the individual, or exclude him or her from conversations rather than learning techniques to enhance the individual's ability to maintain an active role in conversation. In many cases, family members who serve as interpreters for those with hearing loss may begin to resent their role, feeling stifled in social interactions.

■ VOCATIONAL ISSUES IN HEARING LOSS

Individuals with hearing loss face the same issues with regard to employment as others with disability; however, additional special vocational issues must be considered in the former case. Many jobs require individuals to be alert to auditory cues to perform or to maintain safety. Most jobs also require communication with co-workers and/or customers. People who are deaf or hard of hearing may have difficulty receiving instructions or supervision or participating in staff meetings or in-service training. In addition, they may have difficulty interacting as part of work-related social functioning. Assistive devices may be needed to help them with basic communication, or there may be a need for job restructuring, redesigning procedures, or redelegation of assignments to accommodate their communication needs.

Just as there are myths and stereotypes about hearing loss in the social world, so there are myths and stereotypes in the world of work. Employers and fellow workers may not understand hearing loss and may be unaware of the special needs of individuals who are deaf or hard-of-hearing or the special techniques available to enhance communication with those who experience it. Because hearing loss is an invisible disability, co-workers or supervisors may not recognize the need for special accommodations or may feel that individuals with hearing loss are feigning their degree of disability. In some instances, individuals' lack of ability to hear may be interpreted as lack of intellectual ability, and individuals with hearing loss may be relegated to jobs requiring less cognitive ability.

In the work setting, individuals with hearing loss may need special assistive devices, communication aids, and signaling devices. The use of such devices is often dependent on the availability and expense of the purchase and installation of the special items. Equipment may be prioritized according to need if funds are limited. For example, a signaling device that is crucial for safety may be considered vital, whereas equipment that would enhance individuals' performance may not receive as high a priority.

Because visual cues are so important to communication for individuals with hearing loss, good lighting in the workplace is a necessity. Many individuals with hearing loss experience discomfort with loud noises; therefore, noise levels in the environment should be evaluated. In some instances, it may be necessary for individuals to wear ear protectors to prevent further hearing loss. Room acoustics must also be considered, because the reverberation of sound in an environment can interfere with the effectiveness of a hearing aid.

Hearing aids can greatly enhance some performance in the work setting. Although technological advances have made hearing aids more durable, they are intricate devices that may be susceptible to damage from environmental factors. These aids are sensitive to extremes of temperature especially extreme cold and they require protection from perspiration in hot and humid environments.

Individuals with hearing loss are a heterogeneous group and should be considered as such. Although special needs associated with hearing loss should be considered, individuals' unique talents and interests should also be taken into account in helping individuals with hearing loss to adjust to the work environment. With the use of assistive devices, many job opportunities not previously open to individuals with hearing loss are now well within the range of possibilities. Central to success in vocational placement of individuals who are deaf or have hearing loss is employer familiarity with individuals' accommodation needs (Schroedel & Geyer, 2001). In addition, attitudinal barriers still exist and may preclude the individual with hearing loss from obtaining satisfactory employment.

CASE STUDIES

Case 1

Mr. D. is a 35-year-old construction worker who is experiencing moderate bilateral noise-induced hearing loss. He began working in construction while in high school, and has never done any other type of work. Although he had been encouraged to wear hearing protection when at work, especially when using noisy equipment, Mr. D. neglected to take this step, saying that hearing protectors are uncomfortable and make it difficult to talk with other workers.

1. Which specific issues about Mr. D.'s type and level of hearing loss would you address?
2. Which interventions might be helpful for Mr. D. regarding his hearing loss?
3. How would Mr. D.'s hearing loss affect his ability to continue in his current line of work?

Case 2

Ms. N. is a 42-year-old registered nurse who has recently developed hearing loss as a result of Meniere's disease. On audiological evaluation, she was found to have hearing loss in both ears at the 45-decibel range. She currently works as a staff nurse in her local community hospital.

1. To what extent will Ms. N.'s degree of hearing loss impair her ability to continue to function in her current occupation?
2. Given the type and extent of Ms. N.'s hearing loss, which adaptive devices or reasonable accommodations may help her maintain her current employment?
3. What impact will her Meniere's disease have on Ms. N.'s ability to continue in her current line of work?
4. Which other specific issues might you want to address with Ms. N.?

■ REFERENCES

Baloh, R. W. (2004). Hearing and equilibrium. In L. Goldman & D. Ausiello (Eds.), *Cecil textbook of medicine* (pp. 2436–2442). Philadelphia: W. B. Saunders.

Barnett, S. (1999). Clinical and cultural issues in caring for deaf people. *Family Medicine, 31*(1), 17–22.

Berg, A. L., Ip, S. C., Hurst, M., & Herb, A. (2007). Cochlear implants in young children: Informed consent as a process and current practices. *American Journal of Audiology, 16,* 13–28.

Berman, S. (2007). The end of an era in otitis research. *New England Journal of Medicine, 356*(3), 300–302.

Bosman, A. J., Snik, A. F. F., Mylanus, E. A. M., & Cremers, C. W. R. J. (2006). Fitting range of the BAHA cordelle. *International Journal of Audiology, 45,* 429–437.

Chute, P. A. (2004). Cochlear implants: An evolving journey. *ASHA Leader, 9*(3), 7–8.

Claussen, C. F. (2007). Tinnitus. In R. E. Rakel & E. T. Bope (Eds.), *Conn's current therapy.* (pp. 35–40). Philadelphia: W. B. Saunders.

Daniell, W. E., Swan, S. S., McDaniel, M. M., Camp, J. E., Cohen, M. A., & Stebbins, J. G. (2006). Noise exposure and hearing loss prevention programs after 20 years of regulations in the United States. *Occupational & Environmental Medicine, 63*(5), 343–351.

Desselle, D. D., & Proctor, T. K. (2000). Advocating for the elderly hard-of-hearing population: The deaf people we ignore. *Social Work, 45*(3), 277–281.

Edwards, B. (2007). The future of hearing aid technology. *Trends in Amplification, 11*(1), 31–45.

Filer, R. D., & Filer, P. A. (2000). Practical considerations for counselors working with hearing children of deaf parents. *Journal of Counseling and Development, 78,* (1), 37–43

Fischetti, M. (2003). Cochlear implants: To hear again. *Scientific American, 286*(6), 82–83.

Fransman, D., & Walker, S. (2007). Digital hearing aids: A life transformed. *Learning Disability Practice, 10*(3), 16–19.

Gates, G. A., & Miyamoto, R. T. (2003). Cochlear implants. *New England Journal of Medicine, 349*(5), 421–423.

Geers, A. E. (2004). Speech, language, and reading skills after early cochlear implantation. *Archives of Otolaryngology/Head and Neck Surgery, 130,* 634–638.

Gopen, Q. S. (2007). By the way, doctor: What can be done for sudden hearing loss in one ear. *Harvard Health Letter, 32*(6), 8.

Gordon-Salant, S. (2005). Hearing loss and aging: New research findings and clinical implications. *Journal of Rehabilitation Research and Development, 42*(4), 9–24.

Hansson, E. E., & Mansson, N. O. (2005). Treatment for benign paroxysmal positional vertigo: A case study. *Advances in Physiotherapy, 7,* 183–186.

Hendley, J. O. (2002). Otitis media. *New England Journal of Medicine, 347* (15), 1169–1174.

Hodgetts, W. E., Scollie, S. D., & Swain, R. (2005). Effects of applied contact force and volume control setting on output force levels of the BAHAr softband. *International Journal of Audiology, 45,* 301–308.

Kirk, K. I., Firszt, J. B., Hood, L. J., & Holt, R. F. (2006). New directions in pediatric cochlear implantation: Effects on candidacy *ASHA Leader, 11*(16), 6–7, 14–15.

Kovar, M., Jepson, T., & Jones, S. (2006). Diagnosing and treating benign paroxysmal positional vertigo. *Journal of Gerontological Nursing, 32*(12), 22–27.

Lane, H. (1995). Constructions of deafness. *Disability and Society, 10*(2), 171–189.

Lerner, P. K., & Eng, N. (2005). Speech, language, hearing, and swallowing disorders. In H. H. Zaretsky, E. F. Richter III, & M. G. Eisenberg (Eds.), *Medical aspects of disability* (3rd ed., pp. 289–324). New York: Springer.

Levitt, H. (2007). A historical perspective on digital hearing aids: How digital technology has changed modern hearing aids. *Trends in Amplification, 11*(1), 7–24.

Luterman, D. (2007). Technology and early childhood deafness. *ASHA Leader, 12*(6), 43.

McMurray, J. S. (2007). Otitis media. In R. E. Rakel & E. T. Bope (Eds.), *Conn's current therapy* (pp. 228–230). Philadelphia: W. B. Saunders.

Meyer, T. A., & Lambert, P. R. (2007). Meniere's disease. In R. E. Rakel & E. T. Bope (Eds.), *Conn's current therapy* (pp. 237–239.) Philadelphia: W. B. Saunders.

Moore, C. L. (2001). Racial and ethnic members of under-represented groups with hearing loss and VR services: Explaining the disparity in closure success rates. *Journal of Applied Rehabilitation Counseling, 33*(1), 15–20.

Moore, C. L. (2001). *Educating the deaf: Psychology, principles, and practices* (5th ed.). Boston: Houghton Mifflin.

Moores, D. F. (2005). Cochlear implants: An update. *American Annals of the Deaf, 150*(4), 327–328.

Myers, L. L., & Thyer, A. (1997). Social work practice with deaf clients: Issues in culturally competent assessment. *Social Work in Health Care, 26*(1), 61–74.

Nelson, D. I., Nelson, R. Y., Concha-Barrientos, M., & Fingerhut, M. (2005). The global burden of occupational noise-induced hearing loss. *American Journal of Industrial Medicine, 48*(6), 446–458.

Nichols, A. D. (2006). Hearing loss: Perceptions and solutions. *Nursing Homes Magazine,* October, 66–69. www.nursinghomesmagazine.com.

Nicholas, J. G., & Geers, A. E. (2006). Effects of early auditory experience on the spoken language of deaf children at 3 years of age. *Ear and Hearing, 27,* 286–289.

Olson, A. D. (2006). Counseling adults prior to a cochlear implant. *ASHA Leader, 11*(13), 5, 18–19.

Paradise, J. L., Feldman, H. M., Campbell, T. F., Dollaghan, C. A., Rockette, H. E., Pitcairn, D. L., et al. (2007). Tympanostomy tubes and developmental outcomes at 9 to 11 years of age. *New England Journal of Medicine, 356*(3), 248–261.

Phillips, B. A. (1996). Bringing culture to the forefront: Formulating diagnostic impressions of deaf and hard-of-hearing people at times of medical crisis. *Professional Psychology: Research and Practice, 27*(2), 137–144.

Porter, A. (1999). Sign-language interpretation in psychotherapy with deaf patients. *American Journal of Psychotherapy, 53*(2). 163–176.

Rendon, M. E. (1992). Deaf culture and alcohol and substance abuse. *Journal of Substance Abuse Treatment, 9* 103–110.

Robertson, C., Kerr, M., Garcia, C., & Halterman, E. (2007). Noise and hearing protection: Latino construction workers' experiences. *AAOHN Journal, 55*(4), 153–160.

Saxon, J. P., Holmes, A. E., & Spitznagel, R. J. (2001). Impact of a cochlear implant on job functioning. *Journal of Rehabilitation, 67*(3), 49–54.

Schorr, E. A. (2007). Early cochlear implant experience and emotional functioning during childhood: Loneliness in middle and late childhood. *Volta Review, 106*(3) (monograph), 365–379.

Schroedel, J. G., and Geyer, P. D. (2001). Enhancing the career advancement of workers with hearing loss: Results from a national follow-up survey. *Journal of Applied Rehabilitation Counseling, 32*(3), 35–44.

Shafer, D. N. (2006). Early hearing diagnosis key to language skills. *ASHA Leader, 11*(14), 5, 53.

Sherwood, L. (2007) Ear: Hearing and equilibrium. In L. Sherwood (Eds.), *Human physiology: From cells to systems* (6th ed., pp. 208–220). Belmont, CA. Thompson/Brooks-Cole.

Sichel, J. Y., Freeman, S., Eliashar, R., Fleishman, Z., & Sohmer, H. (2004). New approach for implantable hearing aids: A feasibility study. *Annals of Otolaryngology, Rhinotogology, and Laryngology, 113*, 936–940.

Steel, K. P. (2000). New interventions in hearing impairment. *British Medical Journal, 320*(7235), 622–629.

Stenfelt, S. (2005). Bilateral fitting of BAHAs and BAHAr fitted in unilateral deaf persons: Acoustical aspects. *International Journal of Audiology, 44*, 178–189.

Thibodeau, L. M. (2006). Five important questions about FM systems and cochlear implants. *ASHA Leader, 11*(16), 22–23.

Thorp, M. A., & James, A. L. (2005). Prosper Meniere. *Lancet, 366*, 2137–2139.

Tomblin, J. B., Barker, B. A., Spencer, L. J., Zhang, X., & Gantz, B. J. (2005). The effect of age at cochlear implants initial stimulation on expressive language growth in infants and toddlers. *Journal of Speech, Language, and Hearing Research, 48*, 853–867.

Tucker, B. P. (1998), Deaf culture, cochlear implants, and elective disability. *Hastings Center Report, 28*(4), 6–14.

van Cruijsen, N., Jaspers, J. P. C., van de Wiel, H. B. M., Wit, H. P., & Albers, F. W. J. (2006). Psychological assessment of patients with Meniere's disease. *International Journal of Audiology, 45*, 496–502.

Williams, P. J. (2000). Genetic causes of hearing loss. *New England Journal of Medicine, 342*(15), 1101–1109.

Zeng, F. G. (2004). Trends in cochlear implants. *Trends in Amplification, 8*(1), 1–34.

Chapter 7

Intellectual and Developmental Disabilities

The term *developmental disability* was first instituted with the Developmental Disabilities Act of 1975 (PL 94-103). This term was substituted for the categorically defined conditions such as mental retardation, cerebral palsy, and epilepsy. Although the definition, categorization, and classification of developmental disability have changed significantly since 1975, the general term continues to encompasses a wide variety of conditions that occur in childhood, are lifelong, affect intellectual and/or physical functioning, and require ongoing special services and support.

Defining disability can provide guidance for assessment, treatment, or management of specific conditions and can be used to determine eligibility for services. Unfortunately, defining disability can also be a basis for labeling, stereotyping, discrimination, and segregation. In an attempt to avoid such pitfalls, the Developmental Disabilities Assistance and Bill of Rights Act of 1990 emphasized functional capacity rather than categorizations and stressed empowerment of individuals with developmental disabilities (McLaughlin & Wehman, 1996).

The Developmental Disabilities Assistance and Bill of Rights Act of 2000 defines developmental disability as "a severe chronic disability of an individual that:

a) is attributable to mental or physical impairment or combination of mental and physical impairment;

b) is manifested before the individual attains the age of 22;

c) is likely to continue indefinitely;

d) results in substantial functional limitations in three or more of the following areas of major life activity; self-care, receptive and expressive language, learning, mobility, self-direction, capacity for independent living, and economic self-sufficiency,

e) reflects the individual's need for a combination and sequence of special, interdisciplinary, or generic services; individualized support; or other forms of assistance that are of lifelong or extended duration and are individually planned and coordinated" (Developmental Disabilities Assistance and Bill of Rights Act of 2000, Public Law 106-402).

Many of the needs and concerns of individuals with developmental disabilities are the same as those of individuals without disability. No matter how severe the condition, individuals with developmental disability have the capacity to learn, grow, and develop throughout life. A major focus of working with individuals with developmental disability is identifying specific needs, developing strategies that minimize the degree of limitations experienced, and providing necessary supports to enhance functional capacity. Although the family is an important factor when working with individuals with any disability, family context is especially important in the case of individuals with developmental disability.

Although the causes and characteristics of specific developmental disabilities vary, a common feature of developmental disabilities is, functional limitation in one or more areas of function:

- Speech and/or language
- Attention and/or affect
- Cognitive or learning ability
- Self-direction and/or social behavior
- Motor skills and mobility
- Self-care and independence

Developmental disability encompasses a wide range of intellectual and physical disabilities, including conditions such as cerebral palsy (discussed in Chapter 3), spina bifida (discussed in Chapter 4), and epilepsy (discussed in Chapter 3). This chapter focuses on some of the more common intellectual and developmental disabilities classified in the *DSM-IV-TR* as conditions diagnosed in infancy, childhood, or adolescence.

■ INTELLECTUAL DISABILITY

Intellectual disability occurs in about 2% to 3% of the population (Daily, Ardinger, & Holmes, 2000) and is a condition in which there is impairment in both intellectual and adaptive function. In the *DSM-IV-TR*, this condition is termed *mental retardation*. The American Association of Intellectual and Developmental Disabilities (AAIDD; formerly the American Association on Mental Retardation [AAMR]), in an attempt to find a more socially acceptable and less stigmatizing way of describing this multidimensional condi-

tion, has changed the term to *intellectual disability*. Although the change in terminology is not yet reflected in the *DSM* descriptions and classifications, the term intellectual disability is becoming more widely used.

Intellectual disability is characterized by:

> significant limitations both in intellectual functioning and in adaptive behavior as expressed in conceptual, social, and practical adaptive skills. This disability originates before age 18. (AAIDD, 2002)

Many individuals with intellectual disability also have other medical conditions or sensory or motor impairments that further affect their functional capacity. Because both intellectual and adaptive function are considered as essential features in intellectual disability, performance in both areas must be measured before a diagnosis of intellectual disability can be made.

Diagnosis of Intellectual Disability

A diagnosis of intellectual disability is made through measuring both *intellectual function* and *adaptive behavior*. Intelligence refers to individuals' ability to reason, think abstractly, learn, and comprehend complex ideas. Limitations in intellectual functioning are usually measured through administration of individualized standardized intelligence tests such as the *Weschsler Intelligence Scales for Children* or the *Stanford–Binet Intelligence Scale*. The results of these tests are represented as the *IQ* (*intelligence quotient*). Classification of intellectual disability in relation to intellectual functioning is made when the score falls at least two standard deviations below the mean for that instrument, taking into account the standard error of measurement for the test. Consequently, rather than a finite score, scores for classification are reported as ranges (see Table 7-1).

Adaptive behavior is a multidimensional concept, and some behaviors are difficult to

Table 7-1   Classification of Mental Retardation

Classification	IQ
Mild	50–55 to 70
Moderate	35–40 to 50–55
Severe	20–25 to 35–40
Profound	Below 20–25

Source: American Psychiatric Association, 2000.

measure. Adaptive behavior must be considered in the context of the developmental stage of the individual as well as in the context of the individual's specific culture and environment. Three domains of adaptive behavior have emerged from numerous studies that have been conducted to delineate the concept. These domains consist of conceptual, social, and practical skills in the environment, which enable individuals with developmental disability to manage tasks of every day life (Luckasson, Borthwick-Duffy, Buntinx, Coulter, Craig, Reeve, et al., 2002). Examples of conceptual, social, and practical skills can be found in Table 7-2.

A number of standardized tests have been developed to measure adaptive functioning such as the *Vineland Adaptive Behavior Scales* (Carter, Volkmar, Sparrow, Want, Lord, et al., 1998; Sparrow, Balla, & Cicchetti, 1984; Conoley & Kramer, 1989) and the American Association on Mental Retardation Adaptive Behavior Scale (ABS) (Lambert, Nihira, & Leland, 1993; Impara & Plake, 1998). The ABS consists of two versions: A School and Community version (ABS-S: 2) (Lambert et al., 1993) and a Residential and Community version (ABS-RC: 2) (Lambert et al., 1993). The School and Community version measures adaptive behavior as it relates to independence and responsibility, whereas the Residential and Community version relates to problem behaviors.

Rather than relying solely on adaptive test scores, information from additional sources—such as teachers and family members—is typically used to provide a more complete picture of the individual's strengths and limitations. Adaptive behavior is typically assessed through observation of the individual as he or she performs various skills used to function in everyday life. Skills assessed usually include communication, calculation, self-direction, social skills, activities of daily living, and job-related skills.

When individuals 18 years of age or younger demonstrate an intellectual capacity that is below average (below IQ = 70) and when they demonstrate functional impairment in at least two or more areas of adaptive functioning, a diagnosis of intellectual disability (mental retardation) is made (American Psychiatric Association, 2000). Interpretation of scores from testing, whether intelligence testing or testing of adaptive function, should always be made in the context of the individual, including cultural and environmental variations, language ability, and any sensory, motor, and behavioral factors that may affect testing results. Factors such as the individual's environment and the degree of stimulation and support he or she has received within that environment can also affect the person's abilities. For example, individuals who interpret questions or responses differently owing to their cultural background or who are being given a test not in their native language may

---

Table 7-2   Examples of Adaptive Skills

Conceptual Skills

* Receptive and expressive language
* Reading and writing
* Money concepts
* Self-direction

Social Skills

* Interpersonal skills
* Gullibility and naiveté
* Ability to follow rules and laws
* Responsibility

Practical Skills

* Activities of daily living
  - Eating
  - Toileting
  - Dressing
* Instrumental activities of daily living
  - Preparing meals
  - Housekeeping
  - Telephone use
  - Money management
* Job skills
* Maintain safety

---

have scores that are not reflective of their actual intellectual capacity. Likewise, physical discomfort or other medical conditions may affect an individual's ability to perform to maximum capacity during testing. Consequently, test scores alone are not absolute.

Classification of Intellectual Disability

There are varying degrees of intellectual disability. In the past, degrees of severity of intellectual disability were classified through the classification system as outlined in Table 7-1. More recently, the AAIDD has developed another system for conceptualizing levels of severity of intellectual disability. Rather than defining intellectual disability in terms of test scores or impairments, AAIDD defines intellectual disability in terms of the types of supports individuals need to function on a

day-to-day basis. The AAIDD classifications of mental retardation are as follows:

* *Intermittent:* supports required periodically, or on a short-term basis during times of transition or crisis; when supports are needed, they may be either high or low intensity.
* *Limited:* low-intensity, time-limited supports needed for specific needs, such as job training or school transition.
* *Extensive:* ongoing regular supports needed on a low-intensity basis to maintain adequate function in home or work environment.
* *Pervasive:* extensive, ongoing, high-intensity support required for safety and well-being (American Association on Mental Retardation, 1992; Luckasson et al., 2002).

Intellectual disability is a complex and life-long condition. Degrees of severity of intellectual disability can range from mild to profound. Approximately 90% of individuals with intellectual disability are classified in the mild mental retardation range (Volkmar, Klin, & Paul, 2004).

Individuals with intellectual disability have a wide range of abilities as well as disabilities. The extent of support needed varies with the individual and with his or her particular circumstances. Some individuals with intellectual disability may also have delays in motor skills development, speech and language problems, or problems with vision or hearing. In addition, emotional challenges and vulnerabilities may be caused by pathologic or environmental factors. Early intervention, which considers all intellectual, physical, environmental, and social factors, is essential to foster the individual's attainment of his or her full potential.

Causes of Intellectual Disability

The causes of intellectual disability are numerous and can include genetic and/or environmental factors. In approximately 50% of cases of intellectual disability, the cause cannot be determined. Studies indicate that a substantial number of cases of intellectual disability are due to genetic abnormalities, such as *fragile X syndrome* or *trisomy* 21 (Down syndrome) (Boyd, 2005). The most common identified genetic cause of intellectual disability in the United States is Down syndrome (Yang, Rasmussen, & Friedman, 2002).

Intellectual disability can be caused by conditions before or after birth. Congenital causes of intellectual disability include brain malformations (such as *neural tube defects*) or chromosomal abnormalities (such as Down syndrome, fragile X syndrome, or Rett syndrome). Prenatal causes of intellectual disability may include maternal exposure to infections such as rubella or herpes, maternal abuse of drugs or alcohol, maternal exposure to toxic chemicals or radiation, or exposure to prescription drugs that have *teratogenic* (producing abnormal fetal development) effects. Conditions in utero that cause the fetus to experience **hypoxia** (lack of oxygen supply) can also be prenatal causes of intellectual disability.

Intellectual disability can be caused by brain injury to the infant during the birth process or trauma experienced during childhood as a result of accident or abuse. Childhood infections, such as meningitis; exposure to toxic substances, such as lead; metabolic disorders, such as *phenylketonuria* (PKU) or hypothyroidism; malnutrition; and psychological and social deprivation in childhood are additional causes of intellectual disability (Koger, Schettler, & Weiss, 2005).

Functional Ability

Individuals with intellectual disability have below-average general intellectual functioning for their stage of development as well as limitations in adaptive functioning or basic skills needed to manage age-appropriate tasks and demands of everyday life, such as communication, conceptualization, self-care, self-direction, self-sufficiency, and safety. Although actual functional capacity depends on many individual factors, in general functional disability according to level of intellectual functioning can be classified as mild, moderate, severe, or profound.

Mild Intellectual Disability

Generally, individuals with mild intellectual disability are considered capable of attaining a higher level of intellectual functioning. During preschool years, individuals with mild intellectual disability are generally capable of attaining social and communication skills consistent with their peers; consequently, some individuals may not be distinguishable from other children in their age group. Individuals with mild intellectual disability will likely be able to obtain employment and live independently or with minimal support and supervision, although there may be a need for additional support and guidance when individuals are placed in particularly stressful or new situations. Many individuals in this category can live independently in the community.

Moderate Intellectual Disability

Individuals with moderate intellectual disability, in general, may require more supervision in activities of daily living, although they can usually manage self-care. Processing abstract information is generally difficult. Individuals with moderate intellectual disability are usually capable of learning some vocational skills, although they may function best in a semi-independent or partially supervised work environment, such as supported employment. They may have differing degrees of expressive and receptive language skills. They are generally able to live in the community, in a group home, or in a semi-independent setting.

Severe Intellectual Disability

Individuals with severe intellectual disability generally have limited communication skills and poorly developed motor skills. While they are school age, they may attain some elementary self-care skills and may learn to read and write on a limited basis; however, for the most part, individuals with severe intellectual disability will require close supervision for most tasks. In adulthood, they may live in community group homes, in supported apartments or homes, or with their families. Many individuals with severe intellectual disability have an associated medical disability, which compounds their limitations of function. Most individuals at this level respond best to a consistent caregiver and a low-stimulus environment. Because of the severity of the condition, close supervision and support in most daily activities are usually needed.

Profound Intellectual Disability

Individuals with profound intellectual disability often have a number of other medical and physical disabilities that further limit function. For the most part, individuals in this category are dependent on others for all care.

Psychosocial Issues in Intellectual Disability

The diagnosis of intellectual disability in young children is often missed because of misconceptions about the presentation of intellectual disability or the belief that young children cannot be tested (Daily, Ardinger, & Holmes, 2000). Identifying intellectual disability in young children requires a complete child and family history, including information about the pregnancy. Early-intervention programs or rehabilitation services are crucial to enable individuals to reach their optimal level of functional capacity, to build on strengths, and to identify talents. Individuals with intellectual disability may be gifted in areas of art and music, for example.

Activities and Participation in Intellectual Disability

Intellectual disability, although diagnosed in childhood, is not simply a childhood disability. Individuals with intellectual disability live into adulthood and increasingly are living into older age, which may mean an increasing prevalence of chronic disease (Noble, 2001) and multiple and complex health problems that change over the life span (Prater & Zylstra, 2006). Individuals with intellectual disability who develop hypertension, diabetes, or other chronic medical conditions or psychiatric conditions present additional challenges. They may also develop psychiatric diagnoses, which further compound existing problems.

The overall goal is to help individuals attain and maintain an optimal level of health and function throughout the life span within the range of their capacity. Currently, there are glaring health disparities regarding availability of adequate health care for individuals with intellectual disability as compared to that available to the general population (National Institute of Child Health and Human Development, 2001).

Inclusion refers to the integration and full participation of everyone, regardless of special needs and disabilities or the environment (e.g., school, community), with typical peers in the least restrictive setting. The opinions and expectations most people have about themselves are influenced to a great extent by the behavior of those around them. When minimal expectations or lack of belief in individuals' ability to achieve are communicated, the chances for individuals to progress in attaining goals are diminished. Because a number of inaccurate and stereotyped ideas about individuals with intellectual disability still exist, barriers to reaching optimal function and independence continue to be present. Although societal and employer attitudes are changing slowly, there is continued need for education and integration of individuals with intellectual disability into society and into the workplace. Although all individuals with intellectual disability can experience stresses resulting from societal stereotypes and attitudes, individuals with mild intellectual disability may confront specific stresses because they may appear normal to others and, consequently, their limitations may not be recognized as a disability.

The concept of inclusion (being a full participant of the whole) rather than being "in the community" is essential in understanding the expectations of individuals with intellectual disability. Lack of acceptance and devaluation can result in low self-esteem and isolation, which in turn can lead to deviant behaviors or acting out. In more severe cases, a psychiatric disorder may develop as a means of coping.

When evaluating adults with Down syndrome for depression in a recent study, 32% of participants showed elevated depression scores and 40% reported feeling lonely (Ailey, Miller, Heller, & Smith, 2006). The relationship between depression, perceived social support, loneliness, and life satisfaction was statistically significant. The use of such a framework in monitoring depression in individuals with Down syndrome across their life spans could be an asset in early intervention and treatment.

Many individuals with intellectual disability are cared for by others in either their own homes or in residential settings, such as assisted-living or group home environments. The level of stress that may be experienced by caregivers and vulnerability of individuals with intellectual disability raise a concern about the potential for violence, abuse, and neglect toward people with this disability. In 2004, Strand, Benzein, and Saveman reported on the results of a questionnaire that they sent to 164 staff members in 17 different care settings for adults with disabilities in Sweden. In their responses, 74% of respondents reported being involved in or witnessing violent incidents toward clients, and 14% admitted to being the perpetrator of the violent act. Most of the violence occurred on a daily basis, was both physical and psychological, and tended to occur in close caretaking situations. This study indicates the importance of supportive supervision, education and outlets for staff and family members and increasing training of individuals with intellectual disability about reporting abusive situations.

Vocational Issues in Intellectual Disability

The level of occupational functioning for individuals with intellectual disability depends to some extent on the degree of disability. Lack of exposure to or experience in a variety of work settings can be a significant limitation in successful work participation. Because intellectual disability is often accompanied by other medical conditions, the physical limitations associated with any other condition must also be considered. Individuals with intellectual disability usually perform better in a structured environment. Many individuals may need to be taught how to function independently and may need accompanying social skills training.

As with other disabilities, the major barrier to individuals reaching their full potential may be societal stereotypes and prejudice. Although there has been heightened effort toward increasing integrated employment opportunities for individuals with intellectual disability, rehabilitation outcomes—especially for individuals of racial and ethnic under-represented groups—have been less than ideal (Moore, 2001). Consequently, continued equality in service delivery and assurance and education of potential employers may be crucial factors in successful occupational placement. Little information is available in the vocational rehabilitation literature on the pattern of work support and employment success of individuals based on the level and degree of intellectual disability they have. Fewer individuals with severe disabilities have received service because they have been deemed ineligible, based on their recorded level of intellectual disability (Moore, Harley, & Gamble, 2004).

■ PERVASIVE DEVELOPMENTAL DISORDERS

Pervasive developmental disorders is the official diagnostic term used in the *DSM-IV-TR* (American Psychiatric Association 2000) to describe a broad range of developmental conditions that are characterized by impairments in multiple areas of development and that vary in subtype and severity. Two common conditions included in this diagnostic category are autism and Asperger's syndrome. The term *autism spectrum disorders (ASD)* is also often used as a synonym for pervasive developmental disorders (Simpson et al., 2005). ASD is used to describe a broad range of subtypes and levels of severity of conditions included in the spectrum of autism and pervasive developmental disorders.

Autistic Disorder (Autism)

General Description

Autistic disorder or autism is a disorder of brain function that has a broad range of behavioral consequences, including impairment in reciprocal social interaction and impairment in verbal and nonverbal communication, play skills, and cognitive and adaptive functioning (Layne, 2007; American Psychiatric Association, 2000). It is the best known of the Autism Spectrum Disorder (ASD) and has shown a steady increase in reported prevalence since it was first described in 1943 (Merrick, Kandel, & Morad, 2004). Autism is the third most common developmental disability (Goolsby & Blackwell, 2001) and four times more prevalent in males than in females (www.autism-society.org). The estimated prevalence of Autism is 5.8 per 1000 children (Hirtz, Thurman, Gwinn-Hardy, Mohamed, Chaudhuri, & Zalutsky, 2007). Whether the incidence of autism is actually increasing, or whether the reported increase is influenced by heightened awareness by parents and health professionals and/or the epidemiological methods used by different groups to arrive at estimates, is the source of recent controversy (Laider, 2005; Williams, Mellis, & Peat, 2005; Baird et al., 2000). A 2002 report of ASD rates in children in the United States indicated that approximately 1 in 150 children had a form of ASD, a rate consistent with earlier estimates (Centers for Disease Control and Prevention, 2007).

Manifestations of Autism

Autism is characterized by behavioral patterns that most commonly include impairments in communication and social interaction. Kanner was the first to describe children with autism as "having an inability to relate themselves in an ordinary way to people and situations from the beginning of life" (Kanner, 1972, p. 242). Individuals with autism may exhibit symptoms from birth; however, because of the subtlety of early symptoms, the condition may not be diagnosed until symptoms are more noticeable later in development. Onset occurs prior to the age of three (American Psychiatric Association, 2000).

The range and severity of symptoms vary with each individual. Usually parents report that the child, almost since birth, has been perceived as different. Language delays and inability to relate to social cues are often reported. Parents of children with autism may report that their child did not enjoy being cuddled, seldom smiled, and did not respond to games such as "peek-a-boo." These children may remain aloof and have problems throughout childhood, with either an improvement in or an exacerbation of behavior in adolescence. They often prefer solitary behavior, preferring to be left alone rather than engaging in explorative behaviors or other social interaction. They may lack the ability to engage in spontaneous or imaginative play and may show strong attachment to inanimate objects rather than people. In particular, abilities related to attention, empathy, communication, and flexibility are affected (Anckarsater, Stahlberg, Lanson, et al., 2006).

Activity levels of individuals with autism may range from overactive to very passive. Some children display repetitive or stereotypic body movements or behaviors, such as

body rocking, finger flicking, or starring at their hands at close range. In some instances, children may engage in repetitive self-injurious behavior, such as head banging or biting. They may exhibit exaggerated and/or aggressive responses to people or objects. Rituals and the insistence on sameness or resistance to change are common in individuals with autism. Changes in their environment or routine may be very difficult.

Individuals with autism often demonstrate hypersensitivity or disproportionate response to sensory stimuli, including touch or sound; however, in some instances they may show a decreased response to pain. Often communication deficits in verbal or nonverbal behavior exist, including the inability to comprehend verbal communication or decipher nonverbal cues. They may demonstrate difficulty expressing ideas or needs orally or, conversely, be highly verbal. *Echolalia*, in which a word or a phrase is repeated numerous times, may be a feature of the condition. Individuals may also have difficulty integrating cognitive functions. While some individuals with autism have average or above-average intelligence, nearly 70% to 80% to have IQ scores falling into the range of mental retardation (Yeargin-Allsopp, Rice, Karapurkar, Doernberg, Boyle, & Murphy et al., 2003).

If autism accompanies another disorder, such as encephalitis, phenylketonuria (PKU), or fragile X syndrome, corresponding neurological and medical symptoms will be present. Seizures have been noted in as many as 25% of children with autism, with onset often in adolescence. EEG abnormalities are common even without seizures (Brasic, 2006a; Walz, 2002; American Psychiatric Association, 2000).

Causes of Autism

Years ago, autism was attributed to poor parenting skills, and many believed that parents who were emotionally unavailable to their children contributed to the development of symptoms of autism. This belief has now been discredited, and parenting skills are no longer thought to be responsible for the development of autism. Although no definitive cause of autism has yet been found, it is most likely that autism results from a brain function abnormality that is biologically based and arises from a combination of genetic vulnerability and environmental triggers (Blackwell & Niederhauser, 2003).

There has been considerable concern that a link exists between thimerosal, a mercury-based preservative sometimes used in vaccines, and autism. Until 1999, vaccines against a number of infectious diseases contained thimerosal as a preservative. The MMR (measles, mumps, rubella), varicella (chickenpox), inactivated polio (IPV), and pneumococcal conjugate vaccines have never contained thimerosal. Currently, with the exception of some influenza vaccines, none of the vaccines used in the United States to protect children contains thimerosal as a preservative (Federal Drug Administration, 2007).

Diagnosis of Autism

Autism is distinguished from other pervasive developmental disorders by its characteristics and pattern of developmental deficits. Diagnostic criteria, as outlined in *DSM-IV-TR* (American Psychiatric Association, 2000), include abnormal behaviors in the following categories: deficit in social interaction; deficit in communication; and demonstration of restricted repetitive patterns of behavior, interest, or activities. These symptoms must occur before the age of three and must be symptoms that are not accounted for by another pervasive developmental disorder. Screening tools including the *Childhood Autism Rating Scale* (CARS) (Schopler, Reichler, & Renner, 1988) are used to diagnose autism (Matson & Minshawi, 2006). Extensive training and experience are required to administer these tools in a valid and reliable way. Consequently, definitive diagnosis of autism should be made by clinicians who have extensive experience with the screening instruments and with individuals with autism.

Management of Autism

Autism is a lifelong condition. One of the most important aspects in its management is early identification and individualized, intensive behavioral and psychological interventions. In spite of increasing awareness of the prevalence of autism, delays in diagnosis frequently occur due to lack of standardized screening for developmental delays (Filipek et al., 2000). Developmental profiles should focus on speech and language, verbal and nonverbal communication, cognitive function, and motor function. In addition, audiological screening and lead exposure screening should be conducted to rule out other causes of developmental delay.

Communication problems are prevalent in autism. Consequently, there should be a thorough evaluation of how the individual best communicates (Cade & Tidwell, 2001). In assessing individuals with autism, the individual's social, communication, and behavioral strengths and limitations should be incorporated into any rehabilitation plan. As there are frequently both verbal and nonverbal problems in communication, augmentative systems may be needed (such as signing or use of a communication board) to facilitate communication. Provision of an augmentative communication system that can be successfully used requires careful assessment by skilled professionals. Behavioral protocols—including many employing contingent reinforcement, such as use of tokens—have been used successfully and may facilitate interaction.

Other types of therapies, such as auditory integration training or sensory integration therapy, may be helpful to individuals with autism in some instances. Exercise may be therapeutic for individuals with autism. In some instances, physical therapy may be helpful.

Establishment of any treatment or management plan should always include family members as partners to develop a plan that is best suited for the individual and his or her particular circumstances. Treatment planning often involves a multidisciplinary approach, including an audiological exam, speech and language evaluation, occupational therapy evaluation, psychiatric observation and interview, and neurological exam. Each area of function should be measured against standardized norms and the results used to determine the individual's special needs.

Referral to an early-intervention program, which evaluates needs and assists children with developmental disability, is crucial. Early-intervention programs involve the whole family and assist in identifying innovative solutions to both behavioral and medical problems.

While no specific medications are considered standard in management of autistic disorder, a number of medications are used for managing related problems and behaviors. Medications used to reduce aggression and self-injury in children with autism have been used with moderate success (Research Units on Pediatric Psychopharmacology Autism Network, 2002). Other medications are at times used to reduce symptoms of hyperactivity and impulsiveness (Handen, Johnson, & Lubetsky, 2000). When using medications for management of symptoms, careful monitoring of drug interactions or side effects should be part of the general protocol. In instances where other medical conditions coexist with the condition, specific medications for management of those conditions, such as seizure disorder, may be added. When other medications are added to the medication protocol, the potential for drug interaction and subsequent synergistic untoward effects should also be considered.

Behavioral and social skills training has been used extensively in management of specific behaviors in autism (Blackwell & Niederhauser, 2003). The goal of behavioral training and management is to assist individuals with autism to approach normal functioning as closely as possible and to assist them to gain independence. Behavior management helps individuals learn skills to help prevent undesirable behaviors. To be most effective, caregivers must apply behavior management consistently over time. Many parents find that this effort requires significant time commitment, and they may not have the stamina and dedication to maintain the intervention. Although there is no cure or specific treatment for autism, early intervention and special education programs greatly increase the likelihood of reaching optimal level of function and independence. The long-term outcome for individuals with autism is directly related to their intelligence quotient and communication skills (Brasic, 2006a; Howlin, 2000). Specifically, individuals with IQ above 70 appear to have more positive outcomes (Howlin, Goode, Hutton, & Rutter, 2004).

Psychosocial Issues in Autism

The goals for individuals with autism are the same as the goals for most individuals: to live a meaningful, productive adult life, with friends, social outlets, and gainful employment. Individuals' level of achievement often depends not only on limitations associated with the condition, but also on how those limitations have been experienced. Individuals who have been helped to activate their potential and develop skills they are capable of acquiring also experience increased self-worth.

Despite problems with level of intellectual and social functioning, many individuals with autism who are higher functioning continue to live with their parents or with professional support. However, the number of individuals with autism who are higher functioning and who are gainfully employed is lower than might be expected for their level of function (Renty & Roeyers, 2006). As with other disabilities, the extent to which individuals experience disability because of their condition is often influenced their environment and social attitudes, as well as manifestations of the disability itself.

For most families, children leave home to go to college or enter the workforce when they become young adults. In the case of families of individuals with autism, this transition may be postponed indefinitely. Parents may be reluctant to allow the individual to achieve greater independence due to feelings of guilt, or they may believe that in allowing their child to leave they are abandoning their own role as parents and providers of care. In some instances, fear of the individual's vulnerability may be of concern. In other instances, appropriate resources may be lacking. Expectations for achievement may be set inappropriately low.

Although parents play a central role in helping their adult child with autism achieve his or her full life potential, each individual has different strengths, limitations, and life circumstances. As much as possible, individuals should be given opportunities to strengthen their social support network and to receive support that is tailored to their individual needs, thereby enabling them to achieve their greatest level of quality of life.

Sexuality in individuals with autism is often ignored but is of major concern both for individuals with autism and for their family. Age-appropriate sexual behavior may be present in some individuals with autism, while in others it may be inappropriate. Individuals with autism trying to engage another person in sexual contact may have difficulty distinguishing between desired and undesired contact, which may be related to their inability to distinguish social and emotional reciprocity (Hellemans, Colson, Verbraeken, Vermeiren, & Deboutte, 2007).

Vocational Issues in Autism

A recent review of the literature indicates that only a minority of individuals with autism, even if they have a high functional capacity, obtain a college or university degree, live semi-independently, or have a paid job (Tsatsanis, 2003). Although not all adults with autism are able to work, nearly 35% of adults with autism who are higher functioning and 10% of adults who are lower functioning work in a supported work environment (Ganz, 2007). Social deficits and the degree of stereotyped and ritualistic behavior can have a detrimental effect on employment regardless of communication skills or intellectual ability (Tsatsanis, 2003). Until recently, there have not been supported employment programs specifically designed for individuals with autism, although a growing number of programs are being developed (Hagner & Cooney, 2005). However, some studies indicate that supported employment programs not only increase productivity and satisfaction for individuals with autism with both higher and lower levels of functioning (Howlin, Alcock, & Burkin, 2005), but can also increase levels of executive functioning (see Chapter 3) in these individuals (Garcia-Villamisar & Hughes, 2007).

Supported employment, in addition to providing individuals with more opportunities to gain employment and increased independence (Hurlbutt & Chalmers, 2004; Tantam, 2003), has also been shown to decrease psychological distress (Tantam, 2000) and to increase quality of life (Beadle-Brown, Murphy, & Wing, 2005).

Each individual with autism is unique. Consequently, careful appraisal of individual interests, abilities, strengths, and limitations is important to achieve a better vocational outcome.

Asperger's Syndrome (Disorder)

Asperger's syndrome and *Asperger's disorder* are terms used interchangeably. Asperger's disorder was first identified in 1944 by Hans Asperger, a German physician who studied a group of high-functioning children with manifestations similar to those experienced in autism (Volkmar & Klin, 2000). Behaviors characteristic of Asperger's disorder were included in *DSM-III* (American Psychiaric Association, 1987) under the classification of pervasive developmental disorder, not otherwise specified. Not until 1994, however, did Asperger's disorder appear as a diagnostic category in the *DSM-IV*.

There has been some controversy as to whether Asperger's syndrome should be defined as a separate category from autism or defined as high-functioning autism (Klin & Volkmar, 2003; Macintosh & Dissanayake, 2004). The debate over the nature of and relationship between Asperger's syndrome and autism continues. Although there are similarities, the diagnostic criteria are not as clear for Asperger's syndrome (Boggs, Gross, & Gohm, 2006). Some symptoms are common to both conditions, but individuals with Asperger's syndrome show no significant delay in language or cognitive development, although some individuals may demonstrate some cognitive difficulties. Often individuals with Asperger's syndrome are able to function at relatively high levels, establishing careers and living independently (Eisenmajar et al., 1996; Walz, 2002).

Definitive prevalence of Asperger's syndrome is difficult to determine because definitions have varied since it was first defined, and because the diagnostic criteria have changed. Asperger's syndrome appears to be more common in males, with the mean age of diagnosis being approximately 8 years of age (Eisenmajar Prior, Leekam, 1996).

No clear cause of Asperger's syndrome has been established; however, it is thought to be neurologically based (Zaretsky, Richter, & Eisenberg, 2005). The condition appears to occur in families, and a genetic predisposition has been suggested, although no clear genetic marker has been identified (Volkmar et al., 2000).

Manifestations of Asperger's Disorder

Difficulties in social interaction are a central feature of Asperger's syndrome (Goddard, Howlin, Dritschel, & Patel, 2007). Individuals with this syndrome may also demonstrate repetitive behavior patterns and resistance to change, similar to individuals with autism. Many individuals with Asperger's syndrome also exhibit symptoms of hyperactivity and inattention so that this condition is often misidentified as attention deficit/hyperactivity disorder (American Psychiatric Association, 2000).

Intellectual and communication functions are not usually impaired in Asperger's syndrome. Affected individuals often have normal and at times even superior intelligence (Brasic, 2006b; Frith, 2004). Impairments in social interaction and communication may be subtle and, therefore, difficult to diagnose (Portway & Johnson, 2005). Diagnosis of Asperger's syndrome may not be made until individuals reach school age and difficulties with social interaction become apparent. Individuals with Asperger's syndrome may have difficulty recognizing social cues, such nonverbal behavior and body language, so that they are unable to recognize cues indicating that their behavior is inappropriate (Safran, 2002).

Individuals with Asperger's syndrome may not adhere to social conventions, such as respecting others' personal space. They may make remarks that are inappropriate in most social environments or talk loudly, relentlessly pursuing a subject of interest to them, even though others show no interest in what they are saying and show little response to the discussion. Individuals with Asperger's syndrome may be rigid about adhering to strict routines and become upset or agitated if change is necessary. Some individuals may demonstrate poor gross motor function, appear clumsy, or use repetitive behaviors, such as ritualistic walking patterns and obsessive–compulsive routines.

Distinguishing Asperger's syndrome from high-functioning autism remains an unresolved issue (Rourke & Tsatsanis, 2000). Diagnostic criteria for Asperger's syndrome as listed in *DSM-IV-TR* are similar to the diagnostic criteria for autism, with the exception that in Asperger's syndrome there is no delay in language acquisition or in intellectual development (American Psychiatric Association, 2000).

Asperger's syndrome is a lifelong disorder, with social abilities waxing and waning or significantly improving into adulthood. Adolescents often learn to use areas of strength, such as rote verbal skills or savant-like mathematical skills, to compensate for other limitations. Although overall prognosis is better for individuals with Asperger's syndrome than for those with Autism (American Psychiatric Association, 2000), as they reach adulthood, they may experience increasing rejection, social isolation, anxiety, and depression.

Management of Asperger's Syndrome

Even though *DSM-IV-TR* specifies diagnostic criteria for Asperger's syndrome, there are many subtleties of the disorder, such that diagnostic boundaries that are not always clear (Wing, 2000). As a result, the condition may be misdiagnosed or overlooked and hence interventions appropriate to the diagnosis may not be forthcoming. Manifestations may not be immediately apparent during assessment conducted in a one-to-one setting. A full history of the individual's behavior and the means by which he or she interacts with others can be an important diagnostic tool.

Asperger's syndrome is a condition marked by social disability. Referrals and resources to help individuals develop social skills, recognize social cues, and learn socially based communication and language skills can help the individual become more socially adept (Giarelli, Souders, Pinto-Martin, Bloch, & Levy, 2005; Landa, 2000). Because coping with change is difficult, maintaining comfortable routines can be helpful to the individual; when change is necessary, it should be introduced gradually.

Lack of social skills and other social deficits may cause individuals with Asperger's syndrome to experience significant stress. As a result, they may also experience depression, and medications such as antidepressants may be prescribed for associated symptoms (Martin, Patzer, & Volkmar, 2000).

Psychosocial Issues in Asperger's Syndrome

Learning about the symptoms of Asperger's syndrome can help individuals and their families cope with the symptoms and can prevent misunderstanding regarding behavior that others may consider socially inappropriate. Rather than focusing solely on any savant-like behaviors that may be present, families should focus on encouraging age-appropriate skills and behaviors. Because this condition involves social skill deficits, encouragement and feedback that help the individual to recognize social cues and ways in which socially appropriate behavior can be integrated into social interactions can be helpful (Cole Marshall, 2002).

Asperger's syndrome is an invisible disability; individuals with this condition are not obviously different to others. Consequently, when individuals exhibit behaviors associated with the condition, others may not attribute those behaviors to a disability. For this reason, individuals with Asperger's syndrome may not receive the same level of understanding and support experienced by others with more obvious disability. Individuals with Asperger's syndrome may feel they do not fit into many social and work situations. Social deficits may make it difficult for individuals to form intimate relationships with others and to find a life partner. They may have difficulty establishing friendships and finding a confidant.

As a result of social rejection and the characteristics of the condition itself, individuals may lack needed psychological and social resources to cope with continued rejection and isolation. Consequently, individuals with Asperger's syndrome may experience enduring problems related to anxiety and/or depression, which can lead to further functional incapacity. Learning appropriate outlets for stress and anxiety can be helpful, as can support and understanding from family.

Vocational Issues in Asperger's Syndrome

Individuals with Asperger's syndrome usually have typical language and intellectual functioning and may excel in areas not dependent on social interaction. Career choices using computer technology, lab research, or other areas in which there is limited social interaction have been shown to be successful for individuals with this condition.

Social impairment in Asperger's syndrome can be severely debilitating. Despite the capacity of individuals with Asperger's syndrome to be productive and their ability to make significant intellectual contributions, their social insensitivity and indifference can be severely handicapping. Social skills training can be of help in this regard. Given that change is frequently difficult for individuals with Asperger's syndrome to accept, they may perform better in a structured environment with set routines.

■ LEARNING DISORDERS

Learning disorders, as classified in *DSM-IV-TR*, are a group of conditions that affect the individual's ability to acquire and/or use information through sources such as reading, writing, mathematical calculations, listening, speaking, or reasoning in the absence of more global intellectual disability. Learning disorders are present in approximately 2% to 5% of the population in the Western world (Gillberg & Soderstrom, 2003). No specific cause for learning disorders has been identified. Individuals with coexisting neurological disorders, perinatal injury, or genetic predisposition may also exhibit learning disabilities. Nevertheless, many individuals with a learning disorder have no specific identifiable cause to which the condition can be attributed.

As with other developmental disabilities, there are varying degrees of disability associated with learning disorder. Severe learning disabilities affect a large number of academic and functional skills. Although individuals with severe learning disability usually have a lower level of achievement in academic or other areas than would be expected for someone of that age group, it is not indicative of low intellectual ability (Reschly, 2005). Individuals with severe learning disability may have normal or even high levels of intelligence. Nevertheless, the disability can lead to major functional impairment in many areas of daily life (Gillberg & Soderstrom, 2003).

Deficits associated with severe learning disability have negative impacts on academic and general life achievements. They can interfere with the individual's ability to read, to carry out mathematical calculations, or to write. Tasks of everyday life, such as using money, paying bills, reading instructions, or completing applications or forms, may be severely impaired (American Psychiatric Association, 2000).

Manifestations of Learning Disabilities

Learning disabilities can be manifested in any area of information processing. Individuals generally do not have difficulty with all areas of learning, but may have a learning disability specific to one area. For example, **dyslexia** is a specific type of learning disability that affects reading in approximately 5% of all school-aged children (Boyd, 2005); it impairs the individual's ability to interpret written language. Other types of learning disabilities relating to reading affect other parts of the reading process, including the ability to accurately recognize words, reading speed, and the ability to comprehend what is read. Reading disability not only affects academic achievement, but also interferes with many other activities that require reading skills, such as reading notices, understanding forms and applications, and reading labels of medicine bottles.

Other types of learning disabilities may affect writing, which includes impairment in handwriting, spelling, or composition. The term dysgraphia is often applied broadly to this type of learning disability, although **dysgraphia** technically means only difficulty with writing, rather than referring to broader issues such as composition. Individuals may have difficulty organizing thoughts in written composition, make numerous punctuation and spelling errors, or have poor handwriting. Academic achievement and other tasks of daily living that require writing are affected.

Learning disabilities may also affect math skills (*dyscalculia*). Individuals with this type of disability have difficulty with simple calculations and following sequence of steps to solve math problems. They may also have difficulty reading numerical symbols or understanding math terms. This type of learning disability, in addition to affecting academic achievement, implications for other tasks in daily life that utilize mathematical principles and skills, such as counting money, paying bills, and calculating measurements.

Management of Learning Disabilities

Learning disabilities are often not identified early, and they may not be noticed until the individual enters school. When problems are identified, they may be inaccurately interpreted as lack of interest, not trying, or lack of cognitive ability (Dudley-Marling, 2004). Individuals may be labeled as having low intellectual ability and not receive the type of intervention that could accommodate their disability. Although learning disorders are often diagnosed in school, undiagnosed learning disorders may also be identified in adulthood. In adults, learning disorders may not be identified unless it becomes obvious that individuals are unable to read signs, written instructions, or complete forms.

Diagnosis of a learning disability is usually made through standardized tests given by a clinician who has been trained to administer and interpret standardized tests. Because other factors such as inadequate educational opportunities (e.g., deficient teaching, high rate of absenteeism) or sensory impairment (e. g., impaired vision or hearing) may also affect ability to learn or ability to gain specific skills, a diagnosis of a specific learning disorder should not be made until these other factors are identified and, when possible, corrected.

Although learning disability can be managed, it can be managed successfully only when it is accurately diagnosed. Early-intervention programs such as special educational programs to assist individuals (children and adults) to learn alternative ways of processing information can be beneficial. Provision of special accommodations that enable individuals to adapt to limitations they are experiencing is also helpful. Those assistive devices or materials that best accommodate the individual's learning needs should be used. Visual aids, materials written in simple phrases, or use of auditory rather than visual learning modes can all help individuals learn material in accordance with their own needs. The underpinning of effective management is tailoring the interventions to best meet each individual's specific needs (Dudley-Marling, 2004).

Psychosocial Issues in Learning Disabilities

Adults with a learning disability face many challenges in employment and daily routines; however, with appropriate interventions and adjustments, individuals can attain educational and employment success and personal satisfaction. Although early recognition of learning disability and referral to appropriate special education programs can assist many individuals to achieve their full potential, not all individuals are in a situation that affords them this benefit. Individuals who achieve higher levels of success have been found to come from higher socioeconomic backgrounds, have greater social and psychological support systems, and have access to quality special education programs (Greenbaum, Graham, & Scales, 1996).

Individuals with learning disability may experience loss of self-esteem or shame if they are unable to perform learning or other tasks that others take for granted. Self-esteem may be further damaged if the individual is made to feel inadequate or incompetent by others. As adults, these feelings can become internalized and lead to feelings of helplessness. When learning disability is not identified and individuals do not receive appropriate intervention or have adequate levels of support, the picture can be bleak. Individuals may drop out of high school, frustrated by school failure, or obtain entry-level jobs with little hope for advancement. In other instances, individuals may turn to crime or substance abuse.

Early identification of learning problems, determination of appropriate expectations, and identification and coordination of specific support systems and educational interventions are critical factors in assisting individuals with a learning disability to achieve their full potential. Individuals who have not been diagnosed with learning disability in child-hood but continue to experience the manifestations of their disability in adulthood are frequently ashamed of their limitations, and may attempt to hide them and reject services even when they are available. Multitiered academic and behavioral interventions may be of benefit (Reschly, 2005). Providing specific instructional aids, helping individuals identify and acknowledge specific learning needs, and acquiring appropriate supports and resources to meet those needs are examples of interventions that may be instituted.

Vocational Issues in Learning Disabilities

Given the wide variety of limitations experienced by individuals with learning disabilities, they may need to develop a wide range of compensatory skills and abilities to manage their disability effectively. Individuals should be placed in an environment that suits their specific interests and abilities as well as their particular limitations. Appropriate assessment for identification of the specific type of learning disability and associated limitations is the first step of successful intervention. When specific limitations are identified, appropriate accommodations can be provided. Individuals should be helped to understand their condition and identify compensatory strategies and techniques that are most helpful for them.

Attention should also be paid to the individual's ability to deal with pressure and criticism. Because individuals may have a history of isolation and negative experiences, they may be more sensitive to pressure to perform or to feedback or criticism about their work or productivity.

Depending on the type of learning disability, individuals may need accommodations regarding time management, organization, or memory. In other types of learning disabilities, individuals may have difficulty with visual or auditory processing, writing, or reading. Various types of assistive technologies or software, such as personal management software, talking calculators, electronic notebooks, software, display controls, or word processing tools, may also be helpful in enhancing individual performance.

■ PSYCHOSOCIAL AND VOCATIONAL ISSUES IN INTELLECTUAL AND DEVELOPMENTAL DISABILITIES

Psychosocial Issues

Individuals with developmental disabilities can be found in every age, ethnic, racial, and socioeconomic group. Whether the individual has an intellectual disability, a pervasive developmental disability, a learning disability, or a combination of disabilities, his or her needs and concerns may be as diverse as those of the general population. This includes mental health needs.

Individuals with intellectual disabilities or developmental disabilities are generally considered at increased risk for a range of health problems, including mental health problems (Rush, Bowman, Eidman, Toole, & Mortenson, 2004; Gustafsson & Sonnander, 2004). Unfortunately, the same mental health services available to the general population are often not accessed by persons with developmental disability (Stawski & Merrick, 2006). Often mental health problems go undetected because of communication problems present in many intellectual and developmental disabilities, or because symptoms of mental health problems may present differently in this population. At times symptoms are missed because of *diagnostic overshadowing* (the attribution of symptoms to the primary disability rather than to mental health problems). Even when mental health issues are identified, treatment may be unavailable due to the misconception that symptoms aren't treatable or because mental health pro-

fessionals have little training or experience working with individuals with intellectual or developmental disability who also have mental health problems.

The rate of depression in individuals with intellectual or developmental disability is higher than in the general population, (Lunsky, 2004). A number of studies show that suicidal ideation and attempted suicide do occur in individuals with intellectual or developmental disability, but there has been limited research on intervention strategies when suicidal behavior is identified (Merrick, Merrick, Lunsky, & Kandel, 2006).

Communication problems are common in individuals with intellectual or developmental disabilities. For individuals who are unable to communicate adequately, a change in behavior or a demonstration of challenging behaviors may be the first sign of a medical or psychiatric problem. Assessing the meaning of the behavior as well as the cause, rather than jumping to conclusions about the cause and the appropriate treatment, is an important step in appropriate management. Medications should be used only when needed to treat an underlying medical condition—not to control behaviors. Unrecognized medical conditions, psychiatric disorders, or environmental changes can all cause changes or exacerbation of behaviors. Family violence and abuse are also associated with individuals with developmental disabilities and should not be discounted as a potential cause for behaviors exhibited by the individual (Strickler, 2001).

Activities and Participation

Individuals with intellectual or developmental disabilities have, in the past, been labeled as people incapable of determining their own best interests or negotiating to meet their needs. This myth is slowly being dispelled, as there is increased recognition that each person with an intellectual disability has individual strengths that can be utilized to meet life's challenges. Individuals with intellectual or developmental disabilities want the same things that most people want in life, including living in a home environment, having the opportunity for friendship and social interaction, and having the opportunity to fulfill educational and vocational goals to the level of their ability. Identifying intellectual problems as early as possible and implementing appropriate interventions as soon as possible are important to helping meet these goals (Pinto-Martin et. al., 2005).

Like all people, individuals with intellectual or developmental disabilities are sexual persons, and they may voice a desire for sexual expression, marriage, and children. However, owing to misconceptions, stereotypes, and prejudice, health and rehabilitation professionals, family, and the community may be reluctant to discuss sexual issues with them and actively discourage them from sexual practice. Sexuality is more than anatomical or physical functioning, but rather is linked to basic needs of acceptance, affection, value, and self-esteem (Murphy & Elias, 2006). Individuals with intellectual or developmental disability have the same right to information about sexuality, such as attaining and maintaining intimate relationships, and managing complex emotions, as well as information about sexual orientation, sexually transmitted disease, contraception and abstinence, health implications of pregnancy, and prevention of sexual abuse.

Throughout their life spans, individuals with intellectual or developmental disabilities will undoubtedly encounter some of the same challenges that most people encounter. Because of the nature of their disability, however, these individuals are often more vulnerable to a variety of challenges. They should be educated about inappropriate use of illicit drugs and alcohol, development of inappropriate relationships, sexuality, sexual abuse, pregnancy prevention, and prevention of sexu-

ally transmitted disease (American Academy of Pediatrics, 1996). Psychosocial and environmental problems can be a major concern for many individuals with intellectual or developmental disability. These can be related to the following issues:

- The primary support group (e.g., removal from the home, physical or sexual abuse, parental overprotection)
- The social environment (e.g., difficulty with acculturation, discrimination, death or loss of a friend)
- The educational environment (e.g., conflict with teachers or peers, academic problems, restrictive classroom placement that is inappropriate to meet specific needs)
- Work (e.g., unemployment, difficult work conditions, poor matches between the individual and the job; underemployment)
- Housing (e.g., inadequate housing, conflict with neighbors or landlords, overly restrictive environment)
- Money (e.g., inadequate finances, inadequate public support)
- Health care (e.g., unavailable transportation to facilities, inadequate insurance; inability to adequately communicate to participate in diagnosis or treatment)
- The legal and justice systems (e.g., victimization, arrest, exploitation, lack of knowledgeable representation)
- Availability of support services (e.g., conflict with nonfamily caregivers)
- Lack of access to information about assistance available; confusing and uncoordinated service systems

Individuals with an intellectual or developmental disability are likely to experience at least one problem in each of these areas by adulthood (American Psychiatric Association, 1994).

Individuals with intellectual or developmental disability and their families should be helped to identify and eliminate barriers and challenges so that individuals can reach the highest quality of life within the range of their ability. Just as advances in medical technology have increased life expectancy for the general population, so they have also increased life expectancy for individuals with intellectual or developmental disabilities (Horwitz, Kerker, Owens, & Zigler, 2000), who are now living longer and confronting the same chronic illnesses that others encounter in later life, compounding existing impairments (Noble, 2001). In addition, the prevalence of mental health disorders, including dementia, is increased in a number of intellectual disabilities, such as Down syndrome (Cooper, 1998; Fisher, 2004).

Many individuals with developmental disabilities continue to live with their families into adulthood. In families without a family member with intellectual or developmental disability, there is a time when children move out of the parental home to go to school, go to work, or to begin their own families. In families in which a family member has an intellectual or developmental disability, this stage of the family life cycle may be postponed (Krauss, Seltzer, & Jacobson, 2005). In most instances, whether due to illness or death of the primary family caretaker, a decision about moving the individual with intellectual or developmental disability to another setting is made. Such decisions affect both the individual and other family members, and they can cause considerable conflict within and distress for families. Support for families involved in making this type of alternative, residential setting decision should be made available.

Benefits of residential services and supports for individuals with intellectual and developmental disabilities are increasingly being realized. Individuals receiving residential services and supports in the community have been found to experience increased personal freedom and opportunities for social activities as well as development of increased level of func-

tional skills which in turn increases individual independence (Lakin & Stancliffe, 2007).

Vocational Issues

Intellectual and developmental disabilities encompass a wide variety of conditions that occur in childhood and are lifelong conditions, affecting intellectual and social function and requiring ongoing special services and support from a transdisciplinary team to meet those lifelong opportunities and challenges. Knowledge of the specific condition is important to provide the most effective and least obtrusive support and intervention for individuals with intellectual or developmental disability as they go about meeting the challenges in their everyday lives. Understanding the characteristics of specific conditions can promote steps to independence and self-determination.

Although the individual's needs are often related to the type of disability and its manifestations, and needed support is determined by test results and other resources, the affirmation that each person is an individual with unique circumstances is essential in the structure of a plan that is most appropriate for that individual. Working with the individual's strengths, interests, and abilities in creative ways produces a better outcome than trying to treat all individuals with the same disability in the same way (Olney, 2000). Individuals should be assessed in the context of their unique circumstances and preferences. Adequate information should be obtained, which can then be used to make appropriate referrals or to establish plans and interventions to help individuals meet their goals to the best of their ability. Both the strengths and the limitations of the individual serve as a framework for such planning. Services and supports should be identified in conjunction with goals and objectives that have been mutually decided upon by the individual with intellectual disability and his or her family.

Employment has the potential for helping individuals with intellectual or developmental disability achieve independence and social inclusion (Caldwell & Heller, 2007; Cordes & Howard, 2005). Paid and meaningful work can enhance self-image, dignity, and social competence of individuals with intellectual or developmental disability through social integration and help them gain socially valuable roles. Many individuals with intellectual or developmental disability may not be working because of prejudice and stereotypes that they are unemployable.

In many instances, part-time or supported employment options offer opportunities for individuals for whom work was not previously considered an option. Essential factors that help individuals with intellectual or developmental disability obtain the best outcome include a job placement that is in accordance with the individual's interests and skills, appropriate transportation arrangements, ongoing monitoring and communication with the employer, adequate training, and advocacy.

Although work remains a primary goal, some concerns regarding work for individuals with intellectual or developmental disability must also be considered. Individuals with intellectual or developmental disability may be able to perform a certain set of skills at the job site, but other facets of work, such as time constraints or competition, may produce high levels of stress and make maintaining a satisfactory work environment more difficult. Monitoring anxiety levels and helping individuals improve their ability to cope with stress can increase both job satisfaction and productivity. Most essential is a thorough assessment of the individual, his or her strengths and challenges, and the identification of the job, job setting, and type and degree of support needed to achieve a good match. Individuals with intellectual or developmental disability should be exposed to a variety of appropriate jobs. As much as possible, the individual's job interest and top job choices should be honored.

CASE STUDIES

Case 1

Ms. R. is a 26-year-old woman with autism and borderline intellectual disability who is living in a rural community. Her speech production and communication are adequate, although her understanding of language is extremely concrete, and she has difficulty with abstract concepts. Although Ms. R. completed special education, she has lived in a very protected environment with her parents, who have been reluctant to allow her to interact socially with other people of her own age or to explore her own interests or activities. Ms. R. is capable of personal activities of daily living such as grooming, but she has poor judgment and impulse control, and she has not been required to engage in any type of vocational activity. She recently has become aggressive on occasion, and her parents have become increasingly unable to control her behavior. They express concern for her future if they should no longer be able to care for her. Ms. R. has only one other sibling, who currently lives in another state.

1. Which types of alternatives might Ms. R.'s parents explore?
2. What are some particular issues you might anticipate with Ms. R. and her parents?
3. Are there particular resources Ms. R. and her parents may be able to utilize?

Case 2

Mr. D. is a 50-year-old man with moderate intellectual disability. He demonstrates limited communication skills and limited skills in daily living. He has lived in a group residential setting for the last 20 years, but the site of his residence is closing soon. Mr. D. has no living relatives. He has been working as a grocery bagger at the local supermarket for the last five years and says he feels comfortable in both his work and home environment.

1. Which alternatives for a living environment might Mr. D. have after his residential setting closes?
2. Which types of specific needs may Mr. D. have if he must move from his current living arrangement?
3. How might Mr. D.'s move to a different environment affect his ability to continue working?
4. What may be some issues regarding Mr. D.'s ability to continue work?

■ REFERENCES

Ailey, S. H., Miller, A. M., Heller, T., & Smith, E. V. Jr. (2006). Evaluating an interpersonal model of depression among adults with Down syndrome. *Research and Theory for Nursing Practice, 20*(3), 229–246.

American Academy of Pediatrics. (1996). Sexuality education of children and adolescents with developmental disabilities. *Pediatrics, 97,* 275–278.

American Association on Intellectual and Developmental Disabilities (AAIDD). (2002). *Definition, classification, and systems of support* (10th ed.). Washington, DC: Author.

American Association on Mental Retardation (1992). *Mental retardation: Definitions, classification, and systems of support* (9th ed.) Washington, DC: Author.

American Psychiatric Association. (1987). *Diagnostic and statistical manual of mental disorders* (3rd ed., rev.). Washington, DC: Author.

American Psychiatric Association. (1994). *Diagnostic and statistical manual of mental disorders* (4th ed.). Washington, DC: Author.

American Psychiatric Association. (2000). *Diagnostic and statistical manual of mental disorders* (4th ed., rev.). Washington, DC: Author.

Anckarsater, H., Stahlberg, O., Larson, T., Hakanson, C., Jutblad, S. B., Niklasson, L. et al. (2006). The impact of ADHD and autism spectrum disorders on temperament, character, and personality development. *American Journal of Psychiatry, 163,* 1239–1244.

Baird, G., Charman, T., Baron-Cohen, S., Cox, A., Swetlenhan, J., Wheelwright, S. et al. (2000). A screening instrument for autism at 18 months of age: A 6-year follow up study. *Journal of the American Academy of Child and Adolescent Psychiatry, 39,* 694–702.

Beadle-Brown, J., Murphy, G., & Wing., L. (2005). Long-term outcome for people with severe intellectual disabilities: Impact of social impairment. *American Journal on Mental Retardation, 110*(1), 1–12.

Blackwell, J., & Niederhauser, C. (2003). Diagnosis and management of autistic children. *Nurse Practitioner, 28*(6), 36–43.

Boggs, K. M., Gross, A. M., & Gohm, C. L. (2006). Validity of the Asperger's syndrome diagnostic scale. *Journal of Developmental and Physical Disabilities. 18*(2), 163–182.

Boyd, M. A. (2005). *Psychiatric nursing: Contemporary practice.* Philadelphia: Lippincott Williams & Wilkins.

Brasic, J. R. (2006a). Pervasive developmental disorder: Autism. *eMedicine.* Retrieved May 23, 2007, http://www.emedicine.com/ped/topic180.htm.

Brasic, J. R. (2006b). Pervasive developmental disorder: Asperger syndrome. *eMedicine.* Retrieved May 23, 2007, from http://www.emedicine.com/ped/topic147htm.

Cade, M., & Tidwell, S. (2001). Autism and the school nurse. *Journal of School Health, 71*(3), 96–100.

Caldwell, J., & Heller, T. (2007). Longitudinal outcomes of a consumer-directed program supporting adults with developmental disabilities and their families. *Intellectual and Developmental Disabilities, 45*(3), 161–173.

Carter, A. S., Volkmar, F. R., Sparrow, S. S., (1998). The Vineland Adaptive Behavior Scales: Supplementary norms for individuals with autism. *Journal of Autism and Developmental Disorders, 28*(4), 287–302.

Centers for Disease Control and Prevention. (February 9, 2007). New data on autism spectrum disorders (ASDs) from multiple communities in the U.S. *Morbidity and Mortality Weekly Report, 56* (SS-1). Retrieved February 15, 2007, from www.cdc.gov/print.do

Cole Marshall, M. (2002). Asperger's syndrome: Implications for nursing practice. *Issues in Mental Health Nursing, 23,* 606–615.

Cooper, S. (1998). Clinical study of the effects of age on the physical health of adults with mental retardation. *American Journal on Mental Retardation, 102,* 582–589.

Conoley, J. C., & Kramer, J. J. (Eds.). (1989). *The tenth mental measurements yearbook.* Lincoln, NE: Buros Institute of Mental Measurement.

Cooper, S. (1998). Clinical study of the effects of age on the physical health of adults with mental retardation. *American Journal on Mental Retardation, 102,* 582–589.

Cordes, T. L., & Howard, R. W. (2005). Concepts of work, leisure and retirement in adults with an intellectual disability. *Education and Training in Developmental Disabilities, 40*(2), 99–108.

Daily, D. K., Ardinger, H. H., & Holmes, G. E. (2000). Identification and evaluation of mental retardation. *American Family Physician, 61*(4), 1059–1067.

Developmental Disabilities Assistance and Bill of Rights Act of 2000 (114 STAT.1684, Public Law 106-402-October 30, 2000).

Dudley-Marling, C. (2004). The social construction of learning disabilities. *Journal of Learning Disabilities, 37*(6), 482–489.

Eisenmajar, R., Prior, M., Leekam, S., et al. (1996). Comparison of clinical symptoms in autism and Asperger's disorder. *Journal of the American Academy of Child and Adolescent Psychiatry, 35,* 1523–1531.

Federal Drug Administration (2007). Thimerosol in vaccines. Retrieved September 3, 2007, from http://www.fda.org/cber/vaccine/thimfag.htm#q2.

Filipek, P. A., Accardo, P. J., Ashwal, S., Baranek, G. T., Cook, E. H. Jr., Dawson G., et al. (2000). Practice parameter: Screening and diagnosis of autism. *Neurology, 55*(4), 468–479.

Fisher, K. (2004). Nursing care of special populations: Issues in caring for elderly people with mental retardation. *Nursing Forum, 39*(1), 28–31.

Frith, U. (2004). Emanuel Miller lecture: Confusions and controversies about Asperger syndrome. *Journal of Child Psychology and Psychiatry, 45*(4), 672–686.

Ganz, M. L. (2007). The lifetime distribution of the incremental societal costs of autism. *Archives of Pediatrics and Adolescent Medicine, 161*(4), 343–349.

Garcia-Villamisar, D., & Hughes, C. (2007). Supported employment improves cognitive performance in adults with autism. *Journal of Intellectual Disability Research, 51*(Pt 2), 142–150.

Giarelli, E., Souders, M., Pinto-Martin, J., Bloch, J. & Levy, S. E. (2005). Intervention pilot for parents of children with autistic spectrum disorder. *Pediatric Nursing, 31*(5), 389–399.

Gillberg, C., & Soderstrom, H. (2003). Learning disability. *Lancet, 362*(9386), 811–821.

Goddard, L., Howlin, P., Dritschel, B., & Patel, T. (2007). Autobiographical memory and social problem-solving in Asperger syndrome. *Journal of Autism and Developmental Disorders, 37*(2), 291–300.

Goolsby, M. J. & Blackwell, J. (2001) Clinical practice guideline: Screening and diagnosing autism. *Clinical Practice Guidelines, 13*(12), 534–536.

Greenbaum, B., Graham, S., & Scales, W. (1996). Adults with learning disabilities: Occupational and social status after college. *Journal of Learning Disabilities, 29*(2), 167–173.

Gustafsson, C., & Sonnander, K. (2004). Occurrence of mental health problems in Swedish samples of adults with intellectual disabilities. *Social Psychiatry and Psychiatric Epidemiology, 39,* 448–456.

Hagner, D., & Cooney, B. F. (2005). "I do that for everybody": Supervising employees with autism. *Focus on Autism and Other Developmental Disabilities, 20*(2), 91–97.

Handen, B. L., Johnson, C. R., & Lubetsky, M. (2000). Efficacy of methylphenidate among children with autism and symptoms of attention-deficit hyperactivity disorder. *Journal of Autism and Developmental Disorder, 30,* 245–255.

Hellemans, H., Colson, K., Verbraeken, C., Vermeiren, R., & Deboutte, D. (2007). Sexual behavior in high functioning male adolescents and young adults with autism. *Journal of Autism and Developmental Disorders, 37,* 260–269.

Hirtz, D., Thurman, D. J., Gwinn-Hardy, K., Mohamed, M., Chaudhuri, A. R., & Zalutsky, R. (2007). How common are the "common neurologic disorders"? *Neurology, 68*(5), 326–327.

Horwitz, S. M., Kerker, B. D., Owens, P. L., & Zigler, E. (2000). *The health status and needs of individuals with mental retardation.* New Haven, CT: Yale University Press.

Howlin, P. (2000). Outcome in adult life for more able individuals with autism or Asperger syndrome. *Autism, 4*(1), 63–83.

Howlin, P., Alcock, J., & Burkin, C. (2005). An 8 year follow-up of a specialist supported employment service for high-ability adults with autism or Asperger syndrome. *Autism, 9*(5), 533–549.

Howlin, P., Goode, S., Hutton, J., & Rutter, M. (2004). Adult outcome for children with autism. *Journal of Child Psychology and Psychiatry, 45*(2), 212–229.

Hurlbutt, K., & Chalmers, L. (2004). Employment of adults with Asperger syndrome. *Focus on Autism and Other Developmental Disabilities, 19*(4), 212–222.

Impara, J. C., & Plake, B. S. (Eds.). (1998). *The thirteenth mental measurements yearbook.* Lincoln, NE; Buros Institute of Mental Measurements.

Kanner, L. (1972). *Child psychiatry* (4th ed.). Springfield, IL: Charles C Thomas.

Klin, A., & Volkmar, F. R. (2003). Asperger's syndrome: Diagnosis and external validity. *Child and Adolescent Psychiatric Clinics of North America, 12*(1), 1–13.

Koger, S. M., Schettler, T., & Weiss, B. (2005). Environmental toxicants and developmental disabilities: A challenge for psychologists. *American Psychologist, 60*(3), 243–255.

Krauss, M. W., Seltzer, M. M., & Jacobson, H. T. (2005). Adults with autism living at home or in non-family settings: Positive and negative aspects of residential status. *Journal of Intellectual Disability Research, 49*(2), 111–124.

Laider, J. R. (2005). U.S. Department of Education data on "autism" are not reliable for tracking autism prevalence. *Pediatrics 116*(1): Supplement: 120-4.

Lakin, K. C., & Stancliffe, R. J. (2007). Residential supports for persons with intellectual and developmental disabilities. *Mental Retardation and Developmental Disabilities Research Reviews, 13,* 151–159.

Lambert, N., Nihira, K., & Leland, H. (1993). AAMR Adaptive Behavior Scale—School (2nd ed). Austin, TX: Pro-ed.

Landa, R. (2000). Social language use in Asperger syndrome and high functioning autism. In A. Klin, F. R. Volkmar, & S. S. Sparrow (Eds.), *Asperger syndrome* (pp. 125–155). New York: Guilford.

Layne, C. M. (2007). Early identification of autism: Implications for counselors. *Journal of Counseling and Development, 85,* 110–114.

Luckasson, R., Borthwick-Duffy, S., Buntinx, W. H. E., Coulter, D. L., Craig, E. M., Reeve, A. et al., (2002). *Mental retardation: Definitions, classifications and systems of supports* (10th ed.). Washington, DC: American Association on Mental Retardation.

Lunsky, Y. (2004). Suicidality in a clinical and community sample of adults with mental retardation. *Research on Developmental Disabilities, 25,* 231–243.

Macintosh, K. E., & Dissanayake, C. (2004). The similarities and differences between autistic disorder and Asperger's disorder: A review of the empirical evidence [annotation]. *Journal of Child Psychology and Psychiatry, 45*(3), 421–434.

Martin, A., Patzer, D. K., & Volkmar, F. R. (2000). Psychopharmacological treatment of higher functioning pervasive developmental disorders. In A. Klin, F. R. Volkmar, & S. S. Sparrow (Eds.), *Asperger syndrome* (pp. 210–228). New York: Guilford.

Matson, J. L., & Minshawi, N. F. (2006). *Early intervention for autism spectrum disorders, Volume I: A critical analysis—assessment and treatment of child psychopathology and developmental disabilities.* Oxford, UK: Elsevier Science.

McLaughlin, P. J., & Wehman, P. (Eds.). (1996). *Mental retardation and developmental disabilities* (2nd ed.). Austin, TX: Pro-ed.

Merrick, J., Kandel, I., & Morad, M. (2004). Trends in autism. *International Journal of Adolescent Medical Health, 16*(1), 75–78.

Merrick, J., Merrick, E., Lunsky, Y., & Kandel, I. (2006). A review of suicidality in persons with intellectual disability. *Israel Journal of Psychiatry and Related Science, 43*(4), 258–264.

Moore, C. L. (2001). Disparities in closure success rates for African Americans with mental retardation: An ex-post-facto research design. *Journal of Applied Rehabilitation Counseling, 32*(2), 31–36.

Moore, C. L., Harley, D. A., & Gamble, D. (2004). Ex-post-facto analysis of competitive employment outcomes for individuals with mental retardation: National perspective. *Mental Retardation, 42*(4), 253–262.

Murphy, N. A., & Elias, E. R. (2006). Sexuality of children and adolescents with developmental disabilities. *Pediatrics, 118*(1), 398–403.

National Institute of Child Health and Human Development. (2001). *Closing the gap: A national blueprint for improving the health of persons with mental retardation. Report of the Surgeon General's Conference on Health Disparities and Mental Retardation.* Washington, DC: National Institutes of Health.

Nihira, K., Leland, H., & Lambert, N. (1993) AAMR adaptive behavior scales: Residential and community (ABS-RC:2) Austin, TX. Pro-ed.

Noble, J. (2001). *Textbook of primary care medicine.* (3rd ed.). St. Louis: Mosby.

Olney, M. F. (2000). Working with autism and other social communication disorders. *Journal of Applied Rehabilitation Counseling, 66*(4), 51–56.

Pinto-Martin, J. A., Dunkle, M., Earls, M., Fliedner, D., & Landes, C. (2005). Developmental stages of developmental screening: Steps to implementation of a successful program. *American Journal of Public Health, 95*(11), 1928–1932.

Portway, S. M., & Johnson, B. (2005). Do you know I have Asperger's syndrome? Risks of a non-obvious disability. *Health, Risk and Society, 7*(1), 73–83.

Prater, C. D., & Zylstra, R. G. (2006). Medical care of adults with mental retardation. *American Family Physician, 73*(12), 2175–2180.

Renty, J., & Roeyers, H. (2006). Quality of life in high-functioning adults with autism spectrum disorder: The predictive value of disability and support characteristics. *Autism, 10*(5), 511–524.

Reschly, D. J. (2005). Learning disabilities identification: Primary intervention, secondary intervention, and then what? *Journal of Learning Disabilities, 38*(6), 510–515.

Research Units on Pediatric Psychopharmacology (RUPP) Autism Network. (2002). Risperidone in children with autism and serious behavioral problems. *New England Journal of Medicine, 347,* 314–321.

Rourke, B. P., & Tsatsanis, K. D. (2000). Nonverbal learning disabilities and Asperger syndrome. In A. Klin, F. Volkmar, & S. Sparrow (Eds.), *Asperger syndrome* (pp. 231–253). New York: Guilford Press.

Rush, K. S., Bowman, L. G., Eidman, S. L., Toole, L. M., & Mortenson, B. P. (2004). Assessing psychopathology in individuals with developmental disabilities. *Behavior Modification 28,* 621–637.

Safran, J. S. (2002). Supporting students with Asperger's syndrome in general education. *Teaching Exceptional Children, 34,* 60–66.

Schopler, E., Reichler, R. J., & Renner, B. R. (1988). *The Childhood Autism Rating Scale.* Austin, TX: Pro-Ed.

Simpson, R. L., de Boer-Ott, S. R., Griswold, D. E., Smith, M. B. Byrd, S. E., Ganz, J. B. et al., (2005). *Autism spectrum disorders.* Thousand Oaks, CA: Corwin Press.

Sparrow, S., Balla, D. & Cicchetti, D. (1984). Vineland adaptive behavior scales. Circle Pines, MN: American Guidance Service.

Stawski M., & Merrick, J. (2006). Mental health services for people with intellectual disability in Israel: A review of options. *Israel Journal of Psychiatry and Related Science, 43*(4), 237–240.

Strand, M., Benzein, E., & Saveman, B. I. (2004). Violence in the care of adult persons with intellectual disabilities. *Journal of Clinical Nursing, 13*(4), 506–514.

Strickler, H. L. (2001). Interaction between family violence and mental retardation. *Mental Retardation, 39,* 461–471.

Tantam, D. (2000). Psychological disorder in adolescents and adults with Asperger syndrome. *Autism, 4*(1), 47–62.

Tantam, D. (2003). The challenge of adolescents and adults with Asperger syndrome. *Child and Adolescent Psychiatric Clinics of North America, 12*(1), 142–163.

Tsatsanis, K. (2003). Outcome research in Asperger syndrome and autism. *Child and Ado-*

lescent Psychiatric Clinics of North America, 12(1), 47–63.

Volkmar, F. R., & Klin, A. (2000). Diagnostic issues in Asperger syndrome. In A. Klin, F. R. Volkmar, & S. S. Sparrow (Eds.), *Asperger syndrome* (pp. 25–71). New York: Guilford Press.

Volkmar, F. R., Klin, A., & Paul, R. (2004). *Handbook of autism and pervasive developmental disorders* (3rd ed.). New York: Wiley.

Volkmar, F. R., Klin, A., Schultz, R. T., Rubin, E., & Bronen, R. (2000). Asperger's disorder. *American Journal of Psychiatry, 157*(2), 262–267.

Walz, M. (2002). *Autistic spectrum disorders: Understanding the diagnosis and getting help.* Cambridge, UK: O'Reilly.

Williams, K., Mellis, C., & Peat, J. K. (2005). Incidence and prevalence of autism. *Advances in Speech–Language Pathology, 7*(1), 31–40.

Wing, L. (2000). Past and future of research on Asperger syndrome. In A. Klin, F. R. Volkmar, & S. S. Sparrow (Eds.), *Asperger syndrome* (pp. 418–432). New York: Guilford.

Yang, Q., Rasmussen, S. A., & Friedman, J. M. (2002). Mortality associated with Down syndrome in the USA from 1983–1997: A population-based study. *Lancet, 359*(9331), 1019–1025.

Yeargin-Allsopp, M., Rice, C., Karapurkar, T., Doernberg, N., Boyle, C., & Murphy, C. (2003). Prevalence of autism in a U.S. metropolitan area. *Journal of the American Medical Association, 289*, 49–55.

Zaretsky, H. H., Richter, E. F., & Eisenberg, M. G. (Eds.). (2005). *Medical aspects of disability* (3rd ed.). New York: Springer.

Chapter 8

Psychiatric Disabilities

▪ A HISTORICAL PERSPECTIVE

Conceptualizations of psychiatric conditions, as well as strategies and interventions to treat psychiatric symptoms have changed drastically over time as societal views of psychiatric disability have changed. Psychiatric conditions have, in the past, been viewed as a condition in which individuals were possessed by demons, as a form of moral perversion disease, or as a manifestation of extreme emotion and eccentric behavior (Porter, 2001).

Regardless of the conceptualization, historically individuals with psychiatric conditions have been confronted not only with their symptoms, but also with accompanying negative social attitudes and rejection (Gordon, Tantillo, Feldman, & Perrone, 2004: Kahng & Mowbray, 2004). Prehistoric cultures viewed psychiatric symptoms as having a magical or religious basis to be treated with spells or rituals. Ancient Greek and Roman cultures viewed psychiatric disability as a consequence of immorality to be exorcized. In the Middle Ages, individuals with psychiatric symptoms were hospitalized, but often little more than custodial care was provided and individuals were often neglected and mistreated. In the 1800s, the emphasis was on a biological basis of psychiatric symptoms and the development of medical interventions to cure them (Porter, 2001). When no effective treatments were found, psychological rather than biological explanations for the development and treatment of psychiatric symptoms were in vogue. Nevertheless, strictly psychological approaches also proved to be inadequate to explain the development of psychiatric symptoms and for treating more serious psychiatric conditions (Porter, 2001).

In the 1950s the discovery of medications that could control psychiatric symptoms rekindled the conceptualization of psychiatric conditions as a biological entity. Control of symptoms with medication, along with other social factors, led to deinstitutionalization of large numbers of individuals from state hospitals. Deinstitutionalization shifted responsibility of care for individuals with psychiatric conditions into community settings, which necessitated the establishment of services in the community to meet their needs (Pollio, North, Reid, Miletic, & McClendon, 2006). Services frequently came in the form of community mental health centers designed to address these mental health needs. Although community mental health centers monitored medication effectiveness and addressed many short-term needs of individuals, overall long-term needs including ongoing support, access to housing, employment, and education often were ignored. Consequently, individuals with psychiatric disability often needed to be rehospitalized.

Despite the efforts over the years to simplify psychiatric conditions by turning them into medical, psychological, or environmental conditions that can be easily diagnosed and treated, trends suggest that in reality psychiatric conditions are extremely complex and individualized, so that no single approach can be adequate for all individuals. Psychiatric conditions have neurobiological and neurophysiological elements as well as psychological, social, and behavioral elements. The effective management of psychiatric disability requires that all elements, in the context of the individual, be considered.

As with physical conditions, the degree of disability experienced with psychiatric conditions varies. The focus of interventions to manage symptoms of psychiatric conditions has been transformed from the medical model, which focused on curing the psychiatric condition, to a *recovery model*, which fosters hope, autonomy, and empowerment for individuals with psychiatric disability. The recovery model focuses on providing accommodations, supports, and services that enable individuals with psychiatric disability to live full, productive, and dignified lives within the community. Many health professionals working with individuals with psychiatric disability now incorporate a biopsychosocial model, integrating concepts from biological and psychological models along with the effects of the social and interpersonal environment surrounding the individual.

Psychiatric rehabilitation (also referred to as *psychosocial rehabilitation*) is a multidisciplined approach to assist individuals with psychiatric disability develop skills and supports that will enable them to function at their highest capacity in the residential, educational, or vocational setting of their choice. Two overreaching goals of psychiatric rehabilitation are work and independence (Corrigan & McCracken, 2005). Increasingly, emphasis has been placed on treating and managing symptoms through evidence-based interventions

that have been shown to be efficacious relative to placebo or no treatment (Duncan, Miller, & Sparks, 2004).

■ DEFINING PSYCHIATRIC DISABILITY

Psychiatric disabilities have significant societal impact and are leading causes of disability worldwide (Agid, et al., 2007; Andersson, Wiles, Lewis, Brage, & Hensing, 2007). The term psychiatric disability encompasses a broad range of conditions with a wide variety of manifestations and varying degrees of disability. Although manifestations of psychiatric conditions and the degree of associated disability vary widely, generally psychiatric disability is thought to be a condition that blocks individuals' goals and interferes with their ability to function effectively within the community. Manifestations of psychiatric disability can consist of both behavioral actions and subjective feelings. Some psychiatric conditions may be accompanied by limitations in organizational ability, cognitive functions, or social interactions; others are associated with loss of contact with reality (**psychosis**). Still other psychiatric conditions are characterized by significant fluctuations and changes in mood or demonstrations of maladaptive behavior.

The extent of disability experienced by individuals as a result of a psychiatric condition depends, to a great extent, on the degree to which their manifestations:

- Interfere with their ability to function within their environment,
- Cause distress or disruption perceived by others in the environment, or
- Cause subjective distress to the individual.

Unlike many physical conditions, psychiatric conditions are more difficult to define and diagnose. Causes of psychiatric conditions are not always identifiable. There are no laboratory tests readily available to confirm the diagnosis.

Instead the primary basis for diagnosis and prediction of functional capacity is the experienced judgment of professionals conducting the evaluation. Moderating variables, such as the ethnic status, education, and/or socioeconomic status of both the client and the professional, may influence individuals' performance on evaluation as well as professionals' interpretation of the evaluation results.

The Diagnostic and Statistical Manual of Mental Disorders

The need for a systematic, more standardized approach to the diagnosis of psychiatric conditions has been recognized for more than a century. Although initially the classification and definition of psychiatric conditions was codified for the purpose of collecting statistical information, in 1952 the American Psychiatric Association's Committee on Nomenclature and Statistics published the *Diagnostic and Statistical Manual of Mental Disorders* (DSM-I). This book was the first official manual of mental disorders that had clinical utility. Since it's initial publication, there has been continued work to revise and refine the *DSM*.

As more empirical research and field trials have been conducted, reliability, descriptive validity, and performance characteristics for diagnostic criteria have been established. Updated versions of the manual bear the number of the edition (*e.g., DSM-II, DSM-III, and DSM-IV*). The fourth edition of the manual, *DSM-IV*, was published in 1994. In 2000, *DSM-IV-TR* (fourth edition, text-revision) was published, representing the latest effort in empirical documentation on which to base diagnostic decisions.

The *DSM* is an attempt to establish objective criteria for the diagnosis of psychiatric conditions. In addition to providing specific criteria on which to base a diagnosis, it provides consistency among professionals in communicating about psychiatric conditions. The use of the manual for diagnostic purposes requires specialized clinical training, because the criteria within the manual are meant to be guidelines and are not considered absolute. Although professionals working with individuals with psychiatric conditions should be familiar with the manual, responsibility for making a diagnosis most frequently lies with psychiatrists, psychologists, and, in some states, social workers.

The *DSM-IV-TR,* rather than taking a theoretical approach to defining psychiatric conditions, attempts to describe conditions by defining manifestations, which are observed. It should be emphasized that diagnostic criteria should *not* be used to categorize or label people, but rather to assist in treatment planning.

The *DSM-IV-TR* uses a multiaxial system of diagnosis to increase specificity. Given that since psychiatric conditions, like physical conditions, rarely occur in a vacuum and vary from individual to individual, the multiaxial approach helps professionals to avoid focusing only on specific manifestations. Rather, it enables professionals to take a comprehensive approach to identifying other variables that could affect interventions and help to predict outcome.

The *DSM* incorporated multiaxial diagnoses in 1980 in an effort to clarify complexities and relationships of manifestations, thereby assisting professionals in more appropriate management planning. The *DSM-IV-TR* uses five axes:

- Axis I describes clinical syndromes.
- Axis II describes personality disorders and mental retardation,
- Axis III describes medical conditions that may also be present and, consequently, be relevant to individuals' treatment.
- Axis IV describes relevant psychosocial or environmental problems that may have contributed to the development of the condition or may affect individuals' treatment or prognosis.

- Axis V is used for reporting individuals' overall level of functioning in the judgment of the clinician who has done the evaluation, in accordance with the Global Assessment of Functioning scale.

Level of functioning is determined by using the *Global Assessment of Functioning (GAF) scale*, which is a guideline for determining individuals' psychological, social, and occupational functioning along a hypothetical continuum of mental health and illness. Impairment in functioning due to physical or environmental limitations is not considered. Overall level of psychological functioning is rated on a scale of 1 to 100. The scale ranges from superior level of functioning (100) to persistent danger of hurting self or others (1).

Psychiatric conditions are coded according to the *International Classification of Diseases,* ninth revision, clinical modification (*ICD-9-CM*). In reporting evaluation results, the *ICD-9-CM* code precedes the name of the condition. Diagnostic codes are used for record keeping purposes and for reimbursement.

Examples of multiaxial recording of evaluation results with *ICD-9-CM* coding can be seen in Table 8-1.

■ DELIRIUM AND DEMENTIA

Delirium and dementia have in common manifestations in which there is a decrease in cognitive ability or memory from a prior level of functioning. These conditions are characterized by alteration of brain function and are often caused by an identifiable organic factor.

Both conditions can occur at any age. They can be secondary to another medical condition (e.g., heart disease in which circulation

---

Table 8-1   Multiaxial Recording of Evaluation Results

Case I

Axis I	309.81 Post-traumatic stress disorder
	305.0 Alcohol abuse
Axis II	V7.09 No Diagnosis
Axis III	491.20 Bronchitis, chronic obstructive pulmonary disease (COPD), without acute exacerbation
Axis IV	Unemployment
Axis V	GAF = 53 (current)

Case II

Axis I	295.30 Schizophrenia, paranoid type
Axis II	V71.09 No diagnosis
Axis III	250.01 Diabetes mellitus, type I/insulin dependent
Axis IV	Abusive caregiver
Axis V	GAF = 27 (on admission)
	GAF = 52 (on discharge)

Case III

Axis I	296.23 Major depressive disorder, single episode, severe without psychotic features
Axis II	317 Mental retardation
Axis III	None
Axis IV	None
Axis V	GAF = 60 (current)

and consequently oxygen supply to the brain are diminished) or can be caused by a systemic disease (e.g., thyroid disease), injury to the brain itself (e.g., mini-strokes), or toxic substances (e.g., poisons, alcohol, or other drugs). In addition, several causes may be present simultaneously. Manifestations of these conditions may affect psychological, cognitive, or behavioral function. In previous editions of the *DSM,* these conditions were classified as organic mental disorders. The *DSM-IV-TR* no longer uses this term, because it implies that other mental disorders may not have a biological basis.

The diagnosis of mental conditions in this category is usually based on a detailed history of manifestations, findings on physical and neurological evaluation, clinical and laboratory studies, and neuropsychological assessments. These conditions affect a variety of cognitive abilities:

- Memory
- Judgement orientation
- Attention
- Computational and organizational skills

There may also be associated psychomotor or language impairments, sleep disturbances, and other behavioral manifestations. Although some of these conditions remain stable, others are associated with progressive deterioration and decline of function.

Conditions classified in this *DSM* category can be acute or chronic. Manifestations of acute conditions are sudden in onset, such as symptoms caused by generalized infection or intoxication. Manifestations of chronic conditions generally occur more slowly and are characterized by the deterioration of cognitive processes over time, such as manifestations occurring with arteriosclerosis or Alzheimer's disease.

Mental conditions in this category may be either reversible or irreversible. If the underlying cause of the manifestations can be cor-

rected and the brain has not been permanently damaged, the condition is said to be *reversible.* If the underlying cause cannot be corrected or treated, or if the damage to the brain is permanent, the condition is referred to as *irreversible.*

Delirium

Delirium is characterized by difficulty in sustaining attention to external stimuli, difficulty in shifting attention to new stimuli, and difficulty in maintaining a coherent thought process. Manifestations of delirium characteristically develop over a short period of time and include clouded state of consciousness and confusion or disorientation. These manifestations may be caused by any of the following conditions:

- Infection
- Consequences of another medical condition
- Side effects of medication or drug interaction effects
- Substance intoxication or substance withdrawal
- A combination of causes

If the cause of delirium can be identified and is treated appropriately, and if no permanent brain damage has resulted, the condition is reversible.

Dementia

Dementia is a global deterioration of multiple intellectual abilities, including memory. In addition to memory impairment, impairments may occur in other higher intellectual functions, such as the ability to abstract, judgment, and personality variables. There are many causes of dementia, some of which are outlined in Table 8-2.

Some types of dementia are reversible, and some are not. Some potentially reversible dementias are listed in Table 8-3. Dementias such as those observed in Alzheimer's disease,

Table 8-2 Potential Causes of Dementia	
Alzheimer's disease	Infections of the central nervous system
Anemia	Metabolic disorders
Anoxia	Multicerebral infarcts
Binswanger's disease	Multiple demyelinating lesions
Brain tumor	Parkinson's disease
Chronic alcohol/drug use/abuse	Pick's disease
Chronic liver disease	Subdural hematoma
Chronic lung disease	Syphilis
Communicating hydrocephalus	Systemic lupus erythematosus
Creutzfeldt-Jakob disease	Thyroid disorders
Depression	Uremia
HIV infection	Vitamin B_{12} deficiency
Huntington's disease	

multi-infarct dementia, or arteriosclerosis are not reversible. Some conditions responsible for *nonreversible dementia* are described next.

Alzheimer's Disease

Alzheimer's disease is a progressive, degenerative type of dementia. Its onset is generally insidious, with gradual deterioration of cognitive function, eventually resulting in death. The most common and disabling manifestations of Alzheimer's disease are aggression and agitation, delusions, and hallucinations (Karlawish, 2006). Although Alzheimer's disease has commonly been thought of as a condition that occurs in older age groups, it may occur as early as middle life.

Although there are identifiable, structural changes in the brain characteristic of Alzheimer's disease (Goedert & Spillantini, 2006), there is currently no definitive way to make the diagnosis except by direct examination of the brain itself at autopsy. Diagnosis is based on documentation of memory impairment, cognitive testing, detailed personal and social history, progression of symptoms, drug evaluation, and ruling out other causes of manifestations through laboratory, physical, and neurological examinations.

Progression of Alzheimer's disease and the severity of manifestations at different stages vary from individual to individual. Some studies suggest that physical and mental exercise can slow down progression of the disease, so that severe incapacitation may not appear in the individual's lifetime (Marx, 2005). Although several drugs that mitigate manifestations are currently on the market, there is no cure for Alzheimer's disease. Management is directed toward helping individuals maintain general health, well-being, and functional capacity for as long as possible, as well as assisting in support of the family responsible for their care.

Table 8-3   Potential Reversible Causes of Dementia
Thyroid disorder
Anemia
Nutritional deficiencies
Depression

Multi-infarct Dementia

Multi-infarct dementia refers to a phenomenon in which deficits in cognitive function result from small strokes in various locations of the brain. Areas of damage can be identified through use of CAT scan or MRI. Once permanent damage to the brain occurs, functional loss of affected areas of the brain is not reversible. Management is directed toward controlling the underlying condition responsible for the small strokes so as to prevent further damage from occurring.

Dementia Due to Other Causes

Arteriosclerosis can contribute to dementia when vessels supplying blood to the brain become narrowed or occluded, diminishing blood flow and hence delivery of subsequent oxygen to the brain. Larger vessels, such as the carotid arteries in the neck, are often affected by this condition. Arteriosclerosis is a chronic condition (see Chapter 13). Consequently, management of dementia caused by arteriosclerosis is directed toward controlling the underlying disease itself.

Dementia may also be experienced as a result of HIV disease (see Chapter 10). In this type of dementia, destruction of brain tissue results in symptoms of forgetfulness, difficulty with concentration and problem solving, and general slowness. There may also be behavioral symptoms of apathy and social withdrawal, as well as motor symptoms such as tremor or difficulty walking.

Dementia due to brain trauma from a single injury is not progressive, but the damage to the brain and its consequent associated manifestations are permanent (see Chapter 3). Individuals who are exposed to repeated head trauma may have increased manifestations as additional trauma occurs. The degree and severity of manifestations will depend on the extent and location of injury in the brain. Manifestations may range from severe cognitive, motor, and sensory limitations to mild concentration and memory difficulties.

■ SCHIZOPHRENIA

Schizophrenia is a complex, chronic, lifelong condition characterized as a *psychotic disorder*. **Psychosis** is a condition in which there is distortion of reality and disturbances of thought. This neurodevelopmental disorder stems from interactions among genetic and environmental factors (Jarskog, Miyamoto, & Lieberman, 2007). The prevalence of schizophrenia in the general population is about 1%, with 70% of individuals experiencing their first manifestations between the ages of 15 and 35 (Schiffer, 2004). Manifestations of the condition cause impairment in the workplace, in social relationships, and in self-care.

Manifestations may develop slowly and insidiously. Individuals may show increasing lack of interest in their surroundings and gradually withdraw from family and friends. Personal appearance and hygiene may deteriorate over time. Previous level of function may gradually diminish, and the person may begin to demonstrate inappropriate behavior or responses. Although often development of manifestations occurs over time, in many cases manifestations have sudden onset, possibly related to a specific precipitating stress. Characteristic manifestations of schizophrenia include the following:

- Delusions
- Hallucinations
- Disorganized speech
- Disorganized behavior
- Flattening of affect or other negative symptoms (American Psychiatric Association, 2000)

Manifestations are categorized as either positive or negative. *Positive symptoms* include more active symptoms such as **delusions** (false beliefs), **hallucinations** (false perceptions with no relation to reality), or bizarre behavior. *Negative symptoms* refer to more passive manifestations such as social withdrawal, apathy, or inability to experience pleasure (*anhedonia*).

Individuals with delusions may experience beliefs that have no grounding in reality. Prominent delusions involve the false belief that their thoughts, feelings, or actions are being controlled by external forces, that their private thoughts are being transmitted to others *(thought broadcasting)*, and that thoughts are being inserted into their mind by others *(thought insertion)*. Individuals may assign personal significance on events that are unrelated to them, such as the belief that the radio announcer is delivering a special message to them personally *(ideas of reference)*. Individuals may exhibit an exaggerated sense of self such as holding a belief that they alone are able to save the world from disaster *(delusions of grandeur)*.

Although hallucinations are most often auditory, they may involve any of the senses. Individuals with auditory hallucinations may, for example, hear voices that direct them to perform a specific task. Individuals with visual hallucinations may see persons or objects that are not present.

Individuals may have *disorganized speech,* in which there is failure to conform to semantic and syntactic rules governing communication. Ideas and topics are fragmented and unrelated with no logical progression of thought and rapid shifting from one unrelated idea to the other *(loose of association)*. There may be *poverty of speech,* in which words spoken convey little meaning. Individuals may withdraw from involvement with the outside world and exhibit little motivation, having difficulty with self-initiated activity *(volition)*, even to the extent of maintaining a minimum standard of personal hygiene. There may be difficulty with decision making *(ambivalence)*, so that when presented with even a simple choice, such as whether to have orange juice or apple juice, they are unable to make up their mind and become agitated. Motor behavior may also be affected: Movement may be agitated, distorted, or extremely slow. Individuals may also

show *flattening of affect,* in which there is little expression or emotional response.

No specific cause of schizophrenia has been found, although it appears that multiple genetic and environmental factors contribute to disturbances in brain function (Tsuang, 2000). There is some evidence of structural or chemical disturbances in the brain of individuals with schizophrenia (Freedman, 2003).

Subtypes of Schizophrenia

Five subtypes of schizophrenia are described in the *DSM-IV-TR:*

- Paranoid type
- Disorganized type
- Catatonic type
- Undifferentiated type
- Residual type

Each subtype shares common symptoms of schizophrenia but is differentiated by specific symptoms. The *paranoid type* of schizophrenia is characterized by persecutory or grandiose delusions that are often supported by the hallucinations experienced. The *disorganized type* is characterized by incoherence of speech, loosening of associations, grossly disorganized behavior, and flat or inappropriate affect. The *catatonic type* of schizophrenia includes psychomotor behavior that is either agitated or so retarded that the individual appears to be in a stupor. Individuals with *undifferentiated type* have prominent psychotic symptoms, but symptoms do not fall into any specific category of schizophrenia. In the *residual type* of schizophrenia, individuals have experienced at least one schizophrenic episode in the past but have no current prominent psychotic symptoms, although some residual signs may remain.

Functional Issues in Schizophrenia

The acute or active phase of schizophrenia severely impairs personal and social functioning. During this phase, individuals require supervision and direction to meet basic needs and to prevent self-injury. Depending on their particular circumstances and the degree of available support, many individuals are able to function independently and obtain employment after the psychosis has been resolved. The degree of independent function possible depends on the success of the medication management of the condition, the extent of the individual's insight into the condition, and the extent to which he or she continues the management protocol. Some individuals need continued assistance because of repeated exacerbation of symptoms, residual symptoms, or impairment.

Management of Schizophrenia

Although there is currently no cure for schizophrenia, it is a condition from which individuals can recover (Gillam, 2006). Management is directed toward reducing and/or controlling manifestations, assisting individuals to focus on their strengths, and helping them manage difficulties so that they can function more effectively and appropriately within the community. Pharmacologic management and psychosocial interventions are used together to help individuals achieve maximum benefit. Medications are usually needed throughout life (Davis, 2006). The type of medication and the dose are individually determined. Individuals taking antipsychotic medications should be carefully monitored to determine the effectiveness of the medication in controlling manifestations and to identify any side effects or medication-related problems they may be experiencing.

Although antipsychotic drugs help reduce the risk of future psychotic episodes and assist individuals to resume independent function, they are not a guarantee against relapse. Likewise, medications used to treat manifestations of schizophrenia are not without serious side effects. In addition to side effects that cause discomfort (e.g., restlessness, decreased energy, weight gain, muscle spasms or tremors, dry mouth, difficulty with urination, or constipation), some newer atypical antipsychotic mediations have been shown to increase the risk of developing conditions such as diabetes and cardiovascular disease (Law, 2007; Lieberman et al., 2005).

Adherence to medication protocol has been shown to be a major problem for individuals with schizophrenia. Individuals who experience side effects, who fear that side effects may occur, or who may deny their need for medication may discontinue taking their medication (Gillam, 2006; Stroup, et al., 2006). A recent study found that 40% of individuals with schizophrenia discontinued their medication of their own accord (Lieberman et al., 2005). Whether the decision to discontinue medication was due to a lack of objective insight into the person's condition, the financial burden of medication cost or medication side effects is unknown (Dettling & Anghelesu, 2006). Abrupt discontinuation of antipsychotic medication can be potentially dangerous as well as have profound implications for long-term outcomes (Hui et al., 2006). Individuals expressing concerns about their medication should be referred to their physician for advice and monitoring.

In addition to medication, individuals are managed with a variety of psychosocial interventions to improve their functioning. Psychosocial interventions are directed toward improving individuals' coping resources and support systems, thereby minimizing the stress from life events and enhancing individual coping efforts (Beebe, 2007). Counseling and individual and/or group therapy can assist individuals to understand and accept their condition as well as to build self-esteem. Case management, behavioral interventions, social skills training, family groups, and support groups are other interventions that have been used successfully (Revheim & Marcopoulos, 2006).

Psychosocial Issues in Schizophrenia

The severity of manifestations and chronicity of schizophrenia have profound effects on both affected individuals and their families (Rhoades, 2000). The course and outcome for schizophrenia are immensely variable (Gillam, 2006). Individuals and families can experience social stigma and isolation, disruption of activities of daily life, interruption of future goals, financial burden, and other stressors that have effects on health and well-being.

Individuals with schizophrenia tend to have a number of health problems in addition to the symptoms experienced as a result of their condition. They have a 20% shorter life expectancy relative to the general population. People with schizophrenia have a high risk of obesity, twice the risk of developing diabetes, and twice the risk of dying from cardiovascular disease compared to the general population (Klam, et al., 2006). Although the risk is increased to some degree because of medication side effects, some of these excess risks are related to lifestyle, such as unhealthy diet, inactivity, and smoking. Smoking, for example, is twice as frequent in individuals with schizophrenia than in the general population (Klam et al. 2006).

Substance dependence and/or abuse is also a risk for individuals with schizophrenia and is associated with poorer outcomes (Swofford, Scheller-Gilkey, Miller, Woolwine, & Mance, 2000). Other risks include suicide attempts and homelessness.

Individual and family therapy can assist individuals and their families to develop the resources necessary to cope with this chronic lifelong condition as well as facilitate communication and enhance problem solving, which in turn increase the chance of a positive outcome. Although medical management remains key in helping individuals with schizophrenia achieve their optimum functional capacity, psychosocial interventions are the key to helping individuals and families achieve acceptance and ultimately successful outcomes.

Vocational Issues in Schizophrenia

Employment has numerous potential benefits for individuals with schizophrenia, including structure, socialization, increased income, and increased self-esteem (Twamley et al., 2005). Because individuals with schizophrenia generally experience their first symptoms in adolescence or young adulthood, when job and career choices and skill building are major development tasks, individuals may have limited work skills. Likewise, they may have difficulty with social skills. There may be a need for extensive job training, problem-solving, skills, and money management skills; use of public transportation; and social skills training. Individuals with schizophrenia may have difficulty coping with stress. Consequently, the amount of physical and emotional stress in the workplace and individuals' ability to cope with stress should be considered.

■ MOOD DISORDERS

Mood disorders comprise conditions in which the characteristic manifestation is disturbance in mood. While manifestations of mood disorders usually occur when individuals are in their twenties, depressive conditions have also been identified in children in early childhood (Krishnakumar & Geeta, 2006). Hospitalization is frequently necessary during the acute phase of mood disorders because of the severity of the disturbance that the condition creates in interpersonal and/or occupational functioning. In addition, there is a strong association with substance use disorders and mood disorders, which contributes further to disability (Compton, Thomas, Stinson, &

Grant, 2007). Disturbances in mood can be categorized as either *depressive disorders* or *bipolar disorders*.

Major Depressive Disorder

Major depressive disorder is one of the leading causes of functional impairment, second only to heart disease as a major cause of functional disability (Rytsala et al., 2007). It is defined by depressed mood or loss of interest in nearly all activities (or both for at least two weeks), which is accompanied by three or more of the following symptoms:

- Insomnia or *hypersomnia* (sleeping too much)
- Feelings of worthlessness or excessive guilt
- Fatigue or loss of energy
- Diminished ability to concentrate
- Substantial change in appetite or weight
- Psychomotor agitation or retardation
- Recurrent thoughts of death or suicide (American Psychiatric Association, 2000)

Depression imposes an enormous individual and societal burden in terms of economic cost, time lost at work, disability days, and pervasive effects on physical, mental, and social well-being (Lerner et al., 2004). Not only does it exist as a primary disability, but it also has the potential to coexist with any chronic illness or disability (Bishop & Sweet, 2000). Depression is frequently underdiagnosed, because manifestations can be confused with manifestations of other medical conditions (Whooley & Simon, 2000).

Individuals who are in the midst of a major depressive episode experience feelings of hopelessness and discouragement, loss of interest in activities previously found pleasurable, decreased energy levels, and difficulty with memory. They may also express feelings of worthlessness or guilt and have impaired cognitive functions, expressing the inability to concentrate or to make decisions. Other manifestations, such as insomnia or hypersomnia, and appetite disturbances resulting in weight gain or weight loss are called *vegetative signs*.

The degree of impairment produced by major depression varies, although social and occupational activities are usually affected to some degree. Chronic depression causes marked impairment in psychosocial function and work performance (Keller et al., 2000; Scott, 2000). With severe depression, incapacitation can be so great that individuals are unable to attend to their own daily needs, such as basic hygiene and nutrition. Prominent factors that have been found to be predictive of overall degree of disability are the severity, duration, and number of depressive episodes (Rytsala et al., 2005). In addition, older age appears to be a major factor predicting the degree of work disability (Rytsala et al., 2007).

Dysthymia

Dysthymia is a mood disorder characterized by symptoms similar to those experienced in major depression, but in a lesser degree. Although symptoms are not so severe, the chronic nature of the condition may impair social and occupational functioning. The essential distinction between major depressive disorder and dysthymia is the severity and duration of the symptoms. While major depression generally has a more acute onset, individuals with dysthymia may be chronically depressed for months or years.

Bipolar Disorders

Bipolar disorders are found in 2% to 5% of the population and are a common cause of disability (Huxley & Baldessarini, 2007). Each person with a bipolar disorder is affected differently. A range of personal, social, and environmental factors influence how manifestations of bipolar disorder affect each individual (Russell &

Browne, 2005). The condition is marked by *mood instability,* with resulting phases of *mania* (euphoria, increased energy, hyperactivity, irritability, or insomnia), and *depression* (loss of interest, sleep difficulties, despair, hopelessness). When individuals experience manifestations with both manic and depressive features, they are said to have a *mixed episode.* Some individuals have frequent alterations between mania and depression, a manifestation is called *rapid cycling.* Episodes of rapid cycling can take place in any combination or sequence, but usually occur four or more times in 12 months (Antai-Otong, 2006b). Mania may also be accompanied by psychotic manifestations such as psychosis, delusions, and hallucinations (McColm, Brown, & Anderson, 2006). Although both mania and depression can be debilitating, a major portion of the disability occurring with bipolar disorder results from the depressive phase of the condition (Howland, 2006a; Post, 2005; Mitchell & Malhi, 2004).

While the onset of bipolar disorder usually occurs in adolescence or young adulthood, it has been noted as late as in the early forties (Kennedy et al., 2005; Meyer & Quenzer, 2005) and in children younger than the age of 13 (Spearing, 2002; Perlis, Miyahara & Marangell, 2004). Individuals often experience a *prodrome,* or period prior to the development of major symptoms during which there is deviation from previous levels of function but symptoms are not recognized as manifestations of bipolar disorder (Conus, Berk, & McGorry, 2006). Λ high correlation between substance abuse and bipolar disorder has been noted, although the extent to which substance abuse is an attempt at self-medication or precipitates manifestations is unknown (Salloum & Thase, 2000; Strakowski & DelBello, 2000). Anxiety-related disorders, including social phobias, panic disorder, and obsessive–compulsive disorders, have also been found to co-occur with bipolar disorder (Freeman, Freeman, & McElroy, 2002). Individuals with bipolar disorder are at higher risk for suicide, especially

when emerging from depression, and for committing violence against others if experiencing anger and aggressiveness during the manic phase (Murphy, 2006).

There are three major classifications of bipolar disorder:

- Bipolar I disorder
- Bipolar II disorder
- Cyclothymia (American Psychiatric Association, 2000)

Bipolar I Disorder

Bipolar I disorder is the most common of the three major classifications and is characterized by the occurrence of at least one manic episode, which lasts more than one week and interferes with social, interpersonal, or vocational functioning, or by one mixed episode (Montejano, Goetzel, & Ozminkowski, 2005; American Psychiatric Association, 2000). During manic episodes, the person's mood becomes distinctly elevated and behavior becomes hyperactive. Individuals in a manic episode appear flamboyant and overly enthusiastic, often engaging in excessive activity and needing little sleep. Speech becomes rapid, nonstop *(pressured speech),* loud, and difficult to follow because of rapid changes from one unrelated topic to another *(flight of ideas).* A *mixed episode* is characterized by rapidly changing moods alternating between elation and sadness. Individuals with bipolar I disorder also frequently have one or more major depressive episodes (American Psychiatric Association, 2000).

Manic episodes impair social and occupational functioning considerably. During these episodes, individuals may be easily distracted. Their attention shifts rapidly from one activity to another, unrelated activity with little provocation. They may have grandiose delusions in which they believe that they have special skills, knowledge, or relationships. Hallucinations may occur during a manic episode and often relate to the individual's mood or delusions. Poor judgment during the manic phase can lead to catastrophic financial losses or illegal activities.

Bipolar II Disorder

Bipolar II disorder is similar to bipolar I disorder, but is characterized by at least one major depressive episode and milder form of mania (*hypomania*). The presence of the hypomanic episode distinguishes bipolar II disorders from major depressive disorders (American Psychiatric Association, 2000). A major depressive episode is characterized by loss of interest in activities, sadness, and depressed mood. By contrasts a hypomanic episode is characterized by elevated or irritable mood over a period of time. If individuals experience a manic or mixed episode, they are then categorized as having bipolar I disorder rather than bipolar II disorder.

Cyclothymia

Cyclothymia is a mood disorder characterized by manifestations similar to those of bipolar disorders, with both hypomanic manifestations and mild depressive manifestations lasting more than two years (Montejano et al., 2005). Because manifestations are usually milder, cyclothymia causes less impairment in function than does a bipolar disorder. The distinction between bipolar disorders and cyclothymia is not clearly demarcated, and the diagnosis often depends on the judgment of the evaluator regarding the severity of the episode. Owing to the chronic nature of the condition, individuals with cyclothymia can experience manifestations for months or years.

Management of Bipolar Disorders

Bipolar disorders are not always immediately diagnosed, even after manifestations are present. Manifestations may be disguised by alcohol and/or substance abuse or, if manifestations are mild, as in hypomania, they may be denied or ignored. Individuals who experience psychotic manifestations may be diagnosed as having schizophrenia, rather than bipolar disorder. If depressive manifestations are present, individuals may be diagnosed as having major depression rather than bipolar disorder.

Accurate diagnosis of bipolar disorders is crucial because it has important implications for management and prognosis (Bowden, 2005). Although bipolar disorder is a lifelong condition, appropriate treatment can have a significant impact on the individual's quality of life and on his or her ability to work (Montejano et al., 2005). Acute manifestations are usually treated with medications. Once symptoms are stabilized, maintenance management—which may include both medication and psychosocial interventions—is instituted to improve function and to prevent further occurrence of manic or depressive episodes.

In the past, *lithium* was the main drug used in management of bipolar disorders. Today, however, many different drugs may be used depending on the stage and phase of the condition. While in the manic phase, individuals may receive lithium as well as several other medications such as anticonvulsant drugs, which have mood-stabilizing effects. Likewise, antipsychotic drugs are used for management of acute manic episodes. Individuals who experience anxiety may also be given antianxiety medications. If individuals have severe bipolar depression, in addition to lithium or an anticonvulsant drug, an antidepressant may be added. The use of antidepressants for bipolar depression is somewhat controversial however, because there is a risk of mood destabilization (Howland, 2006b; Montejano et al., 2005). When medication does not adequately control symptoms, *electroconvulsive therapy (ECT)* may be indicated.

Although treatment with medication is essential for controlling manifestations in bipolar disorders, nonadherence to medication regimens is high (Consus et al., 2006; Huxley & Baldessarini, 2007). Consequently, effective management of bipolar disorders includes a combination of medication and psychosocial interventions. Strategies that help individuals manage manifestations include psychosocial education in which the individual and their family gain general information the condition, learn to manage symptoms, and identify potential triggers of mood change. Other strategies, such as cognitive-behavioral therapy, may be used to help individuals learn to monitor their behavior and thoughts and develop a plan for handling stress and crisis. Interpersonal and group therapies as well as participation in self-help groups are other interventions that are used to help individuals gain insight into their management, establish healthy thinking styles, maintain interpersonal relationships, and explore the effects of the condition on self-esteem (Frank et al., 2005).

Psychosocial Issues in Bipolar Disorders

Social adjustment, interpersonal relationships, leisure activities, and vocational function may all be impaired in individuals with bipolar disorders (Huxley & Baldessarini, 2007). Accepting and learning about the condition are major steps toward managing it. Individuals with bipolar disorders may be concerned about disclosure regarding their condition, stigma, unpredictability of mood, unstable interpersonal relationships, and potential financial and career loss. Strategies to maintain function and prevent relapses can be developed to help individuals learn to observe small changes in their physical, mental, or emotional status that may be early warning signs of relapse. In this way, individuals become able to implement interventions, that can prevent relapse from occurring. The response to his or her condition is different for each individual. Identification of specific factors, such as fatigue, seasonal changes, or hormonal changes, that serve as triggers for episodes of mania or depression can help each person institute interventions specific to his or her individual response.

Making changes such as maintaining a healthy diet, exercising, getting adequate sleep, taking medication regularly, avoiding alcohol and/or drug abuse, and adopting a less hectic lifestyle may help individuals to avoid relapse.

Maintaining a range of social support networks such as family and friends, community groups or organizations, religious affiliations, or support groups, can also help individuals better manage their condition.

Vocational Issues in Bipolar Disorders

The rates of unemployment and underemployment for individuals with bipolar disorders far exceed the corresponding rates for the general population despite the former's relatively high premorbid academic and vocational functioning (Huxley & Baldessarini, 2007). Lack of understanding of bipolar disorder and manifestations may contribute to these low employment rates, as does the stigma associated with psychiatric disability. Individual and group psychotherapy can have a positive influence on vocational status by helping individuals gain insight into and a sense of control over, management of their condition (Lam, Hayward, Watkins, Wright, & Sham, 2005). Early onset of manifestations and a more severe and longer course of manifestations have both been associated with some cognitive impairments, such as impairment in executive function, attention, and verbal and working memory, which may influence functional ability in individuals with bipolar disorders (Smith, Muir, & Blackwood, 2006). In these instances, cognitive remediation may be helpful in improving functional capacity.

Workplace accommodations may assist individuals with bipolar disorders to continue or obtain employment. The extent of accommodations needed depends on the individual's unique circumstances. Examples of specific workplace accommodations that may be needed include flexible scheduling and minimizing distractions in the immediate work environment

■ ANXIETY DISORDERS

Anxiety disorders are prevalent, disabling, and often not recognized and treated (Kroenke,

Spitzer, Williams, Monahan, & Lowe, 2007). Approximately one-fourth of the U. S. population experiences some type of anxiety disorder over the course of a lifetime (Kessler et al., 2005) and about 17% experience severe anxiety (Antai-Otong, 2006a). A number of different types of anxiety disorders exist:

- Panic disorder
- Agoraphobia
- Phobias
- Social phobia (social anxiety disorder)
- Obsessive–compulsive disorder
- Post-traumatic stress disorder
- General anxiety disorder (Issakidis, Sanderson, Corry, Andrews, & Lapsley, 2004; Roy-Byrne & Wagner, 2004; Gross et al., 2005; Gillock, Zayfert, Hegel, & Ferguson, 2005; Magruder, Frueh et al., 2005).

Common features of these disorders include not only anxiety, but also increased arousal and avoidance of situations that the individual perceives as anxiety provoking. Individuals with anxiety disorders also frequently have a mood disorder, especially depression (Garakani, Mathew, & Charney, 2006).

A number of psychotherapeutic interventions (e.g., exposure therapy, relaxation techniques) and medications are used to treat anxiety disorders. Although benzodiazepines were at one time first-line treatments, selective serotonin reuptake *inhibitors (SSRIs)* are now also frequently used in the treatment of anxiety disorders (Sheehan & Sheehan, 2007).

Panic Disorders

Panic disorders are anxiety disorders in which individuals experience feelings of intense fear or discomfort; they are characterized by **panic attacks,** episodes in which the individual has feelings of intense anxiety or terror, accompanied by a sense of impending doom (American Psychiatric Association, 2000). During a panic attack, an individual experiences physical symptoms, such as shortness of breath, increased heart rate and palpitations, sweat-

ing, and, at times, nausea or other physical discomfort. Panic attacks may occur spontaneously and not be triggered by a certain event (unexpected or uncued panic attack) and, at least initially, are unpredictable and at times irrational. At other times, panic attacks are directly related to different situations or stimuli (situationally bound or cued panic attack). Attacks usually last from a few minutes to a few hours. During attacks, individuals may express fear of losing control, fear of dying, or a feeling of being detached from reality (Antai-Otong, 2006a). Although the panic attack in and of itself may not be disabling, the individual's fears and concerns associated with the attack can cause significant change in behavior, including avoiding certain situations or, in some instances, giving up a job.

Panic disorder is distinguished from generalized anxiety in that individuals with panic disorders become preoccupied with the physical symptoms associated with the panic attack (Mahoney, 2000). Management focuses on amelioration of manifestations through medication and counseling.

Agoraphobia

Panic disorders are sometimes accompanied by **agoraphobia,** the fear of being in a situation or place from which it might be difficult or embarrassing to escape or in which there may be no help available if the individual experiences a panic attack. Although not all individuals who have panic attacks experience agoraphobia, those who do may severely restrict their activity, hampering both social and occupational functioning. They may refuse to venture outside their home alone, or they may be reluctant to travel by car, bus, or other common means of transportation.

Phobias

The term **phobia** refers to fear and anxiety related to specific situations, persons, or objects. Different types of phobias are categorized on the basis of the object of fear.

Impairments resulting from phobias may vary from mild to severe. On the one hand, a phobia may be more of a nuisance than a disability. On the other hand, a phobia may be so disabling that individuals are unable to function effectively in their day-to-day activities if the phobia causes them to avoid particular objects or situations or causes anxiety to the extent that they are unable or unwilling to engage in necessary activities.

Social Phobia (Social Anxiety Disorder)

Social phobia consists of a persistent fear of social situations such as parties or other social gatherings. Individuals with social phobia avoid these situations because of the distress they experience and fear of embarrassment. Social phobia can severely affect individuals, jobs, relationships, and social functioning.

Obsessive–Compulsive Disorder

Obsessive–compulsive disorder (OCD) is a chronic condition that, if not treated, can cause significant disability, with symptoms following a waxing and waning course (Maj, Sartorius, Okasha, & Zohar, 2002). Although OCD usually occurs in late adolescence or early adulthood, its onset can appear any time throughout the life span, from preschool age to older adults (Zohar, Fostick, Black, & Lopez-Ibor, 2007).

Individuals with OCD have recurrent **obsessions** (persistent thoughts) or **compulsions** (persistent actions) that they are unable to control. For instance, individuals may have recurrent thoughts of the death of a loved one, or they may have an irresistible urge to perform repetitively some behavior that seems purposeless, such as turning a light on and off three times before retiring for the night. Attempts by individuals to ignore the compulsions merely increase anxiety, discomfort, and distress. Individuals with OCD may experience considerable shame regarding manifestations

of the condition, and in an attempt to keep manifestations secret, they may not seek help. OCD can cause significant distress and social disability. Individuals may become increasingly reluctant to interact socially and may, in some instances, become housebound.

Cognitive-behavioral therapy is a major intervention for OCD (Foa, Franklin, & Moser, 2002). Medication is often used in combination with cognitive-behavioral therapy, especially for individuals who are unable to function in their job or socially owing to manifestations of the condition (Jenike, 2004).

Post-Traumatic Stress Disorder

Post-traumatic stress disorder (PTSD) is a disabling condition, that is often accompanied by depression (Ipser, Seedat, & Stein, 2006). When depression is present, functional status of PTSD is negatively influenced (Stapleton, Asmundson, Woods, Taylor, & Stein, 2006). PTSD is broadly defined as an anxiety disorder in which symptoms occur after the experience of a traumatic event, such as an automobile accident, plane crash, natural disaster, or act of violence (Hough & Ursano, 2006). Individuals may develop manifestations of the condition after either experiencing a traumatic event themselves or observing a traumatic event. Reactions to a traumatic event vary with the individual, although manifestations of PTSD generally fall into three broad categories (Strauser, Lustig, & Uruk, 2006):

- Persistent recollection of the event; sleep difficulties; difficulty concentrating; hypervigilance or hyperarousal; exaggerated startle responses when exposed to stimuli related to the traumatic event
- Persistent experience of the event; recall of distressing images; nightmares or flashbacks
- Emotional numbing; avoidance of individuals or situations reminiscent of the event; detachment; loss of interest in pre-

viously enjoyed activities or in important close relationships.

PTSD, which may occur at any age, causes varying degrees of impairment. Individuals with a previous history of mental health problems, or with depression or an anxiety disorder at the time of the traumatic event, are at higher risk for development of PTSD (Stevenson, 2005; Freedy & Simpson, 2007). Distress experienced with PTSD can affect mental function, including memory. Individuals with PTSD may have difficulty concentrating. Short-term memory has also been found to be significantly affected in PTSD, which can affect intellectual function (Emdad & Sondergaard, 2006).

Physical manifestations of PTSD may also be present. Individuals may experience vague or severe physical manifestations, such as headache, gastrointestinal upset, fatigue, or muscle tension, which do not have an easily identifiable physical cause (Lincoln et al., 2006). Chest pain related to anxiety may also be present and at times may be misinterpreted so that treatment for what could be a cardiac condition is delayed (Alcaras & Roper, 2006). Emotional manifestations of PTSD such as emotional withdrawal, irritability, and distrust of others are frequently experienced as well (Freedy & Simpson, 2007).

When PTSD is identified and appropriately managed, the prognosis is frequently positive (Stevenson, 2005). Conversely, if PTSD is not identified and manifestations persist, it can be debilitating and require ongoing psychological and pharmacologic intervention (Ursano, 2002).

Education and counseling can help individuals understand the nature of their condition and facilitate their recovery. Psychodynamic therapies may be used to help individuals explore their feelings and behavior. Cognitive therapy and anxiety management therapies can also be helpful. Group therapy and peer counseling groups reduce isolation and

stigma and provide individuals with PTSD the opportunity to discuss and share their experiences with others (Foa, Keane, & Friedman, 2000; Stevenson, 2005). Symptoms of PTSD also affect other family members. So family therapy is helpful to encourage family members discuss specific issues. Medications such as SSRIs are often used in the treatment of PTSD to reduce symptoms, including associated depression (Ipser et al., 2006).

■ SOMATOFORM DISORDERS

Somatoform disorders are conditions in which individuals experience physical symptoms for which no organic cause can be found. These symptoms can cause significant distress and impairment in social, occupational, and interpersonal functioning (American Psychiatric Association, 2000).

Somatization Disorder

Somatization disorder is a somatoform disorder that is characterized by recurrent, multiple physical complaints, for which a medical cause cannot be found. Physical manifestations can be so distressing that they impair social or occupational function. Because physical manifestations are often similar to manifestations of a variety of medical conditions, individuals may receive medical intervention for their manifestations even though no organic cause can be found. Individuals with somatization disorder do not consciously produce the manifestations but truly experience them, although no organic cause of the manifestations is readily identifiable.

Conversion Disorder

Another type of somatoform disorder is *conversion disorder*. In this condition, individuals lose physical function, often related to neurological function (e.g., paralysis, blindness, or numbness of a body part). Manifestations do not typically follow a pattern that would correspond to a specific disease or injury. Again, the individual does not intentionally produce the manifestations.

Hypochondriasis

Hypochondriasis, another type of somatoform disorder, is characterized by preoccupation with physical illness. Individuals with this condition may fear or believe that they have a serious physical illness or, in some instances, may perceive the manifestations of a coexisting disease or condition in an exaggerated way. For example, they may perceive a cough associated with a common cold as a sign of tuberculosis or lung cancer.

◼ PAIN DISORDER

Pain disorder is a preoccupation with pain that is severe enough to cause impairment in function at home, school, or work, although no organic cause can be found to explain the pain manifestation. Individuals with pain disorder do not consciously produce the manifestations of a pain and actually experience the pain reported. This condition can be extremely incapacitating, often severely limiting social and work activities.

◼ FACTITIOUS DISORDERS

Although not severely disabling, a variety of other mental conditions may interfere with effective functioning. **Factitious disorders** are conditions in which individuals *voluntarily* produce psychological or physical symptoms, feigning illness because of a seemingly compulsive need to assume the sick role (American Psychiatric Association, 2000). A factitious disorder differs from **malingering** (in which individuals also produce symptoms intentionally) in that the goal of malingering is usually obvious, such as a desire to receive an insurance settlement or to collect disability payments.

◼ DISSOCIATIVE DISORDERS

Conditions in which individuals experience an alteration in memory, consciousness, or identity for no organic reason are called *dissociative disorders*. *Dissociative fugue* is a condition in which individuals leave their environment and assume a new identity without being able to recall their previous identity. *Dissociative amnesia* is the inability to recall events that occurred within a certain period of time or the inability to recall information regarding one's own identity. *Dissociative identity disorder* (formerly known as multiple personality disorder) is a condition in which at least two personalities exist within the same individual and control the individual's behavior.

◼ PERSONALITY DISORDERS

Everyone has personality traits or characteristics. If these traits are maladaptive, they can interfere with function, especially during times of crisis. **Personality disorders** are characterized by inflexible or maladaptive behaviors, usually characteristic of long-term functioning, which impair interpersonal or occupational functioning or cause subjective distress (American Psychiatric Association, 2000).

Individuals with personality disorders may have no insight into the role that their own behavior plays in creating problems within their environment. They may rationalize their actions, blaming others for their situation or misfortune without examining their own responsibility for the situation at hand.

Many types of personality disorders exist (e.g., *paranoid, antisocial, borderline*), which cause varying degrees of impairment. When a personality disorder exists in combination with other mental conditions, the prognosis is more guarded, and intervention and management of the personality disorder are more difficult. At times, affected individuals may not have a full-blown personality disorder, but rather their maladaptive personality traits may interfere with the management or the diagnosis of the concomitant condition.

■ DIAGNOSTIC PROCEDURES IN PSYCHIATRIC DISABILITY

The diagnosis of mental conditions is as much an art as a science. It requires skill and experience on the part of those evaluating individuals' manifestations and interpreting results of the various tests designed to measure psychological or intellectual function. Many professionals may be involved in testing and evaluation; psychiatrists and clinical psychologists are frequently involved in the diagnosis of mental conditions. Diagnosis is usually based on information gathered from a variety of sources.

Uses of Diagnostic Psychological Testing

Systematic samples of certain types of verbal, perceptual, intellectual, and motor behavior under standardized conditions can be obtained through psychological testing. Psychological tests may be used to evaluate intelligence, personality, or behavior.

Results of psychological tests provide partial information needed for the accurate diagnosis of a mental condition. Note, however, that no single test is adequate to offer a definitive diagnosis in all situations. Because mental conditions often affect a variety of functions, use of several psychological tests that measure different functions is frequently required.

Intelligence Tests

The term *intelligence* is difficult to define. Theoretically, intelligence consists of a number of skills and abilities, some of which have no means of measurement. Intelligence is a combination of individuals' own unique mental structures and processes plus cultural and educational experiences.

Psychological science has developed a number of tests to define intelligence operationally for a variety of capacities. The most commonly used intelligence tests are the *Wechsler Intelligence Scale for Children—Revised (WISC-R), the Wechsler Preschool and Primary Scale of Intelligence (WPPSI), the Stanford–Binet test, and the Wechsler Adult Intelligence Scale—Revised (WAIS-R).*

Limitations of intelligence testing originate from several sources:

- The difficulty of tapping all aspects of intellectual ability
- The effects of individual ability to take the test
- The degree to which the test measures aptitude rather than prior learning and experience
- The effects of cultural variation on test results

One way of classifying levels of intelligence is through a numerical value known as the IQ (intelligence quotient). There is considerable individual variability in abilities, however, and the results of intelligence tests, like the results of other forms of psychological tests, must be evaluated within the context of the individual's cultural and environmental variables. Much intelligence testing involves sampling individuals' intellectual capacity in a variety of different spheres. Many tests focus on cognitive processes, including problem solving, adaptive thinking, and other aspects of performance. Tests alone should not determine a definitive diagnosis.

Mental Status Examination and Assessment Through Interview

The structured interview is one way in which the mental functioning of an individual with a suspected mental condition may be assessed during the initial evaluation. Information obtained in this way may aid in determining the diagnosis, as well as in making plans for future treatment.

Structured interviews provide information regarding individuals' orientation, form and content of thought, speech, affect, and degree of insight. Observations made during the interview of individuals' general appearance, behavior, and emotional state are also relevant.

The *mental status examination* is a specific type of structured interview used as a screening instrument in assessing intellectual impairment. Such an examination may be used to detect dementia or impaired intellectual function, as well as to determine the severity of the impairment. Several mental status examinations of varying lengths have been developed. Although some are part of other instruments that measure functional status, a number of short screening instruments have been devised especially for the purpose of evaluating mental status. One widely used mental status test is the *Short Portable Mental Status Questionnaire (SPMSQ)*, which is used to assess orientation, personal history, remote memory, and calculation. Another short mental status examination is the *Mini-Mental State Examination* (MMSE), which is used to assess orientation, memory, and attention, as well as the ability to write, name objects, copy a design, and follow verbal and written commands.

Personality Assessment

Personality may be assessed by either *objective* or *projective* means. Objective personality assessment instruments are structured, standardized tests for which clear and concise criteria have been established. These tests have undergone research and scientific scrutiny to establish their reliability and validity. Although numerous objective personality tests are available, one of the most commonly used is the *Minnesota Multiphasic Personality Inventory*

(MMPI). The MMPI has a number of clinical scales that can be useful in the diagnosis of a variety of mental disorders, ranging from schizophrenia to depression, social introversion, and substance abuse.

Projective personality tests, such as the *Rorschach inkblot test* and the *Thematic Apperception Test (TAT)*, also have criteria on which interpretations are based, but they are generally more subjective in nature. Projective testing usually consists of asking individuals to describe vague and ambiguous pictures. There are no right or wrong answers. The assumption is that the way in which an individual interprets the pictures is a reflection of his or her personality.

Projective tests may be more time-consuming to administer than are objective tests, and professionals who administer them require special training. As with all other clinical data, the results of personality assessment tests are merely one part of the total information needed for an accurate diagnosis of a particular mental condition. No matter which type of test is used, the accuracy of the results depends on the individual's honesty and care in answering test questions. If the individual answers questions in a socially desirable way rather than as an expression of his or her true feelings, test results can be invalid.

Neuropsychological Testing

Standardized neuropsychological test batteries may be used to assess major functional areas of the brain. These tests make it possible to assess a variety of cognitive, perceptual, and motor skills.

Traditionally, neuropsychological testing has been used to identify or localize brain damage that has behavioral consequences; however, with newer technological advances such as computed tomography (CT) and magnetic resonance imaging (MRI), this function is now not widely promoted. Neuropsychological tests have become increasingly popular to rule out and monitor the progression of the manifestations of mental conditions that have an identified organic basis. Because individual performance on neuropsychological tests changes with brain function, test results provide a baseline against which future impairment of brain function can be measured; they also provide data that can be incorporated into the diagnosis.

A variety of comprehensive standard neuropsychological test batteries are available for adults. Two of the more widely recognized tests are the *Halstead–Reitan Battery* and the *Luria–Nebraska Neuropsychological Battery.*

Behavioral Assessment

Some methods of assessing mental function involve direct, systematic observation of individuals' behavior. Trained observers, family members, or even individuals themselves may monitor and record individuals' behavior. Observation and measurement of behavior may take place in individuals' own environment or in a controlled environment. Behavioral assessment methods are being applied to an increasing number of conditions, because they offer not only information that can be used in diagnosis, but also a method of monitoring improvements in behavior once treatment has been initiated.

■ MANAGEMENT OF PSYCHIATRIC DISABILITY

There is no single therapeutic approach used for treatment of all psychiatric disabilities. Instead, treatment of psychiatric disability is based on a comprehensive assessment of the individual's problems, needs, and strengths. It is usually a collaborative effort involving the individual, the family, and professionals from a variety of disciplines, such as psychiatrists, psychologists, social workers, nurses, and rehabilitation counselors. Interventions may be provided in a variety of settings, depending on the individual's particular condition and specific needs.

Levels of intervention range from the least restrictive, such as that provided in an outpatient setting, to the most restrictive, such as that provided in an institutional setting. Levels of intervention in between these two extremes include intensive outpatient intervention, residential care, and halfway houses.

Intervention in acute episodes of psychiatric conditions may initially focus on alleviating manifestations of the condition. Ongoing intervention is directed toward preventing recurrence of manifestations and helping individuals attain optimal functional capacity. Many psychiatric conditions require ongoing intervention or periodic evaluations of the effectiveness of the intervention prescribed. Some psychiatric conditions, like many physical conditions, require daily medication to control manifestations and are characterized by periods of remission and periods of exacerbation. In many instances, individuals' willingness and ability to adhere to the prescribed intervention can determine the success of intervention.

A variety of intervention modalities, including both nonpharmacologic and pharmacologic methods, may be used to reduce, alleviate, and manage the manifestations experienced in psychiatric disability. More intensive levels of care may include, in addition to psychotherapy and pharmacologic intervention, occupational therapy, art and music therapy, or recreational therapy. Often several different types of interventions are used simultaneously.

Nonpharmacologic Approaches to Management of Psychiatric Disability

Psychiatric Rehabilitation (Psychosocial Rehabilitation)

Accurate *DSM* diagnosis is considered a cornerstone of management of psychiatric disability, as it allows appropriate medications and therapies designed to eliminate and manage manifestations to be prescribed. Many psychiatric disabilities require ongoing medications to control and manage manifestations. Although medications can reduce manifestations and hospitalizations in individuals with psychiatric disability, the most effective intervention typically includes psychosocial interventions in addition to medication management. Psychiatric disabilities, however, affect multiple areas of function. Consequently, a multitude of personal, environmental, and health factors must be considered in helping individual's function to their optimum capacity (MacDonald-Wilson & Nemec, 2005).

Psychiatric rehabilitation (sometimes called psychosocial rehabilitation) is a multidisciplinary approach that assists individuals with chronic psychiatric disability to address specific psychosocial issues not addressed by medication alone. Psychiatric rehabilitation has been conceptualized as a process by which individuals are assisted to develop those skills and supports they need to be successful and satisfied in their chosen environment (Anthony, Cohen, Farkas, & Gagne, 2002). Basic goals of psychiatric rehabilitation include recovery, community integration, and improved quality of life (Pratt, Gill, Barrett, & Roberts, 1999). Psychiatric rehabilitation is community based, client centered, and empowerment oriented (Leech & Holcomb, 2000), and it helps individuals identify and obtain resources and support needed to attain their goals (Garske, 1999).

Community Support Programs

Community support programs encompasss a network of services that are made available to individuals with psychiatric disability living in the community. Services focus on systems of outreach, support, advocacy, and other types of assistance that may be needed by individuals in their daily lives and are directed toward assisting individuals with psychiatric disability to live as independently as possible in the community.

Clubhouse Model

In the 1950s, the *clubhouse model* of psychosocial rehabilitation was created at Fountain House in New York City. This model provides integrated mental health, employment, and peer support services and has become mandated as a mental health service under managed care in several states (Macias, Jackson, Schroeder, & Want, 1999).

In the 1990s, many states shifted to a case management approach. By the end of the decade, independent employment models were being created within clubhouses in an effort to assist members achieve employment with higher wages and more advancement potential (Reed & Merz, 2000). Clubhouses not only provide a central meeting place for individuals with psychiatric disability, but also provide informal and experiential strategies to help individuals gain skills that can be integrated into the workplace. Vocational participation may range from clubhouse members performing chores around the clubhouse to members identifying and obtaining part-time employment within the community. The effectiveness of several of these programs has been evaluated and results are mixed (Reed & Merz, 2000; Pratt et al., 1999). Continued research to assess the efficacy of programs in integrating individuals into both society and the workplace is essential to effective rehabilitation of individuals with psychiatric disability (Accordino, Porter, & Morse, 2001).

Social Skills Training

The purpose of *social skills training* is to identify specific social skills deficits and the circumstances under which these deficits occur. Educational interventions are then directed toward correcting these deficits. Interventions usually begin by targeting small elements of behavior and then gradually adding elements of behavior, working toward the ideal. Through participation in social skills training groups, individuals learn to make specific responses to specific social situations, to recognize relevant social cues, and to determine appropriate action by using the cues. Such training may involve specific interventions, such as role modeling, feedback and reinforcement, and practice, with the goal of helping individuals to perform specified behaviors reliably and to generalize the behavior to other situations.

Specialized Groups

Individuals with some types of psychiatric disability may neglect their own needs of daily living, including personal hygiene, money management, or housing needs. Special groups (e.g., activities of daily living groups) may help individuals learn the specific skills needed for day-to-day functioning.

The popularity of self-help groups that provide support as well as other types of assistance has grown considerably over the last decade. Drop-in centers that offer an opportunity for social interaction with other individuals with psychiatric disability, recreational activities, and other types of practical assistance have become increasingly popular as well. *The National Alliance for the Mentally Ill (NAMI)* is a grassroots organization that is part of this movement; it provides education, support, and advocacy for individuals with psychiatric disability and their families.

Individuals with some types of psychiatric disability may require ongoing supervision, and many require a period of transition from inpatient settings to outpatient settings. A variety of therapeutic living arrangements may be used to meet their needs, including group homes, therapeutic communities, and transitional living centers. Day programs provide a structured environment in which individuals may participate in the program during the day and return to the community setting at night. The goal of day programs is to facilitate the adjustment of these individuals to the com-

munity setting, to help them maintain their optimal level of functioning, and to prevent hospitalization.

Assertive Community Treatment

Assertive community treatment (ACT) programs utilize multidisciplinary teams to provide highly individualized services to individuals with psychiatric disability in an effort to decrease or eliminate their symptoms and to prevent relapse. ACT assists individuals to meet basic needs, improve functioning within the community, and increase their ability to live independently. Rather than using a case management model in which services are distributed among a number of different agencies or services, members of the ACT team work collaboratively to offer direct services to the individual. Members of the ACT team meet the individual in his or her home, providing services and contact based on the individual's unique needs. Team members also monitor the individual's management of symptoms and observe for warning signs of potential relapse.

Family Psychoeducation

Family Psychoeducation is an intervention in which a professional, an individual with psychiatric disability, and his or her family work in partnership to promote recovery. Through this partnership, current information about the individual's psychiatric disability is communicated to the individual and family, and strategies to help the family develop skills for coping with issues involving manifestations of the individual's disability are developed. Interventions can be used with a single family or conducted with a group of families.

Illness Management and Recovery

Illness management and recovery programs are intended to help individuals with psychiatric disability to develop strategies to cope with manifestations of the condition, reduce relapses and hospitalizations, and improve their overall functioning within the community.

Integrated Dual Disorders Treatment

Integrated dual disorders treatment (IDDT) was developed for individuals who have both psychiatric disability and disability related to substance abuse and/or dependence. This approach integrates and blends interventions for both psychiatric disability and substance abuse so that one professional or team provides intervention for both conditions. Techniques used in IDDT programs include individual and group counseling, family psychoeducation, social support, case management, and medication management.

Pharmacologic Approaches to Treatment of Psychiatric Disability

Antipsychotic Medications

Treatment of psychosis may require use of *antipsychotic medications* (see Table 8-4). Antipsychotic medications, sometimes called *narcoleptics* or *major tranquilizers*, do not cure psychosis, but rather control the manifestations. The first antipsychotic drug, chlorpromazine (Thorazine), was developed in the 1950s. Since then, numerous other antipsychotic medications have been developed. Antipsychotic drugs are classified into different chemical groups. Drugs in each group have

varying potency, and individual responses to any of the medications will vary.

Conventional antipsychotic medications were largely replaced by *atypical antipsychotics (second-generation antipsychotics)* that were developed after a 1980s study showed that the medication clozapine controlled treatment-resistant symptoms in schizophrenia without causing the extrapyramidal side effects that were common with the older antipsychotic medications (Gardner, Baldessarini, & Waraich, 2005). Since then, a number of other (atypical or second-generation) antipsychotics have been developed and approved for the treatment of both schizophrenia and acute bipolar episodes/maintenance treatment of bipolar disorders (Masand, 2007). Although the use of atypical antipsychotics is still common, the use of conventional antipsychotic medications has begun increasing after recent studies suggested that the atypical antipsychotics also carry side effects, and that compliance is not improved with the newer medications (Lieberman et al., 2005).

It is believed that the manifestations of psychosis may be due to excessive levels of the neurotransmitter dopamine, although other neurotransmitter systems have also been implicated. In schizophrenia, it is hypothesized that positive symptoms such as delusions and hallucinations are related to overactive dopamine transmission (Stahl, 2004) and that negative symptoms such as depression and

---

Table 8-4   Common Antipsychotic Agents

Trade Name	Generic Name
Clozaril	Clozapine
Haldol	Haloperidol
Loxitane	Loxapine
Mellaril	Thioridazine
Navane	Thiothixene
Prolixin	Fluphenazine
Stelazine	Trifluoperazine

mood instability are due to insufficient dopamine availability (Gardner et al., 2005). It has been postulated that antipsychotic medications reduce positive symptoms by blocking the action or transmission of dopamine.

Blocking of dopamine activity, however, may produce side effects including psychomotor manifestations similar to those seen in Parkinson's disease (see Chapter 4). These are called *extrapyramidal effects*, in recognition of the fact that changes take place in the extrapyramidal tracts of the central nervous system. These side effects are more common in older antipsychotic medications, but may include **dystonia** (abnormal muscle tone), **akinesia** (decreased motor activity and apathy), and **akathisia** (extreme restlessness and inability to sit still or remain in one place for any length of time), all of which have acute onset. The most severe extrapyramidal side effect is *tardive dyskinesia*, which consists of abnormal movements of the mouth, such as chewing motions or thrusting movements of the tongue. The side effect of tardive dyskinesia may not be immediately apparent; indeed, it may not develop until years after treatment. Tardive dyskinesia is often related to drug dosage and is irreversible. Frequent monitoring for early manifestations of tardive dyskinesia is important to prevent permanent damage from occurring. Antiparkinsonian medications, such as benztropine (Cogentin) and trihexphenidyl (Artane), may be prescribed, especially in conjunction with older antipsychotic medications, to prevent extrapyramidal side effects.

Although atypical or second-generation antipsychotics have been thought to be better tolerated and more efficacious than conventional antipsychotics, they are not without limitations (Masand, 2007). *The Clinical Antipsychotic Trials of Intervention Effectiveness (CATIE)* study compared the effectiveness of several atypical antipsychotics and conventional antipsychotics in the treatment of schizophrenia (Lieberman et al., 2005). Although rates of dis-

continuation were slightly lower for individuals taking atypical antipsychotic medications, nearly three-fourths of the individuals discontinued their medications within 18 months, often because of intolerable side effects. Among the side effects associated with antipsychotic medications are weight gain, diabetes, and elevated blood cholesterol, all of which increase the risk of heart disease (Dekker et al., 2005; Sridhar, 2007). In addition, there can be an increased risk of death associated with use of antipsychotic medications in older adults (Wang et al., 2005).

In the CATIE Study (Lieberman et al., 2005), sedation was the side effect that accounted for discontinuation of antipsychotic medication in nearly one-third of the participants. Individuals taking antipsychotic medications may also develop *photosensitivity*, which makes them more sensitive to the effects of the sun and predisposes them to sunburn. Some medications that have potent sedating effects may decrease alertness and produce drowsiness. These symptoms usually subside within two weeks after the individual begins to take the medication; if they persist, alteration in medication may be necessary. Individuals may also experience *orthostatic hypotension*, in which their blood pressure drops when they move from a seated or prone position to a standing position, resulting in dizziness or lightheadedness. Individuals may complain of other uncomfortable side effects, such as dry mouth, after beginning antipsychotic medications. These symptoms generally subside within two weeks, however. Men on antipsychotic medication may become impotent or unable to ejaculate. Reducing the dosage or changing the medication may alleviate this side effect. Any medication change should always be conducted under the direction of a physician.

The duration of treatment with antipsychotic medications is determined individually and based on the individual's specific life situation and condition. These agents may be prescribed for up to a year as a prophylactic measure after psychosis is controlled. All individuals should have their medications reviewed at least annually by a psychiatrist.

Antidepressants

Conditions in which depression is a manifestation may be treated with antidepressants. Although the exact way antidepressants work has not been determined, these medications are thought to block the uptake of the neurotransmitters norepinephrine and serotonin, thereby increasing their concentration. Levels of both of these neurotransmitters appear to be reduced in depression.

The type of depression and the manifestations experienced, as well as other individual factors, determine the type of antidepressant used. In most cases, medication effects are not immediate and may take as long as six to eight weeks to show full therapeutic effect. *Tricyclic antidepressants*, named for their chemical structure, were once widely used to treat depression, This group of medications is not used as frequently today as first-line therapy owing to their unpleasant side effects, such as orthostatic hypotension dry mouth, or urinary retention. A more serious possible side effect is the development of cardiac arrhythmia, which can result in myocardial infarction or, in the case of overdose, death.

Newer second-generation antidepressants are now more frequently prescribed because they work as well as the older medications but have fewer side effects. Some newer antidepressants, named for their action rather than their chemical structure, mainly affect the neurotransmitter serotonin. These medications are called *selective serotonin reuptake inhibitors (SSRIs)*. Newer medications similar to tricyclic antidepressants, which affect both serotonin and norepinephrine, have since been developed. *Monoamine oxidase inhibitors (MAOIs)* are older types of antidepressants that are thought

to act by blocking the action of the enzyme monoamine oxidase (MAO), which normally helps to break down norepinephrine and serotonin. When the action of MAO is inhibited, the concentration of the neurotransmitters increases. MAO is also responsible for the regulation of metabolism of a substance found in many foods called tyramine. When the action of MAO is inhibited and individuals ingest food-containing tyramine, the resulting amount of tyramine in the system can precipitate a severe elevation in blood pressure, causing a *hypertensive crisis* that could result in stroke. To prevent this complication from occurring, individuals on MAOIs must follow a number of dietary restrictions carefully to prevent potentially serious side effects. Examples of foods to be avoided include aged cheese, wine, beer, chocolate, coffee, raisins, and yogurt. In addition, many other medications, including over-the-counter medications such as sinus medications and cold preparations, also can present a hazard. Individuals with chronic alcoholism or liver damage are not good candidates for treatment with MAOIs. Individuals placed on these medications must have the cognitive ability and motivation to precisely follow dietary restrictions so that they can avoid the potentially severe complications with these drugs.

Suicide is always a possibility with individuals who are depressed, and the risk of suicide is influenced by a number of factors (Simon, 2006). The availability of antidepressant medication that could be used in a suicide attempt is a risk that needs to be considered, for example. The risk of attempted suicide may be higher when the antidepressant begins to take effect because suicidal impulses are still present: As individuals' energy returns, so does their motivation to attempt suicide. Suicide is the third leading cause of death among young people (Brent & Mann, 2006). Known risk factors for suicide, especially in young persons with mood disorders, include alcohol abuse, recent loss of a loved one, and a family history of suicidal behavior (Bridge, Goldstein, & Brent, 2006; Friedman, 2006a). Although antidepressants are an important aspect of intervention for depressive disorders, psychotherapeutic modes of treatment should be used in combination with the pharmacologic approach.

Mood Stabilizers

As mentioned earlier, lithium is a medication used to treat bipolar disorder. This element occurs naturally as a salt. Use of lithium for treatment of psychiatric disability in the United States began in the 1970s, and this agent is now widely used in bipolar disorders—both in the treatment of manifestations and in the prevention of recurring manifestations. In some instances, lithium has been used alone or in combination with antidepressants to treat depressive disorders. Because not all individuals respond to lithium in the same way, its use is decided on an individual basis.

The way in which lithium works is unclear. Common side effects include **polyuria** (excessive urination), **polydipsia** (excessive thirst), and, in some individuals, fine hand tremor. Side effects may also include *hypothyroidism* (too little thyroid hormone) or enlargement of the thyroid gland, so individuals should have thyroid function checked regularly. Other side effects may include fatigue, muscle weakness, and weight gain.

Individuals who use lithium should have regular blood tests to measure levels of the medication in the blood and must be regularly monitored by a physician. If the lithium level is too low, the medication will not be effective. If the level is too high, individuals may experience a variety of side effects. The balance of lithium is easily altered by anything that affects the level of sodium in the body. For instance, a reduction of salt intake, exces-

sive sweating, fear, nausea, and diarrhea can all affect the amount of sodium in the body, thereby causing a buildup of lithium and leading to toxicity. Diuretics (substances that cause loss of body fluid) such as medications, coffee, or tea also increase lithium levels and can lead to lithium toxicity. Warning signs of toxicity include nausea and vomiting, confusion or disorientation, slurring of speech, irregular heartbeat, and, in severe cases, seizures. Overdose of lithium can be fatal.

Anticonvulsant Medications

Some individuals with bipolar disorders may take *anticonvulsant medications* (medications typically used to treat seizures), such as valproic acid, especially in the acute mania phase. Because valproic acid may cause liver problems, individuals who are taking this mediation should have liver function tests prior to beginning treatment and then regularly thereafter.

Antianxiety Medications

Antianxiety medications are generally used for conditions in which anxiety is the predominant manifestation. A common classification of antianxiety medications are the benzodiazepines (e.g., diazepam, clonazepam). These medications may have side effects of drowsiness, loss of coordination, or mental slowing, at least initially. Consequently, individuals placed on antianxiety medication should avoid driving or operating certain machinery until they know how they will be affected by the medication. Individuals taking benzodiazepines should also avoid alcohol due to the potential for interaction and possibly life-threatening effects. Because many antianxiety agents also have the risk of abuse or physical dependence, their use should be monitored carefully.

Individuals taking benzodiazepines should never suddenly stop the medications because of the severe withdrawal reaction that could potentially occur. Sudden discontinuation effects may include severe manifestations of anxiety and, in some instances, seizures. Before stopping benzodiazepines completely, dosage is gradually tapered over time under the supervision of a physician.

Electroconvulsive Therapy

Before psychopharmacologic preparations were readily available, Electroconclusive Theory (ECT) was a major mode of treating some types of psychiatric disability. Psychotherapeutic drugs have largely replaced ECT, even though some individuals respond well to ECT. Consequently, most large hospitals or academic medical centers continue to offer an ECT service for individuals who are referred for this type of therapy. It may be especially useful when the long-term administration of medication is contraindicated (Fink, 2000). ECT is often used in the following circumstances:

- Individuals with conditions such as major depression, bipolar depression, or mania who do not respond to medications.
- Individuals' medical health and mental health are threatened without treatment.
- Individuals express a preference for ECT due to its fast-acting nature.
- Individuals have responded favorably to ECT in the past (Lisanby, 2007).

Although ECT does not cure psychiatric disability, it can bring about a remission of symptoms. It may be used either alone or in conjunction with psychotherapeutic medications (Lisanby, 2007).

■ PSYCHOSOCIAL AND VOCATIONAL ISSUES IN PSYCHIATRIC DISABILITY

Psychosocial Issues

Individuals with psychiatric disability experience a wide range of symptoms that affect psychological, cognitive, and social functioning.

The needs of individuals with psychiatric disabilities are multifaceted and complex (Kress-Shull & Leech, 2000). In individuals with a dual diagnosis, problems related to functioning are compounded. Although the benefits of medication in the treatment of psychiatric disability are substantial, medication usually does not cure the condition but rather merely controls the manifestations. Individuals often have residual manifestations, deficits, and impairments as a result of their condition, and many are subject to periodic relapses with recurrence of manifestations.

Manifestations experienced vary with the condition, leading to variable degrees of impairment. Although fear and anger are normal emotional responses, these responses may be acutely disproportionate to the stimuli in some psychiatric disabilities. Some individuals' responses are covert, whereas others' responses are more pronounced. Some individuals manifest their condition through patterns of behavior rather than in emotional forms. Others experience subjective distress, such as an inner sense of weakness, jealousy, or anxiety, although functioning in most of their life is minimally disturbed. Some psychiatric disabilities are characterized by disorganization of mental capacities, which can affect individuals' ability to function in an unstructured environment. Disorders of memory and perception can severely limit independent function. Individuals may fail to carry out age-appropriate role functions and have varying degrees of dependence on others.

Manifestations of the psychiatric disability may cause stress and anxiety, further compounding the disabling component of the condition. Individuals' own anguish over their impoverished life can be devastating. The degree to which psychiatric disability affects individuals' lifestyle depends to a great extent on the nature of the condition. Some psychiatric disabilities so severely impair individuals' ability to carry on the activities of daily living that constant supervision or hospitalization is necessary. In other cases, individuals are able to carry on these activities, but in an altered manner. Awareness of their own impaired function and the impact of their condition both on others and on their own future may cause considerable pain and discomfort. In some instances, individuals with psychiatric disability may be reluctant to seek appropriate help because of their fear of the stigma associated with psychiatric conditions that require professional help. In other instances, individuals may not be aware of their symptoms and the effect of their symptoms on function, further hindering appropriate treatment.

Some individuals with psychiatric disability may be particularly vulnerable to stress and may lack the ability to withstand pressure or to cope with the normal stresses of everyday life. They may have limited problem-solving ability or find it difficult to engage in self-directed activity. Some individuals may become passive, apathetic, or over-submissive as a direct result of repeated hospitalizations or as a result of the condition itself.

Individuals with psychiatric disability frequently have comorbid medical conditions and physical health problems that compound manifestations and intervention (Twigger & Houltram, 2006; O'Day, Killeen, Sutton, & Iezzoni, 2005). In addition to the higher incidence of heart disease, diabetes, and obesity that are often associated with medications used to treat such conditions, tobacco use is higher in individuals with psychiatric disability than in the general population (Osborn, 2001). Individuals with psychiatric disability often also have comorbid substance use disorders, which further compound treatment problems (Magruder, Sonne, Brady, Quello, & Martin, 2005). A number of barriers exist that interfere with these individuals' ability to obtain adequate health care to treat such medical conditions. Individuals may be reluctant to seek care for medical issues, or they

may have inadequate financial resources to do so. In other instances when medical care is sought, emphasis may be placed on the psychiatric condition rather than addressing other medical issues. Developing strategies to identify empathetic health professionals who are also knowledgeable about issues involved with psychiatric disability as well as helping individuals learn to be their own advocates in getting their healthcare needs met can help prevent many physical health problems from occurring (O'Day, et al., 2005).

At times, the management requires lifestyle changes. Individuals with psychiatric disability may need to rearrange their schedules so that they may attend therapy sessions. Some medications used in the management of psychiatric disability may require special lifestyle considerations. For example, the use of MAOIs for depression requires careful monitoring of diet. Other medications have side effects, such as drowsiness and sedation that affect daily function in a detrimental way.

Either the psychiatric disability or its management may alter sexual function. Individuals with a depressive disorder may lose interest in sexual activity, whereas individuals with a bipolar depression may have excessive sexual interests. Side effects of some medications can alter sexual function as well. In addition, subjective manifestations of lowered self-esteem and self-confidence may make it more difficult for individuals to form intimate relationships.

The impact of a psychiatric disability on social function also depends on the nature of the condition and the individual's reaction to it. Low self-esteem frequently accompanies psychiatric disability and, in turn, leads to negative self-concept (Knapen, Vermeersch, Van Coppenolle, Cuykx, Pieters, & Peuskens, 2007). In some individuals, admission of having disability can lead to a sense of futility and hopelessness (Hensley, 2006). Unfortunately, stigma and myths about psychiatric disability persist. While society as a whole has become more accepting of individuals with psychiatric disability, family members may continue to be resistant to recognition of the problem and pursuit of appropriate intervention (Hall & Purdy, 2000). If, individuals manifest bizarre, abusive, or socially offensive behavior, some family members or others within a social group may avoid the individual altogether, leaving him or her socially isolated.

Other psychiatric disabilities may lead to social withdrawal. Families of individuals with psychiatric disability may experience a variety of stresses engendered by the condition. These stresses may be caused by their objective problems in dealing with the individual and his or her condition, as well as by more subjective psychological distress (Hall & Purdy, 2000).

Psychiatric disabilities, especially those in which individuals need close supervision or long-term care and intervention, may place financial hardships on the family because of medical bills, the individual's economic dependency, and special needs related to household functioning. In some instances, demands of caregiving may require family members to curtail their social activities or alter their relationships with friends and acquaintances. Time commitments of caregiving may lead to neglect of other family members' needs, further disrupting the family unit. Increasing family-based services that address ongoing stressors such as financial concerns, housing, and relationship issues promote development of a stronger family unit and ongoing support (Riebschleger, 2004).

Social barriers are frequently erected against individuals with a psychiatric disability and their families. Social stigma may be the result of either ignorance about psychiatric disability or feelings of inadequacy in knowing how to interact with individuals with psychiatric disability. In other instances, there is fear of the potential for individuals with psychiatric disability to become violent. Although most people with psychiatric disability do not commit assaultive acts, the prevalence of violence among people with serious psychiatric disability such as schizophrenia, major depression, or bipolar disorder is 16%, compared to 7% for individuals without psychiatric disability. (Friedman, 2006b). Substance abuse among individuals with psychiatric disability compounds the increased risk for violence (Swanson et al., 2002). If social stigma is already a burden for individuals with psychiatric disability, being perceived as dangerous can have a devastating effect in regard to relationships, housing, and employment. Fear that individuals with psychotic disorders are dangerous can lead to social distancing and further impair social function (Kleinfelder, Telijohann & Price, 2004).

Continuing to educate the public that most individuals with psychiatric disability do not commit violent acts can help to reduce this stigma. It appears that manifestations of the psychiatric condition—rather than the diagnosis itself—contribute to the risk of violence. Consequently, individuals with psychiatric disability who are free of psychotic manifestations have a drastically reduced risk of violent behavior (Friedman, 2006b).

Regardless of the cause of social stigma, the results can be a source of continuing stress for individuals with psychiatric disability and their families, as well as a barrier to social activity and interaction. Social stigma and stereotypes can also influence the extent of limitations that individuals experience. Limitations sometimes occur not because of the psychiatric disability, but rather because of the public's reaction to it (Corrigan & Calabrese, 2001). Other issues such as housing instability and, at times, homelessness further contribute to social stigma, the individual's levels of stress, and overall well-being (Tsemberis, Gulcur, & Nakae, 2004).

Increasing emphasis has been placed on social integration of individuals with psychiatric disability. However, although individuals may be living in the community, frequently they are not part of it (Ware, Hopper, Tugenberg, Dickey, & Fisher, 2007). Full integration includes the individual's participation in the community, including maintenance of reciprocal interpersonal relationships, which extends beyond support mechanisms and interaction with other people with psychiatric disability. It also behooves individuals with psychiatric disability to accept their responsibility and accountability to the community in which they live.

Vocational Issues

Psychiatric disability affects a significant portion of the working-age population in the United States (Donnell, Lustig, & Strauser, 2004). The ability of individuals with psychiatric disability to work depends on the type of disability, the type of work in which they are involved, and the attitudes of those within the work setting. It is important that both professionals and individuals with psychiatric disability keep in mind that symptoms currently being experienced may not be present in the future and that functional capacity can change (Killeen & O'Day, 2004). Even when individuals experience significant disability as a result of their psychiatric condition, as they learn to manage manifestations and medications, their level of functional capacity can increase so that return to regular employment in accordance with their interests, talents, and goals can be achieved.

Although work is important to increase self-esteem for those with a number of disabilities, it can be an especially strong therapeutic tool for those with a psychiatric disability (Tschopp, Bishop, & Mulvihill, 2001). Individuals with psychiatric disability may lack self-confidence, have a poor perception of their own abilities, and feel a high level of vulnerability and fear of failure (Hoekstra, Sanders, van den Heuvel, Post, & Groothoff, 2004). Although the skills, aptitude, motivation, and objective symptoms of individuals with psychiatric disability are important, their ability to endure and cope with stress and to engage in active problem solving also determine their ability to work. Job restrictions may be related to job pressure or the ability to work with others, regardless of the individual's particular level of skill or physical and cognitive ability to perform work-related tasks. As noted earlier, individuals with psychiatric disability are more vulnerable to stress (Dorio & Marine, 2004). Chronic work stress has been found to amplify the disability associated with psychiatric disorders (Dewa, Lin, Kooehoorn, & Goldner, 2007). Consequently, individuals should be assisted to develop effective coping mechanisms at work. Discussion with the employer to identify ways to create a less stressful environment may be needed.

Other considerations may relate to individuals' treatment. It may be necessary to arrange scheduled absences so that individuals can attend therapy sessions. Some medications used in treatment may produce side effects, such as drowsiness or sedation, that could adversely affect work performance. In addition, individuals' level of adherence to the therapeutic regimen is especially important, because failure to do so means possible relapse and recurrence of manifestations.

Individuals' reactions to the work environment, including noise and distractions, should be taken into account, as should their level of personal responsibility and capacity for self-direction and decision making. The existence of limited interpersonal and coping skills may make it difficult for some individuals to adjust to unforeseen circumstances. Individuals' flexibility to take advantage of chance occurrences and their degree of flexibility in the workplace must be taken into consideration (Szymanski, 2000). Some individuals may require a more structured work environment. In some instances, individuals' expectations of work or assessment of their own capabilities may be unrealistic. Unless these unrealistic notions are identified and dealt with before individuals enter (or reenter) the work setting, discouragement, disappointment, or even relapse may occur.

Supported employment has been found to be an important way to foster empowerment in individuals with psychiatric disability (Corrigan, 2004) and to help individuals with psychiatric disability obtain competitive employment (Bond, 2004). It is a commonly adopted method to help people with psychiatric disability achieve better and meaningful quality of life through work (Lee, Chronister, Tsang, Ingraham, & Oulvey, 2005; Morris & Lloyd, 2004). In supported employment, individuals work in integrated settings, with monitoring, support, and follow-up being provided on a regular basis. Supported employment provides permanent jobs that are based on individuals' skills and abilities.

Social skills, aptitude, and the ability to work are not necessarily concurrent in individuals with psychiatric disability. Employment for each individual must be considered in the context of his or her particular manifestations of the condition and feelings and the nature of the work environment. The role that social stigma plays in individuals' perceptions of their own condition and their willingness to accept and follow up with treatment are crucial aspects in the total rehabilitation of individuals with psychiatric disability.

The unemployment and underemployment rates for individuals with psychiatric disabilities remain high (Kress-Shull, 2001; Cook, 2006; Rogers, Anthony, Lyass, & Penk, 2006). Once employment is obtained, maintaining employment may also be a challenge for individuals with psychiatric disability (Auerbach & Richardson, 2005). Although no one factor

accounts for low employment status, several systemic and programmatic barriers exist that may be difficult for individuals with psychiatric disability to overcome (Henry & Lucca, 2004). Predisability occupational experience appears to be a valid predictor of individuals, ability to return to work (Pluta & Accordino, 2006), with low education also predicting unfavorable vocational outcomes for individuals with psychiatric disability (Watzke, Galvao, Gawlik, Huehne, & Brieger, 2006). Given that many individuals are diagnosed with psychiatric disability in adolescence or young adulthood, their lack of opportunities to become established in a career may contribute to their inability to obtain competitive employment. Fewer than 15% of individuals served in the public mental health system are in competitive employment (Gowdy, Carlson, & Rapp, 2004). Low expectations are often imbedded in policies and programs, such that individuals are given negative messages regarding their capacity to work (Killeen & O'Day, 2004). Because of concern that stress may cause relapse, individuals with psychiatric disability may be encouraged to accept unskilled, low-wage positions that are far below their actual skills and capabilities. The amount of stress generated by working for poverty-level wages in a job that does not match the individual's ability is often ignored.

In other instances, financial disincentives may contribute to underemployment or unemployment (MacDonald-Wilson, Rogers, Ellison, & Lyass, 2003; Cook et al., 2006). Often individuals' ability to work is affected by their desire to retain Social Security benefits (Killeen & O'Day, 2004). Individuals may fear that if benefits are relinquished to pursue full-time work, no benefits will be available if they should have a relapse or if they should lose their job. Applying for benefits again after they have been relinquished can be a cumbersome and lengthy process, which individuals with psychiatric disability may choose to avoid.

Consequently, they may remain unemployed or accept low-paying, part-time work rather than lose disability benefits.

Funding of mental health services is often greater than funding for employment services for individuals with psychiatric disability, so that employment outcomes are often not the major focus of services provided (O'Brien, Ford, & Malloy, 2005). Continued advocacy, which includes educating not only employers but also policy makers and individuals with psychiatric disability, is necessary in the ongoing process of reducing unemployment and underemployment for individuals with psychiatric disability. Although a focus on competitive employment and job development is important, emphasis on job retention through job support is equally important to enhance positive employment and quality of life outcomes (Leff et al., 2005).

CASE STUDIES

Case 1

Ms. H. is a 25-year-old female with bipolar disorder. She was first diagnosed one year ago, when she experienced mania and was hospitalized. At the time of her hospitalization, she was in her second year of medical school. After her hospitalization, Ms. H. asked for a medical leave of absence from her medical school responsibilities, which was granted. Since her hospitalization her symptoms have been well managed with medication, and she has stated that she feels ready to continue her medical school studies. Ms. H. wants to work on a plan that will help her manage her symptoms on reentry.

1. Do you believe Ms. H's plan to reenter medical school is feasible? Why or why not?

2. Which factors might you consider in helping Ms. H. develop her plan?
3. Which specific issues regarding her condition might you consider?
4. Are there support strategies that would be particularly helpful to Ms. H.?

Case 2

Mr. B. is a 56-year-old male with schizophrenia. He was first diagnosed at age 17. Since that time, he has had a number of relapses. For the last 10 years, however, he has been able to manage his symptoms well and has not had any recent relapses. Mr. B. has been successfully employed as a certified nursing assistant in a nursing home for the last five years, and he tells you that he would like to go to a community college and work on an associate degree in nursing. Although he has used a number of therapies and approaches to symptom management, Mr. B. has also taken medication for symptom management. He recently told you that he is concerned about the potential long-term effects of the medications and is considering discontinuing them.

1. How would you approach Mr. B.'s desire to discontinue his medication?
2. Which specific issues might you address when working with Mr. B. on his rehabilitation plan?
3. Are there other factors you might consider?

■ REFERENCES

Accordino, M. P., Porter, D. F., & Morse, T. (2001). Deinstitutionalization of persons with severe mental illness: Context and consequences. *Journal of Rehabilitation, 67*(2), 16–20.

Agid, Y., Buzsaki, G., Diamond, D. M., Frackowiak, R., Giedd, J., Girault, J.A., et al. (2007). How can drug discovery for psychiatric disorders be improved? *Nature Reviews Drug Discovery, 6*(3), 189–201.

Alcaras, N. M., & Roper, J. M. (2006). Chest pain among combat veterans: A conceptual framework. *Military Medicine, 717*(6), 478–483.

American Psychiatric Association, (2000). *Diagnostic and statistical manual of mental disorders* (4th ed., Text Revision). Washington, DC: Author.

Andersson, L., Wiles, N., Lewis, G., Brage, S., & Hensing, G. (2007). Can access to psychiatric health care explain regional differences in disability pension with psychiatric disorders? *Social Psychiatry and Psychiatric Epidemiology, 42,* 366–371.

Antai-Otong, D. (2006a). Anxiety disorders. *Nursing, 36*(3), 48–49.

Antai-Otong, D. (2006b). The art of prescribing: Treatment considerations for patients experiencing rapid-cycling bipolar disorder. *Perspectives in Psychiatric Care, 42*(1), 55–58.

Anthony, W. A., Cohen, M. R., Farkas, M., & Gagne, C. (Eds.). (2002). *Psychiatric rehabilitation* (2nd ed.). Boston: Boston University Center for Psychiatric Rehabilitation.

Auerbach, E. S., & Richardson, P. (2005). The long-term work experiences of persons with severe and persistent mental illness. *Psychiatric Rehabilitation Journal, 28*(3), 267–273.

Beebe, L. H. (2007). Beyond the prescription pad: Psychosocial treatments for individuals with schizophrenia. *Journal of Psychosocial Nursing, 45*(3), 35–43.

Bishop, M., & Sweet, E. A. (2000). Depression: A primer for rehabilitation counselors. *Journal of Applied Rehabilitation Counseling, 31*(3), 38–45.

Bond, G. R. (2004). Supported employment: Evidence for an evidence-based practice. *Psychiatric Rehabilitation Journal, 27,* 345–359.

Brent, D. A., & Mann, J. J. (2006). Familial pathways to suicidal behavior: Understanding and preventing suicide among adolescents. *New England Journal of Medicine, 355*(26), 2719–2721.

Bridge, J. A., Goldstein, T. R., & Brent, D. A. (2006). Adolescent suicide and suicidal behvior. *Journal of Child Psychology and Psychiatry, and Alllied Disciplines, 47,* 372–394.

Compton, W. M., Thomas, Y. F., Stinson, F. S., & Grant, B. (2007). Prevalence, correlates, disability, and comorbidity of *DSM-IV* drug abuse and dependence in the United States. *Archives of General Psychiatry, 64*(5), 566–576.

Conus, P., Berk, M., & McGorry, P. D. (2006). Pharmacological treatment in the early phase of bipolar disorders: What stage are we at? *Australian and New Zealand Journal of Psychiatry, 40,* 199–207.

Cook, J. A. (2006). Employment barriers for persons with psychiatric disabilities: Update of a report for the President's Commission. *Psychiatric Services, 57*(10), 1391–1405.

Cook, J. A., Leff, H. S., Blyler, C. R., Gold, P. B., Goldberg, R. W., Clark, R. E., et al. (2006). Estimated payments to employment service providers for persons with mental illness in the Ticket to Work program. *Psychiatric Services, 57*(4), 465–471.

Corrigan, P. W. (2004, Autumn). Enhancing personal empowerment of people with psychiatric disabilities. *American Rehabilitation,* 10–21.

Corrigan, P. W., & Calabrese, J. D. (2001). Practical considerations for cognitive rehabilitation of people with psychiatric disabilities. *Rehabilitation Education, 15*(2), 143–153.

Corrigan, P. W., & McCracken, S. G. (2005). Place first, then train: An alternative to the medical model of psychiatric rehabilitation. *Social Work, 50*(1), 31–39.

Davis, J. M. (2006). The choice of drugs for schizophrenia. *New England Journal of Medicine, 354*(5), 518–520.

Dekker, J. M., Girman, C., Rhodes, T., Nijpels, G., Stehowwer, C. D., Bouter, L. M. et al., (2005). Metabolic syndrome and 10 year cardiovascular disease risk in the Hoorn study. *Circulation, 112,* 666–673.

Dettling, M., & Anghelescu, I. G. (2006). Antipsychotic drugs and schizophrenia. *New England Journal of Medicine, 354*(3), 298.

Dewa, C. S., Lin, E., Kooehoorn, M., & Goldner, E. (2007). Association of chronic work stress, psychiatric disorders, and chronic physical conditions with disability among workers. *Psychiatric Services, 58,* 652–658.

Donnell, C. M., Lustig, D., & Strauser, D. R. (2004). The working alliance: Rehabilitation outcomes for persons with severe mental illness. *Journal of Rehabilitation, 70*(2), 12–18.

Dorio, J., & Marine, S. (2004). A comprehensive look at promoting job retention for workers with psychiatric disabilities in a supported employment program. *Psychiatric Rehabilitation Journal, 28*(1), 32–39.

Duncan, B. L., Miller, S. D., & Sparks, J. A. (2004). *The heroic client.* San Francisco, CA: Jossey-Bass.

Emdad, R., & Sondergaard, H. P. (2006). General intelligence and short-term memory impairments in post traumatic stress disorder patients. *Journal of Mental Health, 15*(2), 205–216.

Fink, M. (2000). Electroshock revisited. *American Scientist, 88,* 162–167.

Foa, E. B., Franklin, M. E., & Moser, J. (2002). Context in the clinic: How well do cognitive-behavioral therapies and medications work in combination? *Biological Psychiatry, 52,* 987–997.

Foa, E. B., Keane, T. M., and Friedman, M. J. (Eds.). (2000). *Effective treatments for PTSD: Practice guidelines from the International Society for Traumatic Stress Studies.* New York: Guilford Press.

Frank, E., Kupfer, D. J., Thase, M. E., Mallinges, A. G., Swartz, H. A., Fagiolini, A. M. et al. (2005). Two year outcomes for interpersonal and social rhythm therapy for individuals with bipolar I disorder. *Archives of General Psychiatry, 62,* 996–1004.

Freedman, R. (2003). Schizophrenia. *New England Journal of Medicine, 349*(18), 1738–1749.

Freedy, J. R. & Simpson, W. M. (2007). Disaster-related physical and mental health: A role for the family physician. *American Family Physician, 75*(6), 841–846.

Freeman, M. P., Freeman, S. A., & McElroy, S. L. (2002). The co-morbidity of bipolar and anxiety disorders: Prevalence, psychobiology, and treatment issues. *Journal of Affective Disorders, 68*(1), 1–23.

Friedman, R. A. (2006a). Uncovering an epidemic: Screening for mental illness in teens. *New England Journal of Medicine, 355*(26), 2717–2719.

Friedman, R. A. (2006b). Violence and mental illness: How strong is the link? *New England Journal of Medicine, 355*(20), 2064–2066.

Garakani, A., Mathew, S. J., & Charney, D.S. (2006). Neurobiology of anxiety disorders and implications for treatment. *Mount Sinai Journal of Medicine, 73*(7), 941–949.

Gardner, D. M., Baldessarini, R. J., & Waraich, P. (2005). Modern antipsychotic drugs: A critical overview. *Canadian Medical Association Journal, 172,* 1703–1711.

Garske, G. G. (1999). The challenge of rehabilitation counselors: Working with people with psychiatric disabilities. *Journal of Rehabilitation, 65,* 21–25.

Gillam, T. (2006). Positive approaches to schizophrenia. *Mental Health Practice, 10*(4), 30–33.

Gillock, K. L., Zayfert, C., Hegel, M. T., & Ferguson, R. J. (2005). Posttraumatic stress disorder in primary care: Prevalence and relationships with physical symptoms and medical utilization. *General Hospital Psychiatry, 27,* 392–399.

Goedert, M., & Spillantini, M. G. (2006). A century of Alzheimer's disease. *Science, 314*(3), 777–784.

Gordon, P. A., Tantillo, J. C., Feldman, D., & Perrone, K. (2004). Attitudes regarding interpersonal relationships with persons with mental illness and mental retardation. *Journal of Rehabilitation, 70*(1), 50–56.

Gowdy, E. A., Carlson, L. S., & Rapp, C. A. (2004). Organizational factors differentiating high performing from low performing supported employment programs. *Psychiatric Rehabilitation Journal, 28*(2), 150–156.

Gross, R., Olfson, M., Gameroff, J. J., Shea, S., Feder, A., Lantingua, R. et al. (2005). Social anxiety disorder in primary care. *General Hospital Psychiatry, 27,* 161–168.

Hall, L. L., & Purdy, R. (2000). Recovery and serious brain disorders: The central role of families in nurturing roots and wings. *Community Mental Health Journal, 36*(4), 427–441.

Henry, A. D., & Lucca, A. M. (2004). Facilitators and barriers to employment: The perspectives of people with psychiatric disabilities and employment service providers. *Work, 22,* 169–182.

Hoekstra, E. J., Sanders, K., van den Heuvel, W. J. A., Post, D., & Groothoff, J. W. (2004). Supported employment in the Netherlands for people with an intellectual disability and a chronic disease. A comparative study. *Journal of Vocational Rehabilitation, 21,* 39–48.

Hough, C. J., & Ursano, R. J. (2006). A guide to the genetics of psychiatric disease. *Psychiatry, 69*(1), 1–20.

Howland, R. H. (2006a). Challenges in the diagnosis and treatment of bipolar depression: Part 1: Assessment. *Journal of Psychosocial Nursing, 44*(4), 9–12.

Howland, R. H. (2006b). Challenges in the diagnosis and treatment of bipolar depression: Part 2: Treatment options. *Journal of Psychosocial Nursing, 44*(5), 9–12.

Hui, C. L. M., Chen, E. Y. H., Kan, C. S., Yip, K. C., Law, C. W., & Chiu, C. P. Y. (2006). Detection of non-adherent behavior in early psychosis. *Australian and New Zealand Journal of Psychiatry, 40*, 446–451.

Huxley, N., & Baldessarini, R.J. (2007). Disability and its treatment in bipolar disorder. *Bipolar Disorders*, 183–196.

Ipser, J., Seedat, S., & Stein, D. J. (2006). Pharmacotherapy for post-traumatic stress disorder: A systematic review and meta-analysis. *South African Medical Journal, 96*(10), 1088–1096.

Issakidis, C., Sandeerson, K., Corry, J., Andrews, G., & Lapsley, H. (2004). Modeling the population cost-effectiveness of current and evidence-based optimal treatment for anxiety disorders. *Psychological Medicine, 34*, 19–35.

Jarskog, L. F., Miyamoto, S., & Lieberman, J. A. (2007). Schizophrenia: New pathological insights and therapies. *Annual Review of Medicine, 58*, 59–71.

Jenike, M. A. (2004). Obsessive–compulsive disorder. *New England Journal of Medicine, 350*(3), 259–265.

Kahng, S. K., & Mowbray, C. (2004). Factors influencing self-esteem among individuals with severe mental illness: Implications for social work. *Social Work Research, 28*(4), 225–236.

Karlawish, J. (2006). Alzheimer's disease: Clinical trials and the logic of clinical purpose. *New England Journal of Medicine, 355*(15), 1604–1606.

Keller, M. B., McCullough, J. P., Klein, D. N., Arnow, B., Dunner, D. L., Gelenberg, A. J., et al. (2000). A comparison of Nefazodone, the cognitive behavioral analysis system of psychotherapy, and their combination for the treatment of chronic depression. *New England Journal of Medicine, 342*(20), 1462–1470.

Kennedy, N., Boydell, J., Kalidindi, S., Fearson, P., Jones, P. B., Van Os, J. et al. (2005). Gender differences in incidence and age at onset of mania and bipolar disorder over a 35 year period in Camberwell, England. *American Journal of Psychiatry,162*, (2), 257–262.

Kessler, R. C., Berglund, P., Demler, O., Jin, R., Merikangas, K. R., & Walter, E. E. (2005). Lifetime prevalence and age-of-onset distributions of DSM-IV disorders in the National Co-morbidity Survey Replication. *Archives of General Psychiatry, 62*(6), 593–602.

Kessler, R. C., Chiu, W. T., Demler O., Merikangas, K. R., & Walters, E. E. (2005). Prevalence, severity, and comorbidity of 12-month DSMIV disorders in the National Comorbidity Survey Replication. *Archives of General Psychiatry, 62*(6), 617–627.

Khouzam, H. R., & Donnelly, N. J. (2001). Post-traumatic stress disorder. *Postgraduate Medicine, 110*(5), 60–62;67–70;77–78.

Killeen, M. B., & O'Day. (2004). Challenging expectations: How individuals with psychiatric disabilities find and keep work. *Psychiatric Rehabilitation Journal, 28*(2), 157–163.

Klam, J., McLay, M., & Grabke, D. (2006). Personal empowerment program: Addressing health concerns in people with schizophrenia. *Journal of Psychosocial Nursing, 44*(8), 20–28.

Kleinfelder, J., Telijohann, S. K., & Price, J. H. (2004). Are university health education programs addressing mental health issues? *American Journal of Health Studies, 19*(4), 226–227.

Knapen, J., Vermeersch, J., Van Coppenolle, H., Cuykx, V., Pieters, G., & Peuskens, J. (2007). The physical self-concept in patients with depressive and anxiety disorders. *International Journal of Therapy and Rehabilitation, 14*(1), 30–35.

Kress-Shull, M. K. (2001). Continuing challenges to the vocational rehabilitation of individuals with severe long-term mental illness. *Journal of Applied Rehabilitation Counseling, 31*(4), 5–10.

Kress-Shull, M. K., & Leech, L. L. (2000). Editorial: Effective psychiatric rehabilitation: A collaborative challenge. *Journal of Applied Rehabilitation Counseling, 31*(4), 3–4.

Krishnakumar, P., & Geeta, M. G. (2006). Clinical profile of depressive disorder in children. *Indian Pediatrics, 43*, 521–526.

Kroenke, K., Spitzer, R. L., Williams, J. B. W., Monahan, P. O., & Lowe, B. (2007). Anxiety disorders in primary care: Prevalence, impairment, co-morbidity, and detection. *Annals of Internal Medicine, 146*(5), 317–325.

Lam, D. H., Hayward, P., Watkins, E. R., Wright, K., & Sham, P. (2005). Relapse prevention in patients with bipolar disorder: Cognitive therapy outcome after 2 years. *American Journal of Psychiatry, 162,* 324–329.

Law, D. (2007). Physical health: How to minimize the risks faced by patients with schizophrenia. *Mental Health Practice, 10*(6), 26–28.

Lee, G. K., Chronister, J., Tsang, H., Ingraham, K., & Oulvey, E. (2005). Psychiatric rehabilitation training needs of state vocational rehabilitation counselors: A preliminary study. *Journal of Rehabilitation, 71*(3), 11–19.

Leech, L. L., & Holcomb, J. M. (2000). The nature of psychiatric rehabilitation and implications for collaborative efforts. *Journal of Applied Rehabilitation Counseling, 31*(4), 54–60.

Leff, H. S., Cook, J. A., Gold, P. B., Toprac, M., Blyer, C., Goldberg, R. W., et al., (2005). Effects of job development and job support on competitive employment of persons with severe mental illness. *Psychiatric Services, 56*(10), 1237–1244.

Lerner, D., Adler, D. A., Cang, H., Lapitsky, L., Hood, M. K., Perissinotto, C. et al. (2004). Unemployment, job retention, and productivity loss among employees with depression. *Psychiatric Services, 55*(12), 1371–1378.

Lieberman, J. A., Stroup, T. S., McEvoy, J. P., Swartz, M. S., Rosenheck, R. A., Perkins, D. O., et al. (2005). Effectiveness of antipsychotic drugs in patients with chronic schizophrenia. *New England Journal of Medicine, 353*(12), 1209–1223.

Lincoln, A. E., Helmer, D. A., Schneiderman, A. I., Copeland, H. L., Prisco, M. K. et al., (2006). The war-related illness and injury study centers: a resource for deployment-related health concerns. *Military Medicine, 171*(7), 577–585.

Lisanby, S. H. (2007). Electroconvulsive Therapy for depression. *New England Journal of Medicine. 357*(19). 1939–1945.

MacDonald-Wilson, K. L., & Nemec, P. B. (2005). The international classification of functioning, disability and health (ICF) in psychiatric rehabilitation. *Rehabilitation Education, 19*(2 & 3), 159–176.

MacDonald-Wilson, K. L., Rogers, E. S., Ellison, M. L., & Lyass, A. (2003). A study of the Social Security work incentives and their relation to perceived barriers to work among persons with psychiatric disability. *Rehabilitation Psychology, 48*(4), 301–309.

Macias, C., Jackson, R., Schroeder, C., & Wang, Q. (1999). Brief report: What is a clubhouse? ICCD 1996 survey of USA clubhouses. *Community Mental Health Journal, 35*(2), 181–190.

Magruder, K. M., Frueh, B. C., Knapp, R. G., Davis, L., Hamner, M. B., Martin, R. H., et al. (2005). Prevalence of posttraumatic stress disorder in Veterans Affairs primary care clinics. *General Hospital Psychiatry, 27*(3), 169–179.

Magruder, K. M., Sonne, S. C., Brady, K. T., Quello, S., & Martin, R. H. (2005). Screening for co-occurring mental disorders in drug treatment populations. *Journal of Drug Issues, 35,* 593–605

Mahoney, D. M. (2000). Panic disorder and self states: Clinical and research illustrations. *Clinical Social Work Journal, 28*(2), 197–212.

Maj, M., Sartorius, N., Okasha, A., & Zohar, J. (Eds.). (2002). *Obsessive–compulsive disorder* (2nd ed.). Chichester, UK: John Wiley.

Marx, J. (2005). Preventing Alzheimer's: A lifelong commitment? *Science, 309*(5), 864–866.

Masand, P. S. (2007). Differential pharmacology of atypical anti-psychotics: Clinical implications. *American Journal of Health-System Pharmacy, 64*(2 suppl 1), S3–8; quiz S24–25.

McColm, R., Brown, J., & Anderson, J. (2006). Nursing interventions for the management of patients with mania. *Nursing Standard, 20*(17), 46–49.

Meyer, J. S., & Quenzer, L. F. (2005). *Psychopharmacology: Drugs, the brain and behaviour.* Sunderland, MA: Sinauer Associates

Mitchell, P. B., & Malhi, G. S. (2004). Bipolar depression: Phenomenological overview and clinical characteristics. *Bipolar Disorders, 6,* 530–539.

Montejano, L. B., Goetzel, R. Z., & Ozminkowski, R. J. (2005). Impact of bipolar disorder on employers: Rationale for workplace interventions. *Disability Management Health Outcomes, 13*(4), 267–280.

Morris, P., & Lloyd, C. (2004). Vocational rehabilitation in psychiatry: A re-evaluation. *Australian and New Zealand Journal of Psychiatry, 38*(7), 490–494.

Murphy, K. (2006). Managing the ups and downs of bipolar disorders. *Nursing2006, 36*(10), 58–63.

O'Brien, D., Ford, L., & Malloy, J. M. (2005). Person centered funding: Using vouchers and personal budgets to support recovery and employment for people with psychiatric disabilities. *Journal of Vocational Rehabilitation, 23*, 71–79.

O'Day, B., Killeen, M. B., Sutton, J., & Iezzoni, L. I. (2005). Primary care experiences of people with psychiatric disabilities: Barriers to care and potential solutions. *Psychiatric Rehabilitation Journal, 28*(4), 339–345.

Osborn, D. P. J. (2001). The poor physical health of people with mental illness. *Western Journal of Medicine, 175*, 329–334.

Perlis, R. H., Miyahara, S., Marangell, L. B., (2004). Long-term implications of early onset in bipolar disorder: data from the first 1000 partipants in the Systematic Treatment Enhancement Program for Bipolar Disorder (STEP-BD). *Biological Psychiatry, 55*(9), 875–881.

Pluta, D. J., & Accordino, M. P. (2006). Predictors of return to work for people with psychiatric disabilities: A private sector perspective. *Rehabilitation Counseling Bulletin, 49*(2), 102–110.

Pollio, D. E., North, C. S., Reid, D. L., Miletic, M. M., & McClendon, J. R. (2006). Living with severe mental illness: What families and friends must know: Evaluation of a one-day psychoeducation workshop. *Social Work, 51*(1), 31–38.

Porter, R. (2001). Mental illness. In: R. Porter (ed.), *The Cambridge illustrated history of medicine* (pp. 278–303). Cambridge, UK: Cambridge University Press.

Post, R. M. (2005). The impact of bipolar depression. *Journal of Clinical Psychiatry, 66*(suppl 5), 5–10.

Pratt, C. W., Gill, K. J., Barrett, N. M., & Roberts, M. M. (1999). *Psychiatric rehabilitation.* San Diego: Academic Press.

Reed, S. J., & Merz, M. A. (2000). Integrated service teams in psychiatric rehabilitation: A strategy for improving employment outcomes and increasing funding. *Journal of Applied Rehabilitation Counseling, 31*(4), 40–46.

Revheim, N., & Marcopulos, B. A. (2006). Group treatment approaches to address cognitive deficits. *Psychiatric Rehabilitation Journal, 30*(1), 38–45.

Rhoades, D. R., (2000) Schizophrenia: A review for family counselors. *Family Journal: Counseling and Therapy for Couples and Families, 8*(3), 258–266.

Riebschleger, J. (2004). Good days and bad days: The experiences of children of a parent with a psychiatric disability. *Psychiatric Rehabilitation Journal, 28*(1), 25–31.

Rogers, E. S., Anthony, W. A., Lyass, A., & Penk, W. E. (2006). A randomized clinical trial of vocational rehabilitation for people with psychiatric disabilities. *Rehabilitation Counseling Bulletin, 49*(3), 143–156.

Roy-Byrne, P. P., & Wagner, A. (2004). Primary care perspectives on generalized anxiety disorder. *Journal of Clinical Psychiatry, 65*(suppl 13), 20–26.

Russell, S. J., & Browne, J. L. (2005). Staying well with bipolar disorder. *Australian and New Zealand Journal of Psychiatry, 39*, 187–193.

Rytsala, H. J., Melartin, T. K., Leskela, U. S., Sokero, T. P., Lestela-Mielonen, P. S., & Isometsa, E. T. (2005). Functional and work disability in major depressive disorder. *Journal of Nervous and Mental Disease, 193*, 189–195.

Rystala, H. J., Melartin, T. K., Leskela, U. S., Sokero, T. P., Lestela-Mielonen, P. S., & Isometsa, E. T. (2007). Predictors of long-term work disability in major depressive disorder: A prospective study. *Acta Psychiatrica Scandinavia, 11*, 206–213.

Salloum, I. M., & Thase, M. E. (2000). Impact of substance abuse on the course and treatment of bipolar disorder. *Bipolar Disorders, 2*(3 Pt 2) 269–280.

Schiffer, R. B. (2004). Psychiatric disorders in medical practice. In L. Goldman & D. Ausiello(Eds.), *Cecil textbook of medicine* (22nd ed., pp. 2212–2223). Philadelphia: Saunders.

Sheehan, D. V., & Sheehan, K. H. (2007). Current approaches to the pharmacolojic treatment of anxiety disorders. *Psychopharmacology Bulletin,* 40(1), 98–109.

Simon, G. E. (2006). The antidepressant quandary: Considering suicide risk when treating adolescent depression. *New England Journal of Medicine, 355*(26), 2722–2723.

Smith, D. J., Muir, W. J., & Blackwood, D. H. R. (2006). Neurocognitive impairment in euthymic young adults with bipolar spectrum disorder and recurrent major depressive disorder. *Bipolar Disorders, 8,* 40–46.

Spearing, M. (2002). *Bipolar disorder.* National Institutes of Health, National Institute of Mental Health. September. NIH publication no. 02-3679.

Sridhar, G. R. (2007). Psychiatric co-morbidity and diabetes. *Indian Journal of Medical Research, 125*(3), 311–320.

Stahl, S. M. (2004). Symptoms and circuits: Part 3. Schizophrenia. *Journal of Clinical Psychiatry, 65,* 8–9.

Stapleton, J. A., Asmundson, G. J. G., Woods, M., Taylor, S., & Stein, M. B. (2006). Health care utilization by United Nations peacekeeping veterans with co-occuring, self-reported, post-traumatic stress disorder and depression symptoms versus those without. *Military Medicine, 171*(1), 562–566.

Stevenson, B. (2005). Post-traumatic stress disorder. *Alberta RN, 61*(10), 10–12.

Strakowski, S. M., & DelBello, M. P. (2002). The co-occurrence of bipolar and substance use disorders. *Clinical Psychology Review, 20*(2), 191–206.

Strauser, D. R., Lustig, D. C., & Uruk, A. C. (2006). Examining the moderating effect of disability status on the relationship between trauma symptomatology and select career variables. *Rehabilitation Counseling Bulletin, 49*(2), 90–101.

Stroup, T. S., Lieberman, J. A., McEvoy, J. P., Swartz, M. S., Davis, S. M., Rosenheck, R. A., et al. (2006). Effectiveness of olanzapine, quetiapine, risperidone, and ziprasidone in patients with chronic schizophrenia following discontinuation of a previous atypical antipsychotic. *American Journal of Psychiatry, 163,* 611–622.

Swanson, J. W., Swartz, M. S., Essock, S. M., Osher, F. C., Wagner, H. R., Goodman, L.A., et al. (2002). The social-environmental context of

violent behavior in persons treated for severe mental illness. *American Journal of Public Health, 92,* 1523–1531.

Swofford, C. D., Scheller-Gilkey, G., Miller, A. H., Woolwine, B., & Mance, R. (2000). Double jeopardy: Schizophrenia and substance use. *American Journal of Drug and Alcohol Abuse, 26*(13), 343–358.

Szymanski, E. M. (2000). Disability and vocational behavior. In R. Frank & T. Elliot (Eds.), *Handbook of rehabilitation psychology* (pp. 499–517). Washington, DC: American Psychological Association.

Tschopp, M. K., Bishop, M., & Mulvihill, M. (2001). Career development of individuals with psychiatric disabilities: An ecological perspective of barriers and interventions. *Journal of Applied Rehabilitation Counseling, 32*(2), 25–30.

Tsemberis, S., Gulcur, L., & Nakae, M. (2004). Housing first, consumer choice, and harm reduction for homeless individuals with a dual diagnosis. *American Journal of Public Health, 94*(4), 651–656.

Twamley, E. W., Padin, D. S., Bayne, K. S., Narvaez, J. M., Williams, R. E., & Jeste, D. V. (2005). Work rehabilitation for middle-aged and older people with schizophrenia: A comparison of three approaches. *Journal of Nervous and Mental Disease, 193*(9), 596–601.

Twigger, M., & Houltram, B. (2006). A weighty problem: Monitoring the side effects of medication. *Learning Disability Practice, 9*(10), 28–31.

Ursano, R. J. (2002). Post-traumatic stress disorder. *New England Journal of Medicine, 346*(2), 130–132.

Wang, P. S., Schneeweiss, S., Avorn, J., Fischer, M. A., Mogun, H., Solomon, D. H., et al. (2005). Risk of death in elderly users of conventional vs. atypical antipsychotic medications. *New England Journal of Medicine, 353*(22), 2335–2341.

Ware, N.C., Hopper, K., Tugenberg, T., Dickey, B., & Fisher, D. (2007). Connectedness and citizenship redefining social integration. *Psychiatric Services, 58,* 469–474.

Watzke, S., Galvao, A., Gawlik, B., Huehne, M., & Brieger, P. (2006). Change in work performance in vocational rehabilitation for people with severe mental illness: Distinct responder groups. *International Journal of Social Psychiatry, 52*(4), 309–23.

Whooley, M. A., & Simon, G. E. (2000). Managing depression in medical outpatients. *New England Journal of Medicine, 343*(26), 1942–1950.

Zohar, J., Fostick, L., Black, D. W., & Lopez-Ibor, J. J. (2007). Special populations. *CNS Spectrums, 12*(2 suppl 3), 36–42.

Chapter 9

Conditions Related to Substance Use

All major population groups since before the beginning of recorded time have developed their own knowledge and use of substances that alter states of consciousness (Weatherall, 2001). Substance use for medicinal, social, psychological, and religious purposes has been part of most cultures and civilizations. Over the years, a wide array of substances, including plants or plant derivatives, alcohol, nicotine, caffeine, inhalants, and tonics, have been condoned and used by different cultures for therapeutic, ritualistic, religious, or recreational purposes (Fabricant & Farnsworth, 2001).

Examples of substance use throughout the ages are numerous. People in ancient civilizations considered alcohol—and wine in particular—as a gift from the gods. Opium has been cultivated for more than 6000 years and was used both for medicinal purposes, such as pain relief, and for psychological effects, such as sedation and euphoria. As early as 2000 B.C., marijuana use has been reported for a variety of medical problems as well as for its hallucinogenic properties. In some cultures, marijuana use was believed to assist religious men to have visions of the gods and reveal future events. Psychedelic plants were also used in ancient religious ceremonies.

In the Middle Ages, various psychoactive substances were used widely by medieval witches and medicine men as a poison for adversaries, as an analgesic for pain, and as a hallucinogen to generate prophesies (Fabricant & Farnsworth, 2001). In addition, stimulants were often used in the Middle Ages, when resources were scarce, to combat fatigue and hunger in soldiers (Inaba & Cohen, 1993).

Tobacco, which was widely unknown in Europe, was introduced by Columbus in 1492 after he noted Native Americans smoking. The practice of smoking the dried leaves of the tobacco plant, *Nicotiana*, was brought to England by Sir Walter Raleigh in the sixteenth century primarily for medicinal use; however, it's use as a social drug quickly spread (Weatherall, 2001).

During the 1800s, inhaled nitrous oxide, also called "laughing gas," was discovered and used for medicinal purposes as well as for recreation. It was frequently used both as anesthetic and as an intoxicant (Fairley, 1978). The hypodermic needle was developed in the 1860s, but its use was soon expanded from medical purposes to injecting heroin. It's availability created an ever-growing population of individuals who used the drug compulsively and became addicted (Inaba & Cohen, 1993). The twentieth century brought about a number of patented medications that could be purchased over the counter and that were used for medicinal purposes as well as becoming sources of abuse (Abbott & Fraser, 1998).

As use and abuse of various substances became viewed as problematic, regulation or prohibition of a number of substances was attempted in an effort to control or prevent their use. When society becomes ambivalent toward use of a substance, when it determines such use to be inappropriate, or when substance use becomes uncontrolled, hazardous, or disruptive to individuals or to others, then substance use is considered to be pathological and in some instances illegal. Pathological use of substance use is referred to in the *DSM-IV-TR* as *substance-related disorders* (American Psychiatric Association, 2000).

Substance-related disorders reflect a complex interaction of biological, psychological, social, cultural, and environmental factors and may involve substances that are *licit, illicit, prescribed,* or *not prescribed* (American Psychiatric Association, 2000). The etiology and treatment of substance-related disorders entail a complex interface among all these factors; no one factor explains the development of substance-related disorders.

Just as all chronic illnesses and disabilities affect physical, social, psychological, and vocational aspects of individuals' lives, so too do conditions related to substance use. Like other chronic, relapsing conditions, substance-related conditions produce a variety of impairments. Implications of these conditions must be evaluated in the context of the individual's specific situation. Conditions related to substance use can occur alone or in combination with one or more other physical or psychiatric disabilities. The effects of substance use combined with manifestation of another disability can cause additional physical, psychological, and social complications, adding to the disabling effects of both.

■ INTOXICATION

Intoxication is a term that describes reversible behavioral or psychological changes related to the effect of a substance on the nervous system (American Psychiatric Association, 2000). The level of intoxication from the substance is determined by the concentration of the substance in the blood. The concentration, in turn, is determined by the amount of substances taken into the body as well as the rate at which the substance is absorbed into the bloodstream. The rate at which substances are absorbed into the bloodstream depends on the route of administration. For instance, substances that are injected directly into a vein (*intravenous injection IV*) have an immediate effect, whereas substances that are ingested orally take longer to be absorbed into the bloodstream and, consequently, exert their effects more slowly. The rate of absorption of substances taken orally is also affected by the presence or absence of food in the stomach and the rate of gastric emptying. Body size also affects concentration of substances in the blood. For instance, blood alcohol levels are proportionately lower in large individuals than in small individuals, even though both might consume equal amounts of alcohol under similar conditions. In addition, gender affects concentration of substances in the blood. Females typically have less of a substance called *alcohol dehydrogenase* than do males, and consequently women are unable to metabolize alcohol (ethanol) as quickly as men. Thus, women would show higher blood alcohol levels than men even though both had consumed the same amount of alcohol.

■ SUBSTANCE ABUSE AND DEPENDENCE

Our culture condones the use of a number of substances, and use of these socially sanctioned substances may have no harmful effects when they are used appropriately and in moderation. Misuse or overuse of substances or use of illegal substances, however, can have severe physical, psychological, or social consequences. Two concepts describing the negative effects of substance use are substance abuse and substance dependence (American Psychiatric Association, 2000). In 2004, approximately 22.5 million people in the United States (9.4% of the population) were classified as engaging in either substance abuse or substance dependence. Some 3.4 million members, of this group was classified as being dependent on or abusing both alcohol and illicit drugs (Substance Abuse and Mental Health Services Administration, 2005).

Substance abuse is defined as a maladaptive pattern of substance use that results in recurrent and significant negative consequences of substance use. These consequences may include any of the following:

- Disruption of work or school, such as repeated absences or declining performance
- Neglect of family obligations
- Repeated hazardous behavior, such as driving a motor vehicle or operating machinery while under the influence of the substance
- Recurrent disorderly conduct or problems with interpersonal relationships owing to substance use
- Recurrent legal problems related to use of the substance
- Continued use of the substance despite the negative consequences related to that use

Substance dependence refers to substance use that results in physical or psychological distress related to substance tolerance, withdrawal, or a pattern of compulsive substance use.

Tolerance

When individuals continue to use a substance over time, they may begin to experience diminished effects with the use of the same amount of the substance. Consequently, the amount of the substance taken to achieve the same effects must be increased. This phenomenon is called **tolerance.** The degree of tolerance experienced varies from individual to individual and with the specific substance being used.

Individuals using substances chronically may adapt their behavior so that they are able to continue functioning at work, at home, or in social situations, even though they are under the influence of a substance. Although tolerance is not always an indication of dependence, it is commonly observed in individuals with substance-related conditions. Furthermore, individuals who develop a tolerance for one substance may also develop higher tolerance for related substances, a condition known as **cross-tolerance.**

Withdrawal

Toxic effects of large concentrations of a substance cause physical disturbances to occur when the amount of the substance is decreased or suspended. As a result, when the substance is absent from the body or when the amount is decreased, individuals experience **withdrawal.** Withdrawal is characterized by physiological or cognitive manifestations and/or maladaptive behavior change resulting in impairment in function. The manifestations of withdrawal depend on the substance and on individual factors, such as the presence of additional medical or psychiatric conditions, and the amount and duration of substance dependence.

Compulsive Behaviors

Substance dependence may also be marked by compulsive substance use or substance-seeking behavior, in which individuals become so preoccupied with the substance that much of their daily activity revolves around using and/or obtaining it. Despite the negative consequences of substance use that individuals with substance dependence may have experienced, such as loss of a job or family, they may persist in using the substance.

Addiction

Although the American Psychiatric Association uses the term "dependence" rather than "addiction," the term *addiction* emphasizes the behavioral component of a substance-related condition rather than physical dependence (Maddux & Desmond, 2000). Addiction comprises a chronic, neurobiological condition that is influenced by psychosocial, genetic, and environmental factors and that is characterized by compulsive substance-seeking behaviors, impaired control over drug use, and continued use of the substance despite negative consequences (Ruiz, Strain, & Langrod, 2007; Adinoff, 2004). The physical and psychological craving for the substance becomes so all-consuming that individuals expend tremendous effort, energy, and financial resources to obtain it, often at the expense of the safety and well-being of themselves and others.

In addiction, substance use evolves into more than merely "wanting" or "liking" the substance. The nervous systems of individuals who are addicted become hypersensitized, which causes pathological craving for the substance, independent of physical signs of withdrawal (Robinson & Berridge, 2001). Compulsive substance-seeking and substance-taking behavior is facilitated by difficulties in decision making and the ability to judge consequences of drug-seeking and drug-taking actions (Robinson & Berridge, 2003).

Several factors appear to predispose individuals to addiction. For instance, a growing body of evidence indicates a genetic predisposition in some individuals for development of alcohol-related conditions as well as dependence on other substances such as nicotine, cocaine, and opioids (Ruiz et al., 2007). Personality traits such as risk-taking or novelty-seeking traits have also been found to be more prevalent in individuals who abuse or are dependent on drugs (Helmus, Downey, Arfken, Henderson, & Schuster, 2001). Individuals with psychiatric disorders—especially schizophrenia, bipolar disorder, and depression—have an increased risk of substance abuse (Leikin, 2007). Individuals with dual diagnosis have also been shown to have a more unfavorable prognosis in terms of management and outcome (Kavanagh, McGrath, Saunders, Dore, & Clark, 2002).

■ WITHDRAWAL

Consumption of large amounts of alcohol or other drugs at frequent intervals for prolonged periods creates a state of physical dependence so that cessation or reduction in the amount consumed produces distressful and incapacitating symptoms, known as substance withdrawal. The symptoms experienced during withdrawal vary in severity. The initial symptoms, regardless of the substance, may consist of dysphoria (exaggerated feelings of depression and unrest), insomnia, anxiety, irritability, nausea, agitation, tachycardia (fast heartbeat), and hypertension (high blood pressure).

Individuals with mild to moderate withdrawal symptoms who have no preexisting conditions and who have adequate social support may have withdrawal managed on an outpatient basis. It is important for health professionals managing withdrawal to know the type of substance abused as there are substantial differences in complications as well as management of withdrawal from specific substances. Individuals who develop more serious withdrawal symptoms such as *delirium tremens* (DTs) associated with alcohol, those who experince psychotic symptoms with withdrawal from stimulants or opioids, or those who have coexisting psychiatric or medical conditions usually require inpatient management of withdrawal (Kosten & O'Connor, 2003).

▣ DETOXIFICATION

Detoxification is the first step in treatment of substance abuse and dependence. The goal of detoxification is to initiate abstinence, reduce symptoms of withdrawal, prevent complications, and retain individuals in treatment (Kosten & O'Connor, 2003). During the detoxification process and when undergoing withdrawal, individuals may experience nausea and vomiting, tachycardia, hypertension fever, and **diaphoresis** (profuse sweating). In more severe withdrawal, individuals may experience disorientation, hallucinations, delirium tremens, and, in some instances, seizures. Withdrawal from some substances, such as alcohol and other sedatives, can be fatal.

Risk factors for more severe withdrawal are older age (40 years or older), high tolerance, other health problems (such as diabetes or cardiovascular disease), and poor nutrition. Individuals who are in lower-risk groups may undergo detoxification at community health settings; by contrast, individuals at higher risk usually require hospitalization. During the detoxification process, medical management may consist of providing adequate hydration, restoring electrolyte balance, providing thiamine and other vitamins, administration of sedatives, and monitoring for possible complications (Brown, 2007). After detoxification, treatment may include medications that act as substitutes for the abused substances. The goal in providing these medications is to gradually reduce the dosage, thereby eventually eliminating dependency.

▣ SUBSTANCE USE AND CHRONIC ILLNESS AND DISABILITY

Individuals with other chronic illnesses and disabilities can also have a condition related to substance use. In some instances, substance abuse may have been a factor in the acquisition of the chronic illness or disability, such as injury sustained in a motor vehicle accident

caused by driving under the influence or HIV infection acquired by sharing contaminated needles. Substance abuse and dependence may also be a maladaptive coping mechanism for an individual who is trying to adjust to chronic illness or disability. In other instances, individuals may become dependent on substances, that were originally prescribed to treat symptoms such as pain or anxiety. Whether substance abuse or dependence was a precursor of an acquired chronic illness or disability, or a coping mechanism employed after chronic illness or disability, a diagnosis of two disabling conditions makes management of both conditions more complex.

A number of factors may place individuals with chronic illness or disability at higher risk for substance-related conditions:

- Medical factors such as easy access to prescription medication to alleviate symptoms, such as chronic pain, making it easier to use the medication excessively; or unnecessary or unwarranted prescription of medication for symptoms that could have been treated by alternative means

- Psychological factors such as depression, boredom, or frustration, so that substances are used as a means of escape from reality

- Social factors such as oppression or alienation, so that substances are used recreationally in an attempt to gain acceptance and normalization (Greer, Roberts, & Jenkins, 1990; Watson, Franklin, Ingram, & Eilenberg, 1998)

The coexistence of a substance-related condition with other chronic illness or disability can exacerbate and accentuate manifestations of the condition as well as increase individuals' vulnerability to medical complications, leading to acquisition of additional disability. Although substance abuse can coexist with any disability, comorbidity between substance abuse and psychiatric disability (*dual diagnosis*) is very common (Allen Doyle-Pita, 2001; Volkow, 2001). Whether a substance-related condition is the primary disability or a secondary disability, appropriate intervention and treatment of substance abuse and dependence are necessary if individuals are to reach their full rehabilitation potential.

■ MEDICAL COMPLICATIONS OF ALCOHOL ABUSE AND DEPENDENCE

The effect of alcohol on the body, like the effect of any drug, depends on the interaction between properties of the specific pharmacologic agent and characteristics of a specific individual. Evidence suggests that women tend to be more sensitive to the effects of alcohol and more susceptible to adverse effects of excessive alcohol consumption than are men (Scott-Lennox, Rose, Bohlig, & Lennox, 2000; Kandall, 1996; Harley, 1995; Blume, Counts, & Turnbull, 1992). A wide range of physical and psychiatric complications is associated with alcohol dependence (Ruiz et al., 2007). Medical complications resulting from alcohol abuse and/or dependence result both from direct effects of alcohol on body tissues and from adaptive responses of the body to excessive exposure to alcohol.

Alcohol has a direct pharmacologic effect on the nervous system; it is a powerful central nervous system depressant. Initially, alcohol acts as a stimulant by suppressing the central nervous system's inhibitory systems. As the alcohol level increases in the body, however, it has a sedative effect and causes **ataxia** (difficulty with muscle coordination) and impaired psychomotor performance (Holdstock & deWit, 1998). Alcohol is rapidly absorbed into the bloodstream from the stomach and intestines and rapidly metabolized, making it a fast-acting drug. Because alcohol diffuses quickly into the water content of all body tissues, blood

concentration of alcohol is an accurate reflection of the concentration of alcohol in other body tissues.

Some alcohol is eliminated through the kidneys and lungs, but the liver metabolizes most of this substance. Although a moderate dose of alcohol is normally cleared from the blood in approximately one hour, only a fixed amount of alcohol can be metabolized at a time. When the rate of alcohol consumption exceeds the body's ability to metabolize it, alcohol accumulates in the bloodstream, elevating the blood alcohol concentration.

The intoxicating effects of alcohol correlate roughly with the alcohol concentration in the blood, which in turn reflects the alcohol concentration in the brain. At low levels of intoxication (0.05%), alcohol may produce a sense of relaxation and well-being. As the concentration of alcohol increases (0.11% to 0.20%), neurological signs of ataxia (especially affecting voluntary movement) occur. Judgment may also be impaired. Continued elevation of blood alcohol concentration (0.31% to 0.41%) can produce confusion, mild stupor, and, ultimately, coma. A blood alcohol level of 0.51% or higher usually leads to death from depression of the respiratory center located in the brain.

Another effect in the spectrum of neurological disturbances associated with intensive alcohol intoxication is the occurrence of blackouts. These periods of amnesia are characterized by an inability to remember events during the time of the blackout.

Alcohol withdrawal can be complicated by seizures and delirium. The most severe form of alcohol withdrawal is delirium tremens. Individuals with delirium tremens experience significant restlessness, gross disorientation, cognitive disruption, elevation of temperature and pulse rate, and, in some instances, psychosis. Although delirium tremens can be fatal, its course is often self-limiting. The acute period of delirium tremens usually lasts from 2 to10 days, but can be more prolonged in case of severe withdrawal.

The withdrawal syndrome may be treated medically by the administration of a cross-tolerant drug, such as a sedative. Initially, sedatives are given in large doses to suppress the withdrawal symptoms. The dose is then reduced, or the interval between doses is increased, or both, so that the dosage progressively tapers off to zero. Because of wide variations in drug tolerance, treatment is individualized.

Management of Alcohol Dependence

Alcohol dependence is a chronic, lifelong condition. It requires long-term management that extends beyond the initial period of detoxification and generally involves a wide variety of services, including individual, group, and family therapy. In addition, self-help groups, such as *Alcoholics Anonymous (AA)* for alcohol-dependent individuals and *Alanon* and *Alateen* for their families, are widely recommended.

Typically, the goal of treatment is abstinence from alcohol and other mood-altering substances. In some circumstances, drugs are used to discourage and inhibit the use of alcohol. One such drug, an aversive substance called disulfiram (Antabuse), interferes with the normal metabolism of alcohol so that individuals who ingest alcohol after taking Antabuse experience severe gastrointestinal distress. Although it has not been shown to have a lasting long-term benefit, this agent may facilitate abstinence in the early recovery phase for individuals prone to impulsive drinking (Brown, 2007). Other drugs, such as naltrexone (ReVia) and acamprosate (Campral), help to reduce cravings for alcohol. A new drug, Baclofen, has recently been developed for both the management of alcohol withdrawal and relapse prevention (Addolorato, Leggio, Abenavoli, et al., 2006; Addolorato, Leggio, Agabio, Colombo, & Gasbarrini, 2006).

Effective management of alcohol dependence consists of both pharmacologic and psychosocial interventions. Psychosocial interventions in the form of counseling, psycho-educational, negotiating behavior change, and specific behavioral agreements are frequently used. Most successful interventions have been demonstrated to consist of a combination of medical, psychosocial counseling, and support networks (Brown, 2007).

Alcohol-Related Illness

Medical conditions that can result from chronic alcohol abuse, other than those caused by trauma due to intoxication are generally caused by dietary insufficiency, the direct toxic effects of alcohol on body tissue, or both. These conditions can involve all organ systems. The prognosis of alcohol-related medical illness depends on the nature of the illness and its severity. Although some alcohol-related medical illnesses are reversible, almost no alcohol-related illness can be cured if the individual continues to abuse alcohol.

Nervous System Conditions

Korsakoff's Syndrome

Associated with an excessive intake of alcohol, chronic malnutrition, and a deficiency of the B vitamins (thiamine, in particular), *Korsakoff's syndrome* is characterized by short-term memory impairment. The use of **confabulation**, in which individuals make up experiences to fill in memory gaps, is a common characteristic of those with Korsakoff's syndrome. In addition to abstinence, treatment consists of the administration of *thiamine*. Some cognitive improvement is possible, but full recovery is unlikely. Several months may be required before improvement is noticeable.

Wernicke's Encephalopathy (Wernicke's Disease)

Wernicke's encephalopathy is a condition caused by thiamine deficiency. Although it can occur in other conditions, it is most commonly associated with chronic alcohol abuse (Agronin, 2007). This potentially life-threatening condition is characterized by the sudden onset of confusion, **nystagmus** (involuntary eye movements), and ataxia. Management of Wernicke's encephalopathy consists of the replacement of thiamine. Early intervention is mandatory to prevent permanent deficits. Prompt intervention resolves many of the symptoms.

Wernicke's encephalopathy often occurs in combination with Korsakoff's syndrome. *Wernicke–Korsakoff's syndrome* is characterized by learning and memory impairment that persists. This syndrome is observed when the initial symptoms are not treated rapidly (Agronin, 2007).

Peripheral Neuropathy

Although many causes of peripheral neuropathy exist (see Chapter 4), a number of individuals who chronically abuse alcohol develop disorders of the **peripheral nerves** (nerves outside the central nervous system).

Peripheral neuropathy associated with chronic alcohol abuse is thought to be the result of inadequate nutrition—specifically, inadequate amounts of thiamine and the other B vitamins. This condition affects the extremities and includes symptoms such as numbness, painful sensations, weakness, and muscle cramps. Burning pain of the feet may also occur. Good nutrition and the administration of supplemental B vitamins can bring about improvement, albeit slowly.

Cardiovascular System Conditions

Cardiomyopathy

Alcoholic cardiomyopathy occurs after long-term, chronic use of alcohol. It results from the direct toxic effects of alcohol on the heart muscle itself. The heart may become enlarged (**cardiomegaly**), and the heart muscle may become more fibrous. The heart's ability to pump effectively may be compromised so that symptoms of congestive heart failure, such as difficulty in breathing and swelling (see Chapter 13), may occur as the cardiac damage progresses.

Beriberi Heart Disease

A deficiency in thiamine is thought to contribute to the development of beriberi heart disease. Individuals with this condition have a high cardiac output, even at rest, because of the dilation of the peripheral small blood vessels. Beriberi heart disease responds well to the administration of supplemental thiamine.

Alterations in Heart Rate and Rhythm

Alcohol can affect both the speed at which the heart beats and the rhythm that it maintains. The direct, long-term effect on blood pressure varies, however. Withdrawal from alcohol dependence can put a heavy load on the heart, sometimes compromising cardiac function so severely during detoxification that death can result. Consequently, detoxification should be conducted under careful medical supervision.

Hypertension

Individuals who drink excessively may develop hypertension (high blood pressure). Hypertension can bring about serious consequences such as stroke or **myocardial infarction** (heart attack). (See Chapter 13.)

Alterations in Blood

Alcohol can have a direct and adverse effect on the development of red blood cells, white blood cells, and platelets, resulting in anemia, lower resistance to infection, and interference with blood clotting. One of the mechanisms by which alcohol affects blood cell formation is by altering with the use of folic acid, a nutritional substance that bone marrow requires to manufacture healthy cells effectively.

Megaloblastic anemia (the presence of large abnormal red blood cells) with *leukopenia* (an abnormal decrease in the number of white blood cells) and *thrombocytopenia* (an abnormal decrease in the number of platelets) occurs frequently in individuals with low folic acid intake. Treatment with the administration of supplemental folate, proper nutrition, and abstinence from alcohol can generally reverse these abnormalities.

Respiratory System Conditions

Alcohol has a direct toxic effect on lung tissue. In combination with cigarette smoking, a higher incidence of *chronic obstructive pulmonary disease* (COPD; see Chapter 14) can result from chronic alcohol abuse. In addition, because chronic alcohol abuse affects some of the lungs' natural defenses, individuals who abuse alcohol have a greater tendency to develop lung infections.

Musculoskeletal System Conditions

Regardless of the person's nutritional status, alcohol has a direct toxic effect on skeletal muscle by destroying muscle fibers, leading to weakness, pain, tenderness, and swelling of affected muscles. **Myopathy** (disease of the muscles) related to alcohol abuse may be acute or chronic. The more common form is *chronic alcoholic myopathy,* which evolves over months to years. Pain may be less severe in chronic myopathy, although muscle cramps can occur. In addition, muscles may **atrophy** (shrink or become smaller) and weaken. Most manifestations of myopathy improve with the cessation of alcohol abuse, whereas continued alcohol abuse leads to continued deterioration. Excessive alcohol consumption can also contribute to **osteoporosis** (a reduction in bone mass), causing bones to become weakened, fragile, and easily broken (see Chapter 16). Osteoporosis occurs not only because calcium intake is insufficient, but also because alcohol interferes with the absorption of calcium from the intestines.

In addition to having a direct effect on the musculoskeletal system, alcohol can contrib-

ute to major injury. Individuals under the influence of alcohol may have decreased balance and coordination as well as demonstrate impaired judgment. As a result, individuals may experience injuries in falls, fires, or motor vehicle or pedestrian accidents.

Gastrointestinal System Conditions

Alcohol may affect almost every organ of the gastrointestinal tract. Individuals who consume alcohol excessively have an increased incidence of cancer of the throat and esophagus (see Chapter 12) as well as colorectal cancer (Cho, Smith-Warner, Ritz, van den Brandt, Colditz, & Folsom, 2004). Whether the increased incidence of cancer is attributable to direct contact of alcohol with the tissues, the presence of carcinogenic substances in some alcoholic beverages, or a combination of the two is unknown. Despite the fact that alcohol is considered a **hepatotoxin** (a substance that is harmful to the liver), individuals who chronically abuse alcohol differ widely in their susceptibility to liver disease.

Esophagitis and Gastritis

Esophagitis and **gastritis** are inflammations of the esophagus and of the stomach respectively. Both can occur with acute or chronic abuse of alcohol. The severity of these conditions depends on the individual. In some instances, these conditions produce only mild discomfort; in other instances, the irritation and inflammation lead to ulceration and bleeding. Intervention is directed toward reducing the inflammation. Obviously, abstinence from alcohol is a major treatment objective.

Alcoholic Hepatitis

During the process of alcohol metabolism, fat is deposited in the liver. When individuals consume excessive amounts of alcohol, accumulation of fat enlarges the liver, a condition called *fatty liver.* If individuals continue to consume alcohol, liver cells may die, causing the liver to become inflamed. This inflammatory condition, in which the liver is usually enlarged and painful, is known as *alcoholic hepatitis.* Alcoholic hepatitis is an inflammation of the liver brought about by alcohol; it is *not* a contagious form of hepatitis.

Abstinence from alcohol can reverse the effects of both fatty liver and alcoholic hepatitis. Individuals who continue to abuse alcohol, however, have a high chance of developing cirrhosis.

Cirrhosis

Cirrhosis is a condition that involves **fibrosis** (formation of fibrous tissue) of the liver. It can be caused by a variety of conditions, but is most frequently attributable to either hepatitis C or alcoholism (Ginés, Cárdenas, Arroyo, & Rodés, 2004). When alcohol injures the liver repeatedly over an extended period of time, fibrous tissue replaces liver cells. Circulation within the liver becomes less efficient, resulting in obstructions and ultimately increasing pressure in the vessels.

All blood from the gastrointestinal tract, spleen, pancreas, and gallbladder is carried to the heart through the liver by the *portal system.* As a result of the fibrous changes that occur in the liver with cirrhosis, pressure increases in the portal vein, a condition known as *portal hypertension.* The backflow of blood results in the enlargement of the spleen (**splenomegaly**), accumulation of fluid in the abdominal cavity (**ascites**), and development of esophageal varices (discussed in the next section).

Some individuals with cirrhosis experience no symptoms, especially in the disease's early stages. As the condition progresses, however, individuals may experience weakness, nausea, loss of appetite (**anorexia**), and **jaundice** (yellow discoloration of the skin and whites of the eyes from to the accumulation of bile pigments in the blood).

Diagnosis of cirrhosis is based on symptoms; results of blood tests; imaging via ultrasound, CT, or MRI; and liver biopsy. When standard medical therapy has failed to control the complications of cirrhosis, individuals may be referred for liver transplantation. Several scores have been developed to categorize the severity of cirrhosis and consequently allocation of transplantation (Heidelbaugh & Sherbondy, 2006). The *Child–Pugh* score incorporates three laboratory values and two clinical features experienced by the individual. The Child–Pugh score of cirrhotic severity may be used as an indication of whether individuals should be referred for liver transplantation evaluation. The MELD *(Model for End-stage Liver Disease)* score is also used as an indication of severity of liver damage in individuals being considered for liver transplantation.

Treatment of cirrhosis is largely symptomatic, but abstinence from alcohol is a necessity for survival. Individuals with cirrhotic changes in the liver have an increased risk of liver cancer as well as a higher risk of a number of other complications. Those who continue to abuse alcohol despite cirrhotic changes in the liver or other complications have a significantly decreased survival rate.

Esophageal Varices

Esophageal varices is a condition in which veins in the esophagus become dilated and tortuous as a result of portal hypertension, a complication of cirrhosis of the liver. Approximately 60 to 80% of individuals with cirrhosis develop esophageal varices (Chen & Jutabha, 2007; Heidelaugh & Sherbondy, 2006). Varices may bleed periodically and then stop spontaneously. Individuals with esophageal varices may experience **hematemesis** (vomiting of blood) and **melena** (dark, tarry bowel movements caused by digestion of swallowed blood). Bleeding esophageal varices can be life-threatening. High portal pressure may cause them to burst, resulting in hemorrhage and requiring emergency attention to stop the bleeding.

Management is directed toward controlling hemorrhage. The two major interventions for esophageal varices involve *endoscopy*, in which a tube is inserted into the esophagus. The most common of the two, *endoscopic band ligation*, involves placing elastic bands around the esophageal varices (Heidelbaugh & Sherbondy, 2006; Krige, Kotze, Bornman, Shaw, & Klipin, 2006). The other procedure, *endoscopic sclerotherapy* involves injection of a substance into the varices, that *scleroses* (hardens) and stops the bleeding. In instances in which endoscopic procedures do not stop the bleeding, more invasive surgical intervention may be needed. In some instances, a temporary measure to control acute bleeding may involve insertion of a special tube (*Sengstaken-Blakemore tube*) into the esophagus. A balloon on the tube is then inflated to exert pressure against the bleeding vein.

Pancreatitis

A variety of conditions other than alcohol abuse may cause **pancreatitis** (inflammation of the pancreas). *Alcoholic pancreatitis*, however, is a form of pancreatitis that develops in susceptible individuals after chronic alcohol abuse. In this condition, the pancreatic ducts become obstructed. Normally, the pancreas secretes enzymes into the small intestine to aid in digestion. In alcoholic pancreatitis, however, the enzymes become active while they are still in the pancreas (see Chapter 12) so that the pancreas essentially begins to digest itself, causing progressive degeneration with scarring and calcification of pancreatic tissues. Pancreatic function is often severely curtailed. Chronic pancreatitis can lead to severe disability from pain, malaborption of nutrients resulting in weight loss, and diabetes mellitus secondary to the destruction of cells in the pancreas that secrete insulin *(islets of Langerhans)* (see Chapter 11).

Management of pancreatitis is directed toward halting destruction of tissue and alleviating the manifestations. As with other conditions affecting the gastrointestinal tract, effective management requires that individuals abstain from alcohol. If they no longer consume alcohol, many will recover from alcoholic pancreatitis to live a normal life. If they continue to drink, however, the prognosis is generally poor.

Reproductive System Conditions

Excessive alcohol use has been found to lower the level of the male hormone *testosterone*, which in turn has been related to decreased libido and, in some instances, impotence. Excessive alcohol intake also increases the level of *epinephrine* and other hormones.

The toxic effects of alcohol on the developing fetus during pregnancy can result in a deformity of the infant called **fetal alcohol syndrome**. The amount of alcohol that pregnant women must consume before the fetus is injured is unknown and appears to vary with the individual. Fetal alcohol syndrome is characterized by prenatal and postnatal growth retardation, **microcephaly** (abnormal smallness of the head), abnormalities of the nervous system, and facial disfiguration. Other congenital anomalies may include mental retardation, musculoskeletal abnormalities, and cardiac abnormalities.

■ USE AND ABUSE OF OTHER SUBSTANCES

Caffeine

Although *caffeine* is not commonly thought of as a substance of abuse and dependence, individuals who consume large amounts may exhibit signs of dependence on caffeine including tolerance and withdrawal symptoms (Juliano & Griffiths, 2004; American Psychiatric Association, 2000). Caffeine is commonly obtained from coffee or tea, but it may also be consumed in soft drinks, chocolate, and over-the-counter drugs, such as weight loss aids and antidrowsiness medications.

Caffeine acts primarily as a stimulant (Chou, 1992). Low to moderate doses of caffeine have been shown to produce subjective effects that include positive effects such as increased alertness, greater energy, and feelings of well-being (Strain & Griffiths, 1995). While moderate caffeine use appears to pose few health risks for most healthy individuals, overuse of caffeine can produce caffeine intoxication, which can lead to symptoms of anxiety, insomnia, tachycardia (rapid heartbeat), hypertension (elevated blood pressure), and gastric distress (American Psychiatric Association, 2000). Caffeine can also exacerbate existing disabling conditions and may aggravate preexisting conditions, such as ulcer disease, hypertension, or heart conditions (Ochs, Holmes, & Karst, 1992). It's use can be associated with several psychiatric syndromes, such as caffeine-induced sleep disorder, caffeine-induced anxiety disorder, and caffeine dependence (Ruiz, Strain, & Langrod, 2007; American Psychiatric Association, 2000).

Caffeine also interacts with a number of medications and can interfere with their effectiveness. For example, caffeine and sedative drugs such as benzodiazepines have antagonistic effects, so that the sedative effect of a drug, such as Valium, may be blocked when taken with caffeine. Caffeine has also been shown to interfere with metabolism of some antipsychotic drugs and brochodilating drugs, interfering with their effectiveness (Ruiz et al., 2007).

If caffeine use is found to cause or exacerbate medical or psychiatric problems or interfere with medication efficiency, individuals may need to reduce or eliminate their use of this stimulant. Individuals with caffeine dependence may experience withdrawal symptoms such as fatigue and difficulty concentrating. Gradual reduction of caffeine consumption along with social support can be helpful in this regard. The availability of a large number of decaffeinated products makes it possible to decrease caffeine consumption, if necessary.

Nicotine

Nicotine has been identified as the most widely used substance of abuse (Maseeh & Kwatra, 2005). This substance is a highly dependence-producing drug found in tobacco and tobacco products (Christen & Christen, 1994). Although tobacco use in the United States has decreased in recent years, many individuals in the general population remain dependent on it. In addition, individuals with psychiatric disability and/or substance use disorders have a prevalence of tobacco use that is two to four times more than the prevalence in the general population (Lasser et al., 2000).

Nicotine dependence, like other conditions characterized by dependence, is viewed as a chronic disease that requires ongoing attention (Tinsley, 2007). Nicotine consumed through smoking, chewing, or snuffing tobacco is absorbed through the mucous membranes or surfaces of the lung, producing an immediate reward effect (Maseeh & Kwatra, 2005). When taken into the body, nicotine produces initial stimulation, followed by sedation. In addition, many individuals who smoke cigarettes become dependent on the ritual of smoking, which includes the process of opening the cigarette packet, lighting the cigarette, and seeing and smelling the smoke (Peters & Morgan, 2002).

The health consequences of tobacco use can be severe. It is well documented that tobacco use increases risk of heart disease, cancer, lung disease, and a number of other chronic, disabling, and fatal conditions (Ruiz, Strain, & Langrod, 2007; Kalman, Morissette, & George, 2005). Tobacco use has also been linked to higher infant mortality and lower birth weights (Kellogg, 2002). In a study of all causes of death in the United States in 2000, the leading cause of death was tobacco, which accounted for 18.1% of total deaths (Mokdad,

Marks, Stroup, & Gerberding, 2004). Cigarette smoking, in particular, has been found to be the leading cause of death and disability in the United States (USDHHS, 2004).

Nicotine dependence can interfere with treatment of other smoking-related diseases. A 1985 study reported that at least 50% of individuals recovering from surgery for a smoking-related condition such as lung cancer or cardiovascular disease continued to smoke while they were hospitalized or resumed smoking shortly after they were discharged (Burling, Stitzer, Bigelow, & Mead, 1985). Although smoking was once socially acceptable, pressure from various groups and public awareness of the health hazards of smoking have resulted in sanctions on public smoking behavior.

Individuals who have developed nicotine dependence experience both physiological and psychological withdrawal symptoms within hours after they are deprived of nicotine (Brown, Lejuez, Kahler, Strong, & Zvolensky, 2005). These withdrawal symptoms can include insomnia, irritability, anxiety, depressed mood, increased appetite, and weight gain. Although most manifestations associated with withdrawal are related to deprivation of nicotine, a number of social factors, such as conditioning and expectancy, also contribute to perception of manifestations and craving for nicotine (Ruiz, et al., 2007).

Interventions for nicotine dependence vary widely and consist of pharmacologic and psychosocial approaches.

Pharmacologic Approaches

Pharmacologic approaches include a number of medications used in nicotine replacement therapy. *Nicotine gum* contains small amounts of nicotine and requires a special chewing technique to derive optimal therapeutic effect. The gum is used by individuals regularly throughout the day to provide one-third to two-thirds the level of nicotine that would have been obtained through smoking.

Nicotine patches are transdermal patches that are placed on the skin and are designed to release nicotine slowly and steadily. Patches are available in different strengths of dosage and deliver the dosage over the course of 16 to 24 hours. Patches are generally used over a period of 8 weeks, with a gradual tapering of the dose of nicotine.

Of all other nicotine replacement therapies, *nicotine nasal sprays* provide the most immediate and highest level of nicotine, albeit not as high as would be obtained from cigarettes. Individuals usually initially use the spray one to two times per hour, and then gradually titrate the dose up to a maximum of 40 mg of nicotine per day for 6 to 8 weeks. After this time, there is a gradual tapering off of use over the next 3 to 6 months.

Oral forms of pharmacologic therapy include *nicotine tablets,* which are placed under the tongue, and *nicotine lozenges,* which are sucked until a strong taste is emitted and then placed between gum and cheek until the flavor fades. Both are absorbed directly into the mucous membranes of the mouth; neither should be chewed or swallowed. Because tablets deliver a lower dose of nicotine, they can be taken more frequently than the lozenges. On average, individuals use seven to eight lozenges per day, with a maximum of 25 lozenges per day. The program lasts about 12 weeks, with gradual tapering of use of lozenges.

Non-nicotine drugs, such as Bupropion, nortriptyline, and other antidepressant drugs are also used to treat nicotine dependence. In some instances, antidepressants may be used to reduce the symptoms associated with withdrawal.

Psychosocial Approaches

Counseling to help individuals reduce the stress associated with smoking cessation and a number of behavioral approaches have been used in smoking-cessation programs. Cognitive-behavioral therapies that identify cues for smoking and then develop techniques to break the association between the cues and smoking are frequently used. In addition, a number of alternative interventions, including acupuncture and exercise programs, have been used with varying success (Maseeh & Kwatra, 2005).

Overall, the success rates for pharmacologic and psychosocial approaches to cessation of tobacco use appears to be directly related to the smoker's motivation to stop. Nicotine withdrawal is a major obstacle to smoking cessation (Tinsley, 2007). However, emerging evidence suggests that the factor significantly affecting an individual's ability to stop smoking is how he or she responds to discomfort and distress related to withdrawal, rather than the physical withdrawal symptoms alone (Brown et al., 2005).

Sedatives

Sedation implies calmness and tranquility. *Sedatives* are classified according to the pharmacologic action they produce—namely, depression of the central nervous system. Examples of sedative drugs are alcohol, barbiturates, and benzodiazepines such as diazepam (Valium), and alprazolam (Xanax). If taken in higher doses to produce sleep, these medications are called *hypnotics*. Whether they have been prescribed for treatment of a specific condition or symptom, or whether they have been obtained illegally, sedatives may be associated with abuse, tolerance, and dependence.

Individuals commonly combine substances—for example, they may use sedatives with alcohol, or opiates with stimulants. Commonly abused sedatives include barbiturates (e.g., secobarbital and amobarbital sodium),

benzodiazepines (e.g., chlordiazepoxide hydrochloride [Librium], diazepam [Valium], and chlorzepate dipotassium [Tranzene]), as well as other central nervous system depressants (e.g., methaqualone [Quaalude] and etchlorvynol [Placidyl]).

Withdrawal from sedatives is similar to withdrawal from alcohol. Some sedatives, such as benzodiazepines, may have a delayed withdrawal effect, beginning several days after the person stops taking the drug. If individuals have become sedative dependent on lower doses of the drug, withdrawal symptoms may consist of only irritability, sleep disturbance, and generalized anxiety. If, however, individuals became dependent on higher doses, withdrawal can be life-threatening (Tinsley, 2007). Sudden withdrawal, especially in the face of barbiturate dependence, can result in acute psychosis, seizures, and death.

Therapeutic withdrawal from a sedative, like therapeutic withdrawal from alcohol, usually involves administration of a cross-tolerant drug to suppress withdrawal symptoms with gradual tapering of the dosage. The drug being withdrawn determines the length of time required for tapering. For some sedatives 7 to 10 days is sufficient for detoxification. Longer-acting drugs that have been used at high dosages may require 14 or more days for detoxification.

Opioids

Because *opioids* (narcotic drugs such as morphine, meperidine [Demerol], hydromorphone [Dilaudid], oxycodone [OxyContin], and codeine) are frequently prescribed for pain, addiction can occur through regular prescription use. In other instances, these medications are obtained illegally. One commonly used illegal opioid is heroin.

In addition to delivering pain relief, narcotics produce euphoria, sedation, and a feeling of tranquility. At first, individuals may take illegal narcotics primarily for the feeling of euphoria. Repeated administration rapidly produces tolerance and intense physical dependence. Eventually, as the dosage and/or frequency of drug administration increases, individuals need to continue to take the drug regularly to avoid manifestations of withdrawal.

Numerous negative health consequences are related to opiate use, and especially long-term use of heroin (Gonzalez, Oliveto, & Kosten, 2002; Fiellin & O'Connor, 2002), including lethal respiratory depression with overdose. Drugs that are injected increase individuals' risk of contracting HIV infection or hepatitis C, if needles are shared (Cunningham, Sohler, Berg, Shapiro, & Heller, 2006). Addition of adulterants to substances or use of nonsterile techniques of injection may also produce medical complications (Ponton & Scott, 2004). Skin abscesses, **cellulitis** (inflammation of tissues), **thrombophlebitis** (inflammation of a vein with associated clot formation), **septicemia** (presence of toxins in the blood), and bacterial **endocarditis** (inflammation of the inner lining of the heart) are all potential complications.

Withdrawal symptoms vary in severity and duration, depending on the particular drug abused. Withdrawal from narcotics is generally not life-threatening. Many manifestations of withdrawal are flu-like, although manifestations may also include anxiety, irritability, and restlessness.

Opiate substitution drugs are sometimes used in treatment of opiate addiction and may be used for either detoxification or maintenance. *Methadone*, an opiate, and Clonidine (Catapres), a non-opiate, may be used during the detoxification process to help block withdrawal symptoms. When used for detoxification, the drug dosage is gradually tapered during the withdrawal period.

Methadone maintenance is a mainstay of treatment to reduce use of illicit opiates and high-risk behaviors associated with such drug use

(Fudala et al., 2003; O'Connor, 2000). It is provided only in a strictly regulated environment in which the medication is taken under clinical observation and supervision (Clark, 2003). Methadone maintenance has been found to be effective in decreasing risk of HIV and hepatitis acquired through needle sharing, reducing criminal activity associated with drug-seeking behavior, and helping individuals return to a socially rehabilitated state (Tinsley, 2007).

Buprenorphine is a new product that has been recently approved for opiate addiction. Although the extent of its effectiveness in treating opiate addiction is not known at this time, one potential advantage of buprenorphine is that it can be prescribed by office-based clinicians (Brown, 2007; Mintzer, Eisenberg, Terra, MacVane, Himmmelstein, & Woolhandler, 2007; Moore et al., 2007; Donaher & Welsh, 2006).

Cocaine and Other Stimulants

Acting directly on the central nervous system, *stimulants* create an increased state of arousal and concentration, and speed up mental and motor activity. Individuals may take stimulants for such effects as increased alertness, increased sense of well-being, increased confidence, reduction of fatigue, or decrease in appetite. Amphetamines (e.g., Benzedrine or Dexedrine), methylphenidate (Ritalin), cocaine, and caffeine are all stimulants. In addition to exerting their central nervous system effects, stimulants have generalized systemic effects, including an increase in heart rate, an increase in blood pressure, a rise in body temperature, and the constriction of peripheral blood vessels (Sarnyai, Shaham, & Heinrichs, 2001).

Cocaine is a highly addictive neurostimulant (Pilon & Scheiffle, 2006; Chan, Camprodon, Kane, & Scott-Coombes, 2004). Although it has been used medically as a local anesthetic (especially for ear, nose, and throat procedures), cocaine also is a drug of wide abuse and an important public health hazard (Leikin, 2007). As with other stimulants, its physical effects may include elevated heart rate, elevated blood pressure (Tinsley, 2007), and increased respiratory rate (Kloner & Rezkalla, 2003). Immediate effects of cocaine produce subjective feelings of increased alertness and energy, enhanced confidence, and enhanced physical and mental ability (Ruiz et al., 2007).

In recent years, cocaine has become one of the most widely abused stimulants in the United States (Leikin, 2007). It may be taken orally, used intranasally (snorted), smoked, or injected intravenously. The technique of *free-basing* cocaine, which gained popularity in the 1980s, involves heating a flammable solvent such as petroleum or ether, and then using it to heat the cocaine. This process "frees" cocaine hydrochloride from its salts and adulterants, converting it to a form of cocaine that will vaporize. The free-base cocaine can then be inhaled or smoked, usually with a water pipe, for direct absorption through the alveoli in the lungs. The technique rapidly delivers high concentrations of cocaine to the brain and results in blood levels as high as those achieved with injection.

The free-basing technique can cause additional disability due to burns from fires started during the free-basing process. Because of the concerns regarding the dangers of combustion and injury in free-basing, *crack cocaine* has become increasingly popular.

Crack, a solid form of free-base cocaine is an alkaloid form of cocaine obtained by "cooking" cocaine hydrochloride with bicarbonate of soda (Baldwin et al., 2002). Dependence occurs very rapidly with this form of the drug. Crack is smoked rather than sniffed. Its concentrated form and its route of administration make its potency many times greater than that of cocaine alone. The euphoric effect produced by crack lasts only a matter of minutes, however. To achieve the same euphoria, users may engage in repeated use or binge on large quantities followed by periods of non-use (Henskens, Mulder, Garretsen, Bongers, & Sturmans, 2005; Hope, Hickman, & Tilling, 2005). Crack cocaine can also be injected, and it is frequently injected in combination with other drugs such as heroin. Crack cocaine is associated with a number of criminal and health-related problems (Holloway, Bennett, & Lower, 2004), and crack cocaine injections are associated with increased risk of transmitting HIV and hepatitis C (Judd et al., 2005).

Individuals using cocaine, especially at higher dosages, may use depressant drugs in an attempt to counterbalance the former substance's stimulant effects. For example, alcohol and cocaine are commonly combined for this purpose. The simultaneous injection of cocaine and heroin (*speedballing*) is another combination used by some individuals.

Aside from its psychological, social, and vocational consequences, cocaine use can have serious medical consequences. Free-basing or smoking crack cocaine can lead to pulmonary complications, including hemorrhage in the lungs (Baldwin et al., 2002). Chronic use of intranasal cocaine may cause ulceration or perforation of the nasal septum. Cocaine intoxication can produce neurological effects, such as confusion, anxiety, hyperexcitability, agitation, and violence.

More serious effects are the result of acute *cocaine toxicity*, which is dose related, in which individuals can experience stroke or seizures, severe **hyperthermia** (increased body temperature), **arrhythmia** (irregular heartbeat) (Hsue et al., 2007), **myocardial infarction** (heart attack), and, in some instances, sudden death. Another side effect of excessive cocaine use, *cocaine psychosis*, is manifested as paranoia, panic, hallucinations, insomnia, and picking at the skin. The psychotic episode can last from 24 to 36 hours. Individuals with this condition are usually hospitalized and treated with antipsychotic medication.

The substances sometimes added to adulterate cocaine to increase its weight, thereby increasing profit on its sale, may cause additional medical complications. Problems can result from the nature of the substance used to mix with the cocaine or from the dosage taken. Adulterants such as talc or cornstarch can cause complications ranging from inflammation to **embolus** (matter traveling in the blood) (Low, Jenkins, & Prendergast, 2006).

Adverse behavioral effects are also common with cocaine use. For example, a high prevalence of anger, impulsivity, and violence is associated with cocaine addiction (Goldstein et al., 2005), and chronic use can result in paranoid psychosis (Floyd, Boutros, Struve, Wolf, & Oliwa, 2006; Camí & Farré, 2003).

Procaine, PCP, or heroin, which also may be added to cocaine, may potentiate the drug's effects. Because the user can never be certain of the cocaine's potency, however, the effects are not always predictable. The withdrawal syndrome from cocaine consists of a craving for more cocaine, depression, irritability, sleep disturbances, gastrointestinal disturbances, headaches, and, possibly, suicidal ideation. Because it is not unusual for individuals who are cocaine dependent to be dependent on other drugs as well, a withdrawal reaction from other substances may also be experienced.

Amphetamines are used in medical settings to treat conditions such as attention-deficit disorders. The potential for abuse of these prescribed drugs is continually present. A newer street drug classified as an amphetamine is *crystalline methamphetamine (ice)*, which is highly addictive, both physically and psychologically (Lukas, 1997). Like crack, ice can be heated and inhaled in a technique similar to that used when smoking free-base cocaine. Ice has greater strength and longer duration of effects, lasting from 8 to 24 hours. Methamphetamine increases energy and alertness and decreases appetite. Its greater stimulation of the brain makes it more dangerous mentally,

creating craving that can continue for years after cessation of use (Wermuth, 2000). Toxic levels can produce severe paranoid thinking with hallucinations. There is also greater risk of suicidal depression. Chronic use of methamphetamine in any form can result in serious psychiatric, cardiovascular, metabolic, and neuromuscular changes. Side effects include shaking, seizures, *cardiac arrhythmias* (irregular heartbeat), and hyperthermia (elevated body temperature). Long-term use can lead to a feeling that skin is "crawling," anxiety, and insomnia, as well as addiction (Leikin, 2007).

Management of stimulant abuse, and crack/cocaine abuse in particular, involves management of the manifestations, rather than alternative prescribing options such as those available for opiate abuse. Antidepressants are sometime prescribed if the person has manifestations of depression, and sedatives such as benzodiazepines are sometimes prescribed for manifestations of agitation and insomnia. Because of their potential for addiction, these medications are used sparingly and for short periods of time (Harniman, 2006).

Psychosocial interventions include counseling such as motivational interviewing, cognitive-behavioral therapy, and group and family counseling. Other psychosocial interventions such as stress management skills training and support groups are beneficial as well.

Cannabis

When *cannabis* (*marijuana*) is smoked, the psychoactive compound (THC) that it contains produces euphoria, relaxation, dream-like states, and sleepiness. It can also impair cognitive function and performance of psychomotor tasks (Camí & Farré, 2003). Some individuals report enhanced perceptions of colors, tastes, and textures.

The use of marijuana for medicinal purposes remains controversial, although it has been reported to reduce pain, spasms, nausea, and a variety of other symptoms in a number of medical conditions, including multiple sclerosis (Page & Verhoef, 2006).

The psychoactive response to the drug depends to a great extent on the dose, the personality and experience of the user, and the environment in which the drug is used. Often, users report a sense of the slowing of time and impairment in their ability to learn new facts while they are under the influence of this drug.

Overdose can produce anxiety, panic states, and psychosis (Hall & Solowij, 1998). On a systemic level, cannabis produces an increase in heart rate, dilation of the bronchioles, and dilation of the peripheral blood vessels. Because of its stimulatory effect on the heart, cannabis use may also lead to cardiac complications in individuals with heart disease (Fisher, Ghuran, Vadamalai, & Antonios, 2005).

Chronic smoking of cannabis produces inflammatory changes in the lungs that contribute to the development of chronic conditions such as emphysema (see Chapter 14). Furthermore, the use of other drugs, including alcohol and tobacco, may compound the adverse effects of cannabis. For example, the combination of tobacco and cannabis use is thought to increase the risk of development of lung cancer. Chronic marijuana use on its own or in association with other drugs may also cause alterations in liver enzymes (Borini, Guimaraes, & Borini, 2004)

Although cannabis is usually smoked, it may be ingested orally. Oral consumption can delay its effects for up to an hour, and the effects are less potent. *Hashish*, the concentrated form of THC, is also smoked and has considerably higher potency than cannabis.

Some individuals use cannabis only on special occasions, but others become compulsively preoccupied with its daily use. The long-term effects of cannabis use remain controversial. The degree to which cannabis creates physical dependence has not been established; however, it is possible to develop psychological dependence (Hall & Solowij, 1998). Symptoms of withdrawal including restlessness, irritability, and insomnia have been noted in heavy users (Budney, Hughes, Moore, & Novy, 2001).

There is no specific medical treatment for cannabis abuse. When cannabis use severely hampers individuals' functioning, treatment most often involves psychotherapeutic techniques directed at underlying problems. Because cannabis may be abused in combination with other drugs, management may be multifocal in nature.

Hallucinogens

Sometimes called *psychedelics, hallucinogens* are drugs that, at some dosage, produce hallucinations or distortions in perceptions or thinking. Individuals under the influence of hallucinogens report increased awareness of sensory input and a subjective feeling of enhanced mental activity. Common hallucinogens are LSD, psilocybin, PCP (angel dust), and mescaline.

Substance analogues, or *designer drugs,* can have dangerous, permanent effects. Users of one class of these drugs, the methamphetamines, which include MDMA (ecstasy) and MDEA (Eve), may be especially susceptible to permanent brain damage because the amount that produces psychological effects is not far from the dosage that produces neural damage (Liechti, Kuntz, & Kupferschmidt, 2005). The designer drug MPPP is associated with a parkinsonian syndrome (see Chapter 4) in some individuals. Designer derivatives of amphetamines produce euphoria, but can also have hallucinogenic effects, and may cause cardiac arrhythmias (irregular heartbeat), *cerebral hemorrhage* (stroke), hyperthermia (elevated body temperature), altered mental status, panic, and psychosis. Individuals with PCP intoxication are especially prone to agitation and violence (Leiken, 2007).

Hallucinogens are usually taken orally. Although the use of these substances has declined somewhat in recent years, patterns of their use vary widely. Their use is now often concurrent with the use of other drugs. One of the most powerful hallucinogens is *LSD* (*lysergic acid diethylamide*). Its effects vary with the individual, the dose, and the environment in which the drug is used. Generally, the effects develop within several hours and last as long as 12 hours. Individuals may report heightened sensitivity and clarity, increased insights, a sense of time moving more slowly, and distortions of visual images. Some individuals experience adverse effects from LSD, such as a panic state with severe anxiety.

The physical consequences of abuse of most hallucinogens in and of themselves are not significant. The psychological consequences, however, can be severe. Adverse effects of hallucinogens vary from acute psychosis to self-mutilation or suicide. Accidents can result from misjudgment or impairment. Some individuals experience "flashbacks" in which hallucinations reappear briefly even months after the last drug dose. An overdose of hallucinogens can result in exceedingly high body temperatures, seizures, and shock.

Because hallucinogens produce no physical dependence, no specific medical regimen for treatment exists. Adverse effects such as panic episodes are usually treated with a supportive environment and observation.

Inhalants

Substances that cause perceptible changes in brain function when they are administered through inhalation are called *inhalants*. Inhalants are generally classified into four categories:

- Aerosols
- Gases
- Solvents
- Nitrites (Ballard, 1998)

A wide variety of substances are abused in this way, often because they are readily accessible and inexpensive. For example, commonly used inhalants include airplane glue, typewriter correction fluid, marking pencils, industrial and household chemicals, paint thinners, gasoline, nitrites (poppers, snappers, or rush), and nitrous oxide. Although individuals of all age groups practice inhalant abuse, it is especially prevalent among adolescents and preadolescents (Leikin, 2007).

Although the effects of inhalants are brief, they can be serious, especially with prolonged or long-term use. Adverse effects of inhalants vary according to the type of substance inhaled. Organic solvents such as airplane glue can produce cardiac arrhythmia, bone marrow depression, damage to the kidney and liver, and, in some instances, death.

Prolonged use of *nitrites* is thought to suppress the immune system, thereby increasing the individual's susceptibility to infection. Nitrites are frequently used to enhance sexual pleasure; consequently, individuals who use nitrites in this way and engage in unsafe sex practices may be at greater risk for developing HIV infection owing to the suppression of the immune system and subsequent increased vulnerability to infection.

Chronic abuse of *nitrous oxide* can result in nerve damage, seizures, bone marrow changes, respiratory depression, or death. Because nitrous oxide distorts the senses, driving during intoxication with this substance is hazardous. Even though the effects of inhalants are brief, their use can result in dependence. No specific medical treatment is usually indicated for inhalant abuse, although specific psychotherapeutic measures may be used to prevent relapse and to help individuals discontinue inhalant use.

OxyContin

Although addiction is often assumed to be associated with illicit or illegal drugs, a growing number of people have become addicted to legal or prescription drugs (Smith, 2005). OxyContin (oxycodone) is one medication that is prescribed for pain control, but it has become increasingly more popular as a drug of abuse and addiction. Its popularity is, in part, due to its availability; it also provides an instant euphoria and is cheaper than drugs such as heroin. The medication is taken orally for prescription purposes, but those individuals using the drug for illicit reasons tend to crush it and then swallow or snort the powder, or inject the drug after it has been dissolved in water.

■ MEDICAL CONSEQUENCES OF SUBSTANCE ABUSE AND DEPENDENCE

Not only does substance abuse cause psychological, social, and vocational impairments, but it can also lead to criminal activity as users try to obtain drugs or get money to buy additional drugs. Substance abuse also has serious medical consequences.

Dermatologic Complications

Many of the medical complications related to drug abuse result from nonsterile injections or from adulterants, rather than from the drug itself.

Abscess

Bacterial infection may cause pus to collect in the tissues, forming an abscess. In association with drug use, improper cleansing of the skin before injection or the use of a nonsterile needle may lead to an abscess. In this situation, skin at the site becomes warm, red, swollen, and painful with a **purulent** (pus) discharge. Skin around the area frequently becomes **necrotic** (dies). If the abscess goes untreated, individuals may develop systemic symptoms

of fever, loss of appetite, and fatigue. Infection may spread to the bloodstream, creating a generalized systemic infection (**bacteremia**).

Treatment of an abscess consists of draining the purulent material and **debriding** (removing) the area of dead tissue. Antibiotics are usually prescribed, especially if individuals demonstrate systemic symptoms.

Cellulitis

An acute inflammation of the tissues without **necrosis** (tissue death) is called cellulitis. When associated with intravenous drug abuse, cellulitis is caused by the invasion of a variety of organisms or by irritation of the tissues from the drug itself. The tissue becomes red and tender, and **adenopathy** (swelling of lymph nodes) may occur.

Treatment of cellulitis depends on the cause. Occasionally, cellulitis progresses to abscess formation.

Other Dermatologic Complications

Injections with nonsterile needles or injections of drugs that have been contaminated by adulterants may leave needle track scars. Injections cause a mild inflammatory reaction and, with subsequent injections, produce scarring at the injection site. Injection of a drug into an artery instead of a vein can cause an extreme reaction of intense pain, swelling, and coldness of an extremity. If this condition is not treated properly, gangrene may develop, necessitating amputation.

Cardiovascular Complications

Other than direct effects on the heart from the drug itself, most cardiovascular complications that result from drug use are related to the use of nonsterile injection techniques or to contamination of the drug with adulterants. One potential complication is **endocarditis** (inflammation of the inner lining of the heart), which affects the valves of the heart and can have potentially serious consequences (see Chapter 13).

Some drugs have a direct toxic effect on the heart muscle or directly affect heart rhythm. In some instances, inflammation of the veins with clot formation (thrombophlebitis) may occur because of the toxic effects of the drug.

Pulmonary Complications

The intravenous injection of drugs to which adulterants such as talc, starch, or baking soda has been added may result in pulmonary complications. Because these "filler" substances do not dissolve, they circulate in the blood and may become lodged in lung tissue. The lodged particles cause an inflammatory reaction in the lungs, resulting in **fibrosis** of the lung tissue. If the fibrous changes are extensive, they may affect the oxygen-exchanging ability of the lungs. Symptoms similar to those of emphysema may develop. Changes in lung elasticity can eventually result in pulmonary hypertension and subsequent heart failure. (See Chapter 14 for a discussion of the manifestations of emphysema and Chapter 13 for a discussion of pulmonary hypertension and heart failure.)

Lung infections or lung abscesses may occur if infectious organisms become localized in the lungs after the nonsterile injection of a substance. *Aspiration pneumonia,* an inflammation of the lungs, may result from the inhalation of foreign substances or chemical irritants. Aspiration of gastric contents is also a common cause of aspiration pneumonia. Individuals who become unconscious because of a drug overdose may, in their unconscious state, vomit and subsequently inhale the vomitus. If they inhale a large quantity, the results can be fatal.

Individuals, who abuse drugs, including alcohol, may also develop *tuberculosis* (see Chapter 14). Rather than being a direct result of drug use, tuberculosis is more likely to be the consequence of the general lifestyle and living conditions of individuals who abuse drugs. Malnourishment, poor hygiene, and overcrowding all contribute to development of this infectious disease. In addition, because some drugs have an immunosuppressant effect, individuals may be more susceptible to the infection. An overdose of narcotics or sedative/hypnotics can severely depress the respiratory center, causing cessation of breathing and consequent death. Overdoses of narcotics have also been associated with development of severe **pulmonary edema** (collection of fluid in the lungs), which, without treatment, can result in death.

Gastrointestinal Complications

Because the liver acts as the detoxification center for the body, individuals who chronically abuse drugs may damage this organ. Some substances appear to be more directly harmful to the liver than others. Chronic, excessive abuse of solvents, for example, can cause liver **necrosis** (tissue death). Other substances may cause liver abnormalities such as inflammation or fibrosis.

Hepatitis is a common complication of drug abuse. *Hepatitis A* may be related to poor hygiene habits and poor environmental conditions. More commonly, *hepatitis B* (*serum hepatitis*) occurs as the result of nonsterile or contaminated intravenous injections. (See Chapter 12 for a discussion of hepatitis A and hepatitis B.)

Hepatitis C is caused by infection with the hepatitis C virus (HCV). HCV causes what was previously called *non-A, non-B hepatitis* and is transmitted through infected blood. Consequently, individuals who use intravenous drugs and share needles are at high risk for developing this disease. Hepatitis C generally becomes a chronic disease and can predispose the individual to development of cirrhosis (Ginés et al., 2004). The only treatment currently used for hepatitis C consists of injections of interferon and ribavirin; even with treatment, approximately half of all patients will experience a relapse.

Neurological Complications

Seizures may result from an overdose of drugs or a hypersensitivity to adulterants. They are especially prevalent after an overdose of amphetamines or cocaine. In some instances, stroke may also accompany an overdose. Toxic effects of adulterants on the nervous system can lead to blindness and peripheral nerve damage.

Other Complications

The chronic use of some drugs may result in **nystagmus** (involuntary eye movement). Use of solvents can produce bone marrow changes and aplastic anemia (see Chapter 10). An overdose of drugs can result in acute renal failure, which can progress to permanent kidney damage (see Chapter 15). Individuals who abuse drugs also have a higher incidence of venereal disease, such as gonorrhea, syphilis, and chlamydia related to their general lifestyle and sexual practices. One of the most serious and hazardous complications of drug use is infection with HIV (see Chapter 10), a risk that is related to both intravenous drug use and unsafe sexual practices. Heavy use of some drugs, such as ecstasy, has been shown to induce vulnerability for cognitive disorders, and in some cases affective and anxiety disorders that may persist for more than five months after cessation of the drug's use (Thomasius, Petersen, Zapletalova, Wartberg, Zeichner, & Schmoldt, 2005).

Drug abuse during pregnancy has serious implications for the offspring. Some fetal hazards are related to lifestyle of the drug-abusing mother, which tends to result in poor prenatal care, poor nutrition, and a generally poor health status. The direct toxic effects of drugs on the developing fetus (tetratogenic effects) can include neurological and/or physical abnormalities, as well as pose dangers related to withdrawal syndrome to the infant after birth.

■ DIAGNOSTIC PROCEDURES

Diagnosis of a substance use disorder is often delayed or symptoms overlooked, contributing to the disorder's continued disabling effects, development of medical complications, and progression of dependence. Denial and resistance to acknowledging the problem are universal manifestations of substance abuse/dependence. Consequently, even if family members or associates have identified a substance use problem, the individual who abuses substances may not acknowledge the condition and refuse to seek treatment.

Conditions related to substance use are frequently associated with health and personal concerns. Consequently, many individuals presenting at health or counseling facilities may have coexisting or secondary substance use problems that have not been identified or diagnosed. Some professionals may feel uncomfortable questioning or confronting individuals about substance use disorders, so that diagnosis or management of the problem is further delayed. Undetected substance use problems have significant effects on the health and well-being of individuals as well as the health and well-being of their family and others.

Screening Instruments

Routine screening of individuals presenting for health care or counseling helps professionals determine whether a problem exists and whether a more in-depth assessment is needed. Several types of screening instruments are available for this purpose. One of the best-known and widely used instruments is *CAGE*. Others include *MAST (Michigan Alcoholism Screening Test)*, *T-ACE*, TWEAK, Alcohol Use Disorders Identification Test (AUDIT), *Substance Abuse Life Circumstances Evaluation (SALCE)*, *MacAndrew Scale (MAC)* and *MacAndrew Scale—Revised (MAC-R)*, and the *Substance Abuse Subtle Screening Inventory (SASSI)* (Piazza, Martin, & Dildine, 2000). Each screening test has its own benefits and limitations. The type of screening test used should be based on the circumstances under which the test is used as well as on specific factors related to the individual.

Direct Drug Screening

Direct testing for the presence of the substance in the body may involve *breath analyzers* and *blood alcohol tests*. Both tests serve as a measurement of intoxication, but they do not reveal the extent of abuse or dependence. Screening of blood or urine samples is also used to verify suspected substance use. As with any laboratory test, there is a possibility of false-negative or false-positive results. Newer screening methods are designed to be more sensitive and produce more accurate results.

Drug testing results are valid only if the testing is accomplished under strictly controlled conditions. Many individuals who abuse or are dependent on drugs are aware of a variety of methods to invalidate test results, such as substituting a specimen from a drug-free individual for their own specimen. The appropriate methods and times of drug screening are highly controversial. Routine screening for drugs without the individual's knowledge and consent evokes a variety of legal and ethical concerns.

Medical Evaluation

Medical diagnosis of substance use may rely on information obtained from several sources. Physical manifestations of substance abuse/dependence may include a variety of conditions. Questions about substance use practices should be routinely asked in the examination of individuals with gastrointestinal disturbances, hypertension or heart disease, liver disease, neurological changes, or a history of traumatic injuries. Blood cell abnormalities, such as a decreased number of platelets or signs of bone marrow depression (see Chapter 10), or other indirect clinical laboratory signs, such as elevated levels of *gamma-glutamyltransferase (GGT)*, *gamma-glutamyltranspeptidase (GGTP)*, and elevated *red blood cell mean corpuscular volume (MCV)* may suggest problems with substance abuse. Elevated levels of enzymes such as *serum glutamic oxaloacetic transaminase* and (SGOT) *serum glutamic pyruvic transaminase* (SGPT) may also be associated with substance abuse, although increased concentrations of SGOT and SGPT can be associated with other conditions (e.g., myocardial infarction) as well.

Behavioral and Psychological Screening

Investigation of subtle psychological or behavioral symptoms is also important in diagnosis of a substance use disorder. Depression, hyperactivity, sleeps disturbances, anxiety, sexual problems, or personality changes are common manifestations of substance use disorders. In addition, the incidence of accidents and injury is often increased.

■ MANAGEMENT OF SUBSTANCE USE DISORDERS

The first step in the management of a substance-related disorder is the identification and acknowledgment of the problem. Screening may be hampered by several barriers:

- Denial of the problem by the individual or family members
- Reluctance of medical and mental health personnel to confront or discuss the problem

Once the problem is identified and confronted, individuals should be assessed for the medical and psychosocial problems that typically accompany it and the level of the individual's motivation for change determined (O'Connor, 2000). Successful intervention for substance use disorders generally requires more than one level of care during the long recovery process. Specifically, intervention may involve outpatient or inpatient care along with continued outpatient care. Most individuals receiving intervention for substance use consider themselves as "recovering," denoting the long-term, chronic nature of the recovery process. Relapse is a common part of recovery. Rather than being thought of as failure, it can be viewed as an opportunity for learning and growth (American Academy of Pediatrics, 2000).

Many individuals with substance-related conditions eventually experience physical, social, or psychological crises that require inpatient or residential treatment. The precise treatment received varies greatly from facility to facility and depends on the particular type of crisis experienced. Some facilities provide treatment for substance use disorders solely on an outpatient basis. Others provide a combination of inpatient or residential and outpatient intervention.

Management usually begins with detoxification, which may or may not involve inpatient or residential intervention, depending on the individual, the specific substance of abuse, and the presence of additional complications. Detoxification is merely the initial step in the management of substance use disorders, however. Ongoing therapy that includes a variety of rehabilitation strategies, such as psychotherapy, family therapy, and self-help programs (e.g., *Alcoholics Anonymous* or *Narcotics Anonymous*), is often necessary to prevent relapse. Several psychotherapeutic approaches to the management of substance abuse exist. The specific type of therapy used often depends on the facility in which the individual is being treated and the overall philosophy of the professionals conducting the intervention. In almost all instances, however, abstinence is a management goal.

In some instances, drugs are prescribed in the ongoing management of substance dependence. Antabuse and methadone (or another opiate substitute), which were discussed earlier, are drugs commonly used in the management of alcohol dependence and opiate dependence, respectively.

Individuals with a substance use disorder may also require ongoing medical intervention for any medical complications that have resulted from the substance use. Because nutritional deficiencies frequently accompany substance use disorders, most detoxification centers and residential facilities provide nutrition therapy as a part of the management plan. Educational programs that stress the importance of nutrition and other aspects of a healthy lifestyle are often incorporated into the general management program.

■ PSYCHOSOCIAL AND VOCATIONAL ISSUES IN SUBSTANCE ABUSE AND DEPENDANCE

Psychosocial Issues

The extent to which psychological disability is the direct *result* of a substance-related disorder versus the *cause* of the disorder is not easily determined. Individuals with substance use disorders frequently have low self-esteem and experience depression. They may have feelings of inadequacy, loneliness, and isolation that lead to increased substance use. Individuals, when influenced and controlled by the substance used, may rely on it rather than on their own resources. They may doubt that they have the ability to cope without the substance. Consequently, their self-confidence and self-esteem may be eroded even more.

Individuals who are psychologically dependent on a substance feel a need and longing for the substance and become irritable, depressed, anxious, and resentful when the substance is not available. Individuals with a psychological craving for a substance may attribute their need to a personal flaw in their character or may consider their need to be a negative reflection on themselves. Either interpretation further contributes to lowered self-esteem and self-deprecation.

Individuals may use denial or rationalization as a form of self-protection and as a way to minimize substance use problems. They may deny that a substance use problem exists, or they may rationalize their behavior by redefining their substance use so that it appears to be acceptable. Some individuals become aggressive or perform violent acts when they are under the influence of certain substances. Those who are predisposed to this type of reaction may become involved in criminal acts, such as brawls, homicide, rape, or child abuse.

As individuals become increasingly dependent on the substance, the concept of living without it produces fear and dread. Individuals interpret removal of the substance as removal of all joy and excitement from life. As with all types of perceived loss, individuals may experience grief and bereavement.

Recovery from a substance use disorder involves restoration of self-esteem and confidence, and it requires a willingness to accept responsibility for one's personal behavior. Individuals need assistance to accept losses that they have experienced and to develop skills for coping in the future. Recovery is a continuing process that incorporates long-term vigilance and a continuing commitment to remain drug-free.

A substance-related condition affects every aspect of an individual's daily life. As dependence on the substance becomes more pronounced; individuals may lose interest in self-care, show a decreased desire for food,

and experience a variety of sleep disturbances, resulting in sleep deprivation. Daily activities may become focused on obtaining more of the substance. Activities once enjoyed may offer little joy or inspire little interest.

Substance use can also affect individuals' ability to drive a motor vehicle. Poor driving performance can result in accidents or arrests, which can in turn lead to the loss of the person's driver's license. Therefore, transportation may become a problem if individuals must depend on others for their transportation needs.

Sexual dysfunction is common in individuals with substance use disorders. Women may experience decreased libido or become promiscuous. Men may experience not only decreased libido, but also adverse effects on sexual performance, including impotence—a common side effect of chronic alcohol abuse. Individuals recovering from a substance use disorder may need to learn or relearn components of a healthy lifestyle such as self-care, including hygiene and grooming, proper diet, and the importance of exercise. These aspects of daily living may be a vital part of an individual's rehabilitation.

Social effects of substance-related disorders are widespread, touching family relationships, relationships with friends and associates, and general functioning as a member of society. Individuals' ability to function as a member of a social group may gradually deteriorate as substance use increases. To some extent, social factors may determine the social implications of substance use. For example, the availability of substances within a group or as part of a social event may determine whether individuals with a condition related to substance use participate in the activity.

The extent of social tolerance of individuals' behavior while intoxicated may either curtail or enhance substance use at first. As individuals become increasingly dependent on the substance, however, the substance takes on an increasing importance. Conversely, the importance assigned to individuals' social contacts and activities declines.

Individuals with a substance-related condition may be unable to function within their social network. Repeated, heavy use of the substance often leads to upheavals in relationships. Social and family relationships are strained and often destroyed if individuals become abusive, or violent, or if they engage in socially unacceptable behavior while under the influence of the substance. Individuals' behavior often alienates others, leading to social isolation. Decreasing reliability in performance of social roles and inability to maintain commitments cause those affected by the individual's deterioration in behavior to feel disappointed and angry. Others in the social environment may have to alter their own roles to assume duties that the individual once fulfilled. This shifting of responsibilities places additional burdens on all concerned and may eventually lead to resentment or even banishment of the individual from the group. Family members and associates may begin to withdraw from the individual emotionally. As individuals become increasingly more isolated, feelings of self-loathing, guilt, and shame may develop. Feeling rejected by family and associates, individuals may limit their social contacts to relationships with others who also engage in substance use.

The broader social consequences of substance-related conditions may have legal and even criminal implications. As mentioned earlier, there is a strong correlation between substance use disorders and a variety of accidents rates. Motor vehicle accidents, for example, can lead to physical disability not only for the individual with the substance use disorder, but also for others. Thus the loss of a driver's license and the threat of more serious criminal charges are potential outcomes of substance use disorders. Furthermore, individuals who become dependent on illegal substances may engage in illegal activities to obtain money with which to purchase additional drugs. Even if individuals do not face criminal charges, they can become overly focused on obtaining the drug rather than on functioning in a productive social role.

In some cases, family and social relationships can be salvaged in the recovery process. In other instances, loss of these relationships is permanent. Depending on individual circumstances, therapeutic recovery may involve the development of new social roles and relationships or the reestablishment of old ones.

Vocational Issues

In the early stages of a substance-related condition, individuals may be concerned that the use of the substance will interfere with their work. If substance uses progresses to abuse or dependence, however, concern may be reversed such that individuals become more concerned that their work will interfere with their use of the substance. The substance assumes a penultimate role in the person's life, drastically affecting his or her work performance.

Although early identification of and intervention with workers with a substance use disorder are most desirable, the problem may not be recognized until a progressive deterioration of work performance, increased absenteeism, or an increase in job-related accidents occurs. Fear that they will lose their jobs if their employers become aware of these indicators may motivate individuals with a substance use disorder to seek treatment.

The ability of individuals to return to their former employment after intervention for a substance use disorder depends on the circumstances. In some instances, the stress and tension associated with the job may be beyond individuals' stress tolerance and coping ability. It may be beneficial to find a less stressful work setting, especially in the early stages of recovery, until the individual's tolerance for stress gradually increases. Physical disability resulting from a substance use disorder must also be considered when evaluating vocational potential.

It is essential to identify past work problems, which may extend beyond issues of substance abuse/dependence. Some individuals may need to learn social skills, work-appropriate behaviors, or good hygiene or grooming practices; some need to improve their work skills. Individuals who began abusing substances at an early age may not have developed sufficient work skills or work history to obtain employment. These individuals in particular may require additional education or job training. If individuals return to the same work setting that originally precipitated feelings of inadequacy, which in turn contributed to development of substance abuse/dependence, the return to work may increase the risk of relapse. In some cases, learning new skills or coping strategies may enable individuals to return successfully to the same work setting. In other instances, however, a new work environment may be necessary.

Loss of a driver's license because of a substance-related condition may make transportation to and from work more difficult. In addition, if driving a motor vehicle had been part of the former employment, job restructuring or job change may be necessary. Some occupations require professional licensure, therefore, revocation of an individual's license as a result of a substance use disorder may limit his or her ability to work in that occupation. Many professional licensing boards have provisions for the reinstatement of licensure after documented rehabilitation. If the professional license is reinstated, there may be a probationary period in which the individual's work performance is closely observed and monitored.

Conviction on criminal charges—especially felony charges—may disqualify individuals from employment in some occupations.

Although decisions may be made on a case-by-case basis, such charges and their impact on employment in different fields and in different locations must be considered. As with most disabilities, the attitudes and concerns of employers must be addressed, especially given the social stigma that is often attached to substance use disorders. Employers may require particular encouragement to reinstate or hire individuals who have been convicted of criminal charges. Recognizing the potential for rejection by employers based on these attitudes, recovering individuals may be reluctant to share their complete history with employers or may become defensive when asked questions about substance use. Fear of rejection because of prejudice must be considered when the individual returns to work. With increasing awareness of substance use disorders, and with educational efforts directed toward employers, however, individuals may encounter decreasing levels of prejudice.

Many individuals who are recovering from substance use disorders return to their original employment and lead full productive lives. In all instances, however, abstinence is a prerequisite for continuing productivity. Ongoing long-term treatment or involvement with self-help groups may also be necessary to prevent relapse.

CASE STUDIES

Case 1

Mr. K. is a 42-year-old male with a high school education. He is a construction worker who has been a social drinker since his early twenties. His drinking has gradually intensified over the years, and family and friends have repeatedly confronted him about his drinking. On several occasions, Mr. K. was inebriated on the job, and his employer asked him not to return to work. He is divorced from his first wife, with whom he has two children, and is responsible for child support. His second wife of five years recently left him and is seeking a divorce. After being convicted on a DUI charge and being arrested for disorderly conduct, Mr. K. was referred to a residential treatment facility. He is now in outpatient treatment.

1. When working with Mr. K. to develop a rehabilitation plan, which significant factors would you consider about Mr. K.'s situation?
2. How will social factors influence Mr. K.'s effective rehabilitation?
3. Which additional information would you want to know about Mr. K. to work with him on his rehabilitation plan?
4. Which types of services might be effective for Mr. K.'s rehabilitation?

Case 2

Ms. B. is a 27-year-old schoolteacher who began using cocaine several years ago when she started dating her current boyfriend. Her use of the drug increased, and she has begun to use crack cocaine along with alcohol. Ms. B. was recently dismissed from her job when she was caught stealing money from her office mate's purse. She sought treatment and is currently in counseling. She is very concerned about her future with regard to work.

1. Which factors would you consider when working with Ms. B.?
2. Given Ms. B.'s education and past work history, which specific issues must you consider?
3. What specific information might you want to obtain when helping Ms. B. develop a rehabilitation plan?

■ REFERENCES

Abbott, F. V., & Fraser, M. I. (1998). Use and abuse of over-the-counter analgesic agents. *Journal of Psychiatry and Neuroscience, 23*(1), 13–34.

Addolorato, G., Leggio, L., Abenavoli, L., Agabio, R., Caputo, F., Capristo, E., et al. (2006). Baclofen in the treatment of alcohol withdrawal syndrome: A comparative study vs. diazepam. *American Journal of Medicine, 119*(3), 276.

Addolorato, G., Leggio, L., Agabio, R., Colombo, G., & Gasbarini, G. (2006). Baclofen: A new drug for the treatment of alcohol dependence. *International Journal of Clinical Practice, 60*(8), 1003–1008.

Adinoff, B. (2004). Neurobiologic processes in drug reward and addiction. *Harvard Review of Psychiatry, 12*(6), 305–320.

Agronin, M. E. (2007). Delirium. In: R. E. Rakel, & E. T. Bope (Eds.), *Conn's current therapy* (pp. 1294–1300). Philadelphia: W. B. Saunders.

Allen Doyle-Pita, D. (2001). Dual disorders in psychiatric rehabilitation: Teaching considerations. *Rehabilitation Education, 15*(2), 155–165.

American Academy of Pediatrics. (2000). Indications for management and referral of patients involved in substance abuse. *Pediatrics, 106*(1), 143.

American Psychiatric Association (2000). *Diagnostic and statistical manual of mental disorders* (4th ed., text revision). Washington, DC: Author.

Baldwin, G. C., Choi, R., Roth, M. D., Shay, A. H., Kleerup, E. C., Simmons, M. S., et al.(2002). Evidence of chronic damage to pulmonary microcirculation in habitual users of alkaloidal ("crack") cocaine. *Chest, 121*(4), 1231–1238.

Ballard, M. B. (1998). Inhalant abuse: A call for attention. *Journal of Addictions and Offender Counseling, 19,* 28–32.

Blume, S. B., Counts, S. J., & Turnbull, J. M. (1992, July 15). Women and substance abuse. *Patient Care,* 141–145; 148–151; 154–156.

Borini, P., Guimaraes, R. C., & Borini, S. B. (2004). Possible hepatotoxicity of chronic marijuana usage. *Sao Paulo Medical Journal, 122*(3), 110–116.

Brown, R. L. (2007). Psychiatric disorders. In R. E. Rakel & E. T. Bope (Eds.), *Conn's current therapy* (pp. 1273–1317). Philadelphia: W. B. Saunders.

Brown, R. A., Lejuez, C. W., Kahler, C. W., Strong, D. R., & Zvolensky, M. J. (2005). Distress tolerance and early smoking lapse. *Clinical Psychology Review, 25*(6), 713–733.

Budney, A. J., Hughes, J. R., Moore, B. A., & Novy, P. L. (2001). Marijuana abstinence effects in marijuana smokers maintained in their home environment. *Archives of General Psychiatry, 58,* 917–924.

Burling, T. A., Stitzer, M. L., Bigelow, G. E., & Mead, A. M. (1985). Smoking topography and carbon monoxide levels in smokers. *Addictive Behavior, 10,* 319–323.

Camí, J., & Farré, M. (2003). Drug addiction. *New England Journal of Medicine, 349*(10), 975–986.

Chan, Y. C., Camprodon, R. A., Kane, P. A., & Scott-Coombes, D. M. (2004). Abdominal complications from crack cocaine. *Annals of the Royal College of Surgeons of England, 87*(1), 72–73.

Chen, G. C., & Jutabha, R., (2007). Bleeding esophageal varices. In R. E. Rakel & E. T. Bope (Eds.), *Conn's current therapy* (pp. 587–593). Philadelphia: W. B. Saunders.

Cho, E., Smith-Warner, S. A., Ritz, J., van den Brandt, P. A., Colditz, G. A., Folsom, A. R., et al. (2004). Alcohol intake and colorectal cancer: A pooled analysis of 8 cohort studies. *Annals of Internal Medicine, 140*(8), 603–613.

Chou, T. (1992). Wake up and smell the coffee: Caffeine, coffee, and the medical consequences. *Western Journal of Medicine, 157,* 544–553.

Christen, A. G., & Christen, J. A. (1994). Why is cigarette smoking so addicting? An overview of smoking as a chemical and process addiction. *Health Values, 18*(1), 17–24.

Clark, H. W. (2003). Office-based practice and opioid use disorders. *New England Journal of Medicine, 349*(10), 928–930.

Cunningham, C. O., Sohler, N. L., Berg, K. M., Shapiro, S., & Heller, D. (2006). Type of substance use and access to HIV-related health care. *AIDS Patient Care and STDs, 20*(6), 399–407.

Donaher, P. A., & Welsh, C. (2006). Managing opioid addiction with buprenorphine. *American Family Physician, 73*(9), 1572–1580.

Fabricant, D. S., & Farnsworth, N. R. (2001). The value of plants used in traditional medicine for drug discovery. Environmental health perspectives. *Reviews in Environmental Health, 109*(1), 69–75.

Fairley, P. (1978). *The conquest of pain.* London: Michael Joseph.

Fiellin, D. A., & O'Connor, P. G. (2002). Office-based treatment of opioid-dependent patients. *New England Journal of Medicine, 347*(11), 817–823.

Fisher, B. A. C., Ghuran, A., Vadamalai, V., & Antonios, T. F. (2005). Cardiovascular complications induced by cannabis smoking: A case report and review of the literature. *Emergency Medicine Journal, 22,* 679–680.

Floyd, A. G., Boutros, N. N., Struve, F. A., Wolf, E., & Oliwa, G. M. (2006). Risk factors for experiencing psychosis during cocaine use: a preliminary report. *Journal of Psychiatric Research, 40*(2), 178–182.

Fudala, P. J., Bridge, P., Herbert, S., Williford, W. O., Chiang, C. N., Jones, K. et al. (2003). Office-based treatment of opiate addiction with a sublingual-tablet formulation of buphernorphine and naloxone. *New England Journal of Medicine, 349*(10), 949–958.

Ginés, P., Cárdenas, A., Arroyo, V., & Rodés, J., (2004). Management of cirrhosis and ascites. *New England Journal of Medicine, 350*(16), 1646–1654.

Goldstein, R. Z., Alia-Klein, N., Leskovjan, A. C., Fowler, J. S., Wang, G. J., Gur, R. C., et al. (2005). Anger and depression in cocaine addiction: Association with the orbitofrontal cortex. *Psychiatry Research, 138*(1), 13–22.

Gonzalez, G., Oliveto, A., & Kosten, T. R. (2002). Treatment of heroin (diamorphine) addiction: Current approaches and future prospects. *Drugs, 62,* 1331–1343.

Greer, B. G., Roberts, R., & Jenkins, W. M. (1990). Substance abuse among clients with other primary disabilities: Curricular implications for rehabilitation education. *Rehabilitation Education, 4*(1), 33–44.

Hall, W., & Solowij, N. (1998). Adverse effects of cannabis. *Lancet, 352,* 1611–1666.

Harley, D. A. (1995). Alcohol and other drug use among women: Implications for rehabilitation counseling. *Journal of Applied Rehabilitation Counseling, 26*(4), 38–41.

Harniman, B. (2006). Substance misuse: An overview of assessment and treatment options. *Nurse Prescribing, 7*(5), 180–183.

Heidelbaugh, J. J. & Sherbondy, M. (2006). Cirrhosis and chronic liver failure: Part II. Complications and treatment. *American Family Physician, 74*(5), 767–776, 781.

Helmus, T. C., Downey, K. K., Arfken, C. L., Henderson, M. J., & Schuster, C. R. (2001). Novelty seeking as a predictor of treatment retention for heroin dependent cocaine users. *Drug and Alcohol Dependence, 61,* 287–295.

Henskens, R., Mulder, C. L., Garretsen, H., Bongers, I., & Sturmans, F. (2005). Gender differences in problems and needs among chronic, high-risk crack abusers: Results of a randomized controlled trial. *Journal of Substance Use, 10*(2–3), 128–140.

Holdstock, L., & deWit, H. (1998). Individual differences in the biphasic effects of ethanol. *Alcoholism, Clinical and Experimental Research, 22,* 1903–1911.

Holloway, K., Bennett, T., & Lower, C. (2004). *Trends in drug use and offending: Results of the NEW-ADAM Programme 1999–2002.* Finds 219. London: Home Office.

Hope, V. D., Hickman, M., & Tilling, K. (2005). Capturing crack cocaine use: Estimating the prevalence of crack cocaine use in London using capture–recapture with covariates. *Addiction, 100,* 1701–1708.

Hsue, P. Y., McManus, D., Selby, V., Ren, X., Pillutia, P., Younes, N. et al. (2007). Cardiac arrest in patients who smoke crack cocaine. *American Journal of Cardiology, 99*(6), 822–824.

Inaba, D. S., & Cohen, W. E. (1993). *Uppers, downers, all arounders: Physical and mental effects of psychoactive drugs.* Ashland, OR: CNS Productions.

Judd, A., Hickman, M., Jones, S., McDonald, T., Parry, J. V., & Stimson, G. V. (2005). Incidence of hepatitis C virus and HIV among new injecting drug users in London: Prospective cohort study. *British Medical Journal, 330,* 24–25.

Juliano, L. M., & Griffiths, R. R. (2004). A critical review of caffeine withdrawal: Empirical validation of symptoms and signs, incidence, severity, and associated features. *Psychopharmacology (Berl), 176*(1), 1–29.

Kalman, D., Morissette, S. B., & George, T. P. (2005). Co-morbidity of smoking in patients with psychiatric and substance use disorders. *American Journal of Addiction, 14*(2), 106–123.

Kandall, S. R. (1996). *Substance and shadow: Women and addiction in the United States.* Cambridge, MA: Harvard University Press.

Kavanagh, D. J., McGrath, J., Saunders, J. B., Dore, G., & Clark, D. (2002). Substance misuse in patients with schizophrenia: Epidemiology and management. *Drugs, 62,* 743–755.

Kellogg, J. H. (2002). Tobaccoism. *American Journal of Public Health, 92*(6), 932–934.

Kloner, R. A., & Rezkalla, S. H. (2003). Cocaine and the heart. *New England Journal of Medicine, 348*(6), 487–488.

Kosten, T. R., & O'Connor, P. G. (2003). Management of drug and alcohol withdrawal. *New England Journal of Medicine, 348*(18), 1786–1795.

Krige, J. E. J., Kotze, U., Bornman, P. C., Shaw, J. M., & Klipin, M. (2006). Variceal recurrence, rebleeding, and survival after endoscopic injection sclerotherapy in 287 alcoholic cirrhotic patients with bleeding esophageal varicies. *Annals of Surgery, 244*(5), 764–770.

Lasser, K., Boyd, J. W., Woolhander, S., Himmelstein, D. U., McCormick, D., & Bor, D. II. (2000). Smoking and mental illness: A population-based prevalence study. *Journal of the American Medical Association, 284,* 2606–2610.

Leikin, J. B. (2007). Substance-related disorders in adults. *Disease-a-Month, 53,* 313–335.

Liechti, M. E., Kuntz, I., & Kupferschmidt, H. (2005). Acute medical problems due to Ecstasy use: Case-series of emergency department visits. *Swiss Medical Weekly, 135*(43–44), 652–657.

Low, G. S., Jenkins, N. P., & Prendergast, B. D. (2006). Needle embolism in an intravenous drug user. *Heart, 92,* 315.

Lukas, S. E. (1997). *Proceedings of the National Consensus Meeting on the Use, Abuse, and Sequelae of Abuse of Methamphetamine with Implications for Prevention, Treatment, and Research.* Substance Abuse and Mental Health Services Administration and Center for Substance Abuse Treatment. DHHS Pub. No. (SMA) 96-8013.

Maddux, J. F., & Desmond, D. P. (2000). Addiction or dependence. *Addiction, 95,* 661–665.

Maseeh, A., & Kwatra, G. (2005). A review of smoking cessation interventions. *Medscape General Medicine, 7*(2), 24–39. Retrieved July 7, 2007, from http://www.pubmedcentral.nih.gov.libproxy.lib.unc.edu/articlerender

Mintzer, I. L., Eisenberg, M., Terra, M., MacVane, C., Himmelstein, D. U., & Woolhandler, S. (2007). Treating opioid addiction with buprenorphine-naloxone in community-based primary care settings. *Annals of Family Medicine, 5*(2), 146–150.

Mokdad, A. H., Marks, J. S., Stroup, D. F., & Gerberding, J. L. (2004). Actual causes of death in the United States, 2000. *Journal of the American Medical Association, 291*(10), 1238–1245.

Moore, B. A., Fiellin, D. A., Barry, D. T, Sullivan, L. E., Chawarski, M. C., O'Connor, P. G. et al. (2007). Primary care office-based buprenorphine treatment: Comparison of heroin and prescription opioid dependent patients. *Journal of General Internal Medicine, 22*(4), 527–530.

Ochs, L. A., Holmes, G. E., & Karst, R. H. (1992). Caffeine consumption and disability: Clinical issues in rehabilitation. *Journal of Rehabilitation, 58*(3), 44-

O'Connor, P. G. (2000). Treating opoid dependence:New data and new opportunities. *New England Journal of Medicine, 243*(18), 1332–1334.

Page, S. A., & Verhoef, M. J. (2006). Medicinal marijuana use: Experiences of people with multiple sclerosis. *Canadian Family Physician, 52,* 64–65.

Peters, M. J., & Morgan, L. C. (2002). The pharmacotherapy of smoking cessation. *Medical Journal of Australia, 176,* 486–490.

Piazza, N. J., Martin, N., Dildine, R. J. (2000). Screening instruments for alcohol and other drug problems. *Journal of Mental Health Counseling, 22*(3), 218–228.

Pilon, A. F., & Scheiffle, J. (2006). Ulcerative keratitis associated with crack-cocaine abuse. *Contact Lens and Anterior Eye, 29*(5), 263–267.

Ponton, R., & Scott, J. (2004). Injection preparation processes used by heroin and crack cocaine injectors. *Journal of Substance Use, 9*(1), 7–19.

Robinson, T. E., & Berridge, K. C. (2001). Incentive-sensitization and addiction. *Addiction, 96,* 103–114.

Robinson, T. E., & Berridge, K. C. (2003). Addiction. *Annual Review of Psychology, 54,* 25–53.

Ruiz, P., Strain, E. C., & Langrod, J. G. (2007). *The substance abuse handbook.* Philadelphia: Lippincott Williams & Wilkins.

Sarnyai, Z., Shaham, Y., & Heinrichs, S. C. (2001). The role of corticotrophin-releasing factor in drug addiction. *Pharmacological Reviews, 53,* 209–244.

Scott-Lennox, J. S., Rose, R., Bohlig, A., & Lennox, R. (2000). The impact of women's family status on completion of substance abuse treatment. *Journal of Behavioral Health Services and Research, 27*(4), 366–379.

Smith, L. (2005). Oxycontin litigation. *Journal of Legal Nurse Consulting, 16*(4), 11–13.

Strain, E. C., & Griffiths, R. R. (1995). Caffeine dependence: fact or fiction? *Journal of the Royal Society of Medicine, 88,* 437–440.

Substance Abuse and Mental Health Services Administration. (2005), National survey on drug use and health. Retrieved October 30, 2007 from http: \\www.oas.samhsa.gov/gov/nhsda.htm.

Thomasius, R., Petersen, K. U., Zapletalova, P., Wartberg, L., Zeichner, D., & Schmoldt, A. (2005). Mental disorders in current and former heavy ecstasy (MDMA) users. *Addictions, 100,* 1310–1319.

Tinsley, J. A. (2007). Drug abuse. In R. E. Rakel & E. T. Bope (Eds.), *Conn's current therapy* (pp. 1279–1285). Philadelphia: W. B. Saunders.

U.S. Department of Health and Human Services (USDHHS). (2004). The health consequences of smoking: A report of the Surgeon General. Department of Health and Human Services, Centers for Disease Control and Prevention, National Center for Chronic Disease and Prevention and Health Promotion. Atlanta, GA: Office on Smoking and Health.

Volkow, N. D. (2001). Drug abuse and mental illness: Progress in understanding co-morbidity. *American Journal of Psychiatry, 158*(8), 1181–1183.

Watson, A. L., Franklin, M. E., Ingram, M. A., & Eilenberg, L. B. (1998). Alcohol and other drug abuse among persons with disabilities. *Journal of Applied Rehabilitation Counseling, 29*(2), 22–29.

Weatherall, M. (2001). Drug treatment and the rise of pharmacology. In R. Porter (Ed.), *Cambridge illustrated history of medicine* (pp. 246–277). Cambridge, UK: Cambridge University Press.

Wermuth, L. (2000). Methamphetamine use: Hazards and social influences. *Journal of Drug Education, 30*(4), 423–433.

Chapter 10

Conditions of the Blood and Immune System

■ STRUCTURE AND FUNCTION

Blood circulates continuously through the body and is essential for life. Blood is composed of liquid and a combination of several types of specialized cells:

- Red blood cells (RBC), also called erythrocytes
- White blood cells (WBC), also called **leukocytes**
- Platelets, also called **thrombocytes**

The liquid portion of the blood is a watery, colorless fluid called **plasma.** It contains no blood cells but is essential for carrying blood cells and nutrients through the circulation, as well as for transporting wastes from the tissues. It also contains vital plasma proteins and other important substances.

The total blood volume accounts for approximately 7% of human body weight. Under usual conditions, the quantity of blood in the adult body remains constant. The RBC, WBC, and platelets account for approximately 45% of the total blood volume, while plasma accounts for the other 55%. More than 99% of the cells in the blood are red blood cells.

Blood has many important functions:

- It carries oxygen and nutrients to the body tissues.

- It facilitates communication between the endocrine glands and other body organs by transporting hormones.
- It carries waste products from the tissues to the organs of excretion, such as the lungs and the kidneys.
- It protects the body from dangerous organisms.
- It promotes clotting to minimize excessive bleeding.
- It helps regulate body temperature.

Blood cells are formed by a process called **hemopoiesis** or *hematopoiesis*. Tissues that produce blood cells are said to be *hematopoietic*. Blood cells are produced in the bone marrow as well as in lymphoid tissue and organs. Special cells called *stem cells* are the sources from which all blood cells are formed. Bone marrow is especially rich in stem cells.

Structure and Function of Red Blood Cells

Red blood cells (**erythrocytes**) carry oxygen to the tissues. When mature, they are devoid of a nucleus. These cells are usually disk shaped, with a thin center and thicker edges. They are flexible, which allows the cells to adapt their shape to fit through blood vessels of differing sizes. **Hemoglobin** is the red-pigmented protein contained within the erythrocytes and is the specific part of the red blood cell that carries oxygen; hemoglobin also contains iron.

Special cells in the bone marrow produce erythrocytes. Several vitamins, such as vitamin B_{12} and folic acid (which is part of the vitamin B complex), are necessary for the formation of erythrocytes. These vitamins are obtained from the diet. Iron, which is also obtained from the diet, is important for the formation of hemoglobin. Excess amounts of iron and vitamin B_{12} are stored in the liver.

New red blood cells are constantly being formed. Although most erythrocytes are released into the blood, some are taken up by the spleen to be stored for emergency use when the RBC count drops significantly below regular levels, such as during excessive bleeding (*hemorrhage*). Newly formed red blood cells enter the bloodstream before they are totally mature. At this stage, they are called **reticulocytes**. Within several days, reticulocytes mature to become erythrocytes. The life cycle of erythrocytes is approximately 120 days. As the erythrocytes reach the end of their lives, they become more fragile and rupture. In addition, some of the old erythrocytes are destroyed in the **spleen**. Special cells within the spleen and liver absorb the old erythrocytes, making room for more new cells.

When the quantity of oxygen supplied to body tissues decreases, the body increases the number of red blood cells produced. For example, at higher altitudes, where less oxygen is available in the air, the bone marrow reacts by producing more red blood cells, even if there is an adequate number of red blood cells in the circulation.

Structure and Function of White Blood Cells

White blood cells (**leukocytes**) are important to the body's ability to resist or destroy foreign materials and organisms; that is, they are an important component of immune system function. The five types of leukocytes play different roles in defending the body from infection (see Table 10-1).

Under normal circumstances, blood contains a fairly consistent number of circulating white blood cells. When there is an infection or when some other foreign stimuli are in the body, white blood cells proliferate so that large numbers of them circulate in the bloodstream; this condition is called **leukocytosis**.

White blood cells are formed in the bone marrow and play the predominant role in the body's defense system. These leukocytes take action when body tissues have been damaged or invaded by organisms or other foreign materials. Any infection or invasion by foreign substances causes a dramatic increase in the number of white blood cells in the blood. Some leukocytes—called **phagocytes**—are scavengers and have the ability to destroy and ingest bacteria or foreign particles; the pro-

Table 10-1   Types of Leukocytes

Type	Function
Neutrophils	Engulf and destroy foreign substances
Eosinophils	Are involved in allergic reactions
Basophils	Secrete histamine and are involved in allergic reactions
Monocytes	Become macrophages, which destroy foreign substances
Lymphocytes	
B lymphocytes (B Cells)	Become cells that secrete antibodies to destroy foreign substances
T lymphocytes (T Cells)	Release chemicals that destroy cells invaded by viruses

cess of ingesting cells and foreign objects is called **phagocytosis**. White blood cells' role in immunity is discussed later in this chapter.

Structure and Function of Platelets and Coagulation

Platelets (**thrombocytes**) are disk-shaped cells that are formed by special cells in the bone marrow. The smallest of the cells in the blood, they contain no hemoglobin. The number of platelets circulating in the blood usually does not change. If the number of platelets should decrease, however, the condition is called **thrombocytopenia**; an increase in the number of platelets is called **thrombocytosis**.

Platelets play a crucial role in blood clotting and are involved in an important first step in preventing excessive bleeding after an injury. Approximately one-third of platelets are stored in the spleen for emergency use.

The term **hemostasis** refers to the series of events that stop bleeding from damaged vessels. When bleeding occurs, the damaged blood vessel immediately constricts, going into spasm in an effort to minimize blood loss. The walls of the vessels become sticky, causing the walls to adhere to each other and further restrict blood flow. This sticky surface of the vessels activates platelets so that they group together and adhere to the wall, forming a plug. The plug, in addition to stopping the bleeding momentarily, releases other chemicals that in turn enhance blood coagulation.

Platelets alone cannot stop bleeding indefinitely. Instead, the formation of the plug activates *clotting factors* (coagulation factors from the liver, plasma, and other sources) so that a clot forms to control the bleeding. Clotting involves turning blood from a liquid into a more solid form. The platelet plug acts as a base, allowing the clot to attach and seal the break. For a clot to form, *fibrinogen*, a substance that is formed in the liver and present in the plasma, is converted into *fibrin*. Fibrin forms a matrix at the site that collects blood cells and platelets, resulting in clot formation.

The conversion of fibrinogen to fibrin takes place because of an enzyme called *thrombin*. Thrombin is formed only when needed from a precursor called *prothrombin*, which is found in the plasma. This conversion is made possible by a plasma-clotting factor, *factor X,* which becomes activated because of another plasma clotting factor.

These are *intrinsic* and *extrinsic blood clotting factors*, most named by Roman numerals designated from I to XIII, in which different sets of substances play major roles. Intrinsic clotting factors precipitate clotting by making contact with substances contained in the blood. Extrinsic clotting factors precipitate clotting by interacting with substances in the tissues outside the blood. For instance, thrombin activates factor XIII, thereby stabilizing the fibrin matrix, whereas other substances in the clotting mechanism may be activated because of substances that have leaked from tissues outside the vessel. Vitamin K is necessary for the formation of some clotting factors and is essential to clot formation. To prevent excessive clotting, other body mechanisms are activated as well.

■ THE IMMUNE SYSTEM

The immune system is a complex organization of specialized cells and organs. Although it is constantly bombarded by microorganisms or trauma that can result in infection or injury, because of actions of the immune system, the body has specific defenses to protect it against such invasions. The immune system distinguishes between self and non-self, defending the body against "foreign" materials. Although the body is exposed to a number of microorganisms each day, the immune system helps the body fight off invasion by these organisms and, when injury occurs, helps the body in the healing process.

The primary microorganisms that the immune system defends against are *bacteria* and *viruses*. Bacteria, which are harmful, secrete materials that destroy the tissues they invade. Bacteria are capable of living and reproducing on their own. In contrast, viruses are unable to survive or reproduce without invading another cell, called a *host cell*. Because the virus enters the host cell and utilizes that cell's genetic properties for its own survival, the body may not recognize the cell and may produce defenses against it. During the life cycle of the virus, the host cell may become so depleted that it produces substances that cause damage to the cell.

The immune system can be divided into two component systems: the *innate immune system* and the *adaptive* or *acquired immune system*. The latter system is further subdivided into *antibody* or *humoral immunity* and *cell-mediated immunity*. Each component has a different role and function (Medzhitov & Janeway, 2000).

Innate Immunity

The body's first line of defense against foreign material is called *nonspecific* or *innate immunity*. Innate immunity provides a nonselective response and requires no previous exposure to a foreign substance or recognition of any specific properties of foreign material. This type of immunity includes several mechanisms of protection:

- Protection provided by the skin, which acts as a barrier to organisms
- Protection by the mucous membranes, gastric secretions, and tears, all of which contain special chemicals that destroy potentially harmful organisms

The response of innate immunity is extremely rapid. When, despite external and chemical barriers, an organism or other foreign material gains entry into the body, an *inflammatory response* results. The main purpose of this inflammation is to bring **phagocytes** (cells that destroy and ingest foreign material) to the area to destroy and remove foreign substances so that tissue repair can begin. As a result of the inflammatory process, the affected area becomes red, warm, and swollen, and the inflamed area becomes walled off to prevent or delay bacteria from spreading.

Adaptive (Acquired) Immunity

White blood cells called lymphocytes fight infection through a process called acquired immunity (the ability of cells to recognize an organism to which there has been previous exposure and to neutralize or destroy a later-invading organism of the same type). This is part of the adaptive component of the immune system. Lymphocytes are formed by the lymph nodes, spleen, thymus, and bone marrow, and they circulate throughout the bloodstream and the lymphatic system.

The two major types of lymphocytes are *B lymphocytes* and *T lymphocytes*. B lymphocytes migrate to lymphoid tissue, such as the lymph nodes and spleen. These lymphocytes have the capability of recognizing and selectively responding to foreign substances (**antigen**). In response to recognition of an antigen, special substances called *antibodies* (immunoglobulins) are produced. The antibodies, in turn, enter the bloodstream, recognize and bind to the antigen, and destroy it. This type of immune response is called *humoral immunity*. Thus antibodies do not penetrate cells, but rather interact with circulating antigens. When antibodies are produced because of exposure to an antigen, such that the body generates its own antibodies, the process is described as *active immunity*. If antibodies from another person or animal are introduced into an individual, the process is called *passive immunity*.

T lymphocytes are the regulators and controllers of the immune system. When these lymphocytes are exposed to an antigen, rather than producing antibodies, they react to the antigen directly, attacking body cells that have been invaded by the foreign substance or malignancy. This response is called *cellular immunity*.

T cells comprise several different subsets of cells that behave differently. Killer T cells (CD8 or *cytotoxic* T cells) release chemicals that destroy the targeted cell. Helper T cells (CD4) help coordinate the immune response, activating B cells to make antibodies against antigens, as well as activating and enhancing the activity of cytotoxic cells and macrophages. A subset of helper cells, called regulatory T cells or suppressor T cells, inhibit both the innate and the adaptive immune responses as a way of minimizing harmful effects of the immune response.

Usually, helper cells outnumber "killer" cells by a 2:1 ratio. After the initial insult from a foreign material, T cells form a "memory." If that specific organism invades the body again, it is "remembered" and, consequently, the immune response is more intense. Killer T cells, in addition to working to rid the body of infected cells, attack cancer cells and are responsible for the rejection of grafts or transplants.

The Lymphatic System

The lymphatic system is crucial to the body's defenses against invading organisms and other foreign substances. The lymphatic system is a special circulatory system that is distinct from the general blood circulation. It depends on muscle movement to circulate the fluid within it. This system consists of *lymph vessels, circulating lymph fluid* (clear fluid that bathes the body's tissue), and *lymph nodes* (small glands of the immune system that are located throughout the body and act as filters). Lymph nodes also serve as temporary storage reservoirs for lymphocytes (white blood cells that fight infection) and, with appropriate stimulus, as manufacturers of lymphocytes.

Lymphoid Tissues

Lymphoid tissues are those tissues in the body that produce, store, or process lymphocytes (see Figure 10-1). Although lymphoid tissues include the tonsils, adenoids, appendix, and special tissues in the lining of the gastrointestinal tract, the major organs that are important in the body's defense from microorganisms include the spleen, thymus, and bone marrow.

The spleen, which is located in the upper left quadrant of the abdomen, filters blood and helps to destroy microorganisms. It also disposes of aged blood cells and lymphatic tissue. The **thymus,** which lies in the upper portion of the chest between the lungs, is important in controlling the development of T lymphocytes. *Bone marrow* also produces lymphocytes and, consequently, is also classified as a lymphoid organ.

■ CONDITIONS AFFECTING THE BLOOD (HEMATOLOGICAL CONDITIONS)

Hematological conditions—conditions affecting the blood—may be caused by a number of factors, may arise from many different sources, and may be manifest in many different ways. They include all of the following:

- Irregularities of blood cells
- Overproduction or underproduction of blood cells
- Destruction of blood cells
- Irregularities of clotting mechanisms

Anemia

Anemia is characterized by a reduced capacity of the blood to carry oxygen owing to excessive loss of red blood cells, underproduction or destruction of red blood cells, or deficiency in the components of red blood cells that affects their ability to bind to oxygen. The conditions that fall under the general term "anemia" are characterized by a reduction in the amount of hemoglobin (the molecule in the blood that carries oxygen and is available for oxygen transport to all of the body tissues).

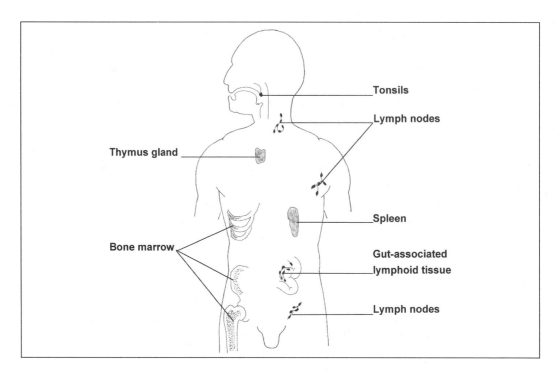

Tonsils

Lymph nodes

Thymus gland

Spleen

Bone marrow

Gut-associated
lymphoid tissue

Lymph nodes

Figure 10-1   The immune system

Anemias are sometimes classified by the size and color of the red blood cells when the condition is present. For example, healthy, uniform sized cells are called *normocytic* uniform-sized cells that are of characteristic color are called *normochromic*. Anemias in which the color of the red blood cells is paler than usual are called *hypochromic anemias*. Anemias in which the red blood cells are larger than usual are called *macrocytic anemias,* while those in which cells are smaller than usual are called *microcytic anemias.*

Although anemia is not considered a disability per se, it is associated with a number of chronic conditions and their management, such as cancer (see Chapter 18); (Bokemeyer & Foubert, 2004; gastrointestinal conditions (see Chapter 12); (Andres, Loukili, Ben, & Noel, 2004; Bodemar, Kechagias, Almer, & Danielson, 2004), and chronic kidney disease (see Chapter 15); (Sherwood, 2007).

Anemia can also derive from other causes:

- Nutritional anemia, in which there is a dietary deficiency in nutrients that contribute to the production of red blood cells
- Anemia due to the body's inability to absorb certain vitamins that are essential for production of red blood cells
- Failure of the bone marrow to produce enough red blood cells
- Hemorrhage
- Destruction of red blood cells

An example of nutritional anemia is *iron-deficiency anemia* (Shah, 2004). Iron-deficiency anemia is one of the most common types of anemia and is caused by a shortage of iron in the diet. It can also result from the body's failure to absorb iron, excessive or chronic blood loss, or an increase in the body's iron requirements.

Pernicious anemia is an example of anemia caused by the body's inability to absorb certain vitamins needed for red blood cell production. This chronic condition is caused by the inadequate secretion by the stomach of a substance (*intrinsic factor*) that is necessary for the intestines to absorb vitamin B_{12}. It may also be caused by dietary deficiency of vitamin B_{12}, especially in vegetarianism (Stabler & Allen, 2004). Deficiency of vitamin B_{12} impairs production and maturation of blood cells. Consequently, the body is unable to produce adequate numbers of red blood cells, resulting in anemia.

Aplastic anemia (sometimes called *pancytopenia*) is an example of the body's inability to manufacture enough red blood cells and is caused by inadequate functioning of the bone marrow. Aplastic anemia can occur spontaneously, or it can be the result of damage to the bone marrow produced by drugs, toxic chemicals, or ionizing radiation. It may also be caused by invasion of the bone marrow by cancer or by the chemotherapy used to treat cancer.

Hemorrhagic anemia refers to anemia resulting from significant blood loss and subsequent diminished volume of circulating blood (*hypovolemia*). When significant blood loss occurs, there are not enough red blood cells (and consequently not enough hemoglobin) to carry adequate amounts of oxygen to body tissues. Blood loss resulting in hemorrhagic anemia can be acute (such as from an injury) or chronic (such as from slow and chronic bleeding from the intestines).

Hemolytic anemia is a type of anemia caused by excessive and/or premature destruction of red blood cells (**hemolysis**). Hemolytic anemia may occur in association with some infectious conditions (such as *malaria*) or with certain inherited red blood cell conditions (such as **sickle cell disease**, discussed later in this chapter). It may also develop as a response to drugs or other foreign or toxic agents. The spleen usually becomes enlarged (**splenomegaly**) in chronic hemolytic conditions because of the need to remove an excessive number of damaged red blood cells.

The degree of anemia reflects the ability of the bone marrow to produce red blood cells or to increase the production of red blood cells enough to keep up with their loss or destruction. Regardless of the cause, anemia disrupts the transport of oxygen to tissues throughout the body, resulting in a number of systemic symptoms. For instance, severe anemia increases the workload of the heart. To compensate for decreased oxygen in the tissue, the heart pumps at a more rapid pace in an attempt to increase the oxygen supply to body tissues. As a result, individuals experience rapid heartbeat (**tachycardia**). As a result of the inadequate number of red blood cells circulating throughout the body, individuals with anemia may have pale skin (**pallor**), weakness, or difficulty in breathing (**dyspnea**). Inadequate oxygen supply to the brain in anemia may cause the individual to be unable to concentrate or to experience irritability.

Fatigue is a major symptom of anemia and may prove debilitating. It can reduce the individual's ability to work, by decreasing physical and emotional well-being, as well as interfere with cognitive ability. As a result, individuals may experience anxiety and depression, which can further interfere with the individual's ability to work (Bokemeyer & Foubert, 2004). Individuals with anemia may also be more susceptible to infection, thus adding to the disabling effects the initial anemia may have caused.

The first step in treating anemia is to identify the cause and correct it if possible. When the cause is identified, management is specific to the cause. If anemia is the result of blood loss, blood replacement through transfusion may be necessary. In other instances, only dietary, vitamin, or iron supplements may be necessary. Management of anemia associated with chronic conditions such as sickle cell disease is discussed later in the chapter.

Thalassemia

Thalassemia is one of the most common genetic conditions in the world (Rund & Rachmilewitz, 2005) and is common in individuals with heritage from the Mediterranean region, Africa, the Middle East, India, Southeast Asia, and Indonesia (Olivieri, 1999). This group of inherited anemias results from defective hemoglobin production (Higgs, Thein, & Woods, 2001). Almost 5% of the world's population carries a gene variant that causes thalassemia, including two common forms (α-thalassemia, β-thalassemia), as do almost 2% of individuals who carry sickle hemoglobin (Angastiniotis & Modell, 1998). Sickle cell disease is discussed later in the chapter.

Thalassemias range from mild to severe and are characterized by the production of thin, fragile, red blood cells and defective hemoglobin synthesis. As a result, the hemoglobin content of the red blood cells is inadequate. In addition, there is often some interference with erythrocyte metabolism, which causes the red blood cells to be deformed and decreases their survival time. Thus anemia associated with thalassemia can result both from the increased destruction of red blood cells and from the impaired production of hemoglobin.

The anemia associated with thalassemia may be severe. Transfusion therapy is the mainstay of management. Because impairment in growth in children is a common feature of thalassemia, early diagnosis is imperative so that regular transfusion therapy can be implemented, allowing for standard growth and development (Rund & Rachmilewitz, 2005).

Individuals with thalassemia may experience underdevelopment or decreased function of testes or ovaries. Hormone replacement therapy in males may help to correct gonadal function. Females may be able to become pregnant with assisted reproductive techniques (De Sanctis, 2002). Older adults may experience bone conditions such as *osteopenia* (decreased bone density) or **osteoporosis** (increase in the porous nature of bone), which may make them more susceptible to fractures and subsequent pain.

Iron overload is a frequent problem for individuals with thalassemia because of the breakdown of red blood cells and increased absorption of iron from the gastrointestinal tract. The accumulated iron forms deposits in various organs of the body, including the heart, liver, and endocrine glands, which damages the organs so affected. Consequently, in addition to transfusion therapy, iron chelation therapy is often necessary to prevent iron overload (Rodgers, 2004). Iron chelation therapy can be painful and expensive, but it can significantly extend the life expectancy of individuals with severe thalassemia (Hoffbrand, Cohen, & Hershko, 2003).

Individuals with thalassemia must also make lifestyle adjustments, including increasing their calcium intake, participating in regular physical activity, and quitting smoking. Although thalassemia can be cured by bone marrow transplantation and gene therapy (Rund & Rachmilewitz, 2005), both therapies require that individuals be compliant with management recommendations.

Polycythemia (Erythrocytosis)

In **polycythemia** (also called *erythrocytosis*), there is an increase in the number of red blood cells, as well as in the concentration of hemoglobin, within the blood. Several types of polycythemia are distinguished. For example, *polycythemia vera* is associated with an overproduction of both red and white blood cells. The cause of polycythemia vera is unknown. Because of the increased number of cells in the blood, individuals with this condition may experience hypertension, congestive heart failure, heart attack (see Chapter 13), or stroke (see Chapter 3). They may also experience hemorrhage if congestion in the blood vessels causes the vessels to rupture.

Secondary polycythemia occurs in conjunction with another condition or, sometimes, as a result of living at high altitudes. When the body's demand for oxygen increases, the bone marrow produces additional red blood cells to meet the increased demand. Chronic obstructive pulmonary disease (see Chapter 14) is one such condition in which secondary polycythemia may occur. Management focuses on the underlying condition.

Individuals with conditions characterized by a loss of plasma without a loss of red blood cells, such as burns, may develop a state similar to polycythemia. Although there is no actual increase in the number of red blood cells, the loss of fluid increases the proportion of red blood cells in the blood. In these cases, management involves fluid replacement to decrease the viscosity of the blood.

Agranulocytosis (Neutropenia)

Agranulocytosis is a marked reduction in the level of a specific type of leukocyte. This reduction in leukocytes is called **leukopenia**. A common cause of agranulocytosis is toxic reaction to certain medications used in the management of chronic conditions, such as medications used to treat epilepsy or medications used to treat certain psychiatric conditions. Agranulocytosis may also result from exposure to certain chemicals or ionizing radiation.

Because white blood cells are important to fight infection, a reduction in the number of these cells increases an individual's susceptibility to infection. Agranulocytosis is a potentially serious condition and, without prompt intervention, can result in death. Management is directed toward removing the toxic agent responsible and providing medications (e.g., antibiotics) to treat resulting infections.

Purpura

Purpura is a condition characterized by hemorrhage of small blood vessels into the skin. With this condition, small amounts of blood leak into various tissues of the body. It can be caused by an allergic response or a deficiency in platelets, or it may be associated with other conditions in the body.

Leukemia

The leukemias are caused by overproduction of various types of white blood cells. They are discussed in greater detail in Chapter 18.

Hemophilia

Hemophilia is one of several inherited, chronic bleeding conditions characterized by a deficiency or absence of one of the clotting factors (Bolton-Maggs & Pasi, 2003). It is an X-linked recessive condition in which males inherit the condition and females have no symptoms but are carriers of the affected chromosome.

In most instances, hemophilia is transmitted when a mother who carries a hemophilia gene and an unaffected father have a son. Under these circumstances, there is a 50% chance that their sons will have hemophilia and a 50% chance that their daughters will be carriers. If the father has hemophilia but the mother is unaffected, none of the sons will be affected, but all daughters will be carriers. Although hemophilia can occur in women, it is extremely rare. If the mother is a carrier and the father has hemophilia, each of their daughters will either have hemophilia or be a carrier, while sons will have a 50% chance of having hemophilia or being unaffected (Pruthi, 2005). In some instances, individuals are born with hemophilia when there is no family history. In these instances, the condition is thought to have been caused by a spontaneous mutation rather than heredity (Britton, 2003).

The degree of severity varies for hemophilia. With new prophylactic infusion therapy, and without complications, individuals with hemophilia now have a life expectancy of approximately 72 years (Plug et al., 2006). Overall, however, hemophilia has the potential to be a disabling condition and is typically associated with high financial costs (Beeton, 2002).

Types of Hemophilia

Several types of hemophilia exist, which are differentiated by the specific clotting factor that is deficient. The most common type of hemophilia is *hemophilia A*, caused by a deficiency in blood coagulation factor VIII. The next most common type is *hemophilia B*, in which *clotting factor IX* (also called *Christmas factor*—named after an individual with the condition) is defective (Pruthi, 2005).

The manifestations of hemophilia A and hemophilia B are indistinguishable. Both are characterized by the development of excessive bleeding precipitated by even minor incidents. In most instances, the condition is recognized in infancy or childhood when, for example, excessive bleeding occurs after circumcision or spontaneous or easy bruising is identified. In mild cases of hemophilia, individuals may not be diagnosed until adulthood.

Manifestations of Hemophilia

Although individuals with hemophilia do not initially bleed faster, the clotting mechanism is disturbed so that bleeding is prolonged or the oozing of blood may persist after injury. Because the platelet count is decreased in hemophilia, bleeding from a small cut or scratch does not pose a severe problem. How-

ever, deficiency in clotting factors can pose danger of internal bleeding into the internal organs, joints, or brain.

The severity of hemophilia varies along a continuum from a tendency toward slow, prolonged, persistent bleeding to a tendency toward severe hemorrhage, and is categorized as *mild, moderate,* or *severe* depending on level of clotting factor present. Individuals with the mild from of hemophilia usually do not experience spontaneous bleeding or excessive bleeding after minor injury, but develop prolonged bleeding only after major injury or after surgery. Individuals with the moderate form of the condition not only experience spontaneous bleeding, but also have prolonged bleeding after minor injury. In the most severe form of the condition, individuals may experience spontaneous bleeding into the joints (**hemarthrosis**) or brain (*intracranial hemorrhage*), severe nosebleed (**epistaxis**), severe bruising (**ecchymosis**), or **hematoma** (a sac filled with an accumulated mass of blood).

Bleeding into the joints (**hemarthrosis**) is extremely painful and can cause significant joint destruction (Elander & Barry, 2003; Shapiro & Hoots, 2000). Knees and ankles are affected most frequently, although elbows may become involved later. Joint deformity and crippling may result from damage to the joint structure and from **atrophy** (wasting) of surrounding muscles. Bleeding into the muscles, if severe, may exert pressure on nerves and cause a temporary sensory loss. If the hemorrhage damages muscle tissue, fibrous tissue may form, causing varying degrees of functional loss.

Management of Hemophilia

Hemophilia is not curable and requires management of bleeding problems throughout the individual's life. With proper care and management, however, individuals with hemophilia can control their condition, and their life expectancy approaches that of individuals without hemophilia (Teitel, Barnard, Israels, Lillicrap, Poon, & Sek, 2004).

The cornerstone to management of hemophilia is prophylaxis and prompt intervention when bleeding occurs. To prevent damage from bleeding, significant blood loss, and joint damage, all bleeding must be detected early and treated promptly. More than 100 comprehensive hemophilia treatment centers are available throughout the United States, all of which help individuals with hemophilia manage their conditions physically and psychologically. These care centers emphasize early intervention for bleeding episodes and train individuals to administer infusion therapy at home, thereby markedly improving school attendance and minimizing absences from work (Teitel et al., 2004).

Because there is no cure for hemophilia, management is directed toward preventing any injury that could precipitate bleeding, and toward controlling bleeding episodes when they do occur. The mainstay of management of hemophilia is replacement therapy with plasma or plasma concentrates that contain the clotting factors in which the individual's blood is deficient. Management of hemophilia with factor concentrates must be individualized for each person and for each bleeding episode (Robinson, 2005). Because of the higher concentrations of clotting factors, plasma concentrates are given more frequently than is fresh plasma. Clotting factors are usually replaced through intravenous infusion (infusing substance directly into a vein). The amount, type, and duration of the infusion depend on the individual's clotting deficiency, his or her size, and the severity of the bleeding problem. Infusions may be instituted prior to surgery to prevent excessive bleeding.

Early management of bleeding helps to prevent complications. Consequently, learning to administer clotting factor concentrates at home is of major benefit. To do so, however, individuals must be able to calculate the appropriate dose and mix, and administer the concentrate intravenously. Home therapy is appropriate for mild bleeding but is not sufficient when major bleeding occurs. Major bleeding requires medical evaluation.

Complications of Hemophilia

Several complications are associated with infusion therapy. As with all therapies that involve intravenous infusion, there is the chance of the transmission of blood-borne viruses such as the hepatitis B and C viruses (HBC and HCV, respectively) and human immunodeficiency virus (HIV) (Yee & Lee, 2005; Parish, 2002). Although identification of viruses, improved purification methods, and development of newer factor concentrates have mainly eliminated this problem in developed countries, other countries do not have access to these resources. Consequently, individuals who have been exposed to hepatitis B or C may experience liver damage, and those exposed to HIV have increased risk of developing associated complications and shortened life expectancy.

Another potential complication of hemophilia is the development of antibodies against factor concentrates that are infused (Pruthi, 2005).

Individuals with bleeding into a joint may require joint immobilization for several days in addition to replacement therapy. Joint pain may be treated with anti-inflammatory medications and analgesics. Medications that contain aspirin should be avoided, however, because aspirin interferes with platelet function and can increase an individual's susceptibility to bleeding. Physical therapy or prescribed exercise carried out at home may be necessary to maintain the range of motion of the affected joints. If the joints undergo severe degeneration, reconstructive orthopedic surgery, such as joint replacement, may also be necessary (see Chapter 16). Individuals with hemophilia should always wear a Medic-Alert identification bracelet or necklace to alert others to their condition in case of an emergency.

Psychosocial Issues in Hemophilia

How individuals respond to having hemophilia as adults depends to a great extent on their experiences with the condition during childhood. Because hemophilia is present from birth, attitudes displayed by parents and significant others during individuals' development significantly affect their self-view and view of their condition. If parents were overprotective, individuals' social and psychological development may have been stunted so that the individual lacks self-confidence and remains overly dependent. If many hospitalizations were required due to the condition, individuals may have experienced multiple school absences, and consequently their educational achievement may also be lower than that of other members of their peer group.

Activities and Participation

Physical activity has benefit for everyone, including individuals with hemophilia. Because of a fear of injury, however, individuals may have not have participated in sports or other activities in which physical and motor skills are learned and mastered. With increased understanding of hemophilia and its management, more athletes with hemophilia are participating in competitive sports (Fiala, Hoffmann, & Ritenour, 2003). Primary considerations in determining the extent of participation are the severity of the hemophilia, the type of sport in which the individual wishes to participate, and the person's level of awareness of his or her condition. Individuals with hemophilia who do not take unnecessary risks are more likely to be able to participate in sports without consequence than those who are risk

takers and more likely to sustain injury (Fiala & Ritenour, 2004). Noncontact sports, such as track and field or tennis, or contact sports, such as basketball and soccer, are less likely to pose a threat of injury than collision sports, such as football, hockey, or rugby, though this point may not be important for individuals with hemophilia.

In some instances, and especially for those individuals with the severe form of hemophilia, inability to predict when bleeding may occur or fear of being unable to control bleeding may result in passivity and inactivity. At other times, if individuals have had difficulty adjusting to the condition, uncertainty about the future, or denial of the seriousness of hemophilia or denial of precautions that need to be taken to control it, excessive risk taking may result.

Although replacement therapy and home infusions have done much to improve the lives of individuals with hemophilia and mitigate the consequences resulting from the condition, therapies are very expensive. Expense of management of the condition may be an additional source of stress. Individuals with inadequate resources to pay for infusions may neglect them altogether or under treat their condition in an attempt to decrease its cost. The long-term effects of inadequate management of hemophilia can cause increased functional limitations.

Individuals with hemophilia may experience both acute and chronic pain if there has been bleeding into the joints. Consequently, pain medications are frequently used. If medications are not carefully used and monitored, there is the potential for the development of drug dependence, sometimes to the extent that drug rehabilitation is required. Individuals who have not adjusted well to their condition and self-medicate to alleviate their emotional discomfort may be at particular risk.

Although exposure to HIV or HCV as a result of infusion therapy is rare today, individuals who were exposed to and contracted HIV or HCV as a result of infusion therapy prior to 1985 may now be living with two chronic, lifelong conditions. As a result, they may experience not only stress and anxiety, but also anger, resentment, and depression. Some individuals may feel stigmatized by their condition, and especially by the public's awareness of the link between hemophilia and HIV, and attempt to hide their condition.

Long-term survivors of HIV infection associated with hemophilia are a small group within the HIV-positive community and may not feel the same sense of support from that community as do other members of this group. Individuals with HIV infection may be living beyond their expectations and, therefore, may need to reevaluate their short- and long-term goals. Those individuals who have contracted HCV may have increased anxiety because of the knowledge that HCV may progress to cirrhosis or liver cancer (Taylor, 2004). Whether individuals have HIV or HCV infection, they may face issues of disclosure, stigma, and uncertain prognosis. Individuals' ability to establish or maintain sexual relationships may also be affected by a diagnosis of HIV or HCV infection.

Sexual issues may likewise be of concern for individuals with hemophilia even in the absence of concomitant HIV or HCV infection. Complications associated with hemophilia may affect sexual activity. Joint damage, medication side effects, and other complications can also interfere with sexual function (Parish, 2002). Because hemophilia is a hereditary condition, individuals may experience guilt or fear, and may grapple with the decision of whether to have children. The potential impact on long-term relationships and the decision whether to have children may be troublesome.

In some instances, there may be avoidance of developing close, meaningful relationships because of the individual's discomfort with having a hereditary condition.

Vocational Issues in Hemophilia

Improved medical technology and the availability of self-infused coagulation factors have greatly increased the ability of individuals with hemophilia to decrease manifestations and consequences of their condition and maintain employment in a variety of settings (Teitel et al., 2004). Individuals with severe hemophilia may also be able to perform a variety of job tasks without limitations; however, in severe manifestations of the condition, there is the increased unpredictability of when the bleeding will occur.

When bleeding does occur, individuals should be able to self-infuse the concentrates in 15 to 30 minutes; however, they will need to take a break from work to perform the replacement therapy. A semiprivate place to perform the infusion, as well as a place to store the equipment and concentrate, will also be needed.

Usually, individuals with hemophilia have few functional limitations in the vocational setting, unless they experience joint complications. Obviously, individuals with hemophilia—especially those with moderate to severe manifestations of the condition—should avoid employment in which there is a direct threat of physical injury. Injuries that may be minimal by most standards can have serious implications for individuals with more severe forms of hemophilia. Joint damage and subsequent joint replacement owing to complications of hemophilia may impose the same limitations as does joint damage from other causes. In some instances, surgical correction of damaged joints may be indicated (see Chapter 16). For the most part, however, primarily their abilities and interests determine the vocational functioning of individuals with hemophilia.

One barrier to employment may be lack of understanding on the part of the employer about the few limitations that are actually associated with hemophilia. Because the public has now connected hemophilia and the potential for HIV infection there may be fear and anxiety from co-workers when working with individuals with hemophilia, especially if a bleeding episode occurs. Likewise, co-workers who observe individuals administering self-infusing concentrates, and who do not understand replacement therapy, may draw false conclusions about the activity, causing further discrimination. Educating employers and co-workers about hemophilia and its management may be one of the most crucial links to vocational success for the individual with hemophilia.

Sickle Cell Disease

Sickle cell disease is a nonspecific, general term used to describe a genetic condition of the blood that affects approximately 2000 infants per year in the United States (Wilson, Krishnamuri, & Kamat, 2003). It is passed on by an autosomal recessive gene and occurs most often in individuals of African descent, although it can also occur in individuals of Hispanic, Mediterranean, Middle Eastern, and Near Eastern ancestry (Perry, 2005). In the United States, 8–10% of African American newborns are born with sickle cell trait and nearly 60,000 individuals are living with sickle cell disease (Embury, 2004).

Sickle cell disease occurs in several forms:

- Sickle–hemoglobin C disease
- Sickle–β-thalassemia (two types)
- Sickle cell anemia

Sickle cell disease occurs because of a genetic mutation of hemoglobin, a component of red blood cells. Hemoglobin that is not affected by a mutation is called hemoglobin A. Individuals with sickle cell disease have a mutation on a part of hemoglobin A that results in the development of sickle cell hemoglobin (*hemoglobin S*).

Inheritance Patterns

Hemoglobin genes are inherited in much the same way as other inherited traits such as blood type, hair color, and eye color. Individuals inherit one hemoglobin gene from each parent. If one parent has the hemoglobin S gene but the other parent has the regular hemoglobin gene, their offspring will have a 50% chance of inheriting the hemoglobin S gene and consequently becoming a carrier of the gene. When hemoglobin S is present, individuals are said to have **sickle cell trait**. Individuals with sickle cell trait will have no symptoms, but will pass the gene to their offspring.

When both parents have sickle cell trait, the chances with each pregnancy are 1 in 4 that the baby will have regular hemoglobin without the mutation, 2 in 4 that the baby will have sickle cell trait, and 1 in 4 that the baby will have sickle cell disease (Wang, Grover, & Gallagher, 1993). If one parent has sickle cell disease and the other has regular hemoglobin, all of their offspring will have sickle cell trait. When one parent has sickle cell trait and the other has sickle cell disease, there is a 50% chance with each pregnancy that the child will have sickle cell trait and a 50% chance that the child will have sickle cell disease. If both parents have sickle cell disease, so will all of their children (Lukens, 1993).

Manifestations of Sickle Cell Disease

Manifestations of sickle cell disease are caused by the rigidity of the sickled red blood cell, the increased adhesiveness on its surface, and decreased red blood cell survival. Sickle cell disease is characterized by lifelong hemolytic anemia (i.e., anemia caused by destruction of RBC) and a wide variety of painful and debilitating vaso-occlusive events (Mentzer & Kan, 2001). This chronic, lifelong condition is unpredictable and has symptoms that can range from mild to severe (Cooper-Effa, Blount, Kaslow, Rothenberg, & Eckman, 2001). It can result in significant physical consequences, including death.

The course of sickle cell disease includes periods of acute and chronic hematological crisis (**sickle cell crisis**) that cause considerable physical pain and psychological distress, and can result in death. These hematological events occur because sickle-shaped red blood cells obstruct vessels and prevent blood flow to surrounding tissue. When the oxygen concentration in the blood is low, the red blood cells' surfaces become sticky and the cells become deformed so that, instead of being disk shaped, they assume the shape of a crescent or sickle. Because of this distortion, the red blood cells become rigid and are unable to adapt their shape to fit through tiny blood vessels. These misshaped red blood cells interact with one another and become stacked up. The sickled cell is very fragile and is easily destroyed, which severely curtails its average life span. As a result, the bone marrow dramatically increases its production of red blood cells in an effort to keep pace with the rate of destruction. Because the rate of production cannot keep pace with the rate of destruction, individuals with sickle cell disease can become severely anemic (**sickle cell anemia**).

The specific causes of sickle cell crisis are unknown; however, certain factors—such as heavy exertional stress, mental stress, infection, dehydration, high altitudes, or extremes in temperature—may precipitate a crisis (Dorman, 2005). During vaso-occlusive crisis, the affected body part does not receive adequate oxygen, resulting in intense pain. If blood flow is severely diminished, the affected tissue may undergo **necrosis** (tissue death). Any part of the body, including any organs, may

be affected; the resulting damage may range from mild to severe, depending on the degree of blockage and the length of time the blockage exists.

Pain is the hallmark of vaso-occlusive events. When blood, and consequently oxygen, is unable to reach a body part, severe pain is the result. These painful episodes occur frequently, on an unpredictable schedule. Although all body parts may be affected, the hands and feet, back, legs, knees, and chest are common sites of pain. The pain some individuals experience can be managed with oral analgesics; in other cases, it becomes severe enough to warrant hospitalization and administration of narcotics and intravenous hydration therapy.

Individuals with sickle cell disease have lived with their chronic condition throughout life and consequently are frequently familiar with the types and dosages of medication required to relieve pain. Because pain intensity is difficult to assess by the outside observer, health professionals may interpret requests for specific pain medications and dosages as drug-seeking behavior. Consequently, pain in sickle cell disease is often undertreated by health professionals because of fear of addiction or perceived drug-seeking behavior (Dorman, 2005), despite the fact that the reported incidence of addiction in individuals with sickle cell disease is only 3% (Marlowe & Chicella, 2002). There is no evidence to suggest that individuals with sickle cell disease will become drug dependent owing to management of their pain with narcotics (Alao, Westmoreland, & Jindal, 2003).

Fatigue is a common manifestation of sickle cell disease owing to the decrease in the body's oxygen supply caused by the chronic anemia. Because fatigue is not a life-threatening manifestation of sickle cell disease, it often doesn't receive the same attention as other symptoms related to sickle cell disease. It can, however, affect individuals' functional capacity and interfere with both daily activities and work-related functioning. In addition to generalized fatigue, some individuals experience difficulty breathing on exertion (**exertional dyspnea**).

Complications of Sickle Cell Disease

Individuals with sickle cell disease are at high risk for damage to many organs (Wilson et al., 2003). Vaso-occlusive events, if severe and prolonged, can cause permanent and life-threatening consequences (Bridges, 2007; Assanasen, Quinton, & Buchanan, 2003; Gebreyohanns & Adams, 2004). This section describes a number of common complications of sickle cell disease.

Complications Related to Abdominal Organs

The spleen is frequently affected during sickle cell crisis and may be permanently damaged over time due to vaso-occlusive crisis. In some instances, *splenic sequestration crisis* may occur, in which there is acute, painful enlargement of the spleen so that the individual's abdomen becomes very bloated and hard. Splenic sequestration is an acute complication of sickle cell disease and can result in death if it isn't immediately recognized and treated. Individuals with severe spleen involvement may have a **splenectomy** (removal of the spleen) or may require chronic transfusion support.

Because the spleen is important in immune function, damage to or removal of this organ can cause increased risk of infection (Wilson et al., 2003; Kizito, Mworozi, Ndugwa, & Serjeant, 2007). In addition, the chronic anemia associated with sickle cell disease lowers resistance and increases individuals' susceptibility to infection.

Individuals with sickle cell disease may be placed on prophylactic antibiotics to decrease their chances of developing an infection that could precipitate sickle cell crisis. Immuniza-

tions, avoidance of contact with individuals with infectious conditions, good nutrition, and general health maintenance are extremely important to prevent infections from occurring in individuals with sickle cell disease.

Aplastic Crisis

Aplastic crisis refers to an acute and temporary worsening of the individual's anemia caused by an abrupt decrease of red blood cell production by the bone marrow. Because individuals with sickle cell disease already have decreased numbers of red blood cells by virtue of their condition, the decreased production of red blood cells in aplastic anemia can be a life-threatening event. Aplastic crisis may be triggered by an infection (Wilson, Krishnamurti, & Kamat, 2003). Recovery from aplastic crisis may be spontaneous or, in some instances, transfusion of red blood cells may be needed.

Pulmonary Complications

Acute chest syndrome is a condition characterized by fever, chest pain, and **dyspnea** (difficulty breathing). It is associated with many causes in sickle cell disease (Johnson, 2005), including pulmonary infection and vaso-occlusive events that involve the lungs. Approximately 30% of individuals with sickle cell disease develop acute chest syndrome, which can be a life-threatening event (Embury, 2004; Vichinsky, 2004). If the lungs are the site of repeated vaso-occlusive events or recurrent lung infections, pulmonary function may be compromised and individuals will experience related functional limitations. (See Chapter 14.)

Cardiac Complications

Chronic anemia associated with sickle cell disease causes the heart to pump faster in an attempt to supply additional oxygen to the tissues (Weiss & Goodnough, 2005). Increased heart action can contribute to enlargement of the heart (**cardiomegaly**) and decreased cardiac efficiency. If vessels of the heart become occluded during vaso-occlusive crisis, permanent damage to the heart muscle (**myocardial infarction**) may result (see Chapter 13).

Neurological Complications

Occlusion of vessels in the brain can result in a stroke and resulting limitations such as **dysphagia** (difficulty swallowing), **dysarthria** (difficulty in coordination and accuracy of muscles, lips, tongue, or other parts of the speech mechanism), **aphasia** (inability to comprehend or use language), **hemiparesis** (paralysis on one side of the body), and other consequences of stroke (see Chapter 3). Stroke occurs in approximately 10% of individuals with sickle cell disease (Wilson et al., 2003) and, in addition to causing permanent neurological damage, can result in death (Adams & Brambilla, 2005; Pratt, 2005).

Skeletal Complications

Occlusion of blood flow during a sickle cell crisis can result in *osteonecrosis* (bone death) and consequent damage to the bones and joints, especially those that are weight bearing, leading to pain, swelling, and limited mobility of joints and resulting deformity and decreased mobility (see Chapter 16).

Occular Complications

Increased blood **viscosity** (thickness) may cause sickle cell **retinopathy** (damage to the retina of the eye), resulting in diminished vision and possibly retinal detachment (see Chapter 5).

Kidney Complications

Sickle cell disease can cause **hematuria** (blood in the urine). In addition, vaso-occlusion can cause severe kidney damage, which then results in chronic kidney failure (see Chapter 15).

Genital Complications

A condition called priapism may occur in males who have sickle cell disease. *Priapism* is a sustained, unwanted erection. The condition requires immediate medical attention to prevent permanent nerve damage and consequent impotence.

Dermatologic Complications

Some individuals develop leg ulcers because of the interruption of circulation during sickle cell crisis. Ulcers may not heal and may become infected, leading to systemic infection. Because leg ulcers are frequently resistant to healing, individuals may need to be on bed rest to facilitate healing of the ulcers.

Complications Related to Growth and Development

There may be varying physical limitations from sickle cell disease at each developmental stage (Westerdale & Jegede, 2004). The growth and development of individuals with sickle cell anemia are significantly impaired, although the exact way the disease contributes to delayed growth is still unclear. Although there is delay in physical and sexual maturation, individuals do eventually reach full maturity (Embury, 2004).

Diagnosis of Sickle Cell Disease

Routine infant screening for sickle cell disease is now required in many states so that early diagnosis and management are possible. Definitive diagnosis of sickle cell disease or sickle cell trait is based on a blood test called *hemoglobin electrophoresis*. If initial blood tests appear to be irregular, confirmatory blood tests are performed.

Management of Sickle Cell Disease

Sickle cell disease is a chronic, lifelong condition. Management is directed toward controlling symptoms and preventing complications. The life expectancy of individuals with sickle cell anemia has increased dramatically in recent years thanks to early detection of complications and improved management of the condition (McKerrel, Cohen, & Billett, 2004).

Individuals with sickle cell disease and their families should be educated about the genetics of sickle cell disease as well as the importance of regular health maintenance, and the importance of seeking prompt medical evaluation for any infection or other acute illness should be emphasized. Although health maintenance is important to all individuals, it is especially important to individuals with sickle cell disease so as to prevent sickle cell crisis. Individuals should have regular, scheduled medical evaluations to monitor the course of their condition and to evaluate the effectiveness of the management plan.

In addition, individuals should be aware of factors that can precipitate a crisis so they can take steps to avoid a crisis from occurring. Triggers such as dehydration, infection, high altitudes, strenuous exercise, or extreme hot or cold weather can all precipitate a crisis (Dorman, 2005).

Good nutrition is essential to combat anemia and to maintain the body's resistance to infection. Because of the propensity of those who have sickle cell disease to develop infections, routine immunizations, including administration of pneumonia vaccines, are crucial. Prophylactic antibiotics are often given as well.

Maintaining adequate fluid intake is also important for individuals with sickle cell disease. Adequate hydration can minimize the sickling of red blood cells and decrease blood viscosity. Adequate hydration is especially important in situations in which individuals may be exposed to high environmental temperatures.

Anemia associated with sickle cell disease may necessitate transfusion therapy. One medication used to treat cancer, *hydroxyurea*,

has recently been tested for use in the management of sickle cell disease and has been found to prevent sickling of red blood cells in some individuals (Lewing & Woods, 2000). Other therapies include the use of antisickling agents and bone marrow transplantation.

Individuals who experience sickle cell crisis usually require hospitalization. During the crisis, management focuses on restoring fluids if dehydration has occurred and relieving pain associated with the crisis, usually through administration of narcotics. Adequate pain management is a crucial part of management of sickle cell crisis. Pain in individuals with sickle cell disease is often undertreated owing to concerns about narcotic addiction or suspicion of drug-seeking behavior, even though the incidence of addiction in individuals with sickle cell disease is relatively low (Dorman, 2005). Individuals may continue to experience residual pain after leaving the hospital.

If significant organ or bone damage has occurred as a result of the crisis, individuals may need referral to a pain clinic to help them learn how to manage chronic pain. If infection or another condition precipitated the crisis, interventions directed toward treating the underlying condition are instituted. Organ damage as a result of sickle cell disease is managed in a similar fashion to management of organ damage that may be present in other chronic conditions, such as chronic kidney disease (see Chapter 15) and chronic lung disease (see Chapter 14).

Bone marrow transplant and gene therapies offer hope for cure of sickle cell disease. As yet, however, the procedures are not readily available to all individuals with the condition. When the procedures are available, they are most often applied to children (Embury, 2004).

Prognosis

The prognosis of individuals with sickle cell disease depends on the individual and the degree of organ damage experienced. In the past, many individuals with sickle cell disease did not live to adulthood; over the past few decades, however, both mortality and morbidity have declined thanks to early detection and management of the disease. Consequently, the life expectancy of individuals with sickle cell disease has increased significantly and now averages 42 years for males and 48 years for females (Barakat, Lutz, Smith-Whitley, & Ohene-Frempong, 2005; McKerrel et al., 2004).

Psychosocial Issues in Sickle Cell Disease

Sickle cell disease usually manifests itself in childhood, necessitating medical attention and, possibly, frequent hospitalizations. Although many individuals with sickle cell disease adjust and cope with their condition, factors related to their condition may disrupt social development and educational progress in other individuals. Psychological coping patterns are relevant both to the experience of pain and to broader adjustment issues (Lutz, 2004). Prolonged periods of hospitalization or illness during childhood can lead to social deprivation, deficit of interpersonal skills, or delayed academic progress (Edwards, Scales, Loughlin, Bennett, Harris-Peterson, et al., 2005).

Transition for any adolescent may be challenging due to disruption of previously established relationships or other life changes as youth move from a more protected environment into the adult world. For adolescents with sickle cell disease, prolonged illness and hospitalization may disrupt the formation of sense of self and contribute to difficulty in forming substantive peer relationships. Adherence to a prescribed therapeutic regimen to prevent crisis or complications, such as drinking recommended daily quantities of water or taking prophylactic penicillin may be especially difficult and require significant support (While & Mullen, 2004). Adolescents may be reluctant to disclose their condition to avoid the marginalization they may associate with their condition or to avoid being seen as "different" by their peers.

Many adults with sickle cell disease have learned to manage their condition and cope with factors related to it. Adults who do experience poor psychosocial adjustment, however, have been found to have increased incidence of depression, employment difficulties, and psychiatric symptoms (Edwards et al., 2005).

Because sickle cell disease is hereditary, parents of children with sickle cell disease may experience guilt or fear the loss of their child. As a result, they may become overly protective, promoting dependence in the child. At the same time, the child may learn manipulative behaviors to gain attention. These maladaptive means of coping may persist throughout life, creating a greater barrier to social relationships and work than does the condition itself.

Sickle cell disease carries the additional stress of unpredictability. Although some factors that provoke a sickle cell crisis may be identifiable, crises are often unpredictable and beyond the individual's control. Not only are the crises painful and debilitating, but there is also the potential for organ damage each time a crisis occurs. Lack of control over the frequency or severity of sickle cell crises and not knowing the extent of damage that each crisis may inflict can lead to feelings of hopelessness and depression.

Activities and Participation

Individuals with sickle cell disease can usually maintain regular schedules and do not need to alter their activities, unless specific activities are found to precipitate a sickle cell crisis. Most activities, if performed in moderation, can be tolerated. Owing to the unpredictability of sickle cell crisis, however, sometimes a crisis may necessitate unplanned hospitalization, disrupting work schedules and interfering with participation in social events. The role of stress as a precipitating factor in sickle cell crisis must also be considered. Although stress is frequently associated with negative events, it can also be associated with positive events, such as a graduation celebration or a wedding.

Sickle cell disease affects the entire family. Individuals with sickle cell disease may require significant attention, which may create tension and anxiety. How the family members react to the individual and the degree of support they provide will greatly influence the individual's self-concept and development of social skills.

Vocational Issues in Sickle Cell Disease

Individuals with sickle cell disease often have a lifelong pattern of disruption caused by repeated hospitalizations, which may in turn have affected their academic achievement, job training opportunities, and acquisition of job skills. The degree of physical consequences individuals experience as a result of sickle cell disease depends on whether organ damage has been experienced. If specific organ or joint damage has been inflicted as a result of repeated sickle cell crises, the individual will have many of the same limitations as individuals who have similar conditions for other reasons. Problems with ambulation, vision, or neurological function can occur if damage to specific areas of the body has occurred, for example. Without organ damage, the physical consequences of the disease will affect the individual's capacity for exertion and strenuous activity. Individuals with sickle cell disease must consider not only the physical demands of a job as related to stamina, but also the role that strenuous exertion has in precipitating sickle cell crisis. Because sickle cell disease is a lifelong condition, over the years most individuals learn which types of activities and how much activity they can usually tolerate.

Despite the potential relationship between overexertion and sickle cell crisis, most individuals with sickle cell disease are able to perform moderate work. In instances where individuals with sickle cell disease experience fatigue and chronic pain, a realistic vocational goal may be part-time employment or a more sedentary type of work. Environmental factors such as extremes of temperature, high altitudes, and potential for exposure to infection should also be avoided. Because dehydration can precipitate a crisis, individuals should have ready access to water or other fluids in their work environment. Likewise, because of their increased fluid intake and consequently high urine output, access to restrooms is also required.

Stress in the work environment, including its contribution to the development of sickle cell crisis, is another factor individuals with sickle cell disease must consider. Not all individuals react to stress in the same way, nor are perceptions of stress always the same. Consequently, the importance of stress must be determined on an individual basis. The degree to which absences due to sickle cell crises become a hindrance to work performance depends on the individual, the frequency of such crises, and the seriousness of the crises when they occur.

The potential for sickle cell crisis and subsequent absences from work should be considered and discussed with employers in advance. Individuals may be reluctant to reveal their condition to the employer because of fear that repeated absences may jeopardize employment. Nevertheless, adequate preparation of employers in advance for potential absences can alleviate problems if absences do occur.

Psychosocial factors and their impact on vocational function cannot be dismissed. The unpredictability of the condition and the continued potential for sudden death as the result of sickle cell crisis may precipitate depression and affect motivation to seek work. If the individual has not developed adequate social skills, social skills training may be needed.

■ CONDITIONS AFFECTING THE IMMUNE SYSTEM

Cells carry specific protein markers to ensure that the body recognizes its own tissue as self and not foreign. Sometimes, however, the immune system becomes unable to recognize the body's own tissues and begins to produce antibodies and T cells that attack the body's own cells. When the immune system directs a response to attack the body's own cells as if they were foreign substances, individuals are said to have an *autoimmune condition*. Examples of autoimmune conditions are systemic *lupus erythematosus* and **rheumatoid arthritis** (see Chapter 16).

A variety of other conditions can alter the body's immune response and leave individuals more susceptible to developing a number of other conditions. Individuals receiving an organ transplant must have their immune system suppressed to prevent rejection of the donor tissue. As a result, they are more prone to infections. Individuals with certain types of cancers, such as lymphoma and leukemia (see Chapter 18), may become *immunodeficient* and develop serious infections. In addition, management of cancer with chemotherapy or radiation therapy may weaken the immune system. Individuals who overuse or abuse narcotics or steroid drugs can also alter the immune response, leaving them more prone to infections. Although there are a number of other conditions in which immunodeficiency is the key characteristic, the most widely known condition affecting immunity is HIV infection.

Human Immunodeficiency Virus Infection

Not all viruses are harmful to humans, although some viruses can cause illness. Conditions that result from viruses range from the common cold and common childhood illness to more serious conditions, such as poliomyelitis and *acquired immune deficiency syndrome* (AIDS).

A virus can be defined as an infectious organism that cannot grow or reproduce outside living cells. To survive, it must enter a living cell and use the reproductive capacity of that cell for its own replication. Consequently, when a virus enters a cell, it instructs the cell to reproduce the virus. Usually, the body recognizes viruses as foreign and activates the immune system to attack and destroy the offending agent.

Of those viruses that are not destroyed, some remain inactive (**dormant**) for long periods without causing problems; however, they remain integrated within the genetic material of the cell and are capable of replicating when triggered to do so. The direct damage the virus does to the cell itself may vary from slight to total destruction. Some cells are able to reproduce after being damaged, but others—especially the cells of the nervous system—are not able to reproduce and, consequently, are not replaced after invasion by a virus.

HIV infection is caused by a retrovirus called human immunodeficiency virus (HIV). A retrovirus uses a complicated process called *reverse transcription* to reproduce itself. This process uses a viral enzyme called *reverse transcriptase* to integrate the virus's genetic material into the genetic material of other cells. In so doing, HIV essentially takes over these cells—primarily the CD4 cells—to produce more HIV. The virus multiplies extremely rapidly, and errors that are caused by this rapid generation of cells are not corrected, so there are constant mutations of the virus. Some of the cells containing the virus burst, releasing HIV directly into the blood. Consequently, there can be both infected cells and virus in the blood traveling to other sites. This characteristic of the virus— that is, its rapid generation and the constant mutations—makes it very hard for the body to kill HIV. It also explains why the virus rapidly becomes resistant to medications that are used to kill it.

There are two viruses that cause HIV infection: HIV-1 and HIV-2. HIV-1 is the most common and is responsible for most cases of HIV infection (Kilby & Eron, 2003). HIV-2 is confined largely to western Africa (Shaw, 2004).

HIV destroys a subset of helper T cells (CD4+) and impairs the cells' ability to recognize antigens. As a result, there is profound deterioration of the immune system so that the body has no defense against even the least aggressive organism. The virus reproduces within the T cell itself, producing additional HIV, which in turn invades other T cells. Over time, the 2:1 ratio of helper cells to suppressor cells becomes reversed. The increased number of suppressor cells severely limits B-cell function, so that the B cells fail to respond to new antigens. In this way, the immune response becomes dysfunctional.

Most individuals with HIV infection exhibit no symptoms until the later stages of the condition. AIDS is the final stage of HIV infection and is characterized by symptoms of severe failure of the immune system.

Transmission of HIV

When a person is infected with HIV, the virus is found in the blood as well as in body secretions such as sperm. Transmission can occur in a variety of ways:

- Infusion of infected blood or blood products
- Accidental stick with an infected needle
- Intravenous drug use and sharing of equipment
- Anal, oral, or genital intercourse
- Contact with a cut or open wound on the skin
- Fetal transmission from a woman with HIV infection to her unborn child

- Transmission of HIV from mother to infant through breast milk (Steinbrook, 2004)

There is no evidence that transmission can occur in any way other than direct blood-to-blood or sexual contact with an infected individual. For example, the virus does not appear to be transmitted through coughing, sneezing, or casual contact. Moreover, because all viruses require living tissue to survive and multiply, the virus dies quickly once outside the body.

Education is an important component of preventing HIV transmission. A large percentage of individuals are unaware of their HIV infection until symptoms appear in the later stages of the condition (Paltiel, Weinstein, Kimmel, Seage, Losina, Zhang, Freedberg, & Walensky, 2005). Early identification can help reduce transmission of HIV through changes in risk behavior as well as provide opportunity for early intervention, which can help delay progression of the condition (Sanders, Bayoumi, Sundaram, Bilir, Neukermans, et al., 2005). In the United States, HIV infection is often not diagnosed until it is at the advanced stage (Bozzette, 2005), so many individuals affected may not take precautions to prevent transmission.

Scientists continue to work on developing an effective vaccine against HIV. Although enormous progress has been made in our understanding of HIV, the unique characteristics of this virus continue to pose challenges and obstacles to vaccine development (Johnston & Fauci, 2007; Saag, 2004).

Diagnosis of HIV/AIDS

Serological status of individuals is required to implement appropriate interventions, including management of HIV/AIDS, notification and testing of partners, and education of individuals and family members about methods of preventing transmission of HIV. Knowledge of HIV status has been associated with reduction in high-risk behaviors and subsequent decrease in risk of transmission (De Cock, Bunnell, & Mermin, 2006).

The procedures most commonly used to diagnose HIV infection are blood tests that identify not the virus itself but rather the presence of antibodies that the body has produced against the virus. The enzyme immunoassay (*EIA*), which is a blood test, is usually performed first. It contains antigens of HIV. If the EIA test is positive, it is repeated, in duplicate. If the EIA tests are positive, the results are then confirmed by using another procedure, the *Western blot*. A positive Western blot confirms the diagnosis of HIV infection. AIDS is usually diagnosed when HIV is present and the individual has developed an opportunistic infection and/or has a CD4 cell count that has fallen below a certain level.

Because most individuals with HIV in the United States do not receive testing for this infection until they become symptomatic, CDC has issued new recommendations that would integrate screening into routine healthcare services, include testing of all pregnant women unless they request not to be tested, and annually screen those individuals at high risk (Bayer & Fairchild, 2006; Wright & Katz, 2006). In an attempt to minimize barriers to testing for HIV, rapid tests that use a finger stick or salivary testing, with results becoming available in 20 to 40 minutes, have been approved by the FDA (Wright & Katz, 2006). Whether these rapid tests should be made available to consumers for home use has been widely debated. Concerns over misuse or misinterpretation of test results, the consequences of false positives or false negatives, and the subsequent costs are all currently issues under scrutiny.

Phases of HIV/AIDS

Infection with HIV can be separated into several phases, although there are no firm guidelines that distinguish the different phases. During the early or acute phase, symptoms may be subtle or nonexistent. Initially, some individuals may experience mild flu-like symptoms that subside, leaving them symptom free, although the virus is still transmissible to others. Although most complications of HIV occur in the later phase, some reports indicate that neurological symptoms such as **ataxia** (impairment in muscle coordination), **meningitis** (inflammation of the membrane covering the brain and spinal cord), and other nervous system manifestations may occur with early HIV infection (Price, 2004).

As the HIV infection progresses, levels of circulating virus increase. At the same time, there is a decline in the number of CD4+ T-lymphocyte cells. Given that the risk of HIV-related complications correlates strongly with absolute CD4 count and percentage of CD4+ lymphocytes, it is generally recommended that individuals have a blood test to determine this number at the time of diagnosis and then every three to four months thereafter, in conjunction with measurement of viral load (Sax & Walker, 2004). As the condition progresses, infected individuals may experience some or all of the following symptoms:

- Weight loss of 10 or more pounds in less than two months for no apparent reason
- Loss of appetite
- Unexplained persistent fever
- Drenching night sweats
- Severe fatigue that is unrelated to exercise, stress, or drug use
- Persistent diarrhea
- Swollen lymph nodes (**lymphadenopathy**)
- As the CD4 cell count declines, the individual's resistance to infectious organisms decreases until the count falls below a critical level, making the individual susceptible to infections that individuals without compromised immunity are able to fight off easily. Generally when the CD4 count falls below 200, the individual is classified as having advanced HIV or AIDS (Sax & Walker, 2004).

Symptoms of Advanced HIV and AIDS

Infection with HIV affects all body systems. Consequently, symptoms and complications of advanced HIV can affect all body systems both in terms of function and in terms of susceptibility to opportunistic infection and malignancy. An **opportunistic infection** is one that would not occur in individuals with immune system function. Many organisms commonly found in the environment pose no threat under usual circumstances, because the functioning immune system resists them. When individuals have HIV infection, however, the immune system is no longer able to act as a defense and there is no resistance to these organisms. Without this protection from the immune system, individuals are left susceptible to developing opportunistic conditions and infections that under usual circumstances would not become full-blown. In fact, death from AIDS is not caused by the dysfunction of the immune system per se, but rather by complications of conditions that develop because of inadequate immune system function. Common complications associated with advanced HIV are described next.

Neurologic Complications

Many individuals with HIV infection develop neurological symptoms. HIV invades the central nervous system early in the development of the condition, causing a variety of neurological conditions during the course of the illness. One neurologic condition frequently associated with HIV infection is a type of dementia called AIDS *dementia complex*. Approximately 20% to 30% of individuals with AIDS develop AIDS dementia complex, which may include cognitive decline, poor concentration, or forgetfulness (Dave & Pomerantz, 2005). As the symptoms progress individuals' motor, bowel, and bladder function may also be affected (Price, 2004).

Opportunistic infections of the nervous system in late HIV infection may include encephalitis (inflammation of the brain) or **meningitis** (encephalitis of the membranes surrounding the brain or spinal cord). Individuals may also be more prone to develop opportunistic **neoplasms** (tumors) of the brain.

Other nervous system manifestations may consist of headache, seizures, or **peripheral neuropathy** (a condition involving the peripheral nerves). Individuals with peripheral neuropathy may experience symptoms ranging from numbness of extremities to burning of the feet and legs, progressing to severe pain. Individuals may develop **ataxia** (impairment in muscle coordination), spasticity, and bladder and bowel difficulty as a result of nervous system involvement as well.

Dermatologic Complications

Skin complications associated with advanced HIV may include infections such as *herpes zoster*, inflammatory conditions such as **psoriasis** (see Chapter 17), or a rare form of cancer called *Kaposi's sarcoma*. Kaposi's sarcoma—an opportunistic type of cancer that is not usually seen in individuals with healthy immune systems—is characterized by pink, brown, or purplish blotches on the skin.

Pulmonary Complications

Respiratory complications are common in individuals with advanced HIV infections. One opportunistic infection of the lungs often associated with advanced HIV infection is *Pneumocystis carinii* pneumonia (Thomas & Limper, 2004). This parasitic infection of the lung is highly uncommon in healthy individuals, although it may be found in other immunocompromised individuals, such as in those who have cancer or those who have received immunosuppressants in association with organ transplantation. Symptoms usually begin with a dry cough and **dyspnea** (difficulty in breathing).

Other pulmonary complications include other types of pneumonia, tuberculosis, or chronic obstructive pulmonary disease (see Chapter 14). Tuberculosis is often fatal in people with AIDS (Sepkowitz, 2006). A major issue facing individuals with tuberculosis is the increasing incidence of drug-resistant tuberculosis (Kim & Farmer, 2006).

Cardiac Complications

HIV-related heart disease, including **pericarditis** (inflammation of the outer lining of the heart), *myocarditis* (inflammation of the heart muscle), or *endocarditis* (inflammation of the inner lining of the heart), may result from an opportunistic infection or malignancy (Saag, 2004) (see Chapter 13). In addition, interventions using antiretroviral drugs may cause a modest increase in the individual's risk of cardiac conditions such as **myocardial infarction** (heart attack).

Gastrointestinal Complications

The opportunistic infection **candidiasis** (yeast infection) occurs in about 80% to 90% of all individuals with advanced-stage HIV (Bartlett, 2004). The fungus *Candida* frequently invades the oral cavity of HIV-infected individuals, causing a superficial infection in the mouth and throat, which is manifested by pain and white plaques. This condition, known as *oral thrush*, may be the first clue that an individual is infected with HIV even though he or she is in the advanced phase of this disease. Although candidiasis is uncomfortable and difficult to cure, infection with *Candida* is not likely to be fatal. Individuals with debilitating conditions other than HIV infections may also develop candidiasis.

Individuals with advanced HIV may develop **esophagitis** (inflammation of the esophagus) and consequent *dysphagia* (difficulty swallowing). Other gastrointestinal problems may arise as a reaction to some of the medications used to treat HIV. Acute or chronic diarrhea occurs frequently in individuals with HIV infection and may be caused by medications or by an opportunistic infection. A variety of tumors may also develop in the gastrointestinal tract as a result of HIV infection. Hepatitis C and hepatitis B (see Chapter 12) are both common in individuals with HIV infection (Koziel & Peters, 2007). As a result, HIV-infected individuals are at risk for developing liver damage and/or cancer of the liver, which can result in death (Merchante, Giron-Gonzalez, Gonzalez-Serrano, Torre-Cisneros, Garcia-Garcia, Arizcorreta, et al., 2006; Pineda & Macias, 2005).

Most individuals in the late phase of HIV infection lose 15% to 20% of their body weight (Bartlett, 2004). This weight loss is a result of not only the condition itself (wasting due to metabolic changes associated with condition), but also difficulty eating or swallowing because of oral thrush or other gastrointestinal infection, side effects of medications used for treating HIV, or depression. As individuals lose weight and become increasingly malnourished, their susceptibility to opportunistic infection increases.

Ophthalmologic Complications

Complications affecting the eye may be infectious or non-infectious and can lead to severe visual impairment. Individuals may experience small hemorrhages of the retina or may develop **retitinis** (inflammation of the retina), which can predispose them to retinal detachment (see Chapter 5).

Kidney Complications

Individuals with HIV infection may experience kidney conditions of a variety of forms, ranging from increased incidence of *renal calculi* (kidney stones) to acute renal failure (see Chapter 15). Some dysfunction of the kidney, which occurs with HIV infection, may be associated with the medications used to treat the condition, while other problems may be related to opportunistic infection. In other instances, HIV-associated *nephropathy* (disease of the kidney) is caused by the direct effect of the HIV on the kidney.

Musculoskeletal Complications

A variety of symptoms relating to the musculoskeletal system may be present in individuals with HIV. These symptoms range from **arthralgias** (painful joints) to severe and debilitating arthritis (see Chapter 16). In addition, individuals may experience muscle weakness or muscle wasting.

Management of HIV/AIDS

Approximately 40,000 new cases of HIV infection occur each year (Wright & Katz, 2006), and 40 million people worldwide are now living with HIV (Assan & Kraszewski, 2006). Currently, there is no means of restoring damaged immune function and hence no cure for the disease. Advances in the medical management of HIV infection have, however, improved the life expectancy of individuals living with HIV (Scosyrev, 2006; Sackoff, Hanna, Pfeiffer, & Torian, 2006). Since 1995, the number of deaths from AIDS in the United States has declined so significantly that HIV/AIDS is no longer treated as a terminal illness but rather as a chronic condition to be managed (Oursler, Goulet, Leaf, Akingicil, Katzel, Justice, & Crystal, 2006; Zetola & Klausner, 2006; Merson, 2006; Frieden, Das-Douglas, Kellerman, & Henning, 2005).

Antiretroviral therapy (ART) is the mainstay of management of HIV/AIDS (Masur, 2004). Management with antiretroviral drugs is directed toward maintaining the individual's CD4 cell count and lowering the viral load (Hammer, 2005). Initially single drugs, such as *zidovudine*, slowed the progression of HIV and decreased the incidence of opportunistic infections. Although zidovudine was effective initially, after 6 to18 months the virus became resistant to it. *Viral loads* (the amount of virus present) again increased, and individuals once again became susceptible to opportunistic infections (Masur, 2004).

As newer drugs were developed, it was recognized that using combinations of drugs that acted on different parts of the virus replication cycle were more effective and longer lasting in preventing viral replication. The combination of these antiretroviral drugs called *highly active antiretroviral therapy* (**HAART**), has produced a remarkable effect in controlling progression of HIV and prolonging life expectancy of those affected (Clavel & Hance, 2004; Huang, Quartin, Jones, & Havlir, 2006). Antiretroviral drugs directly inhibit HIV by disrupting its replication cycle or by interrupting the ability of HIV to bind with other cells. Currently, four distinct classes of antiretroviral drugs exist, each of which attacks HIV in a different way. (See Table 10-2 for examples of medications included in each classification.) Using drugs from different classes has been found to control the development of resistance, which is discussed later in the chapter. HAART regimens generally consist of three or more antiretroviral drugs. To be effective, they must be taken daily for the rest of the individual's life.

Resistance to antiretroviral drugs, however, is a growing problem for individuals with HIV (Gilliam, Chan-Tack, Qaquish, Rode, Fantry, & Redfield, 2006; Haubrich, 2005; Gerberding, 2003). Although the virus may mutate spontaneously to produce drug resistance, the cost of medications, the number of drugs that need to be taken daily, and the possible toxicity of the drugs that causes intolerable side effects may contribute to an individual's lack of compliance with the medication regimen—which can also lead to drug-resistant viruses.

Typically, viral load and CD4 tests provide critical information that is used to make decisions about antiretroviral therapy. Goals of therapy are to reduce the viral load, preserve the immune system as much as possible, and reduce the side effects associated with the drug regimen to increase the individual's quality of life. To realize the maximum effectiveness of the drugs and protect against organism resistance to the medications, individuals must take medications correctly and consistently

Table 10-2 Classification and Action of Antiretroviral drugs	
Nucleoside/nucleotide reverse transcriptase inhibitors (NRTIs)	
	Zidovudine
	Stavudine
	Didanosine
Nucleotide analogue	
	Tenofovir
Non-nucleoside reverse transcriptase inhibitors (NNRTIs)	
	Nevirapine
	Efavirenz
	Delavirdine
Protease inhibitors (PI)	
	Saquinavir
	Ritonavir
	Indinavir
Fusion or entry inhibitors	
	Enfuvirtide

(Currier & Baden, 2006). Recent studies have indicated that episodic use of antiretroviral drugs can be deleterious (SMART Study Group, 2006).

Antiretroviral regimens are complicated and difficult for many individuals to follow. In addition, many of the medications used to treat HIV have serious side effects and dangerous drug toxicities (Lesho & Gey, 2003). Some antiretroviral drugs cause accumulation of body fat, as well as elevated cholesterol, triglyceride (Stein, 2007), and glucose levels (Tashima & Carpenter, 2003). **Hepatotoxicity** (destruction of the liver by an agent or chemical) can be a severe complication of some antiretroviral drugs, while others cause gastrointestinal distress such as **dyspepsia** (indigestion), nausea and vomiting, or diarrhea. Headache, severe skin rash, and bone demineralization with associated decrease in bone density may also be experienced as side effects of antiretroviral drugs.

HAART regimens in the management of HIV infection can be cumbersome as well as expensive, making the medications inaccessible to many individuals with HIV infection who are without insurance or who are underinsured. Newer antiviral drugs can cost as much as $20,000 per year, which is more than twice the cost of the next most expensive antiretroviral drug (Steinbrook, 2003). Although newer medications require fewer pills to be taken, some HAART regimens may require individuals to take more than 20 pills per day.

When HAART regimens are instituted, it is of paramount importance that individuals comply with the regime prescribed (Gallant et al., 2006). If the drugs are not taken correctly, they may lose their effectiveness. Although many of the newer antiretroviral drugs have no specific food requirements, some of the drugs still need to be taken on an empty stomach or their concentration may be significantly reduced. Other drugs require that the individual drink a certain amount of water every hour for three hours after each dose of medication to reduce the risk of kidney damage. Individuals on antiretroviral therapy may also be taking other medications that interact with the antiretroviral agent, thereby decreasing its effectiveness. For example, medications such as Dilantin for epilepsy can significantly decrease concentrations of antiretroviral drugs, lowering their effectiveness (Dybul, Fauci, Bartlett, Kaplan, & Pau, 2002).

In addition to medication, much of the management of HIV infection is geared toward supportive care and prevention of opportunistic infections. Individuals should have adequate rest, should engage in a program of moderate exercise, and should maintain adequate nutrition. Some studies suggest that taking multivitamin supplements may help to delay the progression of HIV (Fawzi, Msamanga, Spielgelman, Wei, Kapiga, Villamor, Mwakagile, Mugusi, Hertzmark, Essex, & Hunter, 2004). As the condition progresses, individuals may need to modify their exercise program and allow for more frequent rest periods to conserve energy. As much as possible, individuals with HIV infection should attempt to prevent opportunistic infection. In addition to maintaining good health practices, they should avoid crowds and people with known infections such as colds and flu. If they develop symptoms of infection, they should consult a physician immediately.

In the later stages of HIV infection, when opportunistic and/or neurologic symptoms occur, management is directed toward the specific infection or symptom manifestation. It is not unusual for individuals with later stages of HIV infection to experience a number of hospitalizations for acute opportunistic infections.

Individuals with HIV infection should take precautions not to transmit the virus. They should fully understand the importance of practicing safe sex; of informing sexual partners of their condition prior to sexual activity; and of not sharing needles, razors, toothbrushes, or any other item that could be contaminated with blood. Education and support are crucial interventions to reduce the risk of HIV transmission, as well as increasing individuals' willingness and ability to adhere to medication management guidelines (Okie, 2007; Balfour, Kowal, Silverman, Tasca, Angel, MacPherson, et al., 2006).

Psychosocial Issues in HIV/AIDS

Individuals who received a diagnosis of HIV infection are confronted with the knowledge they have a lifelong condition that can be incapacitating and life threatening, and that has no cure. As the condition progresses, they also may experience the stress of increasingly noxious symptoms, therapies with unpleasant side effects and potentially toxic medications, periods of physical manifestations, potential loss of employment, possible rejection by family or friends, and economic stress. In addition, they must cope with the knowledge that they may transmit HIV to intimate partners.

Psychological reactions to having HIV are diverse and often vary with the phase of the condition and with the individual's circumstances. Although many individuals with HIV show resilience to stress associated with HIV and adapt well, others experience severe emotional distress. Studies indicate that almost 48% of individuals with HIV infection report symptoms of depression, generalized anxiety, or panic disorder (Orlando, Burnam, Beckman, Morton, Longdon, et al., 2002). Other studies report that nearly 20% of individuals with HIV infection have a diagnosis of substance abuse or dependence (Pence, Gaynes, Whetten, Eron, Ryder, & Miller, 2005).

While depression, anxiety, or substance use may be the direct result of reaction to the stress associated with having HIV infection, psychiatric manifestations or substance abuse or dependence may have been preexisting conditions and may have contributed to the individual's exposure to HIV owing to increased vulnerability or lifestyle practices. Regardless of the nature of these co-occurring conditions, psychiatric or substance-related conditions have implications not only for quality of life, but also for effective management of HIV/AIDS. Because the major focus is often on management of HIV itself, psychiatric diagnosis or substance abuse/dependence issues may not be appropriately addressed or treated.

Stress occurs throughout the course of HIV infection. Uncertainty can be a major source of stress, for example, in HIV infection and can lead to anxiety or depression. It is impossible to predict when or how rapidly the infection will progress to the later phase. Following periods of being very unwell, individuals with HIV infection may then recover and experience periods of well-being, followed by development of another infection, placing them again in an illness state (Cochrane, 2003). Given this type of unpredictability, individuals may find it difficult to set goals for the future, or they may abandon personal aspirations.

Activities and Participation

The social stigma associated with HIV infection may also contribute to stress. This stigma may be based on misinformation about how HIV is transmitted, prejudicial attitudes about groups perceived to be linked to HIV transmission, or generalized fear or avoidance of individuals with chronic or perceived terminal illnesses. Misinformation about how HIV is transmitted can affect social interactions at school, at work, or in the general community. People may avoid individuals with HIV infection due to fear of exposure to HIV through even casual contact. As a result, individuals with HIV may find themselves socially isolated, which also contributes to depression.

Social prejudice regarding individuals with HIV infection may be related to perceptions of the individual's group affiliation. When HIV infection first emerged more than a quarter of

a century ago, those affected were frequently among already-stigmatized populations such as homosexual men, injection drug users, or immigrants from developing countries (Frieden et al., 2005). Although HIV infection exists in every segment of society, affected individuals may still be socially marginalized owing to preexisting prejudicial attitudes against some groups. Some segments of society may view HIV infection as retribution for behaviors they view as morally unacceptable. These social judgments may contribute to discriminatory behaviors toward and social ostracizing of individuals with HIV infection. Although public education about HIV and its modes of transmission has helped to change some attitudes of the general population, individuals with HIV infection still often bear the additional stress of the stigma and fear associated with the condition. The resulting feelings of rejection and abandonment by others may contribute to their feelings of depression and despair.

Individuals with HIV infection may also experience anger and resentment toward the society-imposed isolation that hampers HIV-infected individuals in their efforts to obtain social support and, at times, even the medical care afforded to individuals with other life-threatening conditions. Individuals who have become infected with HIV through interventions, such as blood transfusions, may experience additional anger at contracting the condition as "innocent victims." Those infected through contact with others may direct their anger against the individual or individuals from whom they contracted the condition.

If past behavior or lifestyle contributed to contracting HIV infection, individuals may experience guilt because of the fear that they have been the source of contagion to others and may experience guilt and self-incrimination. Self-blame and guilt can lead to self-destructive behaviors, including drug use or attempted suicide. For individuals whose families and friends had not been aware of their lifestyle, exposure may result in increased anxiety and, in some instances, abandonment. Individuals with HIV infection may be left with little social support at a time when they need it most. Support groups, although beneficial in many chronic conditions, are even more important for individuals with HIV infection.

Although physical function may decline as the HIV infection progresses, in most instances individuals living with this disease are able to continue most activities of daily living (Oursler, Goulet, Leaf, Akingicil, Katzel, Justice, et al., 2006). Individuals with HIV infection require a balance of periods of activity and rest to prevent over-fatigue. A moderate, regular program of exercise can help them maintain optimal emotional and physical health. As the condition progresses and stamina decreases, activities may need to be modified. Individuals in the later phase of HIV infection often need assistance with everyday activities, including at first housekeeping chores and later extending to personal care.

Vocational Issues

Maintaining vocational roles despite significant health issues is important in meeting individuals' emotional and economic needs (Conyers, 2005; Lynch Fesko, 2001). Work, in addition to meeting financial needs, is a source of social contact and offers a sense of belonging. With the advent of new therapies to treat HIV infection and the associated increase in life expectancy for some as a result, HIV-infected individuals may also gain a more positive outlook. Despite increased functional capacity and longevity, however, many individuals living with HIV/AIDS remain unemployed or lose their jobs (Glenn, Ford, Moore, & Hollar, 2003). Barriers to returning to or maintaining employment are numerous and require motivation and commitment to over-

come (Maticka-Tyndale, Adam, & Cohen, 2002).

Many factors—including psychosocial, financial, medical, and legal factors—may affect individuals' ability and willingness to maintain employment (Kohlenberg & Watts, 2003). Individuals are frequently confronted with conflicting pressures about whether they should continue to work (Nixon & Renwick, 2003). Contextual factors, such as disability and health insurance or drug plans, often influence individuals' decisions in this regard (Ferrier & Lavis, 2003).

For individuals with HIV infection, the most serious impediments to successful functioning in the workplace are the fear, discrimination, and prejudice that they encounter. Many HIV-positive individuals face discrimination at work and, as a result, may withdraw from the workplace altogether (Hunt, Jaques, Niles, & Wiezalis, 2003). Individuals with HIV infection frequently fear that they will lose their jobs as a result of their diagnosis, regardless of their continued mental and physical ability to work.

When HIV-infected individuals do maintain their employment, there are usually no special restrictions, especially in the early stages of the condition. Because of the mode of transmission of the virus, however, they should avoid occupations in which their blood may contaminate the blood of others. Because infection can have such serious consequences for individuals with HIV infection, they should also avoid job situations in which they are likely to be exposed to infection. As the HIV infection progresses and individuals experience increasing fatigue, they may need to undertake less strenuous work or arrange for shorter work schedules or more frequent rest periods. In the later stages of the condition, cognitive changes, motor incoordination, or other neurological complications associated with HIV may affect an individual's capacity to function in the work setting.

◼ DIAGNOSTIC PROCEDURES FOR CONDITIONS AFFECTING THE BLOOD OR IMMUNE SYSTEM

Standard Blood Tests

The diagnosis of many blood conditions is made through laboratory analysis of the blood itself. *A complete blood count (CBC)* is a test used to evaluate a number of different components in the blood. Sometimes various components measured in a complete blood count may also be measured separately. The components of a complete blood count include the following:

- *Red blood cell count*: measurement of the total number of red blood cells in one cubic millimeter of blood
- *White blood cell count*: measurement of the total number of white blood cells in one cubic millimeter of blood
- *Differential*: measurement of the proportion of each type of white blood cell (i.e., neutrophils, eosinophils, basophils, lymphocytes, monocytes) in a sample of 100 white blood cells
- *Hemoglobin*: evaluation of the amount of hemoglobin content in erythrocytes in 100 milliliters of blood
- *Hematocrit*: measurement of the percentage or proportion of red blood cells in the plasma; it is based on the assumption that the volume of plasma is within expected limits

Other types of blood tests used to measure specific components of blood are as follows:

- *Reticulocyte count*: assessment of bone marrow function by measuring its production of immature red blood cells (**reticulocytes**)
- *Platelet count:* measurement of the number of platelets in one cubic millimeter of blood
- *Mean corpuscular volume (MCV)*: calculation of the volume of a single red blood cell; found by dividing the hematocrit by the red blood cell count
- *Mean corpuscular hemoglobin concentration*: calculation of the amount of hemoglobin in each red blood cell; found by dividing the hemoglobin concentration by the hematocrit

Bleeding Time

Bleeding time is a test that measures the length of time it takes for bleeding to stop after a small puncture wound; it determines how quickly a platelet clot forms. An extended bleeding time would indicate a tendency toward prolonged bleeding such as that found in conditions in which there is a low number of platelets circulating in the blood.

Prothrombin Time

Prothrombin time (PT, pro time) is a blood test that measures the length of time that a blood sample takes to clot when certain chemicals are added to it in the laboratory. It tests for very specific factors involved in clotting and may be used diagnostically to identify pathologic clotting conditions, such as may be found with liver dysfunction or in the absence of vitamin K. The PT test may also be used to monitor the effectiveness of certain anticoagulant medications, which are used in the management of conditions in which clot formation is or has been a problem. Prolongation of clotting time indicates that individuals may be prone to bleeding. If the test indicates that clotting time is reduced, there may be hypercoagulability of blood, contributing to the formation of blood clots.

Partial Thromboplastin Time

Partial thromboplastin time (PTT) is a blood test that is used to evaluate a special part of the clotting mechanism not evaluated by prothrombin time. As in the prothrombin time test, chemicals are added to a blood sample in the laboratory and the amount of time it takes a clot to form is measured. Prolongation of the time in which it takes a clot to form is indicative of a bleeding condition, such as that found in hemophilia. Prolongation of clot formation may also be found with the use of the anticoagulant heparin, which affects a specific part of the clotting mechanism that is not measured by the prothrombin time test.

Bone Marrow Aspiration

Bone marrow aspiration involves removal of a sample of bone marrow by inserting a special needle into the marrow space of the bone and then aspirating a small sample. The bone marrow is then examined microscopically for irregularities in the number, size, and shape of the precursors of red blood cells, white blood cells, and platelets.

Enzyme Immunoassay (EIA) and Western Blot

Both the EIA and Western blot are blood tests for antibodies to HIV antigens. If the initial screening with the EIA produces positive results, the test is again performed in duplicate. If the results of the second test are negative, the test result is considered negative. If the results of the second round of EIA tests are positive, the Western blot is usually performed as a confirmatory test. If the result of the Western blot is positive, it confirms that the HIV antibody is present and that the individual has been exposed to HIV.

Hemoglobin Electrophoresis

Hemoglobin electophoresis is a blood test used to make a definitive diagnosis of sickle cell disease or sickle cell trait.

HIV Viral Load Assay

The viral load assay is a blood test that measures the amount of circulating HIV per unit of blood.

Sickle Cell Prep

Sickle cell prep is a blood test used in sickle cell screening. It can detect the presence of irregular hemoglobin but cannot distinguish between sickle cell disease and sickle cell trait.

■ GENERAL MANAGEMENT OF CONDITIONS AFFECTING THE BLOOD OR IMMUNE SYSTEM

For many conditions of the blood, management is directed toward alleviating symptoms and/or eliminating the underlying cause. If a blood condition is caused by a toxic substance, the first line of management is to remove the offending agent. Anemia that is caused by a deficiency may be treated by supplementation or replacement therapy. For instance, iron-deficiency anemia may be treated by the administration of oral or injectable iron preparations. Pernicious anemia may be treated with injections of vitamin B_{12}. When there is an overproduction of red blood cells, as in polycythemia, management may involve the removal of blood; venesection (**phlebotomy**) is a procedure in which quantities of blood are removed to reduce the volume.

Transfusion

Part of the management for a number of blood conditions may consist of transfusion of whole blood or a blood component, such as packed red blood cells, plasma, or platelets. Because blood is living tissue, transfusion can be thought of as a form of transplantation, carrying the same risks of immune response as do other types of transplantation. For this reason, the exact matching of a number of factors in the blood between the donor and the recipient is crucial to prevent serious allergic reactions, which could prove fatal. In addition to the risk of such a reaction, there is a risk that a blood transfusion will transmit an infectious condition such as hepatitis or HIV, although careful screening of blood by blood banks has significantly reduced this risk.

Bone Marrow Transplant

Bone marrow transplant is a procedure in which individuals' bone marrow is eradicated and healthy bone marrow is inserted to replace it. Bone marrow transplants are used when the immune system is severely deficient or for conditions such cancers (see Chapter 18), sickle cell anemia, or thalassemia. Bone marrow cells are obtained from a donor who is carefully matched with the recipient to decrease the chances of rejection of the transplant, as well as to prevent a reaction in which the transplanted cells attack the cells of the individual who has received the transplant.

■ PSYCHOSOCIAL ISSUES IN CONDITIONS AFFECTING THE BLOOD OR IMMUNE SYSTEM

Psychological Issues

Conditions of the blood and immune system have a variety of psychological implications. The specific implications for a particular individual depend on the condition. Some conditions may be controlled relatively easily, whereas others may require constant vigilance. Although some conditions may be treated and, in some instances, cured, others require lifelong management and carry a more ominous prognosis.

Individuals with conditions affecting the blood and immune system generally have no visible reminders of their condition. Without external adaptive devices, such as wheelchairs, crutches, or canes, or any other signs of disability, individuals may react by denying the seriousness of their condition and resist medical directives. For example, individuals with hemophilia may engage in risk-taking behaviors, even though injury and subsequent bleeding could occur. Individuals with sickle cell anemia may engage in a flurry of activity, even though the associated stress and fatigue may precipitate a sickle cell crisis. Individuals with HIV infection may withhold their diagnosis from others with whom they engage in sexual

activity, even though their behavior could put their partners at risk.

Some blood- and immune-related conditions occur later in life, necessitating adjustment at the time the condition and any associated limitation occurs. Conditions such as sickle cell anemia and hemophilia are lifelong, however. Consequently, individuals with these conditions have coped with their condition in one way or another from childhood into adulthood. Most individuals with either sickle cell anemia or hemophilia experience frequent illness and medical care throughout their childhood and adolescence. Although these experiences can build confidence in the ability to cope with adversity, they may also have a negative impact on development. Individuals may carry the coping behaviors and attitudes learned in childhood into the adult years, where they continue to affect the individuals' perceptions of themselves, their condition, and their abilities. Depending on the constructiveness of the coping strategy used, such behaviors may be either an asset or a hindrance.

The possibility of early death—a source of anxiety and depression for those with any chronic condition—is a reality for individuals with hemophilia, sickle cell anemia, and HIV infection. Although hemophilia can be controlled to some degree, there is always the fear that an accident or traumatic event may occur in which bleeding may not be controlled. Individuals with sickle cell anemia are aware of the possibility that sudden death will occur as a result of a sickle cell crisis or complications. Individuals with HIV infection know that their progression to AIDS will probably result in death. Individuals may cope with the threat of early death in a variety of ways, ranging from the adoption of a philosophical view toward life to passivity and withdrawal.

The way, in which individuals cope with a condition they have had since childhood depends on a wide variety of factors, some of which reflect the coping mechanisms learned in childhood. Individuals' reactions as adults to their condition depend to some extent on how well their psychological adjustment was managed throughout development. Children who were encouraged to live as regular a life as possible, despite their condition, may exhibit a greater sense of self-esteem and autonomy as adults than do individuals who were kept in a dependent, overprotected state.

Activities and Participation

Different conditions affecting the blood or immune system affect activities of daily living in varying degrees, depending on the associated symptoms. Symptoms of fatigue or difficulty in breathing with exertion may require individuals to pace their activities throughout the day to conserve energy. Individuals may need more frequent rest periods, or they may need to divide activities into smaller steps, which they perform throughout the day, rather than completing a task all at once.

Good health practices are important to everyone. Because of the increased susceptibility to infection that is part of many conditions affecting the blood or immune system (especially HIV infection), however, individuals with these conditions must take extra care to have well-balanced diets and well-balanced regimens of rest and activity. Exercise is especially important to individuals with hemophilia. Regular, moderate exercise can build the muscles that protect joints and decrease the incidence of bleeding into the joints. Activities that carry a higher probability of injury, such as contact sports, should be avoided.

The degree to which individuals with conditions affecting the blood and immune system can maintain routine daily schedules depends on the specific condition, its progression, and complications. For the most part, individuals with hemophilia need not interrupt their daily schedules. The use of home self-infusion therapy has greatly reduced their incapacity by providing prompt and early management of spontaneous bleeding.

Although neither hemophilia nor sickle cell anemia alters sexual function, both are inherited conditions, and individuals may wish to consider genetic counseling before deciding to have children. There is no direct effect on sexual function associated with HIV infection; however, because of the possibility of transmission of the virus to others, individuals with HIV infections should inform their sexual partners about their diagnosis prior to sexual contact and should engage only in safe sexual practices. When a woman with HIV infection becomes pregnant, her child may be born HIV infected.

Social effects of conditions affecting the blood or immune system vary with the condition, the individual, and the particular circumstances. Fatigue and susceptibility to infection—which are characteristics of many conditions affecting the blood or immune system—may alter social functioning to some degree.

Because many conditions affecting the blood or immune system have no readily observable outward cues and signs, and because symptoms are often intermittent, others may not understand why individuals with these conditions must adhere to certain restrictions or why they are under continuing medical care. Because these individuals do not appear to be "legitimately ill" and, in many instances, have little physical impairment, they may receive less social support and understanding than individuals with more visible disabilities.

Conditions that are hereditary and those that occur in childhood can alter the socialization process necessary for social functioning in adulthood. Recurrent hospitalizations may affect a child's school performance and, consequently, his or her sense of industry and achievement. In addition, frequent school absences, hospitalizations, or the inability to engage in some activities may affect a child's interactions and relationships with peers, which in turn could affect the child's self-esteem and sense of self-worth.

Some children, as a means of dealing with the stress inherent in their condition, may learn to use their condition to manipulate and control the behaviors of others. Each of these possible effects of childhood illness can determine individuals' ability to function in the social world as an adult. Parents of a child with an inherited condition, such as hemophilia or sickle cell anemia, may experience guilt, react with over-protectiveness, or foster a sense of dependency in the child. They may adopt a permissive or indulgent attitude toward their child, rather than correcting the child when he or she misbehaves. They may also excuse the child from the responsibilities or the limits established for the child's siblings. Such parental reactions can impede the child's ability to function adequately as an adult in society.

Vocational Issues

The cause and symptoms of a condition affecting the blood or immune system determine its vocational impact. If, for example, the condition has been caused in part by exposure to toxic substances within the environment, hazards should be removed before individuals return to the workplace. If fatigue or dyspnea is a symptom of the condition, as in anemia, it may be necessary to consider the physical demands of the job and the need for more frequent rest periods. When infection is a potential complication of the condition, individuals should avoid exposure to factors and environments that may precipitate infection.

The functional impact of immune conditions also depends on the stage of the condition. With HIV infection, for example, prior to the development of severe immunodeficiency, no limitations may be present. In the milder stages of the condition, individuals may be able to perform all but the most demanding tasks at work. As the immune system becomes more compromised, however, opportunistic infections may result in prolonged periods of illness and hospitalization, interfering with individuals' ability to work. In addition to the physical manifestations resulting from opportunistic infections, individuals with HIV infections may develop central nervous system symptoms, which can affect cognitive, motor, and behavioral abilities.

CASE STUDIES

Case 1

Ms. S. is a 19-year-old African American female with sickle cell disease. She is a high school graduate and is currently enrolled in a junior college, where she is studying to be an x-ray technician. Since entering school at the junior college, she has had a number of sickle cell crises that have necessitated hospitalization. Ms. S. has developed severe damage to joints in her lower extremities as a result of her condition. Although her physician has recommended that Ms. S. reconsider her occupational goal given her series of sickle cell crises since being in school, she is determined to pursue her education and to become an x-ray technician. She continues to push herself even when she does not feel well.

1. How would you approach Ms. S. about her vocational plans given her physician's recommendation?
2. How realistic is Ms. S.'s vocational choice?
3. What medical, physical, and psychological issues would you consider when working with Ms. S. to develop her rehabilitation plan?
4. What is the general prognosis for Ms. S.'s condition?
5. What general lifestyle issues might you address with Ms. S. that could contribute to her rehabilitation potential?

Case 2

Mr. G. is a 26-year-old male who is HIV positive. He contracted HIV from his partner, who died of the disease last year. Mr. G. has a high school education and is a certified nursing assistant working in a nursing home, where he performs routine care for nursing home residents, such as bathing, lifting, turning, and feeding. He has been employed at the nursing home for the past 10 years. He tells you he loves his work and very much wants to continue as long as possible, both for financial reasons and because his health insurance is tied to his employment. He also tells you that work has been therapeutic for him after the loss of his partner. Mr. G. states that his employer is unaware of his condition because it has not interfered with his job performance; however, lately he states he has had more difficulty keeping up with the physical demands at work because of fatigue and in the past few weeks he has developed lymphadenopathy. He has begun a new experimental medication that he also believes might have some side effects that could interfere with his ability to work. He has a strong support group of friends; however, his family has severed all ties with him.

1. Is it appropriate for Mr. G. to withhold information about his diagnosis, and to continue to work in the current setting? Why or why not?
2. What is Mr. G.'s rehabilitation potential?
3. What factors will influence Mr. G.'s rehabilitation potential?
4. What medical factors related to Mr. G.'s condition would you consider when helping him develop a rehabilitation plan?

■ REFERENCES

Adams, R. J., & Brambilla, D. (2005). Discontinuing prophylactic transfusions used to prevent stroke in sickle cell disease. *New England Journal of Medicine, 353*(26), 2769–2777.

Alao, A. O., Westmoreland, N., & Jindal, S. (2003). Drug addiction in sickle cell disease: Case report. *International Journal of Psychiatry in Medicine, 33*(1), 97–101.

Andres, E., Loukili, N. H., Ben, A. M., & Noel, E. (2004). Pernicious anemia associated with interferon-alpha therapy and chronic hepatitis C infection. *Journal of Clinical Gastroenterology, 38*(4), 382.

Angastiniotis, M., & Modell, B. (1998). Global epidemiology of hemoglobin disorders. *Annals of New York Academic Science, 850*, 251–259.

Assan, S. & Kraszewski, S. (2006). Sexually transmitted infections: HIV/AIDS in primary care. *Practice Nurse, 32*(6), 1–7.

Assanasen, C., Quinton, R. A., & Buchanan, G. R. (2003). Acute myocardial infarction in sickle cell anemia. *Journal of Pediatric Hematology and Oncology, 25*(12), 978–981.

Balfour, L., Kowal, J., Silverman, A., Tasca, G. A., Angel, J. B., Macpherson, P. A. et al. (2006). A randomized controlled psycho-educational intervention trial: Improving psychological readiness for successful HIV medication adherence and reducing depression before initiating HAART. *AIDS Care, 18*(7), 830–838.

Barakat, L. P., Lutz, M., Smith-Whitley, K., Ohene-Frempong, K. (2005). Is treatment adherence associated with better quality of life in children with Sickle Cell disease. *Quality Life Research, 14*(2), 407–414.

Bartlett, J. G. (2004). Gastrointestinal manifestations of AIDS. In L. Goldman & D. Ausiello, *Cecil textbook of medicine*. (22nd ed., pp. 2168–2170). Philadelphia: W. B. Saunders.

Bayer, R., & Fairchild, A. L. (2006). Changing the paradigm for HIV testing: The end of exceptionalism. *New England Journal of Medicine, 355*(7), 647–649.

Beeton, K. (2002). Evaluation of outcome of care in patients with haemophilia. *Haemophilia, 8*(3), 428–434.

Bodemar, G., Kechagias, S., Almer, S., & Danielson, B. G. (2004). Treatment of anaemia in inflammatory bowel disease with iron sucrose. *Scandinavian Journal of Gastroenterology, 39*(5), 454–458.

Bokemeyer, C., & Foubert, J. (2004). Anemia impact and management: Focus on patient needs and the use of erythropetic agents. *Seminars in Oncology, 31*(3 suppl 8): 4–11.

Bolton-Maggs, P. H., & Pasi, K. J. (2003). Haemophilias A and B. *Lancet, 361*(9371), 1801–1809.

Bozzette, S. A. (2005). Routine screening for HIV infection: Timely and cost-effective. *New England Journal of Medicine, 352*(6), 620–621.

Bridges, K. R. (2007). Management issues in sickle cell disease. In R. Rakel & E. T. Bope (Eds.), *Conn's Current Therapy*. Philadelphia: Sanders. p. 475–484.

Britton, B. (2003) About hemophilia. *Nursing 2003. 33*(12), 78.

Clavel, F., & Hance, A. J. (2004). HIV drug resistance. *New England Journal of Medicine, 350*(10), 1023–1035.

Cochrane, J. (2003). The experience of uncertainty for individuals with HIV/AIDS and the palliative care paradigm. *International Journal of Palliative Nursing, 9*(9), 382–388.

Conyers, L. M. (2005). HIV/AIDS as an emergent disability: The response of vocational rehabilitation. *Journal of Vocational Rehabilitation, 22,* 67–75.

Cooper-Effa, M., Blount, W., Kaslow, N., Rothenberg, R., & Eckman, J. (2001). Role of spirituality in patients with sickle cell disease. *Journal of the American Board of Family Physicians, 14*(2), 116–122.

Currier, J. S., & Baden, L. R. (2006). Getting smarter: The toxicity of undertreated HIV infection. *New England Journal of Medicine, 355*(22), 2359–2361.

Dave, R. S., & Pomerantz, R. J. (2005). HIV neuropathogenesis: Persistent infection, persistent questions. *Science and Medicine, 10*(2), 112–123.

De Cock, K. M., Bunnell, R., & Mermin, J. (2006). Unfinished business: Expanding HIV testing in developing countries. *New England Journal of Medicine, 354*(5), 440–442.

De Sanctis V. (2002). Growth and puberty and its management in thalassaemia. *Hormone Research. 58*(suppl 1), 72–79.

Dorman, K. (2005). Managing the pain. *RN, 68*(12), 33–36.

Dybul, M., Fauci, A. S., Bartlett, J. G., Kaplan, J. E., & Pau, A. K. (2002). Guidelines for using antiretroviral agents among HIV-infected adults and adolescents. *Annals of Internal Medicine, 37*(5 pt 2), 381–433.

Edwards, C. L., Scales, J. J., Loughlin, C., Bennett, G. G., Harris-Peterson, S., De Castro, L. M. et al. (2005). A brief review of the pathophysiology, associated pain, and psychosocial issues in sickle cell disease. *International Journal of Behavioral Medicine, 12*(3), 171–179.

Elander, J., & Barry, T. (2003). Analgesic use and pain coping among patients with haemophilia. *Haemophilia, 9*(2), 202–213.

Embury, S. H. (2004). Sickle cell anemia and associated hemoglobinopathies, In L. Goldman & D. Ausiello (Ed9.), *Cecil textbook of medicine.* (22nd ed., pp. 1030–1039). Philadelphia: W. B. Saunders.

Fawzi, W. W., Msamanga, G. I., Spiegelman, D., Wei, R., Kapiga, S., Villamor, E., et al. (2004). A randomized trial of multivitamin supplements and HIV disease progression and mortality. *New England Journal of Medicine, 351*(1), 23–32.

Ferrier, S. E., & Lavis, J. N. (2003). With health comes work? People living with HIV/AIDS consider returning to work. *AIDS Care, 15*(3), 423–435.

Fiala, K., Hoffmann, S., & Ritenour, D. (2003). A survey of team physicians on participation status of hemophiliacs in NCAA Division I athletics. *Journal of Athletic Training, 38*(3), 245–251.

Fiala, K., & Ritenour, D. (2004). Medical care for athletes with hemophilia. *Athletic Therapy Today, 9*(2), 16–19.

Frieden, T. R., Das-Douglas, M., Kellerman, S. E., & Henning, K. J. (2005). Applying public health principles to the HIV epidemic. *New England Journal of Medicine, 353*(22), 2397–2402.

Gallant, J. E., DeJesus, E., Arribas, J. R., Pozniak, A. L., Gazzard, B., Campo, R. E., et al. (2006). Tenofovir DF, emtricitabine, and efavirenz vs. zidovudine, lamivudine, and efavirenz for HIV. *New England Journal of Medicine, 354*(3), 251–260.

Gebreyohanns, M., & Adams, R. J. (2004). Sickle cell disease: Primary stroke prevention. *CNS Spectrum, 9*(6), 445–449.

Gerberding, J. L. (2003). Occupational exposure to HIV in health care settings. *New England Journal of Medicine. 348*(9), 826–832.

Gilliam, B. L., Chan-Tack, K. M., Qaqish, R. B., Rode, R. A., Fantry, L. E., & Redfield, R. R. (2006). Successful treatment with atazanavir and lopinavir/ritonavir combination therapy in protease inhibitor-susceptible and protease inhibitor-resistant HIV-infected patients. *AIDS Patient Care, 20*(11), 745–759.

Glenn, M. K., Ford, J. A, Moore, D., & Hollar, D. (2003). Employment issues as related by individuals living with HIV or AIDS. *Journal of Rehabilitation, 69*, 30–36.

Hammer, S. M. (2005). Management of newly diagnosed HIV infection. *New England Journal of Medicine, 353*(6), 1702–1710.

Haubrich, R. H. (2005). HIV resistance: Improving interpretation and recent insights. In J. P. Phair, D. M. Heier, & E. King (Eds.), *HIV/AIDS annual update 2005: Clinical care options* (pp. 33–52). clinicaloptions.com/ccohiv2005.

Higgs, D. R., Thein, S. L., & Woods. W. G. (2001). The molecular pathology of the thalassaemias. In D. J. Weatherall & B. Clegg (Eds.), *The thalasemia syndromes* (4th ed., pp. 133–191). Oxford, UK: Blackwell Science.

Hoffbrand, A. V., Cohen, A., & Hershko, C. (2003). Role of deferiprone in chelation therapy for transfusional iron overload. *Blood, 102*, 17–24.

Huang, L., Quartin, A., Jones, D., & Havlir, D. V. (2006). Intensive care of patients with HIV infection. *New England Journal of Medicine, 355*(2), 173–181.

Hunt, B., Jaques, J., Niles, S. G., & Wiezalis, E. (2003). Career concerns for people living with HIV/AIDS. *Journal of Counseling & Development, 8*, 55–60.

Johnson, C. S. (2005). The acute chest syndrome. *Hematolology and Oncology Clinics of North America, 19*(5), 857–879, vi–viii.

Johnston, M. I., & Fauci, A. S. (2007). An HIV vaccine: Evolving concepts. *New England Journal of Medicine, 356*(20), 2073–2081.

Kilby, J. M., & Eron, J. J. (2003). Novel therapies based on mechanism of HIV-1 cell entry. *New England Journal of Medicine, 348*, 2228–2238.

Kim, J. Y., & Farmer, P. (2006). AIDS in 2006: Moving toward one world, one hope? *New England Journal of Medicine, 355*(7), 645–647.

Kizito, M. E., Mworozi, E., Ndugwa, C., & Serjeant, G. R. (2007). Bacteraemia in homozygous sickle cell disease in Africa: Is pneumococcal prophylaxis justified? *Archives of Disease in Childhood, 92*(1), 21–23.

Kohlenberg, B., & Watts, M. W. (2003). Considering work for people living with HIV/AIDS: Evaluation of a group employment counseling program. *Journal of Rehabilitation, 69*, 22–29.

Koziel, M. J., & Peters, M. G. (2007). Viral hepatitis in HIV infection. *New England Journal of Medicine, 356*(14), 1445–1454.

Lesho, E. P., & Gey, D. C. (2003). Managing issues related to antiretroviral therapy. *American Family Physician, 68*(4), 675–686.

Lukens, J. N. (1993). Hemoglobinopathies, S, C, D, E, and O and associated disease. In G. R. Lee, T. C. Bithell, & J. Foerster (Eds.), *Wintrobe's clinical hematology* (9th ed., pp. 1061–1101). Philadelphia: Lea & Febiger.

Lutz, M. L., & Barakat, L. P. (2004). Psychological adjustment of children with sickle cell disease: Family functioning and coping. *Rehabilitation Psychology, 49*(3), 224–232.

Lynch Fesko, S. (2001). Workplace experiences of individuals who are HIV+ and individuals with cancer. *Rehabilitation Counseling Bulletin, 45*(1), 2–11.

Marlowe, K. F., & Chicella, M. F. (2002). Treatment of sickle cell pain. *Pharmacotherapy, 22*(4), 484.

Masur, H. (2004). Treatment of HIV infection and AIDS. In L. Goldman & D. Ausiello (Eds.), *Cecil textbook of medicine* (22nd ed., pp. 2183–2191). Philadelphia: W. B. Saunders.

Maticka-Tyndale, E., Adam, B. D., & Cohen, J. J. (2002). To work or not to work: Combination therapies and HIV. *Qualitative Health Research, 12*(10), 1353–1372.

McKerrel, T. D., Cohen, H. W., & Billett, H. H. (2004). The older sickle cell patient. *American Journal of Hematology, 76*(2), 101–106.

Medzhitov, R., & Janeway, C. (2000). Innate immunity. *New England Journal of Medicine, 343*(5), 338–343.

Mentzer, W. C., & Kan, Y. W. (2001). Prospects for research in hematologic disorders: Sickle cell disease and thalassemia. *Journal of the American Medical Association, 285*(5), 640–642.

Merchante, N., Giron-Gonzalez, J. A., Gonzalez-Serrano, M., Torre-Cisneros J., Garcia-Garcia J. A., Arizcorreta A., et al. (2006). Survival and prognostic factors of HIV-infected patients with HCV-related end-stage liver disease. *AIDS, 20*, 49–57.

Merson, M. H. (2006). The HIV-AIDS pandemic at 25: The global response. *New England Journal of Medicine, 354*(23), 2414–2417.

Nixon, S., & Renwick, R. (2003). Experiences of contemplating returning to work for people living with HIV/AIDS. *Qualitative Health Research, 13*(9), 1272–1290.

Olivieri, N. F. (1999). The β-thalassemias. *New England Journal of Medicine, 341*(2), 99–109.

Orlando, M., Burnam, M. A., Beckman, R., Morton S. C., London A. S., Bing E. G., et al. (2002). Re-estimating the prevalence of psychiatric disorders in a nationally representative sample of persons receiving care for HIV: Results from the HIV Cost and Services Utilization Study. *International Journal of Methods in Psychiatric Research, 11*, 75–82.

Oursler, K. K., Goulet, J. L., Leaf, D. A., Akingicil, A., Katzel, L. I., Justice, A., et al. (2006). Association of comorbidity with physical disability in older HIV-infected adults. *AIDS Patient Care, 20*(11), 782–791.

Paltiel, A. D., Weinstein, M. C., Kimmel, A. D., Seage G. R., III, Losina, E., Zhang, H., et al. (2005). Expanded screening for HIV in the United States: An analysis of cost-effectiveness. *New England Journal of Medicine, 352*(6), 586–594.

Parish, K. L. (2002). Sexuality and haemophilia: Connections across the life-span. *Haemophilia, 8*(3), 353–359.

Pence, B. W., Gaynes, B. N., Whetten, K., Eron, J. J., Ryder, R. W., & Miller, W. C. (2005). Validation of a brief screening instrument for substance abuse and mental illness in HIV-positive patients. *Journal of Acquired Immune Deficiency Syndrome, 40*(4), 434–444.

Perry, V. (2005). Myths and facts about sickle-cell disease. *Nursing, 35*(12), 27.

Pineda, J. A., & Macias, J. (2005). Progression of liver fibrosis in patients coinfected with hepatitis C virus and human immunodeficiency virus undergoing antiretroviral therapy. *Journal of Antimicrobal Chemotherapy, 55*, 417–419.

Plug I., Van Der Bom, J. G., Peters, M., Mauser-Bunschoten, E. P., De Goede-Bolder, A., Heinen, L., et al. (2006). Mortality and causes of death in patients with hemophilia, 1992–2001: A prospective cohort study. *Journal of Thrombosis and Haemostasis, 4*(3), 510–516.

Pratt, O. S. (2005) Preventing stroke in sickle cell anemia. *New England Journal of Medicine, 353*(26), 2743–2745.

Price, R. W. (2004). Neurologic complications of HIV type 1 infection. In L. Goldman & D. Ausiello (Eds.), *Cecil textbook of medicine.* (22nd ed., pp. 2153–2158). Philadelphia: W. B. Saunders.

Pruthi, R. K. (2005). Hemophilia: A practical approach to genetic testing. *Mayo Clinic Proceedings, 80*(11), 1485–1499.

Robinson, P. (2005). Is surgery safe for a patient with hemophilia? *Nursing 2005, 35*(5), 1–3.

Rund, D., & Rachmilewitz, E. (2005). β-thalassemia. *New England Journal of Medicine, 353*(11), 1135–1146.

Sackoff, J. E., Hanna, D. B., Pfeiffer, M. R., & Torian, L. V. (2006). Causes of death among persons with AIDS in the era of highly active antiretroviral therapy: New York City. *American College of Physicians, 145*(6), 397–406.

Saag, M. S. (2004). Prevention of HIV infection. In L. Goldman & D. Ausiello (Eds.), *Cecil textbook of medicine* (22nd ed., pp. 2149–2153). Philadelphia: W. B. Saunders.

Sanders, G. D., Bayoumi, A. M., Sundaram, V., Bilir, S. P., Neukermans, C. P., Rydzak, C. E., et al. (2005). Cost-effectiveness of screening for HIV in the era of highly active antiretroviral therapy. *New England Journal of Medicine, 352*(6), 570–585.

Sax, P. E, & Walker, B. D. (2004). In L. Goldman & D. Ausiello (Eds.), *Cecil textbook of medicine* (22nd ed., pp. 2137–2139). Philadelphia: W. B. Saunders.

Scosyrev, E. (2006). An overview of the human immunodeficiency virus featuring laboratory testing for drug resistance. *Clinical Laboratory Science, 19*(4), 231–245.

Sepkowitz, K. A. (2006). One disease, two epidemics: AIDS at 25. *New England Journal of Medicine, 354*(23), 2411–2414.

Shah, A. (2004). A. Iron deficiency anemia—Part III. *Indian Journal of Medical Science, 58*(5), 214–216.

Shapiro, A. D., & Hoots, K. (2000). Hemophilia and related conditions. In R. Rakel (Ed.), *Conn's current therapy* (52nd ed.). Philadelphia: W. B. Saunders.

Shaw, G. M. (2004). Biology of human immunodeficiency viruses. In L. Goldman & D. Ausiello (Eds.), *Cecil textbook of medicine* (22nd ed., pp. 2139–2144). Philadelphia: W. B. Saunders.

Sherwood, L. (2007). *Human physiology: From cells to systems.* Belmont, CA: Thomson BrooksCole.

Stabler, S. P., & Allen, R. H. (2004). Vitamin B_{12} deficiency as a worldwide problem. *Annual Review of Nutrition, 24*, 299–326.

Stein, J. H. (2007). Cardiovascular risks of antiretroviral therapy. *New England Journal of Medicine, 356*(17), 1173–1175.

Steinbrook, R. (2003). HIV infection: A new drug and new costs. *New England Journal of Medicine, 348*(22), 2171–2172.

Steinbrook, R. (2004). The AIDS epidemic in 2004. *New England Journal of Medicine, 351*(2), 115–117.

Strategies for Management of Antiretroviral Therapy (SMART) Study Group. (2006). CD4+ count-guided interruption of antiretroviral treatment. *New England Journal of Medicine, 355*(22), 2287–2296.

Tashima, K. T., & Carpenter, C. C. J. (2003). Fusion inhibition: A major but costly step forward in the treatment of HIV-1. *New England Journal of Medicine, 348*(22), 2249–2250.

Taylor, G. (2004). Challenges for social work in hemophilia care. *Health and Social Work, 29*(2), 149–152.

Teitel, J. M., Barnard, D., Israels, S., Lillicrap, D., Poon, M. C., & Sek, J. (2004). Home management of haemophilia. *Haemophilia, 10*(2), 118–133.

Thomas, C. F., & Limper, A. H. (2004). *Pneumocystis* pneumonia. *New England Journal of Medicine, 350*(24), 2487–2498.

Vichinsky, E. P. (2004). Pulmonary hypertension in sickle cell disease. *New England Journal of Medicine, 350*(9), 857–859.

Wang, W. C., Grover, R., & Gallagher, D. (1993). Developmental screening in young children with sickle cell disease. *American Journal of Pediatrics and Oncology, 15*, 87–91.

Weiss, G., & Goodnough, L. T. (2005). Anemia of chronic disease. *New England Journal of Medicine, 352*(10), 1011–1023.

Westerdale, N., & Jegede, T. (2004). Managing the problem of pain in adolescents with sickle cell disease. *Professional Nurse, 19*(7), 402–405.

While, A. E., & Mullen, J. (2004). Living with sickle cell disease: the perspective of young people. *British Journal of Nursing, 13*(6), 320–325.

Wilson, R. E., Krishnamuri, L., & Kamat, D. (2003). Management of sickle cell disease in primary care. *Clinical Pediatrics*, November–December, 753–761.

Wright, A. A., & Katz, I. T. (2006). Home testing for HIV. *New England Journal of Medicine, 354*(5), 437–442.

Yee, T. T., & Lee, C. A. (2005). Transfusion-transmitted infection in hemophilia in developing countries. *Seminars in Thrombosis and Hemostasis, 31*(5), 527–537.

Zetola, N., & Klausner, J. D. (2006). HIV testing: An update. *MLO*, September, 58–62. Retrieved July 22, 2007, from http://www.mio-online.com

Chapter 11

Endocrine Conditions

■ STRUCTURE AND FUNCTION OF THE ENDOCRINE SYSTEM

The *endocrine system* is one of the body's two major communication systems. It works together with the other communication system, the nervous system, to regulate or direct various body functions. The endocrine system is composed of ductless glands (*endocrine glands*) scattered throughout the body. The endocrine glands produce chemical substances called *hormones* (Table 11-1), which are secreted directly into the bloodstream and act as messengers on target cells in other parts of the body. Endocrine glands include the following components of the body (Figure 11-1):

- *Thyroid gland*—located in the neck, in front of and on either side of the **trachea** (windpipe).
- *Parathyroid glands*—small, bean shaped glands buried within the thyroid gland.
- *Adrenal glands*—small glands lying on top of the kidneys. Each adrenal gland has two parts, the *medulla* and the *cortex*. Each part has a different function.
- *Pituitary gland*—located in the skull, just above the roof of the mouth, and connected to the brain by a slender stalk. It is divided into two parts, the *anterior lobe* and the *posterior lobe*.

- *Hypothalamus*—an area of the brain that coordinates the functions of the nervous system and the endocrine system.
- *Islets of Langerhans*—special cells embedded in the pancreas.
- *Testes* in males and *ovaries* in females.

The main function of the endocrine system is regulatory, with different hormones altering various body processes so that the body's internal balance (**homeostasis**) is maintained. Although each gland has its own unique and independent function, the endocrine glands often work in concert. Hormones secreted by the endocrine system control and integrate a variety of body activities, establishing a delicate chain of communication between various body systems. Hormones influence a number of physiologic processes throughout the body and regulate a number of body processes:

- Growth and development of the body and brain
- Reproductive maturity and function
- Metabolism
- Adjustment to internal and external stress
- Water and electrolyte balance

Overproduction or underproduction of one hormone can affect a number of other

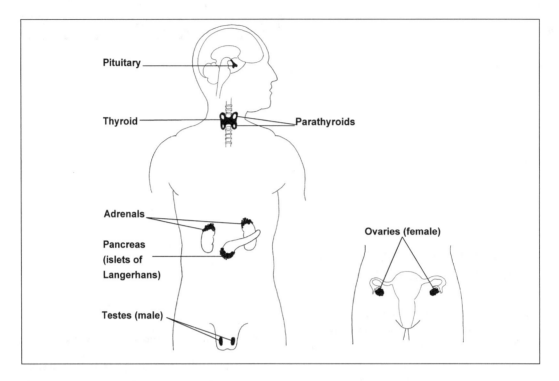

Figure 11-1 The endocrine system

endocrine glands and a variety of body functions. Some hormones have the sole function of regulating the production and secretion of another hormone.

The hormone *thyroxine*, which is secreted by the thyroid gland, regulates the rate of metabolism, influences nervous system maturation, and has profound effects on the heart. When the level of the thyroxine in the blood is high, metabolism speeds up; when it is low, metabolism slows down.

Parathyroid hormone, which regulates the concentrations of calcium and phosphate in the body, is secreted by the parathyroid glands. Excessive amounts of parathyroid hormone in the blood can result in the demineralization of bone, causing bones to become fragile so that they are easily broken. Insufficient amounts of parathyroid hormone in the blood can cause spasm and involuntary contraction of the muscles (**tetany**). If parathyroid hormone is to be effective, vitamin D must be present.

The inner part of the adrenal gland (medulla) secretes the hormones *epinephrine* and, to a lesser extent, *norepinephrine* at times of stress to enable the body to prepare physiologically for emergencies. These hormones increase heart rate, increase muscle tone, and constrict blood vessels in times of stress. The outer portion of the adrenal glands (cortex) secretes hormones called *steroids*, which regulate many essential functions, such as electrolyte and water balance, metabolism, immune responses, and inflammatory reactions. The adrenal cortex is essential to life. If it is dysfunctional, death will occur within a few days unless the hormones that it usually secretes are replaced.

The anterior lobe of the pituitary gland secretes **thyroid-stimulating hormone** (TSH, which is necessary for thyroid function), *growth hormone*, hormones that control reproductive function, and *corticotropin* (a hormone necessary for the function of the adrenal cortex). The posterior lobe of the pituitary gland stores hormones produced in the hypothalamus. *Antidiuretic hormone (ADH)*, which increases water reabsorption by the kidneys, is produced by the hypothalamus but is stored in and secreted by the posterior lobe of the pituitary gland.

Special cells within the islets of Langerhans in the pancreas produce the hormones insulin and glucagon, which are necessary for the metabolism of carbohydrates, proteins, and fats. Hormones produced by the testes and ovaries are important not only to reproductive function, but also to growth and development.

Table 11-1 summarizes the hormones secreted by various endocrine glands.

■ CONDITIONS OF THE ENDOCRINE SYSTEM

A number of medical conditions result from endocrine dysfunction and constitute major health problems (Wilson, 2001). Because manifestations of endocrine conditions are often similar to those associated with a number of psychiatric disabilities, some endocrine conditions may go unrecognized or misdiagnosed as psychiatric disabilities. Likewise, administration of hormones in management of an endocrine deficiency may have side effects similar to the symptoms associated with some psychiatric disabilities. Clearly, the endocrine

Table 11-1   Hormones Produced by Endocrine Glands

Thyroid Gland

Thyroxine
Calcitonin

Parathyroid Glands

Parathyroid hormone

Adrenal Glands

Adrenal Cortex

Cortisol
Aldosterone

Adrenal Medlula

Epinephrine
Norepinephrine

Pituitary Gland

Anterior Pituitary

Luteinizing hormone (LH)
Follicle-stimulating hormone (FSH)
Adrenocorticotropic hormone (ACTH)
Growth hormone (GH)
Thyroid-stimulating hormone (TSH)
Prolactin

Posterior Pituitary

Oxytocin
Antidiuretic hormone (ADH)

Hypothalamus Gland

Corticotropin-releasing hormone (CRH)
Thyrotropin-releasing hormone (TRH)
Growth hormone–releasing hormone (GHRH)
Somatostatin
Gonadotropin-releasing hormone (GnRH)
Dopamine

Pancreas (Islets of Langerhans)

Insulin
Glucagon

Gonads

Testes—Male

Testosterone

Ovaries—Female

Estrogen
Progesterone

system, in addition to regulating internal body functions and maintaining homeostasis, has a role in human behavior and emotions.

Hyperthyroidism (Graves' Disease, Thyrotoxicosis)

Manifestations of Hyperthyroidism

Hyperthyroidism is a term used to describe hyperfunction of the thyroid gland in which there is overproduction of thyroid hormone The term **thyrotoxicosis,** although sometimes used interchangeably with *hyperthyroidism,* actually refers to any condition in which there is excess of thyroid hormone, including overingestion of the hormone or inflammation of the thyroid gland (*thyroditis*) rather than merely overactivity of the thyroid gland itself (Woeber, 2000).

Hyperthyroidism results in *increased* metabolic rate. Manifestations of hyperthyroidism include **palpitations** (feeling the heart beat), **tachycardia** (fast heartbeat) restlessness, irritability, nervousness, difficulty concentrating, insomnia, and increased appetite and weight loss (Burman, 2007). The increased rate of metabolism causes intolerance to heat; thus environmental temperatures that seem comfortable to others seem unbearably warm to individuals with hyperthyroidism. With early diagnosis and appropriate management, hyperthyroidism usually causes no permanent consequences.

Graves' disease, a form of hyperthyroidism that is most likely an autoimmune disorder, is characterized by physical manifestations of exophthalmos and goiter (Dillman, 2004). **Exophthalmos** (protrusion of the eyeball) may also develop with hyperthyroidism. Once exophthalmos develops, the effects are permanent, giving individuals a wide-eyed and startled appearance. The overactive thyroid gland may also become so enlarged that there is a visible swelling in the neck, called a *goiter*. Although management of the condition

is similar to management of other causes of hyperthyroidism (as discussed later in this section), because Graves' disease is most likely an autoimmune disorder, lifelong follow-up is generally recommended (Dillman, 2004).

Management of Hyperthyroidism

In hyperthyroidism, management is directed toward curtailing the secretion of the thyroid hormone. Antithyroid medication that blocks the production of the hormone may be used. Manifestations usually subside within weeks or months after management with medication begins. Medications do not, however, alleviate exophthalmos, which is a permanent manifestation of the condition.

Some physicians recommend oral administration of ^{131}I (radioactive iodine) in cases of hyperthyroidism. Radioactive iodine destroys cells that produce thyroid hormone, and manifestations usually subside within weeks or months. Using radioactive iodine causes some individuals to become **hypothyroid** (too little thyroid hormone), however, which requires that individuals take thyroid medication for life. Surgical intervention for managing hyperthyroidism is sometimes indicated. In these instances, a subtotal thyroidectomy, which involves the removal of most—but not all—of the thyroid gland, is performed. Because some of the thyroid gland is left in place, replacement therapy with thyroid hormone is not usually necessary.

Hypothyroidism (Myxedema)

Manifestations of Hypothyroidism

Hypothyroidism is the most common thyroid condition in the adult population (Wu, 2000). The most common cause of hypothyrodism is chronic autoimmune thyroiditis, in which an autoimmune response causes thyroid failure (Nicoloff & LoPresti, 2007). Individuals with **hypothyroidism** have inadequate production of thyroid hormone. The manifestations of hypothyroidism are, in many ways, the opposite of those of hyperthyroidism. Individuals with hypothyroidism have a slowed metabolic rate; they may feel tired, lack energy, and gain weight. Their hair becomes dry, brittle, and thin, and their voice may be slow, low-pitched, and coarse. Emotional responses are subdued and mental processes slowed. Complications of hypothyroidism include the rapid development of atherosclerotic heart disease, including angina pectoris, myocardial infarction, and congestive heart failure (see Chapter 13). Individuals with severe hypothyroidism can also develop psychosis, with associated paranoia and delusions. Unless complications develop, however, appropriate management usually prevents any permanent consequences.

Management of Hypothyroidism

The goal of management of hypothyroidism is to correct the thyroid hormone deficiency. Consequently, a primary way of managing hypothyroidism is with replacement therapy. The medication of choice for thyroid hormone replacement is levothyroxine (Synthroid), a synthetic thyroid preparation. Individuals with hypothyroidism need to remain on this medication for life. Appearance and level of physical and mental activity usually improve gradually as the level of thyroid hormone rises. Blood levels of thyroid hormone and thyroid-stimulating hormone should be measured regularly when individuals are on thyroid hormone replacement therapy. Individuals who take such therapy should not alter their medication regimen without consulting a physician.

Cushing's Syndrome (Adrenal Cortex Hyperfunction)

Manifestations of Cushing's Syndrome

Overproduction of hormones by the adrenal cortex leads to **Cushing's syndrome,** which is characterized by manifestations including puffiness and a rounded moon face, obesity of the trunk of the body, fat pads at the back of the neck (buffalo hump), and weakness. The skin becomes thin and fragile, wound healing is poor, and the person experiences frequent bruising. Cushing's syndrome is usually accompanied by **hypertension** (high blood pressure) and insulin insensitivity. Women with Cushing's syndrome may have menstrual irregularities and facial hair growth. Mood and mental acuity may also be altered.

Management of Cushing's Syndrome

Management of Cushing's syndrome involves prescription of medication to reduce the body's production of corticosteroids. Depending on the cause of the condition, management can involve surgical intervention, pituitary irradiation, hormone replacement therapy, or other medications to suppress hormone production.

Despite appropriate management, Cushing's syndrome can have profound physical and emotional effects, requiring ongoing assessment of psychological well-being and functional capacity (Sonino, Boscaro, Fallo, & Fava, 2000). Full recovery may be slow, with the individual experiencing neuropsychological (cognitive and emotional) and physical (osteoporosis, hypertension) residual impairments (Boscaro, Barzon, Fallo, & Sonino, 2001).

Addison's Disease (Adrenocortical Insufficiency)

Manifestations of Addison's Disease

In contrast to Cushing's syndrome, **Addison's disease** results from underproduction of hormones by the adrenal cortex. Weakness and fatigue are early manifestations; skin pigmentation may become darker. Individuals with Addison's disease may also experience weight loss, loss of appetite, and decreased cold tolerance. Because hormones secreted by the adrenal cortex play a prominent role in the body's adaptive response to stress, individuals with Addison's disease may have severe, potentially life-threatening reactions such as extremely low blood pressure and severe electrolyte imbalance in situations (e.g., uncomplicated surgical procedures) that do not usually elicit such a response.

Management of Addison's Disease

Although Addison's disease was once fatal, replacement therapy with synthetic corticosteroids now enables individuals with Addison's disease to live full lives. Replacement medication must be taken daily, however. Careful monitoring for the development of the manifestations of excessive corticosteroid ingestion is also necessary.

Diabetes Insipidus

Manifestations of Diabetes Insipidus

Diabetes insipidus is a condition in which there is inadequate secretion of antidiuretic hormone from the hypothalamus. In rarer forms of this condition, the amount of ADH is sufficient but the kidneys do not respond to the hormone. Although diabetes insipidus has a number of causes, the most common cause is damage—due to trauma—to the stalk connecting the hypothalamus to the posterior lobe of the pituitary gland (where ADH is stored), which prevents ADH from being secreted. As a result, excessive water is "lost" by the kidneys (**polyuria**). Excessive and constant thirst (**polydipsia**) is present, with individuals consuming as much as 30 quarts of water per day. Diabetes insipidus may be a temporary condition or it may become chronic. The condition is permanent, but manifestations can be controlled with medication, enabling individuals in most instances to live full lives.

Management of Diabetes Insipidus

Depending on the cause, different hormonal preparations may be used to correct diabetes insipidus or to treat manifestations of the condition. Although the scenario is rare, if the condition has been caused by a pituitary tumor, surgical resection of the tumor may be indicated.

Diabetes Mellitus

Defining Diabetes Mellitus

Diabetes mellitus is a major threat to current and future human health (Steinbrook, 2006). The number of individuals worldwide with this kind of diabetes in 2000 was estimated to be between 151 million and 171 million. By 2030, this number is expected to rise to 366 million (Kasuga, 2006).

Over the last two decades, the prevalence of diabetes in the United States has doubled (Centers for Disease Control and Prevention, 2004). More than 18 million individuals (6.3% of the population) in the United States have diabetes (American Diabetes Association, 2004a).

Diabetes mellitus is a chronic, incurable condition of carbohydrate metabolism that involves an imbalance of the supply of and demand for insulin; it is the most common of all endocrine conditions (Laffel & Wood, 2007; Olefsky, 2001). Every body system is affected by this condition. The impact of diabetes mellitus is immense: it is a leading cause of heart disease, stroke, hypertension, blindness, kidney disease, amputation, and nervous system damage (American Diabetes Association, 2004a; Taylor, 2004).

The cause of diabetes mellitus is unknown, but there may be a familial tendency to develop the condition, especially with Type I diabetes, which is thought to have an autoimmune component (Melton, 2006). Obesity also greatly increases the risk of diabetes (Tataranni & Bogardus, 2001). Diabetes mellitus can occur as a complication of other conditions, such as **pancreatitis** (inflammation of the pancreas) or tumors of the pancreas;

as a side effect of medications; or as a result of specific conditions that increase the body's demand for insulin, such as *gestational diabetes* (diabetes that occurs during pregnancy). In these cases, the correction of the underlying cause may reverse the diabetes.

Mechanisms of Diabetes Mellitus

Diabetes results when cells in the pancreas are unable to maintain adequate insulin secretion to prevent blood sugar from becoming elevated (Rother, 2007). Food ingested is eventually converted to *glucose* (sugar), which is then carried in the blood to nourish all cells of the body. Certain tissues, such as muscle and fat, need insulin to use glucose as a source of energy and store glucose for future use. In diabetes mellitus, insufficient insulin is available to meet this need for one of these three reasons:

- Failure of the islets of Langerhans to produce enough insulin
- Destruction of insulin before it can be used
- Inability of body tissues to use the insulin that is present

When there is insufficient insulin, cells are unable to utilize glucose, so large amounts accumulate in the blood; this condition is known as **hyperglycemia.**

As blood is filtered by the kidney, glucose is usually channeled back into the blood. Because individuals with diabetes mellitus have such a large amount of glucose in the blood, however, some glucose spills over into the urine (**glycosuria**). Owing to the large concentration of glucose in the urine, the kidney excretes large quantities of water, a symptom called **polyuria**. As a result, individuals drink large quantities of water in an effort to replace the excess fluid lost (**polydipsia**). The body's inability to use glucose means that food or energy available to body tissues is inadequate. To compensate for this condition, individuals

with diabetes increase their food intake dramatically (**polyphagia**). Despite the increased food intake, lack of insulin prevents the body from using food as an energy source. Consequently, individuals begin to lose weight and become increasingly weak. Unless supplemental insulin is available, individuals literally enter a state of starvation.

Because the body's need for energy remains unmet, at this point the body begins to metabolize its own stores of fat and proteins for energy. As a result, **ketones** (the byproducts of fat metabolism) are formed. Usually, ketones are broken down and excreted. In individuals with diabetes mellitus, however, they accumulate more rapidly than they can be excreted. When ketone levels become toxic, a condition called **ketosis** or ketoacidosis (**diabetic coma**) occurs. Having too little or no insulin available for the amount of food ingested may also cause a diabetic coma.

Types of Diabetes Mellitus

Two types of diabetes mellitus are distinguished: *Type I diabetes* (insulin-dependent diabetes mellitus, IDDM) and *Type II diabetes* (non-insulin-dependent diabetes mellitus, NIDDM). Type I accounts for about 10% of all cases of diabetes while Type II accounts for the remainder (about 90%) (Sherwood, 2007; American Diabetes Association, 2004a). In Type I diabetes mellitus, the body produces little or no insulin, so that individuals require external sources of insulin for their survival. In Type II diabetes mellitus, the body produces insulin, but either the amount is insufficient to meet the total body needs or the body is unable to use the existing insulin adequately. External sources of insulin may or may not be taken to control the manifestations of Type II diabetes, but survival does *not* depend on an external insulin source. Obesity is a major risk factor in development of Type II diabetes (Tataranni & Bogardus, 2001; Ludwig & Ebbeling, 2001).

Management of Diabetes Mellitus

There is no cure for diabetes mellitus. In 1993, a landmark study (Diabetes Control and Complications Trial Research Group, 1993) demonstrated that strict control of blood glucose could significantly reduce complications of diabetes. Since then, additional data have substantiated those findings (Diabetes Control and Complications Trial/Epidemiology of Diabetes Interventions and Complications Study Research Group, 2007). Management of diabetes, regardless of type, is directed toward controlling levels of glucose and *lipids* (fats) in the blood, controlling blood pressure, and preventing complications (Mirza, 2007; Hoffman, 2001).

Diet is an important part of management of both Type I and Type II diabetes (Rendell, 2000; Chandalia, Garg, Lutjohann, von Bergmann, Grundy, & Brinkley, 2000). Individuals with Type II diabetes may be able to control their blood glucose level with diet alone or with a combination of diet and oral hypoglycemic agents, and at times, insulin. Individuals with Type I diabetes must control blood glucose levels through diet and the use of insulin injections. Individuals with either type of diabetes must consider the amount of energy expended through exercise and balance it with calories available from food. Diet, in the management of diabetes, is the mainstay of treatment. The less flexible the dietary regimen, the less likely the individual is to follow it. Consequently, emphasis is on maintaining an individualized healthy diet that the individual is more likely to follow (Mirza, 2007).

Pancreas transplantation has been used in some individuals with Type I diabetes with poor glucose control and whose quality of life has been significantly diminished by their condition (Robertson, 2004). Transplantation of islets alone shows promise and can result in insulin independence and good glucose control (Sherwin, 2004; Shapiro et al. 2000), although it is still considered to be experimental and controversial (Seaborg, 2007; Robertson, 2000; Stevens, Matsumoto, & Marsh, 2001).

Type I (Insulin-Dependent Diabetes Mellitus)

Type I diabetes is the most severe form of the condition. Insulin is the primary mode of therapy for all individuals with Type I diabetes. Gastric juices inactivate insulin, so, insulin cannot be taken orally. Consequently, individuals who are insulin dependent must inject insulin into the **subcutaneous** (fatty) layer of tissue.

The goal of insulin therapy is to maintain blood sugar levels as close to the recommended range as possible and to delay or prevent complications of diabetes. A number of different commercial insulin preparations are available from a number of different sources (bovine, porcine, bovine–porcine, or human synthetic insulin). The various insulin preparations differ in their time course of action. Some are *rapid acting*, some *intermediate*, and others *long acting*. *Rapid-acting insulin* usually acts within 30 minutes to 1 hour after injection, while *intermediate-acting insulin* types work within 1 to 2 hours. *Long-acting insulin* works within 4 to 6 hours. Each type of insulin also has a different time of peak action and duration.

There is great variability from individual to individual in terms of response to insulin, because of body-specific responses to insulin, absorption differences, and other factors. Not only does insulin absorption vary from individual to individual, but it can also vary in the same individual from day to day. Most individuals require more than one insulin injection per day. Some individuals may be required to take several different types of insulin.

Individuals must rotate the injection site to avoid a buildup of scar tissue, which can interfere with the absorption of insulin. Individuals may use a regular syringe and needle for insulin injections, or some individuals find it more convenient to use a device called an insulin injector, which resembles a pen. The insulin injector consists of a cylinder into which a cartridge filled with a predetermined dose of insulin and disposable needles are placed. The advantage of this device is that it is relatively reliable and accurate in delivering the amount of insulin injected; it is also convenient. Such a device may be carried unobtrusively in a purse or pocket for use away from home. Individuals using the insulin injector do not need to carry extra syringes and insulin bottles. When at a social event, business meeting, or family outing, individuals can easily give themselves injections with minimal disruption.

Disposable syringes eliminate the need for cleaning the syringe between uses and decrease the possibility of contamination and subsequent infection. For the most part, insulin no longer requires refrigeration for storage, but exposure to extremes in temperature and to intense light should be avoided.

Some individuals may choose an *insulin pump*, which provides a slow, continuous subcutaneous infusion of insulin throughout the day, thereby avoiding the need for numerous injections. Insulin is delivered to **subcutaneous** (fatty) tissue in the abdominal wall through a needle and an open-loop delivery device consisting of a small insulin pump (about the size of a pager) that is worn 24 hours a day. Although more expensive than other methods, the pump provides more flexibility relative to meal timing.

Regardless of the method of insulin delivery, the amount and type of insulin are balanced with the number of calories consumed and the amount of physical activity performed daily. Because insulin injected into the body must be balanced with the amount of glucose available, individuals cannot, after receiving insulin, decide to "skip a meal." Likewise, because physical exercise burns glucose for energy, a drastic increase in activity—even though adequate amounts of food were consumed—may

mean that the rapid consumption of glucose for energy will leave too much insulin in the body for the amount of glucose left.

Conditions that increase the metabolism rate or cause the body to consume more of the available glucose—such as stress, illness, infection, and pregnancy—alter insulin requirements and, consequently, may necessitate a modification of an individual's insulin dosage. Consequently, individuals with insulin-dependent diabetes who become ill with flu, fever, or other types of illnesses should consult their physician regarding adjustments to their regular insulin dosage.

Dietary management is also an integral part of controlling diabetes. The primary goal of diet therapy is to optimize blood levels of glucose. Individuals with diabetes mellitus must consider, in addition to proper nutrition, the total number of calories ingested as well as the distribution of calories consumed throughout the day. Because individuals with insulin-dependent diabetes take a predetermined amount of insulin, they must be especially careful to consume a specified number of calories at consistent times throughout the day to maintain the optimal balance of insulin and glucose in the blood. For the most part, calories should be distributed evenly throughout the day so that there is not a large concentration of calories at any one time. Because the only source of insulin for individuals with insulin-dependent diabetes is the insulin that they administer externally, they must pay close attention to the timing of meals and ensure that there is correct timing between the ingestion of food and the time course of action of the insulin they have injected. In addition to being cautious of the caloric value of food, individuals with insulin-dependent diabetes must monitor the types of foods and their balance within the diet, because some types of foods affect the absorption and metabolism of others. Given these concerns, counseling by a *dietitian* or *nutritionist* (individuals who study and counsel individuals on the therapeutic use of food) is imperative in the management of diabetes. Diabetic diets are individualized based on many personal factors, such as weight, age, and type of daily activity (e.g., sedentary, moderately active, very active). Individuals who are overweight may be placed on a low-caloric reduction diet so that the body will need less insulin. Because of their growth needs, adolescents may be placed on a higher-caloric diet than is an older individual of the same size. Individuals who engage in sedentary activities throughout the day do not require as many calories as do individuals who are very physically active in their job or at home. Compliance with the prescribed diet is usually better if lifestyle, religious, and cultural habits are considered as much as possible when dietary recommendations are made.

Exercise is important for the general health and well-being of all individuals. For individuals with diabetes mellitus, however, calories must be balanced with the amount of activity to be performed as well as with the amount of insulin taken. Unplanned exercise that is not coordinated with caloric intake can create an imbalance between the amount of insulin previously taken and the amount of glucose remaining available in the blood. Individuals with insulin-dependent diabetes must learn to balance exercise, insulin, and blood glucose levels to prevent **hypoglycemia (insulin shock)**. Considerable time and effort may be spent in learning how exercise of a given intensity and duration affects blood glucose levels, and which adjustments must be made in eating patterns and insulin dosages to compensate.

Self-monitoring of blood glucose levels is also important in the overall management of diabetes. Monitoring of blood glucose levels helps to determine the efficiency of the insulin dosage prescribed. Individuals who take insulin should monitor their blood glucose levels at least several times each day. Many individuals monitor glucose levels before breakfast, lunch, and dinner, as well as at bedtime. Monitoring gives individuals information about the level of sugar in the blood and, consequently, suggests changes in management that may be appropriate. For instance, if the blood sugar level is too low, the person may need to ingest a "quick" sugar such as orange juice to prevent severe hypoglycemia. If the blood sugar level is too high, the individual may need to inject additional insulin.

Numerous techniques may be used to test blood sugar. Individuals may monitor their own blood glucose levels by lancing their finger and using a small portable machine called a *glucometer* to assess the glucose content of the blood. Blood glucose may also be assessed through a device that provides continuous monitoring of blood glucose levels by using a tiny sensor inserted just beneath the skin, usually on the abdomen. The monitor records as many as 288 readings per day for up to three days. At the end of three days, the sensor is removed and the stored data are downloaded to a computer. The data enable physicians to make appropriate changes in insulin doses based on the glucose readings (Bode, Sabbah, & Davidson, 2001). During the period when the continuous monitoring device is being used, individuals continue to use standard methods of measuring blood glucose because the monitor does not display real-time glucose levels. Individuals may learn to alter their own insulin levels in accordance with their home blood glucose reading; however, such alterations should always be done with the advice and supervision of a physician.

Type II (Non-Insulin-Dependent Diabetes Mellitus, NIDDM)

Although many of the same aspects of management for Type I diabetes also apply to individuals with non-insulin-dependent diabetes (NIDDM), some individuals with NIDDM may control their blood sugar levels with diet alone. In other instances, weight loss may help to control the condition.

When blood sugar levels are not controlled by following a carefully planned diet, individuals may need to take hypoglycemic agents/oral agents (oral medications that are effective in lowering blood sugar). Several types of oral medications are available. Some newer medications developed for use in Type II diabetes have been called into question after it was suggested that individuals taking these medications had an increased risk of myocardial infarction (heart attack) (Home et al., 2007; Drazen, Morrissey, & Curfman, 2007; Psaty & Furberg, 2007; Nathan, 2007). The choice of whether to use these newer medications when older medications with less risk are available remains controversial (Nathan, 2007). When oral medications do not adequately control blood sugar, individuals with NIDDM may need to take supplemental insulin as well.

Diabetic Coma and Insulin Shock

Careful control of blood sugar is important to prevent complications, as discussed later in this chapter. Another major concern is the potentially fatal acute conditions of diabetic coma or insulin shock.

Diabetic coma occurs when there is too much circulating glucose in the blood. It's onset may be gradual, with few manifestations appearing until the blood sugar level becomes severely elevated. Individuals may become confused, seem drowsy, and then eventually slip into unconsciousness. They may have difficulty breathing, or experience nausea, vomiting, and flushing of the skin, which remains dry. Water depletion and dehydration are common. Characteristically, the breath of individuals in diabetic coma has a fruity odor. Diabetic coma is a medical emergency that can result in death if appropriate management isn't initiated quickly. Management is directed toward

lowering the level of blood sugar through the injection of insulin and correcting dehydration and electrolyte imbalance through the intravenous infusion of fluids.

Individuals with diabetes must also be aware of a potentially life-threatening crisis brought on my insulin reactions (Martz, Roessler, & Livneh, 2002). Insulin shock is the opposite of diabetic coma, occurring when there is too much insulin in the blood for the amount of glucose present. Insulin shock may result from injecting too much insulin, from engaging in an unusual amount of exercise that burns up the glucose that is usually available, or from failing to take in sufficient amounts of food for the amount of insulin injected. Individuals going into insulin shock may feel hungry, weak, and nervous. They may perspire profusely, although their skin is cold to the touch. Confusion and personality changes may also occur during insulin shock. If insulin shock is left untreated, individuals may lapse into unconsciousness. If it continues to go untreated, brain damage and eventual death can result. Management of insulin shock is directed toward raising blood sugar levels. If individuals are conscious, simple sugars such as candy, orange juice, or honey may be ingested orally; if individuals are unconscious, glucose must be infused intravenously.

Complications of Diabetes Mellitus

Individuals with diabetes mellitus, whether Type I or Type II, are susceptible to a number of complications that can affect a number of different body systems and result in major consequences (Stevens et al., 2001; Strauss, 2001). The exact reason why individuals with diabetes mellitus develop these complications is unknown; although there does appear to be a link to the length of time individuals have had diabetes mellitus and the degree to which glucose is controlled.

Some complications are related to the circulatory system. Vascular changes can contribute to **myocardial infarction** (heart attack; see Chapter 13) or **cerebrovascular accident** (stroke; see Chapter 3). They may also lead to poor circulation in the extremities (**peripheral vascular insufficiency**; see Chapter 4), so that even minor injuries are prone to become infected and may become so severely infected that **amputation** (see Chapter 16) is necessary. Vascular changes may also deprive the kidney of an adequate blood supply, causing kidney failure requiring dialysis (see Chapter 15). Changes in blood vessels in the retina (**retinopathy**) can result in blindness or cataract formation (Wilson et al., 2007) (see Chapter 5).

Other complications associated with diabetes mellitus may involve changes in the nervous system. Changes in the peripheral nerves (**peripheral neuropathy**) may result in the loss of sensation in the extremities, so that the protective sensation of pain is absent, making them even more prone to injury. Inappropriate footwear is the most common source of trauma to the feet of individuals with diabetes, resulting in foot ulcers, which can lead to the need for amputation (Boulton, Kirsner, & Vileikyte, 2004; Meijer et al., 2001). Consequently appropriate foot care is a necessity to prevent serious complications. Other effects of neuropathy may include sexual impotence in men and decreased genital sensation in women.

Individuals with diabetes mellitus have a higher incidence of surgery (such as cardiovascular surgery, amputation, or ophthalmologic procedures), related to their complications. They are also at higher risk for postsurgical complications because of poor wound healing, increased infection, and increased risk of acute renal failure (Plodkowski & Edelman, 2001).

The risk that individuals with diabetes mellitus will develop complications varies from person to person. Factors such as type of diabetes, age of onset, duration of the condition, and the degree to which individuals follow the prescribed protocol must be considered.

Psychosocial Issues in Diabetes Mellitus

Diabetes mellitus not only involves lifelong multifaceted management, but also has a significant impact on individuals' daily lives and futures, especially if complications develop. Both psychological and physiologic factors frequently determine the course of diabetes mellitus (Martz & Livneh, 2007). Psychological factors may affect management of diabetes directly, by inducing metabolic changes that can affect individuals' ability to control blood glucose levels, or indirectly, by altering the degree to which individuals follow instructions related to medication, diet, and exercise. Motivation to follow the management recommendations is paramount in the control of diabetes mellitus (Dashiff, McCaleb, & Cull, 2006).

Diabetes mellitus is a hidden condition, whose manifestations are not visible. Others may see no indication of a chronic illness or condition that imposes restrictions and may, therefore, have no expectations that individuals may be restricted regarding some aspects of lifestyle or activity. If individuals with diabetes have not adapted to their condition or if they fear social nonacceptance because of their condition, they may attempt to hide their diagnosis of diabetes from others, ignoring dietary restrictions or engaging in activities outside their management plan. Some individuals may believe that following a diabetic diet draws attention to the condition and, therefore, may neglect that diet.

In some instances, the benefit of careful adherence to the recommended regimen is not always apparent to individuals with diabetes mellitus. Even though instructions may have been followed carefully, the blood glucose level may remain elevated or complications may develop. Such occurrences can result in discouragement and depression. If emphasis is placed on restrictions associated with management of diabetes, individuals may feel depressed and hopeless.

Fear of complications that may lead to blindness or possible amputation may create additional anxiety. For some individuals, these feelings are overwhelming. Self-destructive behaviors, such as skipping insulin injections and/or abandoning the diet, both of which can imperil the life of a person with diabetes mellitus, may result.

Many lifestyle changes are necessary for individuals with diabetes mellitus, especially for those with insulin-dependent diabetes. Although diet and insulin dosage can be adjusted to account for different types of activities, advance planning is essential for affected individuals. Activities, including exercise and meal times, should generally be consistent from day to day. Eating on the run or skipping meals is not feasible. If the schedule changes, food intake and insulin dosage must be changed accordingly. If activities involve additional walking, comfortable and well-fitting shoes should be worn to avoid formation of blisters that could become infected.

Individuals with diabetes mellitus should check with their physician about insulin and food schedules before traveling, especially across time zones. If traveling by plane, they should request special meals ahead of time, and they should be served at the time required for the regimen. They should carry insulin with them and should protect insulin against extremes of temperature.

With guidance from physicians or dietitians, individuals can learn to accommodate meals served at restaurants or in other people's homes. The quantity and types of foods must be taken into account, however. Individuals with diabetes must learn to judge calories and portions, and fatty, rich foods should be eliminated from the diet. Although concentrated sweets and alcohol should usually be avoided, planning may permit the incorporation of small quantities into the diet for special occasions.

Diabetes mellitus does not usually affect sexual activity unless there are complications. Neuropathy may be the cause of impotence in men and decreased sensation in women. Frequent vaginal infections in women with diabetes may also alter sexual activity because of the physical discomfort involved. Reproductive function is not affected in men who are not impotent. Women with diabetes mellitus who become pregnant generally have more complicated pregnancies and need special medical attention to monitor progress of the pregnancy and to alter insulin and caloric requirements.

The effects of any chronic condition are not limited to individuals with the condition. This is especially true of diabetes mellitus, because so many lifestyle factors are involved in the adequate management of the condition. Often, the degree to which individuals with diabetes mellitus follow the management recommendations depends on the degree of social support that they receive. Eating habits of family members, as well as their understanding of the importance of the diet prescribed for the individual with diabetes, can contribute significantly to the individual's willingness to adapt to and follow the diabetic diet. Acceptance and understanding of diabetes and its restrictions by friends and colleagues also contribute to individuals' self-concept and subsequent acceptance of their condition.

The effects that the diagnosis of diabetes has on the family of individuals with diabetes depend on the family composition, the family's usual coping mechanisms, the age of the individual at the onset of diabetes, the regimen prescribed, perceptions of future consequences, and functioning of the family before the diagnosis was made. If individuals with diabetes do not control their diet or prepare their own meals, the family member assuming this responsibility has new status and influence. This shift in power can create another source of support or, in some instances, a source of sabotage of the regimen itself.

The effects of diabetes on other social relationships vary. In social situations where food and alcohol are the major focus of activity, individuals with diabetes mellitus may need to modify their participation, although they need not totally avoid such situations. Depending on the individual and others in the social setting, modifications may or may not affect the social relationship itself.

Individuals with diabetes mellitus are constantly aware of the need to comply with dietary restrictions, the need to eat at regular times, the need to balance activity with calories, and the need to stick themselves several times each day to inject insulin or to test the blood glucose level. These factors can make them feel alone and different if they do not have social support at work or home.

Given that diabetes mellitus is an invisible condition, couples planning to marry may not discuss diabetes and its effect on the marital relationship or on plans for children. Depending on the maturity, understanding, and expectations of both individuals in the marital relationship, problems related to the presence of diabetes may emerge later, especially in the decision to have children or in the management of complications, should they arise.

Vocational Issues in Diabetes Mellitus

The type of diabetes, the demands of the job, the person's willingness and ability to carry out management recommendations, and the degree to which the prescribed protocol controls the person's diabetes determine any special needs of individuals with diabetes mellitus in the work environment. Individuals with diabetes tend to report activity limitations and restricted activity days more frequently

than does the general population (Marrero & Guare, 2005). Certain modifications in employment may be necessary to accommodate their condition. In particular, the activity level should be consistent as much as possible, or activity should be planned so that activity is balanced with food intake and insulin or dosage of oral hypoglycemic agents. If at all possible, rotating shifts or irregular schedules should be avoided because of the alterations in insulin (for individuals with Type I diabetes) and food schedules that would be required.

Work in which there is risk of even minor cuts and scratches, especially to the feet, should be avoided owing to the risk of infection. Emotional stress has a direct impact on the blood glucose level. Consequently, individuals with diabetes mellitus should learn coping strategies that enable them to deal effectively with job stress or should avoid overly stressful job situations, if possible.

Despite the ability of many individuals to effectively control their diabetes, discrimination in employment still occurs (American Diabetes Association, 2004b). Owing to employers' perceptions of individuals as a safety risk or fear that fluctuations in blood glucose levels may cause unexpected capacity, individuals may encounter resistance to employment. Many individuals are able to recognize early warning signs of high or low glucose levels and can take steps to counteract their physical reactions so that risk is minimal. Manifestations of insulin reactions are, however, variable from individual to individual. In some instances, individuals may become desensitized to manifestations and, therefore, may not recognize the need to take steps to intervene before the reaction occurs (Martz, 2003).

Employers should generally be informed of an employee's diagnosis of diabetes mellitus so that misunderstandings about the need for regular meal schedules, routine activities, and avoidance of injury do not develop. In addition, employers should be alerted to the manifestations of diabetic coma or insulin shock so that appropriate action may be taken if either of these events should occur.

The potential for complications should be considered in vocational planning. There is no guarantee that even when individuals follow management protocols precisely that complications will not develop. Nevertheless, maintaining good control blood glucose levels can decrease the number of days lost from work because of minor complications. When complications do develop, alterations in employment are specific to the type of complication. For example, individuals with peripheral neuropathy or poor circulation to the lower extremities may need to avoid occupations that require excessive walking or standing. Individuals who develop diabetic retinopathy may require special low-vision aids. Development of peripheral neuropathy of the upper extremities may interfere with sensation and manual dexterity. Because of the possibility of diabetic coma or insulin shock, individuals with diabetes mellitus should not work in isolation.

■ DIAGNOSTIC PROCEDURES FOR CONDITIONS OF THE ENDOCRINE SYSTEM

Blood Tests for Thyroid Function

A number of tests are available to assess thyroid function. Examples of blood tests include *serum thyroxine* (T_4) and *free thyroxine index*. These tests measure either the exact or relative amount of thyroid hormone in the blood. Another type of blood test, which measures the level of thyroid-stimulating hormone in the blood, may also be used and provides accurate assessment of thyroid hormone levels in the blood.

Blood Tests for Diabetes Mellitus

The major blood tests used in the diagnosis of diabetes mellitus are determinations of the fasting blood glucose (FBG) and postprandial plasma glucose (PPG) levels and the oral glucose tolerance test (OGGT). In the fasting blood glucose test, blood is drawn after the individual has not eaten for a number of hours. For a postprandial plasma glucose test, blood is drawn several hours after individuals have eaten. Blood is drawn for the oral glucose tolerance test while individuals are fasting. Individuals are then given concentrated glucose in liquid form to drink, and blood samples are drawn at 1-, 2-, and 3-hour intervals. All three tests make it possible to compare the level of glucose in individuals' blood with the level expected in persons without diabetes mellitus under similar circumstances.

■ GENERAL MANAGEMENT OF ENDOCRINE CONDITIONS

For many endocrine conditions, management involves replacement of hormones, if there is insufficient production, or administration of medication to decrease production of hormones, if hormones are being overproduced. Although in some instances surgery may be indicated, these procedures are not always curative.

■ PSYCHOSOCIAL AND VOCATIONAL ISSUES IN ENDOCRINE CONDITIONS

Psychological Issues

Changes in hormonal patterns associated with conditions of the endocrine system may cause behavioral changes that result in misdiagnosis, delay in initiating treatment, and unnecessary hardships for individuals. Individuals with treatable endocrine conditions have sometimes been diagnosed as having psychiatric conditions, at times being placed in institutions, with the real cause of their manifestations left untreated.

Endocrine conditions can cause a broad range of emotional and psychiatric manifestations (Aslan, Ersoy, Kuruoglu, Karakoc, &

Cakir, 2005). For example, individuals with thyroid conditions may experience emotional outbursts, irritability, or manifestations of anxiety that are not always recognized as manifestations of their condition. Older adults with a thyroid condition may demonstrate memory impairment that is misdiagnosed as Alzheimer's disease or other dementia and that goes untreated. In most cases, changes in behavior are temporary and steadily improve as the endocrine condition is corrected.

In children, unrecognized endocrine conditions can cause permanent consequences, such as intellectual disability. Recognition of the role of the endocrine system and various hormones in cognitive development of children has resulted in earlier recognition and management of endocrine conditions in childhood, in many cases preventing permanent consequences due to hormonal insufficiency from occurring.

Changes in physical appearance, such as the exophthalmos associated with Grave's disease or the physical changes associated with Cushing's syndrome, can disturb individuals' body image, causing subsequent emotional reactions (Bianchi et al., 2004). Management of many endocrine conditions involves long-term or lifelong ingestion of medications. For some individuals, taking medication daily creates frustration and resentment, leading to noncompliance with management recommendations and the development of subsequent complications or a recurrence of the condition.

Activities and Participation

For most individuals, after the endocrine condition has been stabilized and barring complications, primary lifestyle changes involve remembering to take medications at the same time every day. The exception is, of course, diabetes mellitus, in which lifestyle changes are a significant part of the management of the condition and are necessary for survival.

Many social issues associated with endocrine conditions depend on the specific condition. For example, individuals with hyperthyroidism may experience social isolation because of associated behavior changes that occur before management is instituted. Physical changes caused by endocrine conditions, such as those associated with Cushing's syndrome, may lead to self-consciousness and cause individuals to withdraw from social activities. The demands of diabetes can also cause stress in families, especially in siblings of children with Type I diabetes, causing isolation and resentment (Hollidge, 2001).

■ VOCATIONAL ISSUES IN ENDOCRINE CONDITIONS

In most instances, individuals with conditions of the endocrine system, which have been identified and are being treated, have no special vocational needs. When hormone replacement therapy is part of the management, however, the importance of compliance with the prescribed medical regimen cannot be overstated. This is especially true of individuals with diabetes mellitus, the vocational implications of which were discussed earlier in the chapter.

CASE STUDIES

Case 1

Mr. J. is a 52-year-old cabinetmaker. He is moderately overweight. Mr. J. has recently experienced blurring of vision. When he was seen by his physician, his blood sugar level was elevated and he was told that he had Type II diabetes. Mr. J. is concerned about how this diagnosis may affect his ability to continue in his current line of employment.

1. Are there limitations resulting from Mr. J.'s condition that will affect his rehabilitation potential?
2. Which other factors might you consider in helping Mr. J. develop a plan for the future?
3. Which issues in his current line of employment may be important to consider when working with Mr. J. regarding his management plan?

Case 2

Ms. L. is a 30-year-old computer programmer. She recently has experienced significant weight loss, irritability, and inability to sleep. She has had increased difficulty with co-workers, and her employer has asked that she seek medical evaluation. After physical and laboratory evaluation, Ms. L. was told that she had hyperthyroidism.

1. Which factors regarding Ms. L.'s current job would you consider given her condition?
2. Are there limitations regarding her condition that may affect her ability to continue in her current job?
3. What is the likelihood that Ms. L. will be able to continue in her current line of employment?

■ REFERENCES

American Diabetes Association. (2004a). Diabetes statistics. Retrieved May 18, 2004, from http://www.diabetes.org/home.jsp.

American Diabetes Association (2004b) Hypoglycemia and employment and licensure. *Diabetes Care, 27* (suppl1), S134.

Aslan, S., Ersoy, R., Kuruoglu, A. C., Karakoc, A., & Cakir, N. (2005). Psychiatric symptoms and diagnoses in thyroid disorders: A cross-sectional study. *International Journal of Psychiatry in Clinical Practice, 9*(3), 187–192.

Bianchi, G.P., Zaccheroni, V., Solaroli, E., Vescini, F., Cerutti, R., Zoli, M., et al. (2004). Health-related quality of life in patients with thyroid disorders. *Quality of Life Research, 13*, 45–54.

Bode, B. W, Sabbah, H., & Davidson, P. C. (2001). What's ahead in glucose monitoring. *Postgraduate Medicine, 109*(4), 41–49.

Boscaro, M., Barzon, L., Fallo, F., & Sonino, N. (2001). Cushing's syndrome. *Lancet, 357(9258)*, 783–791.

Boulton, A. J. M., Kirsner, R. S., & Vileikyte, L. (2004). Neuropathic diabetic foot ulcers. *New England Journal of Medicine, 352*(1), 48–55.

Burman, K. D. (2007). Hyperthyroidism. In R. E. Rakel & E. T. Bope (Eds.), *Conn's Current Therapy* (pp. 771–775). Philadelphia: W. B. Saunders.

Chandalia, M., Garg, A., Lutjohann, D., von Bergmann, K., Grundy, S. M., & Brinkley, L. J. (2000). Beneficial effects of high dietary fiber intake in patients with Type 2 diabetes mellitus. *New England Journal of Medicine, 342*(19), 1392–1397.

Dashiff, C. J., McCaleb, A., & Cull, V. (2006). Self-care of young adolescents with Type 1 diabetes. *Journal of Pediatric Nursing, 21*(3), 222–232.

Diabetes Control and Complications Trial/ Epidemiology of Diabetes Interventions and Complications (DCCT/EDIC) Study Research Group. (2007). Long-term effect of diabetes and its treatment on cognitive function. *New England Journal of Medicine, 356*(18), 1842–1852.

Diabetes Control and Complications Trial Research Group. (1993). The effect of intensive treatment of diabetes on the development and progression of long-term complications in insulin-dependent diabetes mellitus. *New England Journal of Medicine, 329*(14), 977–986.

Dillman, W. H. (2004). The thyroid. In L. Goldman & D. Ausiello (Eds.), *Cecil's textbook of medicine* (22nd ed, pp. 1391–1411). Philadelphia: W. B. Saunders.

Drazen, J. M., Morrissey, S., & Curfman, G. D. (2007). Rosiglitazone: Continued uncertainty about safety. *New England Journal of Medicine, 357*(1), 63–64.

Hoffman, R. P. (2001). Eating disorders in adolescents with Type I diabetes. *Postgraduate Medicine, 109*(4), 67–74.

Home, P. D., Pocock, S. J., Beck-Nielsen, H., Gomis, R., Hanefeld, M. Jones, N.P. et al. (2007). Rosiglitazone evaluated for cardiovascular outcomes: An interim analysis. *New England Journal of Medicine, 357*(1), 28–38.

Kasuga, M. (2006). Insulin resistance and pancreatic β cell failure. *Journal of Clinical Investigation, 116*, 1756–1760.

Laffel, L. M. B., & Wood, J. R. S. (2007). Diabetes mellitus in children and adolescents. In R. E. Rakel & E. T. Bope (Eds.), *Conn's current therapy* (pp. 682–690). Philadelphia: W. B. Saunders.

Ludwig, D. S., & Ebbeling, C. B. (2001). Type 2 diabetes mellitus in children: Primary care and public health considerations. *Journal of the American Medical Association, 286*(12), 1427–1430.

Marrero, D. G., & Guare, J. C. (2005). Diabetes mellitus. In H. H. Zaretsky, E. F. Richter III, & M. G. Eisenberg (Eds.), *Medical aspects of disability* (3rd ed., pp. 241–265). New York: Springer.

Martz, E. (2003). Living with insulin-dependent diabetes: Life can still be sweet. *Rehabilitation Counseling Bulletin, 47*(1), 51–57.

Martz, E., & Livneh, H. (2007). Do posttraumatic reactions predict future time perspective among people with insulin-dependent diabetes mellitus? *Rehabilitation Counseling Bulletin, 50*(2), 87–98.

Martz, E., Roessler, R., & Livneh, H. (2002). Responses to insulin reactions and long-term adaptation to diabetes. *Journal of Rehabilitation, 68*(2), 14–21.

Meijer, J. W. G., Trip, J., Jaegers, S. M. H. J., et al. (2001). Quality of life in patients with diabetic foot ulcers. *Disability and Rehabilitation, 23*(8), 336–340.

Melton, D. A. (2006). Reversal of Type 1 diabetes in mice. *New England Journal of Medicine, 355*(1), 89–90.

Mirza, S. A. (2007). Diabetes mellitus in adults. In R. E. Rakel & E. T. Bope (Eds.), *Conn's current therapy* (pp. 675–682). Philadelphia: W. B. Saunders.

Nathan, D. M. (2007). Rosiglitazone and cardiotoxicity: Weighing the evidence. *New England Journal of Medicine, 357*(1), 64–66.

Olefsky, J. M. (2001). Diabetes mellitus. *Journal of the American Medical Association, 285*, 628–632.

Psaty, B. M., & Furberg, C. D. (2007). The record on rosiglitazone and the risk of myocardial infarction. *New England Journal of Medicine, 357*(1), 67–69.

Plodkowski, R. A., & Edelman, S. V. (2001). Presurgical evaluation of diabetic patients. *Clinical Diabetes, 19*(2), 92–94.

Rendell, M. (2000). Dietary treatment of diabetes mellitus. *New England Journal of Medicine, 342*(19), 1440–1441.

Robertson, P. R. (2004). Islet transplantation as a treatment for diabetes: A work in progress. *New England Journal of Medicine, 350*(7), 694–705.

Rother, K. I. (2007). Diabetes treatment: Bridging the divide. *New England Journal of Medicine, 356*(15), 1499–1501.

Seaborg, E. (2007). Weighing islet transplants for Type 1 diabetes patients: Still early days. *Endocrine News*, April, 18–24

Shapiro, A. M. J., Lakey, J. R. T., Ryan, E. A., Korbutt, G. S., Toth, E., Warnock, G. L., et al. (2000). Islet transplantation in seven patients with Type 1 diabetes mellitus using a glucocorticoid-free immunosuppressive regimen. *New England Journal of Medicine, 343*(4), 230–238.

Sherwin, R. S. (2004). Diabetes mellitus. In L. Goldman & D. Ausiello (Eds.), *Cecil textbook of medicine* (22nd ed., pp. 1424–1452). Philadelphia: W. B. Saunders.

Sherwood, L. (2007). The peripheral endocrine glands. In *Human physiology* (6th ed., pp. 683–729). Belmont, CA: Thomson Brooks/Cole.

Sonino, N., Boscaro, M., Fallo, F., & Fava, G. A. (2000). A clinical index for rating severity in Cushing's syndrome. *Psychotherapy Psychosomatics, 69*, 216–220.

Steinbrook, R. (2006). Facing the diabetes epidemic: Mandatory reporting of glycosylated hemoglobin values in New York City. *New England Journal of Medicine, 354*(6), 545–548.

Stevens, R. B., Matsumoto, S., & Marsh, C. L. (2001). Is islet transplantation a realistic therapy for the treatment of Type 1 diabetes in the near future. *Clinical Diabetes, 19*(2), 51–59.

Strauss, M. B. (2001). Diabetic foot problems: Keys to effective, aggressive prevention. *Consultant, 11,* 1693–1705.

Tataranni, P. A., & Bogardus, C. (2001). Changing habits to delay diabetes. *New England Journal of Medicine, 344*(18), 1390–1391.

Taylor, R. (2004). Causation of Type 2 diabetes: The Gordian knot unravels. *New England Journal of Medicine, 350*(7), 639–641.

Wilson, J. D. (2001). Prospects for research for disorders of the endocrine system. *Journal of the American Medical Association, 285*(5), 624–631.

Wilson, M. E., Levin, A. V., Trivedi, R. H., Kruger, S. J., Elliott, L. A., Ainsworth, J. R., et al. (2007). Cataract associated with Type-I diabetes mellitus in the pediatric population. *Journal of AAPOS, 11*(2), 162–165.

Woeber, K. A. (2000). Update on the management of hyperthyroidism and hypothyroidism. *Archives of Internal Medicine, 160*(8), 1067–1071.

Wu, P. (2000). Thyroid disease and diabetes. *Clinical Diabetes, 18*(1), 38–42.

Chapter 12

Conditions of the Gastrointestinal System

■ STRUCTURE AND FUNCTION OF THE GASTROINTESTINAL SYSTEM

The primary function of the *gastrointestinal system* is to convert nutrients, water, and electrolytes from food into energy that helps the body function (Sherwood, 2007). The *gastrointestinal tract* (*alimentary canal*) is a hollow, muscular tube approximately 30 feet long (see Figure 12-1). Its principal purpose is to provide a mechanism whereby nutrients and liquids can be taken into the body for energy and tissue growth and through which wastes from the digestive process can be eliminated.

The digestive process begins in the mouth, sometimes called the oral or buccal cavity, where teeth break food into smaller particles. The teeth at the front of the mouth (incisors) provide a cutting action, while the teeth at the back of the mouth (molars) provide a grinding action. Chewing is important to the digestive process. Breaking food into smaller particles not only facilitates the passage of the food into the stomach, but also enlarges the surface area available for the gastric juices to act upon as the digestive process continues in the stomach.

While still in the mouth, smaller particles of food are mixed with saliva, a fluid secretion in the mouth that lubricates and softens food, and facilitates its passage down the throat. Saliva, which is produced by the parotid glands, submaxillary glands, and sublingual glands, contains an enzyme that begins the breakdown of sugars.

Food passes from the throat (**pharynx**) into a muscular tube called the **esophagus,** which leads from the mouth to the stomach. The esophagus and windpipe (**trachea**) have a common opening at the pharynx. Consequently, a flap called the epiglottis closes over the opening to the windpipe when food is swallowed, ensuring that food will pass into the esophagus rather than the windpipe. The esophagus is approximately 10 inches long and moves food along via rhythmic, muscular movements called *peristalsis*.

The esophagus passes through a muscular wall called the diaphragm, which separates the **thoracic** (chest) **cavity** from the **abdominal cavity.** The abdominal cavity contains the stomach, intestines, and other abdominal organs and is lined with a thin membrane called the **peritoneum**. The esophagus passes through the diaphragm to reach the stomach. Food enters the stomach from the esophagus through an opening called the lower esophageal sphincter, sometimes called the *cardiac sphincter*. Pressure gradients around this opening prevent the backflow of food and gastric juices into the esophagus from the stomach.

The stomach is a muscular organ that stores, mixes, and liquefies food. It contains gastric juices, which continue the digestive

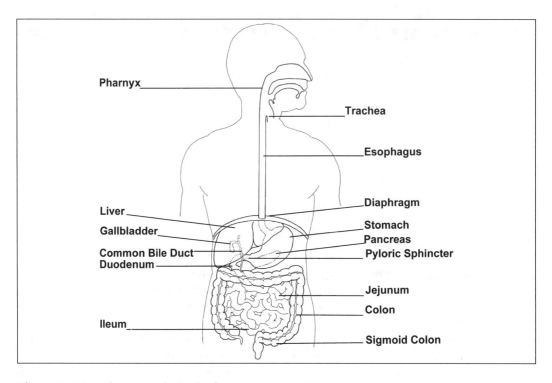

Figure 12-1 The gastrointestinal system

process. One component of gastric juice, hydrochloric acid, has a sterilizing effect; that is, it kills most organisms that enter the stomach. *Pepsin*, the primary enzyme of gastric juice, digests protein in the presence of hydrochloric acid. Also produced in the stomach is intrinsic factor, a substance that is necessary for the absorption of vitamin B$_{12}$. Gastric secretion is stimulated by the vagus nerve as well as by the presence of food in the stomach. The stomach lining is protected from irritation and action of the gastric enzymes by a thin layer of mucus, which is secreted by tiny glands within the stomach's lining. Although some alcohol, water, sugars, and drugs are absorbed in the stomach, most digestion and absorption take place in the small intestine.

From the stomach, food passes through an opening called the pyloric sphincter into the small intestine. The small intestine is approximately 22 feet long and is divided into three

parts. The first part of the small intestine, the *duodenum*, is approximately 10 inches long and is connected to the stomach at the pyloric sphincter. The middle section, the *jejunum*, is approximately 8 feet long. The last part of the small intestine, the *ileum*, connects to the large intestine and is approximately 12 feet long. Digested food continues to move through the gastrointestinal tract by peristaltic movements. Most nutrients are absorbed in the small intestine. Although some fluid is also absorbed in the small intestine, most fluid is absorbed in the large intestine. Thus the contents of the small intestine tend to be liquid in nature.

The small and large intestines are connected by the ileocecal valve, which allows the contents of the small intestine to flow into the large intestine but prevents backflow. The large intestine (**colon**) is only about 5 feet long, but, like the small intestine, it is divided into parts. The part attached to the small intestine at the ileocecal valve is the cecum, to which the appendix is attached. The major portion of the large intestine is divided into the *ascending colon, transverse colon, descending colon*, and *sigmoid colon*. The sigmoid colon leads to the rectum, which leads to the *anus*, the opening through which solid waste is excreted from the body. The large intestine collects food residue and is the site of most water absorption from intestinal contents. Consequently, waste products (**feces**) contained in the large intestine are more solid. The brown color of feces is due primarily to *bile pigments*.

The liver, gallbladder, and pancreas—sometimes called accessory organs of digestion—are located together in the upper abdominal cavity. The liver is the largest single organ in the body and is necessary for survival. In addition to aiding in digestion, the liver is important to carbohydrate, protein, and fat metabolism. The liver performs the following functions:

- Converts glucose, a product of carbohydrate metabolism, into an energy source, glycogen
- Stores glycogen until the body needs it
- Converts the end products of protein metabolism into urea, which is later excreted by the kidneys
- Manufactures and secretes bile for the digestion and absorption of fat
- Breaks down red blood cells
- Produces substances important for clotting of blood
- Acts as a detoxification center of the body, neutralizing poisonous chemicals and drugs

Two major blood vessels enter the liver. The hepatic artery carries oxygenated blood for the liver itself. The portal vein carries blood to the liver from the pancreas, spleen, stomach, and intestine. Blood in the portal vein contains nutrients and toxins for either metabolism or detoxification by the liver. The gallbladder, a small sac that stores bile, is located on the underside of the liver. Bile leaves the liver via the hepatic ducts and enters the gallbladder through the cystic duct. When the gallbladder contracts, bile flows through the common bile duct into the small intestine. Bile, along with bile salts, contains bilirubin, an orange pigment formed from the breakdown of red blood cells. Bile salts are important to fat digestion and absorption.

The pancreas, in addition to its endocrine function of producing the hormones insulin and glucagon (see Chapter 11), also plays an important exocrine function in digestion. The pancreas lies behind the stomach and produces pancreatic juice, which contains enzymes to digest fats, carbohydrates, and proteins. Pancreatic juices enter the common bile duct through the pancreatic duct and then continue to the small intestine.

■ CONDITIONS OF THE GASTROINTESTINAL SYSTEM

Conditions of the Mouth

Although usually not the cause of severe consequences, conditions of the mouth can contribute to development of other conditions by interfering with nutrition. Tooth decay (**dental caries**) and **periodontal disease** (inflammation of the tissues that surround and support the teeth) can lead to the loss of the teeth. Periodontal disease has also been implicated as a contributor to other systemic conditions, such as cardiovascular disease. With periodontal disease, gum tissue may separate from the tooth, leading to the destruction of underlying tissues. The early form of the condition is called **gingivitis** (inflammation of the gums). If it is left untreated, **periodontitis** (a more severe gum condition) may develop.

Periodontitis can affect the supporting structures of the teeth, causing the teeth to become loose and possibly fall out. Loss of teeth has implications not only for cosmetic appearance, but also for nutrition and general health. Inability to chew food adequately may limit food types taken in as well as interfere with the beginning of the digestive process. Although dentures may help cosmetically as well as enhance the ability to chew food, dentures cannot replace the effectiveness of natural teeth for chewing. Dental caries and periodontal disease are best treated through prevention, early detection, and early management.

Other conditions of the mouth that may interfere with proper nutrition include **stomatitis** (inflammation of the mouth) and **parotitis** (inflammation of the parotid glands). Stomatitis can be the result of infection, injury, toxic agents, or systemic illness. Parotitis can result from inactivity of the glands due to lack of oral intake, be caused by infection, or be a side effect of medications or general anesthesia. Management of both stomatitis and parotitis is directed toward correcting or alleviating the underlying cause.

Conditions of the Esophagus

General Conditions of the Esophagus

Dysphagia (difficulty in swallowing) is a major manifestation of a variety of conditions. One cause of dysphagia is *stricture* (narrowing) of portions of the esophagus because of injury or obstruction. When dysphagia is caused by narrowing or constriction of the esophagus, the goal of management is to widen the opening of the passageway. The opening may be dilated repeatedly with a dilating instrument surgical repair may be necessary. When narrowing is caused by a tumor, surgical removal of the tumor or part of the esophagus may be indicated. Dysphagia may also be caused by neurologic conditions, such as stroke or multiple sclerosis, or cardiovascular conditions, such as an enlarged heart.

Achalasia (cardiospasm) is a type of dysphagia believed to be caused by degeneration of the nerves that innervate muscles of the esophagus. As a result, motility of the lower portion of the esophagus is decreased, and food is unable to pass into the stomach efficiently. Food then accumulates within the lower esophagus, causing esophageal irritation (**esophagitis**) and regurgitation. Emotional upsets can aggravate the problem. In addition to the discomforts of esophagitis and the embarrassment of regurgitation, aspiration of undigested food particles into the lungs may occur, resulting in **atelectasis** (see Chapter 14).

Management of achalasia aims to reduce the amount of pressure at the lower end of the esophagus, thereby reducing the extent of the obstruction. The opening between the stomach and the esophagus may be dilated mechanically with the use of a dilating instrument or, in more severe cases, by surgery, which involves cutting the muscle fibers of the sphincter of the lower esophagus.

Dyspepsia (indigestion or discomfort in the upper part of the abdomen) is a common manifestation of conditions of the esophagus. It may be experienced alone or in combination with dysphagia. Among the causes of dyspepsia is **esophageal reflux**, in which stomach contents flow back into the esophagus, irritating the esophageal lining. Esophageal reflux may be treated with medications (e.g., antacids) that decrease acidity, avoidance of smoking, and avoidance of foods or beverages that seem to increase gastric acidity and discomfort. Interventions may include mechanical measures such as sleeping with the head of the bed raised to minimize the amount of reflux by gravity.

Hiatal Hernia (Esophageal Hernia, Diaphragmatic Hernia)

The esophagus passes through an opening in the diaphragm to the stomach. When the opening becomes stretched or weakened, the stomach may protrude through the opening in the diaphragm into the thoracic cavity. This condition, which is called a **hiatal her-**

nia, allows gastric juices to come into contact with the esophageal wall, causing **esophagitis** (inflammation of the esophagus), **dyspepsia** (indigestion), and possibly ulceration of the esophagus. Individuals with a hiatal hernia may experience mild to severe pain and discomfort with the development of esophagitis.

A hiatal hernia may not cause extensive functional consequences, but the resulting discomfort and potential complications may nevertheless interfere with individuals' sense of well-being and subsequent productivity. If manifestations are mild, management of hiatal hernia may be similar to the management of esophageal reflux, as described earlier. To decrease the frequency of manifestations, individuals with a hiatal hernia may need to refrain from any activity that increases intra-abdominal pressure, such as strenuous exercise and bending. In addition, they may need to modify the timing and size of meals (such as having four to six small meals per day) to decrease the amount of gastric acid the stomach produces. Raising the head of the bed by approximately 6 inches while sleeping may also decrease gastric discomfort.

In other instances, hiatal hernia may have to be repaired surgically (Orlando, 2004). Surgery returns the stomach to its regular position and makes the opening in the diaphragm smaller so that the stomach cannot again move above the diaphragm.

Gastroesophageal Reflux Disease (GERD; Reflux Disease)

Gastroesophageal reflux is a condition in which gastric contents move from the stomach to the esophagus. Although reflux occurs in everyone, most individuals have no discomfort or damage associated. When reflux does cause damage and results in discomfort, the condition is called *gastroesophageal reflux disease* (GERD) (Orlando, 2004). In most instances of GERD, the condition involves the lower esophageal sphincter (LES), which connects the esophagus and the stomach. During normal digestion, when food is swallowed, the LES opens to allow food into the stomach. After the food passes the sphincter, the LES usually closes to prevent food and stomach acids from coming in contact with the esophagus. If the sphincter becomes weakened, however, it may not close adequately, allowing stomach contents to flow backward (*reflux*) into the esophagus (acid regurgitation), causing inflammation of the esophagus (esophagitis) When this happens, individuals experience manifestations commonly known as heartburn or acid indigestion. Manifestations cause pressure and burning chest pain, often moving upward to the neck and the throat.

Numerous lifestyle and dietary factors have been implicated as playing roles in the cause of GERD, although there are conflicting data on the impact of most of these factors, including the role of alcohol and tobacco (Meining & Classen, 2000). Fatty meals, sweets, carbonated beverages, juices and citrus products, large meals, and obesity have all been implicated as potential causes. GERD may also be related to hiatal hernia.

In addition to causing significant discomfort, GERD manifestations have been found to precede the identification of cancer in about 60% of individuals with esophageal adenocarcinoma (see Chapter 18) (Lagergren et al., 1999).

Diagnosis is based on manifestations and in some instances *endoscopy* (examination of the esophagus through a hollow tube), which is usually performed by a physician specializing in conditions of the gastrointestinal tract (*gastroenterologist*). Short-term management of GERD usually consists of prescription of medications to reduce stomach acid (Orlando, 2004). Lifestyle modifications may include eating smaller meals, avoiding large meals during the working day, and eating dinner at least 3 hours prior to bedtime. Recommendations may also include avoiding liquids with meals, especially tea, coffee, carbonated drinks, or beer. In some instances, individuals may find raising the head of the bed useful (Marshall, 2007). In general, individuals may be instructed to avoid foods, exercises, or positions that seem to aggravate the condition. Management may be long term in some instances and is directed toward helping individuals control manifestations when they occur (Dent, 2001).

Conditions of the Stomach

Gastritis

Gastritis is an inflammation of the lining of the stomach that can be caused by a variety of irritants or infectious agents. Acute gastritis is of short duration, with manifestations of nausea, vomiting, and pain; it is generally self-limiting, requiring little except for managing manifestations. Chronic gastritis, which is of longer duration, may consist of nondescript upper abdominal distress with vague manifestations. Extensive evaluation may be necessary to identify its causative factors. This type of gastritis may be caused because of irritation of the stomach from medications used to treat another condition (such as aspirin used in the treatment of rheumatoid arthritis, described in Chapter 16) or it may be a manifestation of more serious illness. It may also be caused by infection with the organism *Helicobacter pylori* (Graham & Genta, 2004). If left untreated, chronic gastritis can progress to scarring of the stomach lining, ulceration, or hemorrhage.

Peptic Ulcer

Types of Peptic Ulcers

Peptic ulcer disease (PUD) is a chronic, inflammatory gastrointestinal condition characterized by ulcer (sore) formation in the esophagus, stomach, or duodenum. Peptic ulcers in the upper portion of the small intestine are called **duodenal ulcers**; those in the

stomach are called **gastric ulcers**. Duodenal ulcers occur more frequently than do gastric ulcers.

Until the 1980s, spicy food, acid, stress, and lifestyle were considered major causes of ulcers. In 1982, the bacterium, *Helicobacter pylori* was found to cause more than 90% of duodenal ulcers and as many as 80% of gastric ulcers (Centers for Disease Control and Prevention, 2004). *H. pylori* breaks down the mucosal barrier and seems to increase gastric acid secretions (Barba, Fitzgerald, & Wood, 2007).

After infection with *H. pylori*, the second most common risk factor for developing a peptic ulcer is use of aspirin or nonsteroidal anti-inflammatory drugs (NSAIDs) (Graham, 2004). Although some foods and beverages (e.g., alcohol and caffeine-containing beverages) increase gastric secretion and can irritate the lining of the gastrointestinal tract, there is no evidence to suggest that the intake of these substances causes ulcers.

Another type of peptic ulcer, a **stress ulcer**, may develop after an acute physical crisis, such as a severe injury or a catastrophic illness. Special names are given to stress ulcers that develop with some conditions. For example, stress ulcers associated with burns are called **Curling's ulcers**; those associated with head injury are called **Cushing's ulcers**. The reason that these ulcers develop is unknown; however, they develop rapidly, sometimes within 72 hours of the injury or illness. Manifestations may not appear until the ulcer perforates and massive gastric hemorrhage occurs.

Manifestations and Complications of Peptic Ulcer

The most common manifestations of peptic ulcer are epigastric pain, a gnawing or burning pain located in the lower chest above the heart, and **dyspepsia** (disturbance in digestion), which may include nausea, bloating, or reflux. The terms "gastroesophageal reflux disease," "gastritis," and "dyspepsia" are often used interchangeably (Ryan, 2005).

Pain or discomfort usually occurs several hours after eating, when the stomach is empty, and is relieved by the ingestion of food, especially in the case of a duodenal ulcer. Bleeding of the ulcer may also occur, causing manifestations of **hematemesis** (vomiting of blood) or **melena** (black, tarry bowel movements). In some instances, blood loss may be enough to cause individuals to become anemic.

Peptic ulcers can be life-threatening if complications develop. Two serious complications of peptic ulcer are hemorrhage and perforation, both of which are emergencies. In perforation, erosion of the ulcer through the gastric lining allows the contents of the gastrointestinal tract to escape into the **peritoneal cavity**, causing irritation of the peritoneal lining. The resulting inflammation of the peritoneum (**peritonitis**) can be fatal.

Diagnosis of Peptic Ulcer

Identification of *H. pylori* infection can be determined by invasive techniques, such as endoscopy or biopsy, or by noninvasive techniques, such as blood tests, urea breath test, or stool antigen test (Vaira et al., 2005). For the urea breath test, the individual ingests urea that contains radioactive substances; a short time later the individual's breath is analyzed. This test is used both to make the initial diagnosis of *H. pylori* infection and, after intervention, to confirm eradication of the organism. The stool antigen test involves immunoassay of a fecal sample to detect the presence of *H. pylori*. In some instances, individuals may undergo endoscopy, in which a tube with a camera inside is inserted through the mouth and into the stomach to look for evidence of ulcers; during this procedure, biopsies (tissue samples) of the stomach lining may be obtained and then examined for *H. pylori*.

Management of Peptic Ulcer

The overall goals in the management of peptic ulcer are to relieve discomfort, heal the ulcer itself, and eradicate the organism *H. pylori*. Once the organism is eradicated, reinfection rates are low (Suerbaum & Michetti, 2002).

Antibiotics and medications to suppress stomach acid secretion such as H_2 blockers or proton pump inhibitors (PPIs) are major focuses of peptic ulcer management (Cutler, 2001). Because the *H. pylori* organism is difficult to eradicate, partly because it is protected by the stomach lining, it is especially important that the individual takes medications as prescribed and complete the entire regimen of medication to prevent the organism from developing resistance. Resistance to antibiotics and noncompliance with the management recommendations are the two most common reasons for management failure (Centers for Disease Control and Prevention, 2004).

Little evidence suggests that dietary intake causes peptic ulcer or that dietary therapy is useful in its management. Even so, individuals are generally encouraged to avoid foods that produce discomfort and to use alcohol and coffee only in moderation. Other substances that irritate the stomach lining, such as tobacco, aspirin, and NSAIDs, are generally discontinued as well. Individuals who must continue using aspirin—for example, in the management of arthritis—may be encouraged to use buffered aspirin or aspirin that has a special enteric coating.

Although surgical management of peptic ulcer is rare today, if the ulcer does not respond to therapy or if complications such as uncontrollable bleeding or perforation occur, surgery is indicated. Several types of surgery may be performed (Orloff & Debas, 2004). **Vagotomy,** involves cutting the vagal nerve to eliminate its ability to stimulate acid secretion in the stomach. **Pyloroplasty** involves widening the opening between the stomach and the small intestine to facilitate stomach drainage. In **gastroenterostomy**, the bottom of the stomach and the small intestine are both opened; the two openings are then connected, creating a passage between the body of the stomach and the small intestine to facilitate stomach drainage. In some instances, the acid-secreting portions of the stomach are removed; this procedure is called **antrectomy** or **subtotal gastrectomy**.

Several complications are associated with surgical resection of the stomach. *Dumping syndrome* is a term used to describe manifestations that occur after the individual eats because food enters the small intestine more rapidly and is not adequately mixed. Individuals with dumping syndrome may experience dizziness, sweating, fainting, rapid heartbeat, and nausea 5 to 30 minutes after eating. The management of dumping syndrome involves decreasing the amount of food taken at one time, lying down after meals, and not taking liquids with meals. Dumping syndrome usually subsides 6 months to 1 year after surgery.

Another possible complication of surgical resection of the stomach is **pernicious anemia** (vitamin B_{12} deficiency). Pernicious anemia may occur after the removal of a portion of the stomach because of the absence of the *intrinsic factor*, a substance necessary for the absorption of vitamin B_{12}. In this case, lifelong management with injections of supplemental vitamin B_{12} is necessary. Other nutritional problems, such as reduced absorption of calcium or vitamin D, may also be experienced as a result of the rapid emptying of food into the bowel.

Psychosocial Issues with Peptic Ulcer

In the past, individuals with peptic ulcer were advised to avoid certain foods and were often placed on restricted diets. Evidence now shows that special diets have no greater benefit in the management of peptic ulcer than does consumption of regular meals. Nevertheless, individuals may need to avoid foods or drink that appear to be aggravating manifestations of the condition.

Stress had been viewed as a major contributor to development of peptic ulcer prior to the discovery of the organism *H. pylori* as a causative agent. Although management now focuses on treatment of the condition rather than lifestyle modification, the role of stress as a factor contributing to development of the peptic ulcers is frequently ignored (Levenstein, 1998), but cannot be dismissed. An increase in both gastric and duodenal ulcers has been found in survivors of a number of natural disasters and crisis situations (Aoyama et al., 1998; Nice, Garland, Hilton, Baggett, & Mitchell, 1996). Although *H. pylori* may still be present in these individuals, the effects of the organism and stress may be additive, promoting growth of the organism (Levenstein, Ackerman, Kiecolt-Glaser, & Dubois, 1999). Although stress may be a causative factor in development of peptic ulcers, it can certainly worsen manifestations. Consequently, minimizing stress in general or learning stress-reduction techniques may be an important part of overall management for many individuals with peptic ulcers.

Vocational Issues with Peptic Ulcer

In most instances, long-term vocational consequences of peptic ulcers alone are nonexistent. Now that medications are used predominantly in the management of peptic ulcers (rather than surgery), the incidence of major functional consequences has decreased significantly. Most individuals, with appropriate and timely management, will be able to continue in their employment. Individuals with additional chronic conditions, individuals who do not have access to appropriate health care, or individuals who are nonadherence to management recommendations, however, have a greater chance of experiencing reoccurrence and subsequent complications as a result of their condition.

Conditions of the Intestine

Hernia (Rupture)

Protrusion of an organ through the tissues that usually hold it in place is called **hernia.** The most common types of abdominal hernias are inguinal and femoral hernias, in which the intestine protrudes through a weakened part of the lower abdominal wall. Men are more likely to develop inguinal hernias, whereas women are more likely to develop femoral hernias.

Manifestations are often mild, consisting of little more than a lump or swelling on the abdomen underneath the skin. The protrusion may appear when the individuals cough or lift something heavy, but application of manual pressure over the area often pushes it back into place (reduces it). The protruding structure can become swollen and constricted by the opening, however, making it impossible to move the protrusion back into place. If this condition, called *incarceration*, is not treated, blood supply to the herniated portion of the intestine may be cut off, causing tissue death. This condition, which is called *strangulated hernia*, is a surgical emergency.

Uncomplicated hernias have few long-term consequences, although it may be necessary to avoid activities such as lifting or pushing heavy objects. Even though there may be few significant activity-related consequences of hernia, because of the danger of hernia strangulation it is important for individuals who have a hernia to seek medical attention, even though they have no pain. This is especially true if they engage in strenuous work.

The surgical procedure used to repair hernias is called **herniorrhaphy**. In this surgery, the protruding organs are replaced and the weakened area in the abdominal wall is repaired.

Inflammatory Bowel Disease

Inflammatory bowel disease (IBD) refers to a group of conditions that cause inflammation and/or ulceration in the lining of the bowel. Inflammatory bowel disease is chronic and long term, with an unpredictable course. Two of the most common conditions classified as inflammatory bowel disease are **Crohn's disease** and **ulcerative colitis** (Younge & Norton, 2007; Tanaka & Kazuma, 2005).

Manifestations of inflammatory bowel disease usually consist of fever, weight loss, diarrhea, and tenderness in the abdomen, and sometimes blood in the stool. Some people experience long periods of **remission** (times when manifestations subside), which alternate with **exacerbations** (times when manifestations become worse). The exact cause of inflammatory bowel disease is unknown, but it appears that susceptibility is inherited in at least some cases (Podolsky, 2002). The precise role that psychological factors play in development of the condition is controversial (Hyphantis et al., 2005).

Crohn's Disease (Regional Enteritis, Granulomatous Ileitis)

Crohn's disease is a lifelong, relapsing and remitting condition characterized by inflammation of segments of the **ileum** (small intestine), although it can extend throughout the gastrointestinal tract from the mouth to the anus (King, 2007). It results in scarring, thickening, and small inflammatory nodules of the intestinal wall that can cause **stenosis** (narrowing) of the intestine. It is characterized by chronic diarrhea, abdominal pain, fever, loss of appetite, and weight loss. The condition's manifestations and unpredictable recurrence cause restrictions on lifestyle and can interfere with work attendance. Three interacting factors—genetic susceptibility, environmental triggers, and altered immune response—appear to be indicated in the development of Crohn's disease (Shanahan, 2003).

Crohn's disease may be complicated by obstruction of the intestine because of stenosis or by the formation of abscesses. Bowel obstruction in Crohn's disease is an emergency. Other complications may include formation of an irregular, tube-like passage (**fistula**) between the small intestine and other parts of the abdominal cavity. In both of these instances, surgical intervention may be necessary.

If there are no complications, complete recovery may follow a single isolated attack; however, Crohn's disease is frequently characterized by lifelong exacerbations. Management of the disease is aimed at managing manifestations, improving quality of life, and minimizing complications. The approach taken varies according to the severity of the disease and complications. During severe exacerbations, medications including antibiotics, steroids, and sulfa preparations (to reduce inflammation) are often used in addition to nutrition support through special feedings or *total parenteral nutrition* (TPN) if individuals are unable to tolerate an oral diet for longer than five to seven days (Ireton-Jones, George, Day, & Zeiter, 2000).

Ulcerative Colitis

In contrast to Crohn's disease, which affects segments of the small bowel, ulcerative colitis is an inflammatory condition of the **colon** (large intestine). It starts at the rectum or lower end of the colon and spreads upward, at times involving the entire colon. The colon lining becomes **edematous** (swollen), thickened, and congested with small ulcers that ooze blood. Ulcerative colitis may develop slowly or rapidly. Manifestations usually include crampy abdominal pain and bloody diarrhea. In severe cases, shock may result.

Ulcerative colitis, as a condition characterized by periods of remission and exacerbation, can be a serious condition with systemic complications that range from malnutrition to **arthritis** and **ankylosing spondylitis** (see Chapter 16). Management consists of medications, such as steroids to control inflammation or immunosuppressive drugs to induce remission of the condition (Peppercorn & Moss, 2007). Some individuals with ulcerative colitis eventually require surgical intervention, such as **colectomy** (removal of the colon), which is curative. Removal of the colon does, however, require permanent **ileostomy** or creation of a pouch or reservoir for solid waste (**ileoanal pouch**), both of which are discussed later in this chapter. Because individuals with ulcerative colitis have an increased risk of developing cancer of the colon, regular cancer screening is essential (Ghosh, Shand, & Ferguson, 2000).

Nonsurgical Management of Inflammatory Bowel Disease

The management of inflammatory bowel disease depends on the location, severity, and chronicity of the condition and whether it is Crohn's disease or ulcerative colitis. Steroid therapy may be used to reduce inflammation during an acute exacerbation of the condition. A medication known as *sulfasalazine* is frequently prescribed for individuals with inflammatory bowel disease to prevent or control infections, as the inflamed bowel is susceptible to infection. During acute attacks, individuals with inflammatory bowel disease are directed to keep physical activity to a minimum. They may continue working, but may need rest at frequent intervals. Some individuals with severe manifestations may be debilitated to the extent that bed rest is indicated.

Specific dietary restrictions vary with different individuals. In general, individuals with inflammatory bowel disease need to avoid foods that cause flare-ups. Low-fiber diets may be appropriate for those who have a propensity toward bowel obstruction, while a high-fiber diet that stimulates the bowel may be advisable for other individuals.

Surgical Management of Inflammatory Bowel Disease

When nonsurgical management fails to resolve inflammatory bowel disease or if complications occur, surgery may be indicated. The type of surgery depends on the location and severity of the inflammatory bowel disease. In Crohn's disease, surgery is not curative, but rather is indicated for complications such as obstruction or abscess formation. Surgical management of Crohn's disease may involve removing or resecting the affected portion of the intestine and surgically connecting the two ends of the intestine. This surgical connection is called an **anastomosis**.

The most common surgical procedure for ulcerative colitis is the removal of all or part of the colon, a procedure called a **colectomy**. If removing the entire colon, the surgeon passes a portion of the small intestine (ileum) through a surgically created opening to the outside of the abdomen and establishes an ileostomy. The part of the intestine that is exposed to the outer surface of the abdomen is

called a **stoma**. In this instance, the ileostomy is permanent, and all waste from the small intestine passes through this opening rather than through the rectum. The removal of the entire colon is curative for ulcerative colitis.

If only part of the colon is removed, the surgeon creates an opening between the remaining portion of the colon and the external surface of the abdomen. This opening, called a **colostomy**, is the opening through which solid wastes (**feces**) will be excreted. A colostomy may be either temporary or permanent.

Because the stoma of either an ileostomy or a colostomy has no sphincter, individuals have no control over the elimination of wastes through the stoma. Individuals with an ileostomy have more liquid and more frequent bowel movements than do individuals with a colostomy, because a great deal of liquid is removed from waste products in the large intestine. Thus, although individuals with a colostomy may be able to control the timing of their bowel movements through regular daily colostomy irrigation, individuals with an ileostomy may have more difficulty regulating elimination by this means.

Individuals with either colostomy or ileostomy may wear ostomy pouches, which are small plastic bags placed over the stoma to

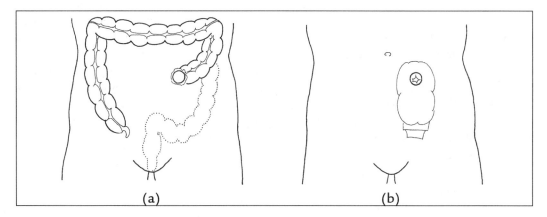

Figure 12-2   (a) Colostomy. (b) Colostomy with bag.

collect fecal waste (see Figure 12-2). The bag is attached by a separate base plate that is individualized to fit snugly around the stoma. A skin barrier paste is typically used to ensure a tight seal and thereby prevent leakage. A variety of products are also available that may be placed in the bag to neutralize odor. For some individuals, especially those with colostomy who are able to control elimination with irrigation, small security pads may be all that are needed over the stoma between irrigations.

Some individuals with an ileostomy have a continent ileostomy in which an intra-abdominal pouch, or *Kock pouch*, is surgically constructed from a portion of the small intestine. Fecal waste collects in the pouch until the individual drains the pouch through the stoma with a catheter. Those who have such a pouch need not wear an external appliance. Individuals insert a catheter three or four times each day, as needed, to remove the waste.

Some individuals are able to have a surgical procedure that creates an *ileoanal pouch*. In this procedure, after the colon is removed, the small intestine is sutured to the anal opening. An internal pouch for storing feces is created from the ileum so that individuals are able to have bowel movements through the anus. A temporary ileostomy may be necessary until the area around the ileoanal pouch heals, but after two to three months the ileostomy may be closed and anal elimination resumed.

Having a colostomy or ileostomy not only alters body function, but also alters body image. Ostomy support groups are useful to help individuals learn to live with a stoma and to overcome self-consciousness, which may be associated with having an ostomy. Ileoanal pouches have gained increasing popularity (Rust & Rose, 2006) and for some individuals have shown to improve quality of life benefits. Nevertheless, individuals weighing the risks and benefits for ileostomy versus ileoanal pouch must consider the higher complication rates associated with the procedure before

making their decision (Seidel, Newman, & Sharp, 2000).

Psychosocial Issues in Inflammatory Bowel Disease

The chronic nature of inflammatory bowel disease, with the associated remissions and exacerbations may cause significant stress, given that individuals are unable to predict flare-ups of their condition. Individuals with ulcerative coltis may experience urgency to defecate along with fecal incontinence to the extent that they find it difficult to function effectively in social or work settings (Stenson, 2004). When surgery is required and a colostomy or ileostomy results, individuals' body image is altered. Because stomas of colostomy and ileostomy have no sphincter, there is no control over elimination. Control over elimination is considered a milestone of childhood maturation, representing competence and health (Gallo-Silver, Maydick-Youngberg, & Weiner, 2005). When control over elimination is altered, not only are self-concept and body image altered, but individuals may also experience shame and self-doubt. They may be concerned about odors or embarrassing sounds when in a social situation and consequently avoid them. Because of the altered body image and fear of an "accident" during sexual activity, individuals may also feel self-conscious and have concerns about sexual encounters. The reactions of significant others, family, and friends greatly influence individuals' adjustment to their condition. An atmosphere of acceptance and support is important to individuals' self-esteem and ability to adjust to their condition.

Vocational Issues in Inflammatory Bowel Disease

When in remission, inflammatory bowel disease should have few effects on vocational function. During an exacerbation, depending on the severity of manifestations, individuals may have repeated absences from work. In some instances, if the condition is severe, repeated hospitalizations may be needed.

Colostomy or ileostomy should have no impact on the ability to work. Even so, the individuals' own level of comfort (or discomfort) with colostomy or ileostomy may be a major determinant of the extent to which they continue in their work.

Diverticulitis

A **diverticulum** is a small balloon-like sac or pouch that develops in the walls of the large intestine. These tiny pouches form when pressure causes the inside wall of the large intestine to bulge out through weak spots in the outer wall of the intestine. One of the major causes of diverticula formation is constipation. Once diverticula have formed, there is no way to reverse the process; however, a diet that contains fiber and bulk to promote regular bowel habits may help to control and minimize the condition. **Diverticulosis** is the presence of numerous such outpouchings in the intestinal wall (see Figure 12-3). Individuals with diverticulosis are often free of manifestations and may be unaware of the condition until it is found accidentally through a radiologic examination for another reason. Diverticula can, however, be a major source of massive hemorrhage in the colon. Collection of fecal matter in the diverticula can erode arteries that are in close proximity, causing massive bleeding (Clearfield, 2007).

Individuals with no manifestations usually experience few consequences and require no special interventions. However, they may be advised to avoid activities that increase intra-abdominal pressure such as bending, lifting, and stooping. They are also instructed to avoid constipation through the ingestion of a high-fiber diet and intake of plenty of fluids.

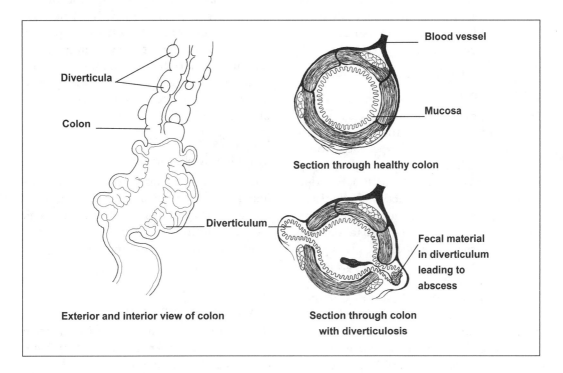

Figure 12-3   Diverticulosis

Some individuals with diverticulosis develop a condition called **diverticulitis** in which there is obstruction, infection, and inflammation of a diverticulum (Wilcox, 2004). Manifestations of diverticulitis include crampy pain in the lower abdomen and, occasionally, mild fever. Management may consist of providing the colon with a period of rest. During this time, individuals are permitted to have nothing by mouth and may be given antibiotics. At times diverticula perforate, such that bowel contents spill into the abdomen. Resulting complications may consist of hemorrhage and **peritonitis** (inflammation of the peritoneum). Individuals who develop complications may require surgery. Surgery usually involves a colon resection, in which the portion of the bowel containing the inflamed diverticula is removed and the healthy portions of the bowel are rejoined (anastomosis). Individuals who undergo surgery for diverticulitis may be able to resume activities within two to four weeks after surgery, but they are usually advised to continue the therapeutic measures recommended for diverticulosis.

Irritable Bowel Syndrome (Spastic Colon)

Irritable bowel syndrome is a chronic or intermittent condition of the gastrointestinal tract in which individuals experience chronic, excessive spasms of the large intestine; cramping abdominal pain; and diarrhea, constipation, or both. It is a functional condition, meaning that it has no identifiable organic cause (Ringel, Sperber, & Drossman, 2001). As a biopsychosocial condition, it is thought to result from interaction of psychosocial factors, altered motility of the bowel, and heightened sensory function of the intestine (Camilleri, 2001; Mach, 2004). Although studies show that individuals with irritable bowel syndrome are more likely to have mood and anxiety disorders (Olden & Brown, 2007), psychosocial factors alone are not the cause of the condi-

tion. Psychological conditions can, however, worsen manifestations of this syndrome and influence the way the condition is experienced by the individual. It is now believed that individuals with irritable bowel syndrome have an irregularity in motor function of the intestinal tract, which renders the intestine more sensitive to a variety of stimuli, including food, some medications, and stress (Talley, 2004). Although irritable bowel syndrome does not cause significant functional consequences, it can affect quality of life and have a large economic impact on healthcare use and indirect costs as a result of absenteeism (Camilleri, 2001).

Manifestations of Irritable Bowel Syndrome

In irritable bowel syndrome, the colon is more sensitive and reacts to mild stimuli more dramatically than the colon of most people, resulting in spasm of the bowel. Individuals may experience cramping abdominal pain and a frequent, urgent need to defecate, especially after meals. Manifestations vary in intensity. Although irritable bowel syndrome can cause significant distress, it does not cause permanent harm to the intestines and does not cause ulceration or bleeding.

Diagnosis of Irritable Bowel Syndrome

Minimal diagnostic tests are advocated in the initial approach to identifying irritable bowel syndrome. Diagnosis is usually made through a detailed history of abdominal pain or discomfort associated with chronic altered bowel habits.

Management of Irritable Bowel Syndrome

Because there is no known cause of irritable bowel syndrome, there is also no cure. Management is directed toward relieving this condition's manifestations and eliminating stress.

Dietary modification may be indicated. Foods and beverages that appear to aggravate the manifestations should be avoided. Individuals who experience constipation may be helped by consumption of a high-fiber diet.

Medications such as laxatives for constipation or antidiarrheal medications for individuals who experience diarrhea may also be prescribed. Medications may also be prescribed to reduce intestinal activity or to relieve tension and anxiety. Antispasmodics for pain and tricyclic antidepressants (see Chapter 8) may be prescribed as well.

Psychosocial intervention, such as counseling, psychotherapy, or hypnotherapy, may be necessary in more severe cases (Sach & Chang, 2002; Alaradi & Barkin, 2002). Individuals may be referred to special programs where they can learn techniques to control emotional tension. Behavioral interventions such as relaxation therapy, hypnosis, biofeedback, and cognitive-behavioral interventions directed toward reduction of anxiety and promotion of healthy behaviors may give the individual a sense of control and help in adaptation to the condition.

Individuals with irritable bowel syndrome always live with the potential for irregular function of the colon. If the individual is able to identify what triggers the manifestations —whether it is a certain food or a stressful situation—it may be helpful in controlling the occurrence of manifestations. Because the bowel responds to stress, individuals with this syndrome should maintain a healthy lifestyle that includes adequate nutrition, rest, exercise, and recreation.

Psychosocial Issues of Irritable Bowel Syndrome

Irritable bowel syndrome can significantly affect individuals' quality of life. Individuals may, as a result of their condition, experience a number of concerns related to their social activities, home life, and work. This condition can have debilitating effects, causing frequent absences from work (Camilleri, 2001).

Because of their frequent, intense need to use the bathroom, individuals may be afraid to go to social events or to travel even short distances because of their manifestations. They tend to be very concerned about their manifestations and may be quite sensitive to the physical discomfort they experience.

Vocational Implications of Irritable Bowel Syndrome

The prognosis for irritable bowel syndrome is often favorable. It is not linked to other serious conditions, and the mortality rate is zero. Distressing manifestations can be relieved or eradicated, increasing the individual's ability to function.

Conditions of the Accessory Organs of the Gastrointestinal System

Pancreatitis

Pancreatitis is an inflammatory process of the pancreas that may be acute or chronic. The most common causes of acute pancreatitis in the United States are gallstones and alcohol abuse (Solorzano & Prinz, 2007; Owyang, 2004). Manifestations of pancreatitis include severe abdominal pain, often radiating to the back and frequently accompanied by nausea and vomiting. Pancreatitis begins with **edema** (swelling) in the tissues surrounding the pancreas and may progress to hemorrhage and **necrosis** (death) of surrounding tissue. Enzymes produced in the pancreas for digestion of food may initiate an autodigestive process, beginning to attack the pancreas itself.

Acute pancreatitis may be mild or may result in complications such as pancreatic abscess and in some situations, death. It may occur after binge drinking, but more often accompanies chronic alcohol abuse (Soloranzo & Prinz, 2007). When acute pancreatitis is precipitated by gallstones, it usually arises because the stone obstructs pancreatic duct flow. Individuals with acute pancreatitis are typically treated in the hospital with intravenous fluids and pain medications during the initial phase of the condition. If there are no complications and early interventions have been implemented, inflammation and manifestations usually subside with no long-term effects.

Chronic pancreatitis is an irreversible, progressive inflammation of the pancreas that involves progressive scarring and calcification of the pancreas. The most frequent cause of chronic pancreatitis in the United States and Europe is alcohol abuse (Solorzano & Prinz, 2007). Manifestations of chronic pancreatitis include pain, which may be worsened by food and alcohol. Individuals may also experience nausea and vomiting. With significant damage to the pancreas, individuals with chronic pancreatitis can develop diabetes mellitus secondary to the pancreatitis (see Chapter 11). Interventions may involve hospitalization for control of pain, although damage to the pancreatic tissue will be permanent. Abstinence from alcohol is crucial. Individuals may experience malnutrition due to poor dietary habits and because they avoid eating due to fear of pain. Parenteral or tube feedings may be give to help individuals improve their nutritional status. In addition, pancreatic enzyme replacements may be needed. Surgical interventions are usually reserved for only the most severe cases (Solorzano & Prinz, 2007).

Cholecystitis

Although **cholecystitis** (inflammation of the gallbladder) can occur in individuals with severe trauma or other critical illness even if they do not have gallstones, an obstruction of the cystic duct by a gallstone is the most common cause of this condition. The presence of gallstones is called **cholelithiasis**. Stones may injure the gallbladder and block passage of bile that is stored there.

Gallbladder conditions can be either acute or chronic. Manifestations of acute cholecystitis include severe pain in the upper abdomen, often with nausea and vomiting. When stones block its passage, bile may back up to the liver, interfering with production of more bile. As a result, the level of bilirubin circulating in the blood becomes excessive, causing **jaundice** (a yellowish appearance of the skin and the whites of the eyes).

Possible complications of cholecystitis include infection and/or perforation of the gallbladder, damage to the liver, and pancreatitis. For individuals with cholecystitis, management may begin with the elimination from the diet of fatty and highly seasoned foods that aggravate the condition. The usual intervention for cholelithiasis is surgical removal of the gallbladder. The curative interventon for cholelithiasis is surgical removal of the gallbladder, a procedure called **cholecystectomy**. Cholecystectomy is often now performed through a small tube called a laparoscope, in a procedure called laparoscopic cholecystectomy. This procedure eliminates the need for large incisions through the muscles of the abdominal wall. Consequently, cholecystectomy is often now performed in an outpatient surgical setting, with individuals going home 24 to 48 hours after surgery (Ruiz, 2007).

Hepatitis

The term **hepatitis** refers to conditions in which there is inflammation of the liver. Although most often hepatitis refers to infectious hepatitis caused by a virus, inflammation of the liver can also be due to noninfectious causes such as alcohol or drug-induced hepatitis, medication-induced hepatitis, hepatitis induced by ingestion of toxic chemicals, or autoimmune hepatitis (O'Brien, 2007). Although manifestations of liver inflammation and subsequent liver damage may be the same in noninfectious causes of hepatitis as in infectious causes, noninfectious hepatitis does not require the same level of precaution to prevent its spread.

Acute Viral Hepatitis

Several viruses can cause acute hepatitis, including the hepatitis A, B, C, D, and E viruses. Viruses are transmitted in different ways, but they all initiate an inflammatory process in the liver that interferes with its effective functioning. Hepatitis is categorized according to the cause.

Hepatitis A

Hepatitis caused by the type A virus is called hepatitis A. It is highly contagious and is usually transmitted through the ingestion of food or water that has been contaminated because of poor sanitation or poor personal hygiene. When spread through direct person-to-person contact, it may be called *infectious hepatitis*. Individuals with hepatitis A usually experience initial weakness, *malaise* (a feeling of general fatigue or discomfort), or body aches.

Hepatitis A is diagnosed through blood tests. There is no specific intervention to eradicate the infection. Acute hepatitis A infection is usually self-limited. Although the infection can persist for months, it does not lead to chronic liver conditions (Hoofnagle & Lindsay, 2004). Vaccination for hepatitis A is available for individuals at high risk for contracting this virus, such as travelers to areas where the rate of infection is high.

There is no specific medication or intervention that directly affects the virus that causes hepatitis A. Usually, hepatitis resolves spontaneously after one to two months. During that interval, management is directed toward alleviating the manifestations and maintaining the individual's state of health so that he or she may withstand the infection. Rest and adequate nutrition are the cornerstones of therapy. Individuals with hepatitis may generally return to work after their jaundice disappears and they feel sufficiently strong to resume their duties.

Hepatitis B

Hepatitis B, sometimes called *serum hepatitis*, is caused by the type B virus (HBV) and is a major health problem. Initial manifestations may consist of flu-like manifestations. Eventually, jaundice may appear because of **hyperbilirubinemia** (an excess of bilirubin in the blood). Individuals may also complain of **pruritus** (itching of the skin).

The hepatitis B virus can live in all body fluids and is transmitted by contact with blood, semen, and vaginal fluids. This virus may be spread through injection with contaminated needles when injecting drugs or through tattooing, ear piercing, electrolysis, or acupuncture. It is also transmitted through contact with contaminated body fluids during sexual intercourse or through sharing personal care items such as toothbrushes.

A pregnant woman can pass the hepatitis B virus to her baby at birth, resulting in lifelong, incurable liver problems for the infant. Diagnosis of hepatitis B is made through a blood test.

Although there is no cure, hepatitis B can be prevented. Because of the potential serious consequences of hepatitis B infection, a comprehensive immunization strategy to eliminate transmission of the hepatitis B virus has been adopted in the United States; it includes routine vaccination of infants and adolescents and vaccination of high-risk adults. Although most individuals recover from the manifestations of hepatitis B in approximately six months, they continue to be carriers of the virus (Zuckerman & Lavancy, 1999). Not all carriers are infectious, but carriers are at higher risk for developing chronic hepatitis, which can be associated with cirrhosis, liver failure, and liver cancer (Lox, 2002).

Hepatitis C

Hepatitis C (formerly called non-A, non-B hepatitis) is caused by the hepatitis C virus (HCV). It is contracted primarily through the transfusion of contaminated blood or blood products or from infected needles. Once an individual becomes infected, the condition is lifelong. A major complication of hepatitis C is chronic hepatitis. Hepatitis C is the most common cause of chronic liver conditions in the United States, and many individuals with hepatitis C go on to develop end-stage liver disease (Gaster & Larson, 2000). Individuals with hepatitis C are also at risk for developing cancer of the liver.

Hepatitis C may be **asymptomatic** (without manifestations), or it may begin with flu-like manifestations, such as **anorexia** (lack of appetite), distaste for cigarettes, chills and fever, nausea and vomiting, or headache.

Management of hepatitis C includes a course of antiviral therapy including a combination of medications such as *interferon* and *ribavirin,* usually three times a week for six months to one year. Although this intervention is not curative, it can have a beneficial effect on survival and development of chronic liver disease (Gaster & Larson, 2000). Medication intervention is expensive, however, and may cause side effects so severe that individuals may be prevented from working during the time they are experiencing the interventions (Yates & Gleason, 1998). Individuals who develop cirrhosis because of hepatitis C may be candidates for liver transplantation. Individuals are usually required to be free of alcohol or illicit drugs for six months prior to being placed on a transplant list.

There is currently no immunization available to prevent hepatitis C infections. Consequently, the best prevention is avoidance of high-risk behaviors.

Hepatitis D

Hepatitis D is spread primarily through injection-drug use and sexual activity. Manifestations of the condition are similar to those seen with other forms of hepatitis. There is no specific treatment for hepatitis D, nor is a specific vaccine against hepatitis D available.

Hepatitis E

Hepatitis E is acquired most frequently when there has been exposure to fecally contaminated food or drinking water in countries in which hepatis E is endemic. It is rarely transmitted from person to person. Manifestations of and treatment for hepatitis E are similar to those for hepatitis A. There is no vaccine available.

Chronic Hepatitis

Chronic hepatitis comprises several conditions that are grouped together because of their similar manifestations and because they can all lead to cirrhosis and end-stage liver disease (Lindsay & Hoofnagle, 2004). When liver inflammation continues longer than three to six months, individuals are said to have chronic hepatitis. This condition may lead to progressive fibrous changes in the liver or cirrhosis. The prognosis is variable, depending on the cause.

Toxic Hepatitis

Because the liver metabolizes and detoxifies many drugs as well as other toxic or poisonous substances, overexposure to or presence of **hepatotoxins** (substances that are harmful to the liver) can cause liver damage and chronic liver disease. The prognosis depends on the extent of the liver damage and the prevention of associated complications.

Cirrhosis

Cirrhosis is a progressive condition of the liver in which liver function is disorganized and altered because of damage that produces fibrous changes in the structure of the liver. Such changes can occur for a wide variety of reasons:

- Infection of the liver, as in viral hepatitis

- Obstruction of bile flow, as in conditions of the gallbladder
- Overexposure to hepatotoxins, such as toxic chemicals
- Alcohol abuse

Manifestations vary widely, ranging from no symptoms to total liver failure (Friedman & Schiano, 2004). As the condition progresses, manifestations may consist of fatigue, weakness, anorexia (lack of appetite) with weight loss, nausea, vomiting, or pruritus (itching of the skin). Individuals with advanced cases of cirrhosis may gain weight because of their retention of fluid and the presence of fluid in the abdominal cavity, a condition called **ascites.** Finally, there may be vomiting of blood (**hematemesis**) and a general bleeding tendency.

Complications of cirrhosis include hemorrhage, coma, and, eventually, death. Management of cirrhosis is based on its cause and any complications that may be present. (Sterling, Mattar, & Kwo, 2007). Management of cirrhosis is discussed in further detail in Chapter 9. The prognosis depends on the severity of the condition and the associated complications.

■ GENERAL DIAGNOSTIC PROCEDURES FOR GASTROINTESTINAL CONDITIONS

Barium Swallow (Upper Gastrointestinal Series)

A radiologic (x-ray) study of the upper gastrointestinal tract, known as a **barium swallow** makes it possible to identify irregularities of the esophagus, stomach, and upper portion of the small intestine. Immediately before the procedure, the individuals drink a white, chalky liquid called barium so that the radiologist can visualize the structures of the upper gastrointestinal tract on x-ray film. The test aids in the identification of structural irregularities, ulcers, and tumors of the upper gastrointestinal tract. The test is usually performed by a **radiologist** (a physician who specializes in diagnostic or therapeutic use of x-ray film).

Barium Enema (Lower Gastrointestinal Series)

Like the barium swallow, a barium enema is a radiologic (x-ray) study. In the case of the barium enema, however, the large intestine is filled by an enema with barium. This procedure enables the radiologist to visualize the large intestine on x-ray film for the identification of structural irregularities, diverticula, and tumors.

Esophageal Manoscopy (Manometry)

Although done infrequently, esophageal manoscopy is a diagnostic procedure to evaluate the function of the sphincter between the esophagus and the stomach. During the procedure, individuals swallow a catheter that has a small instrument or transducer attached to it. When the transducer reaches the lower end of the esophagus, the pressure around the sphincter is measured.

Endoscopy (Gastroscopy)

When there are indications of irregularities in the esophagus, stomach, or small intestine, the walls of these organs may be visualized directly through a specially lighted, flexible tube called a gastroscope or endoscope. This procedure, which is called a **gastroscopy**, is usually performed by a **gastroenterologist** (a physician who specializes in the identification and management of gastrointestinal conditions). During the procedure, the individual's throat is sprayed with an anesthetic medication to numb the gagging reflex. The gastroscope is then inserted through the mouth, into the esophagus, into the stomach, and, at times, into the small intestine. Through the tube, the physician can visualize ulcerations or other irregularities. He or she can also remove stomach contents for analysis, if needed.

Proctoscopy, Colonoscopy, and Sigmoidoscopy

These procedures are performed by a physician—often a gastroenterologist, a family physician, or a general internist—to identify problems of the rectum and large intestine, including tumors, obstruction, and bleeding. The procedure used to detect irregularities of the rectum is called a **proctoscopy**; it involves the direct visualization of the anus and rectum through a special instrument called a proctoscope inserted into the rectum. **Colonoscopy** is a procedure that enables physicians to examine the lining of the colon (large bowel) for irregularities by inserting a flexible tube into the anus and advancing it slowly into the rectum and colon.

Similarly, *sigmoidoscopy* permits direct visualization of the sigmoid colon through a special instrument called a sigmoidoscope inserted through the anus and rectum up into the colon.

Cholecystography

If a condition of the gallbladder is suspected, a **cholecystogram** may be used to detect irregularities, inflammation, or the presence of stones. Before the procedure, the individual swallows special pills or liquid or receives an intravenous injection of a special substance that allows the gallbladder to be visualized on x-ray film. A radiologist usually performs the procedure.

Cholangiography

A study called a **cholangiogram** is used to visualize the bile ducts on x-ray film. Dye is injected into a vein or into a drain called a T tube, which has been inserted into the bile duct (usually after gallbladder surgery). A radiologist performs the procedure to identify any obstruction of the bile ducts.

Ultrasonography (Abdominal Sonography)

In **ultrasonography**, sound waves are passed into the body and converted to a visual image or photograph of a body structure. Abdominal sonograms focus on organs contained within the abdomen and can be used to identify conditions of the pancreas, liver, gallbladder, or any other abdominal organ.

Computed Tomography (CT Scan, CAT Scan)

A special kind of x-ray procedure, **computed tomography** produces three-dimensional pictures of a cross section of a part of the body. The radiologist studies this image to identify problems and determine whether further tests are needed. This procedure can be used to diagnose conditions of the pancreas, tumors, or abscesses in the abdominal area.

Radionuclide Imaging

For radionuclide imaging, individuals are given a small amount of a radioactive chemical (**radionuclide**) that gives off energy in the form of radiation. Different radionuclides concentrate in different organs. Special types of equipment, such as counters, scanners, and gamma cameras, are used to detect the radiation, thereby producing an image on film or on a special type of screen. A physician who specializes in nuclear medicine then examines and evaluates the image. In the gastrointestinal system, radionuclide imaging is helpful in detecting tumors, abscesses, or cirrhosis of the liver and in diagnosing conditions of the gallbladder.

Biopsy

The removal of a specimen of tissue from a specified site for examination is called a **biopsy**.

Common sites of biopsy in the gastrointestinal tract include the esophagus, stomach, rectum, colon, and liver. Biopsies are performed by a physician and can often be performed on an outpatient basis under local anesthesia.

Abdominal Paracentesis

A procedure to remove fluid from the abdominal cavity, abdominal **paracentesis** involves a puncture of the abdominal cavity with a hollow needle through which accumulated fluid can be withdrawn. A physician performs this procedure. It may be done for diagnostic purposes (i.e., to determine the nature of the fluid present) or for therapeutic purposes (i.e., to remove accumulated fluid in the abdominal cavity that may be causing respiratory difficulty, pain, or other problems).

Laparoscopy

Laparoscopy may be conducted for either identification of the condition or for surgical procedures. The abdominal cavity may be directly examined through a hollow tube called a laparoscope or peritoneoscope. This instrument is inserted into the abdominal cavity through a small incision. Individuals who have undergone laparoscopy may remain in the hospital overnight for observation after the procedure.

■ GENERAL MANAGEMENT OF CONDITIONS OF THE GASTROINTESTINAL SYSTEM

Medications

A variety of medications are used in treating conditions of the gastrointestinal system; they may act on either muscular or glandular tissues. Medications frequently used in the management of gastrointestinal conditions are classified as follows:

- Antacids and acid inhibitors to counteract excess acidity.
- Antiemetics to prevent nausea and vomiting. A side effect of these medications may be drowsiness.
- Digestants to replace missing enzyme secretions when there is an enzyme deficiency in the gastrointestinal tract.
- Antidiarrheals to prevent diarrhea.
- Laxatives and cathartics to relieve constipation. Generally, laxatives have mild actions, whereas cathartics have stronger actions.
- Anticholinergics to inhibit the action of the involuntary nervous system. In gastrointestinal conditions, these medications may be given to reduce activity of the intestine or to decrease secretions.
- Histamine H_2 receptor antagonists (e.g., cimetidine) to inhibit cells in the stomach lining from producing acid.
- Proton pump inhibitors.
- Antimicrobials (e.g., sulfonamides) to inhibit the growth of microorganisms.

Hyperalimentation (Total Parenteral Nutrition)

When individuals are unable to take nourishment by mouth, or when their nutritional status is compromised, it is possible to bypass the gastrointestinal tract to provide nourishment. **Hyperalimentation** is the infusion of a special nutritional solution into a vein. Because of the nature of this solution, infusion usually involves a large vessel such as the subclavian vein, located in the upper body. Hyperalimentation may be used in the management of any condition that compromises the individual's nutritional status. It may also be used when there is a need to rest the gastrointestinal tract, as in inflammatory bowel disease, or when there is an obstruction or malabsorption problem in the bowel.

Stress Management

Although stress management may be helpful for a variety of conditions, it is often especially useful in the management of conditions affecting the gastrointestinal tract. Stress itself may not be a direct cause of many conditions of the gastrointestinal tract, but it may exacerbate or prolong an acute episode in some patients with an existing condition.

The body has a number of defensive mechanisms that take actions in the face of threat or danger. When stress is encountered, a variety of physiologic reactions take place in the body, including in the gastrointestinal tract. The digestive system responds differently to different kinds of emotional stimuli. For example, it may become more or less active, and it may secrete more or less gastric juice. The intensity of the physiologic reaction depends on the individual and on the situation.

Stress management helps individuals to control their reactions to stress. Programs in stress management may vary from exercise to techniques that alter the body's response to stress, such as biofeedback.

■ PSYCHOSOCIAL AND VOCATIONAL ISSUES IN CONDITIONS OF THE GASTROINTESTINAL SYSTEM

Psychological Issues

Although they are not a causative factor in all instances, there appears to be at least some association between psychological factors and the gastrointestinal system. Psychological factors that may significantly influence gastrointestinal conditions include nutritional or lifestyle factors, such as alcohol and tobacco ingestion. In some instances, gastrointestinal conditions may also be directly related to the management of another condition, such as intake of aspirin for treatment of rheumatoid arthritis, which in turn results in gastritis.

Conditions that affect the physical processes of eating and elimination have many psychological implications. Throughout life, eating is often associated with pleasure and social interaction. Management of gastrointestinal conditions frequently requires avoidance of substances that irritate the gastrointestinal tract or cause the excessive secretion of gastric juices. When certain types of food and beverages are restricted or when special diets are required, individuals may have difficulty in giving up something that they enjoyed.

Elimination is associated with privacy and personal cleanliness. The modification of elimination habits is learned in childhood as part of the socialization process. Individuals with problems of elimination may fear embarrassment and social ridicule as a result of their condition. Those with an ileostomy or a colostomy may fear the loss of physical and sexual attractiveness because of odor or embarrassing sounds. Individuals who have inflammatory bowel disease accompanied by diarrhea may fear fecal incontinence and concomitant humiliation.

There are other reasons for psychological reactions as well. Individuals with hepatitis may fear transmitting the condition, while individuals with ulcerative colitis may be preoccupied with their increased risk of cancer. Depression is common in individuals with irritable bowel syndrome. The identification and resolution of these reactions may be crucial to rehabilitation.

Emotions affect the involuntary nervous system, which in turn affects the gastrointestinal tract. Thus psychological factors may aggravate conditions of the gastrointestinal tract. For example, anxiety may contribute to flare-ups of inflammatory bowel disease. Although rest and relaxation are of prime importance in the management of many gastrointestinal conditions, individuals may find it difficult to modify their schedules, to adjust to new life patterns, or to alter stressful situations at home or work. Often, directions to "rest and relax" are useless, unless individuals are assisted with education on methods and techniques to do so.

Although many conditions of the gastrointestinal tract do not affect body image, individuals with an ileostomy or a colostomy may encounter problems with both body image and self-concept. Specifically, they may perceive themselves as being different from others. They may also visualize themselves as unattractive and believe that they must wear shapeless, dowdy clothes to hide the ileostomy or colostomy bag. It is often helpful if individuals are able to meet other persons who have a similar condition and are leading active lives.

Many conditions of the gastrointestinal tract require permanent alterations in lifestyle and constant control over emotional tension. At times, individuals with such conditions may exhibit manifestations of the condition that are out of proportion to the objective findings. These individuals should be helped to make the recommended alterations and encouraged to maintain as regular a lifestyle as possible.

Activities and Participation

Individuals with any chronic condition should engage in a healthy lifestyle, including adequate nutrition, rest, and exercise, if they want to reach their maximal functional capacity. This is especially true of gastrointestinal conditions, because stress, fatigue, and emotions appear to have at least some direct effects on the digestive system. Individuals who are accustomed to performing in high-pressure, high-stress situations may need to learn ways either to decrease the stressful aspects of their daily life or work or to cope better with the stress that is present.

Many gastrointestinal conditions carry notable nutritional implications and, in many situations, diet is the cornerstone of therapy. Alterations and restrictions of diet are often based on avoiding foods that appear to cause distress. Depending on the meanings that these foods have for individuals, it may be difficult for them to abide by such restrictions. In most instances, eating well-balanced, regular meals is part of the therapeutic regimen. For individuals whose work or daily schedule is somewhat erratic, even this simple task may be difficult, however.

Alcohol intake should not necessarily be totally restricted, but it may be limited. Tobacco use is restricted for many individuals with gastrointestinal conditions. Depending on the former habits of these individuals, both of these recommendations may be difficult to follow.

In most instances, conditions of the gastrointestinal tract do not directly affect sexual function. Individuals may, however, be reluctant to engage in sexual activity if their gastrointestinal condition affects body image or if they fear fecal incontinence. Those with an ileostomy or a colostomy may have fears of defecation during sexual contact or may be self-conscious about the stoma itself. In some cases, men may become impotent as a result of nerve damage caused by the surgical procedure. Open discussion about such issues is important to uncover such fears and concerns, as well as to provide information that can help individuals and their partners deal with such issues.

Food is a part of celebration and socialization as well as a means of nourishment. When specific conditions of the gastrointestinal system prohibit individuals from eating or from having foods that have typically been part of their social milieu, their social interactions may be adversely affected.

Social situations that are stressful for the individual with a condition of the gastrointestinal system may cause a flare-up the disorder. To avoid such stress, some individuals with gastrointestinal manifestations may withdraw from many social activities.

Individuals with ileostomy or colostomy bags may fear fecal incontinence, odors, or spillage and, for this reason, may withdraw from social interactions to avoid potential embarrassment. For individuals with an ileostomy or a colostomy, problems may arise if family members are repelled by the condition or find it impossible to fit the care of a stoma into the household routine. If these individuals have not accepted responsibility for their own personal care, they may become overly demanding or sloppy in caring for the stoma, antagonizing family members. The acceptance of the individual by family members and friends often determines to a great degree the acceptance of the condition by the individual.

Vocational Issues

In most instances, special work restrictions are not necessary for individuals with gastrointestinal conditions. Those with a diverticular condition or hernia may need to avoid activities that increase intra-abdominal pressure, such as lifting or bending.

Modifications in the work environment or work schedule may occasionally be necessary for those with other gastrointestinal conditions. For example, erratic or rotating schedules may make it difficult for individuals with peptic ulcer to eat regular, well-balanced meals, aggravating the condition. Work situations that cause undue stress may contribute to a flare-up of certain gastrointestinal conditions. If schedules or workload cannot be changed, individuals may need to learn different ways of expressing tension and coping with stress.

Special considerations, such as the ready availability of bathrooms with adequate privacy in the workplace, may be necessary for individuals who experience diarrhea as a manifestation of a gastrointestinal condition or for those who have an ileostomy or a colostomy that may need attention during the day.

CASE STUDIES

Case 1

Ms. B. is a pharmacy technician who has had a number of remissions and exacerbations of ulcerative colitis. Over the past six months, exacerbations of the condition have interfered with her ability to maintain her regular work schedule. As a result of the worsening of her condition, Ms. B. has decided to have a colectomy.

1. Which specific issues would you expect Ms. B. to face as a result of the surgery?
2. Are there specific factors you would need to consider when working with Ms. B. to help her return to employment as a pharmacy technician?

Case 2

Mr. W. has a history of intravenous drug use. Although he is currently in recovery, he has recently tested positive for hepatitis C. You have been working with him to develop a vocational plan.

1. In addition to determining Mr. W.'s interests and abilities, are there factors related to Mr. W.'s hepatitis C that you would need to consider when helping him develop his vocational plan?
2. Is there additional information related to Mr. W.'s hepatitis C that might be helpful when considering his vocational potential?

■ REFERENCES

Alaradi, O., & Barkin, J. S. (2002). Irritable bowel syndrome: Update on pathogenesis and management. *Medical Principles and Practice, 11*(1), 2–17.

Aoyama, N., Kinoshita, Y., Fujimotos, S., Himeno, S., Todo, A., Kasuga, M. et al. (1998). Peptic ulcers after the Hanshin–Awaji earthquake increased incidence of bleeding gastric ulcers. *American Journal of Gastroenterology, 93,* 311–316.

Barba, K., Fitzgerald, P., & Wood, S. (2007). Managing peptic ulcer disease. *Nursing2007, 37*(7), 56hn1-56hn4.

Camilleri, M. (2001). Management of irritable bowel syndrome. *Gastroenterology, 120*(3), 1527-1528.

Centers for Disease Control and Prevention. (2004). Fact sheet for health professionals. http://www.cdc.gov/nchs/hus.htm.

Clearfield, H. R. (2007). Diverticula of the alimentary tract. In R. E. Rakel & E. T. Bope (Eds.), *Conn's current therapy* (pp. 597-602). Philadelphia: W. B. Saunders.

Cutler, A. F. (2001). Eradicating *Helicobacter pylori* infection. *Patient Care,* April 15, 91-92, 94, 97-100.

Dent, J. (2001). The role of the specialist in the diagnosis and short and long term care of patients with gastroesophageal reflux disease. *American Journal of Gastroenterology, 96*(suppl 8), S22-S26.

Friedman, S. L. & Schiano, T. D. (2004). Cirrhosis and its sequelae. In L. Goldman & D. Ausiello (Eds.), *Cecil textbook of medicine* (22nd ed., pp. 936-944). Philadelphia: W. B. Saunders.

Gallo-Silver, L., Maydick-Youngberg, D., & Weiner, M. (2005). Ostomy surgeries. In H. H. Zaretsky, E. F. Richter III, & M. G. Eisenberg (Eds.), *Medical aspects of disability* (3rd ed., pp. 427-441). New York: Springer.

Gaster, B., & Larson, A. (2000). Chronic hepatitis C: Common questions, practical answers. *Journal of the American Board of Family Practice, 13*(5), 359-363.

Ghosh, S., Shand, A., & Ferguson, A. (2000). Ulcerative colitis. *British Medical Journal, 320*(7242), 1119-1123.

Graham, D. Y., & Genta, R. M. (2004). In L. Goldman & D. Ausiello (Eds.), *Cecil textbook of medicine* (22nd ed., pp. 823-827). Philadelphia: W. B. Saunders.

Hoofnagle, J. H., & Lindsay, K. L. (2004). Acute viral hepatitis. In L. Goldman & D. Ausiello (Eds.), *Cecil textbook of medicine* (22nd ed., pp. 911-917). Philadelphia: W. B. Saunders.

Hyphantis, T. N., Triantafillidis, J. K., Pappa, S., Mantas, C., Kaltsouda, A., Cherakakis, P., et al. (2005). Defense mechanisms in inflammatory bowel disease. *Journal of Gastroenterology, 40,* 24-30.

Ireton-Jones, C., George, M. B., Day, L., & Zeiter, T. (2000). Case problem: Medical nutrition therapy for a patient with Crohn's disease/response. *Journal of the American Dietetic Association, 100*(4), 472-475.

King, J. E. (2007). Does my patient have ulcerative colitis or Crohn's disease. *Nursing2007, 37*(3), 30.

Lagergren, J., Bergstrom R., Lingren, A., & Nyren (1999). Symptomatic gastroesophageal reflux as a risk factor for esophageal adenocarcinoma. *New England Journal of Medicine, 340,* 825-831.

Levenstein, S. (1998). Stress and peptic ulcer life beyond *Helicobacter. British Medical Journal, 316,* 538-541.

Levenstein, S., Ackerman, S., Kiecolt-Glaser, J. K., & Dubois, A. (1999). Stress and peptic ulcer disease. *Journal of the American Medical Association, 281*(1), 10-11.

Lindsay, K. L. & Hoofnagle, J. H. (2004). Chronic hepatitis. In L. Goldman & D. Ausiello (Eds.), *Cecil textbook of medicine* (22nd ed., pp. 917-924). Philadelphia: W. B. Saunders.

Lox, A. S. F. (2002). Chronic hepatitis B. *New England Journal of Medicine, 346*(22), 1682-1683.

Mach, T. (2004). The brain-gut axis in irritable bowel syndrome: Clinical aspects. *Medical Science Monitor, 10*(6), RA125-RA131.

Marshall, B. (2007). Gastritis and peptic ulcer disease. In R. E. Rakel & E. T. Bope (Eds.), *Conn's current therapy* (pp. 617-622). Philadelphia: W. B. Saunders.

Meining, A., & Classen, M. (2000). The role of diet and lifestyle measures in the pathogenesis and treatment of gastroesophageal reflux disease. *American Journal of Gastroenterology, 95*(10), 2692-2697.

Nice, D. S., Garland, C. F., Hilton, S. M., Baggett, J. C. & Mitchell, R. E. (1996). Long-term health outcomes and medical effects of torture among

U.S. Navy prisoners of war in Vietnam. *Journal of the American Medical Association, 276,* 375–381.

O'Brien, C. (2007). Acute and chronic viral hepatitis. In R. E. Rakel & E. T. Bope (Eds.), *Conn's current therapy* (pp. 622–632). Philadelphia: W. B. Saunders.

Olden, K. W., & Brown, A. R. (2007). Irritable bowel syndrome. In R. E. Rakel & E. T. Bope (Eds.), *Conn's current therapy* (pp. 610–614). Philadelphia: W. B. Saunders.

Orlando, R. C. (2004). Diseases of the esophagus. In L. Goldman & D. Ausiello (Eds.), *Cecil textbook of medicine* (22nd ed., pp. 814–823). Philadelphia: W. B. Saunders.

Orloff, S., & Debas, H. (2004). Peptic ulcer disease: Surgical therapy. In L. Goldman & D. Ausiello (Eds.), *Cecil textbook of medicine* (22nd ed., pp. 824–838). Philadelphia: W. B. Saunders.

Owyang, C. (2004). Pancreatitis. In L. Goldman & D. Ausiello (Eds.), *Cecil textbook of medicine* (22nd ed., pp. 879–886). Philadelphia: W. B. Saunders.

Peppercorn, M. A., & Moss, A. C. (2007). Inflammatory bowel disease. In R. E. Rakel & E. T. Bope (Eds.), *Conn's current therapy* (pp. 602–610). Philadelphia: W. B. Saunders.

Podolsky, D. K. (2002). Inflammatory bowel disease. *New England Journal of Medicine, 347*(6), 417–429.

Ringel, Y., Sperber, A. D., & Drossman, D. A. (2001). Irritable bowel syndrome. *Annual Review of Medicine, 52,* 319–338.

Ruiz, O. (2007). The digestive system. In R. E. Rakel & E. T. Bope (Eds.), *Conn's current therapy* (pp. 573–577). Philadelphia: W. B. Saunders.

Ryan, S. W. (2005). Management of dyspepsia and peptic ulcer disease. *Alternative Therapies in Health & Medicine, 11*(5), 26–29.

Sach, J. A., & Chang, L. (2002). Irritable bowel syndrome: Current treatment options. *Gastroenterology, 5*(4), 267–278.

Seidel, S. A., Newman, M., & Sharp, K. W. (2000). Ileoanal pouch versus ileostomy: Is there a difference in quality of life? *American Surgeon, 66*(6), 540–548.

Shanahan, F. (2003). Crohn's disease. *Science and Medicine, 9*(1), 48–58.

Sherwood, L. (2007). The digestive system. In L. Sherwood, *Human physiology* (pp. 579–631). Belmont, CA: Thomson Brooks/Cole.

Solorzano, C. C., & Prinz, R. A. (2007). Acute and chronic pancreatitis. In R. E. Rakel & E. T. Bope (Eds.), *Conn's current therapy* (pp. 640–648). Philadelphia: W. B. Saunders.

Stenson, W. F. (2004). Inflammatory bowel disease. In L. Goldman & D. Ausiello (Eds.), *Cecil textbook of medicine* (22nd ed., pp. 861–868). Philadelphia: W. B. Saunders.

Sterling, R. K., Mattar, W. E., & Kwo, P. Y. (2007). Cirrhosis. In R. E. Rakel & B. T. Bope (Eds.), *Conn's current therapy* (pp. 577–587). Philadelphia: W. B. Saunders.

Talley, N. J. (2004). Functional gastrointestinal disorders: Irritable bowel syndrome, nonulcer dyspepsia, and noncardiac chest pain. In L. Goldman & D. Ausiello (Eds.), *Cecil textbook of medicine* (22nd ed., pp. 806–814). Philadelphia: W. B. Saunders.

Tanaka, M., & Kazuma, K. (2005). Ulcerative colitis: Factors affecting difficulties of life and psychological well-being of patients in remission. *Journal of Clinical Nursing, 144,* 65–73.

Vaira, D., Gatta, L., Ricci, C., Tampieri, A., Cavina, M., Bernabucci, V., et al (2005). Symposium on peptic acid disease. Peptic ulcer and *Helicobacter pylori*: Update on testing and treatment. *Postgraduate Medicine, 117*(6), 1–7. Retrieved November 7, 2007, from EBSCO Host, http://web.ebscohost.com/ehost/detail?vid=3&hid=109&sid=7da82cc

Wilcox, C. M., (2004). Appendicitis, diverticulitis, and miscellaneous intestinal inflammatory conditions. In L. Goldman & D. Ausiello (Eds.), *Cecil textbook of medicine* (22nd ed., pp. 869–872). Philadelphia: W. B. Saunders.

Yates, W. R., & Gleason, O. (1998). Hepatitis C and depression. *Depression and Anxiety, 7,* 188–193.

Younge, L., & Norton, C. (2007). Contribution of specialist nurses in managing patients with IBD. *British Journal of Nursing, 16*(4), 208–212.

Zuckerman, A. J., & Lavancy, D. (1999). Treatment options for chronic hepatitis. *British Medical Journal, 319*(7213), 799–800.

Chapter 13

Cardiovascular Conditions

■ STRUCTURE AND FUNCTION OF THE CARDIOVASCULAR SYSTEM

The cardiovascular system consists of the heart and a network of blood vessels, which carry blood throughout the body. Blood vessels in the circulatory system are composed of the following structures:

- *Arteries*, which carry *oxygenated* blood *away* from the heart
- *Veins*, which carry *unoxygenated* blood *to* the heart
- Small branching blood vessels (*arterioles* and *venules*)
- Tiny vessels called *capillaries*, which provide a link between arterioles and venules

The heart, acting as a pump, forces blood through two circuits. One circuit carries blood to and from the lungs (*pulmonary circulation*). The other circuit carries blood throughout the body (*systemic circulation*).

The heart is a strong and powerful muscle located somewhat to the left of the center of the chest. It pumps 5,500 gallons of blood through the body per day and beats about 100,000 times per day. The heart consumes more energy than any other organ in the body (Neubauer, 2007).

The heart muscle itself is called the **myocardium**. It is enclosed in an outer covering (the **pericardium**) consisting of two layers. The space between the two layers of the pericardium contains a small amount of fluid to lessen friction between the two surfaces as the heart beats. The inner surface of the heart is called the **endocardium.**

The myocardium is a special type of muscle that has the ability to work continuously with only brief periods of rest between contractions. This resting period, when the heart is relaxed and the chambers are filling, is called **diastole**. The pumping action, or contraction, of the heart muscle is called **systole**. Diastole and systole produce different pressure gradients; the ratio of these two pressures is called **blood pressure**. The amount of pressure produced depends on the force with which the heart pumps and the degree to which the blood vessels resist blood flow. Blood pressure is expressed numerically as a fraction in which the systolic reading is the numerator and diastolic reading is the denominator. For instance, in a blood pressure reading of 120/80 (measured in units of millimeters of mercury, or mm Hg), the systolic pressure is 120 mm Hg with a diastolic pressure of 80 mm Hg.

Like all muscles of the body, the myocardium requires oxygen and nutrients to survive. A separate network of blood vessels called the *coronary vessels* supply the heart muscle with blood. The coronary vessels consist of **coro-**

nary arteries, which carry oxygen and nutrients *to* the heart muscle, and *coronary veins*, which carry blood used by the heart muscle and containing wastes *away from* the heart muscle. Without blood flow supplied directly to the myocardium, the heart is unable to carry out its function of pumping blood to the rest of the body.

The heart contains four chambers. The two upper chambers are the right and left **atria**, and the two lower chambers are the right and left **ventricles**. Four valves help blood move from chamber to chamber in one direction without backflow. Between the right atrium and the right ventricle is the *tricuspid valve*. Between the left atrium and left ventricle is the *mitral (biscuspid) valve*. The right atrium receives deoxygenated blood from the systemic circulation through a large vein called the vena cava. The deoxygenated blood is pumped from the right atrium to the right ventricle through the tricuspid valve. Blood is then pumped from the right ventricle through the pulmonary (*semilunar*) valve to the pulmonary artery, where it is carried to the lungs (*pulmonary circulation*). The pulmonary artery is the only of artery in the body that carries deoxygenated blood.

In the lungs, wastes, in the form of carbon dioxide, are released from the blood and excreted from the lungs. Oxygen is taken into the blood from the lungs, and the newly oxygenated blood is pumped back to the heart through a vessel called the *pulmonary vein* (the only vein in the body that carries oxygenated blood). Oxygenated blood enters the left atrium of the heart and moves through the mitral valve to the left ventricle where it is pumped out of the heart through the aortic (semilunar) valve to a large blood vessel called the aorta and then into the systemic circulation. (See Figure13-1.)

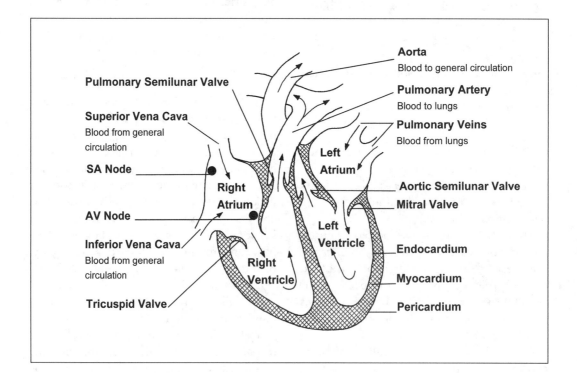

Figure 13-1 The heart

Blood carries oxygen and nutrients to all parts of the body through blood vessels in the **peripheral circulation** (outside the heart). The network of arteries diminishes in size as it branches into the tiny vessels called capillaries. Capillary walls are very thin, allowing for exchange of oxygen and nutrients from the blood with waste products from body tissues. Blood containing waste products is then carried back to the heart through small blood vessels that increase in size until they reach the vena cava, which returns to the heart, and the process begins all over again.

A special nerve conduction system in the heart maintains the regular, rhythmic beating of the heart. Special cells called the *sinoatrial (SA) node* (also called the "pacemaker" of the heart) located within the right atrium initiate the contractions. Impulses from the SA node spread over both atria, causing them to contract simultaneously. The impulse then reaches special cells in the lower right atrium, the *atrioventricular (AV) node*. From the AV node, impulses are transferred to special muscle fibers (*bundle of His*) located on the right and left sides of the septum separating the two ventricles. The bundles branch out to Purkinje fibers, which spread over both ventricles, causing them to contract. At this point, the cycle starts over.

Conduction of these nerve impulses throughout the heart occurs involuntarily. Through communication from the central nervous system, the heart adjusts to the changing needs of the body, speeding or slowing the heart rate as needed.

◾ CONDITIONS OF THE CARDIOVASCULAR SYSTEM

Cardiovascular disease, including stroke, is the leading cause of illness and death in the United States. An estimated 62 million people in this country have cardiovascular disease, and an additional 50 million people have hypertension (Nabel, 2003). Prevention of cardiovascular disease and its resulting complications is a significant part of decreasing associated disability.

Arteriosclerosis (Atherosclerosis)

Arteriosclerosis and **atherosclerosis** are terms often used interchangeably to refer to a condition in which the walls of the arteries become thickened or less elastic, thereby obstructing circulation and diminishing blood flow to various parts of the body. This condition is caused by buildup of *plaques* along the interior vessel wall, causing **stenosis** (narrowing) of the vessel and impeding blood flow.

Arteriosclerosis is generally associated with elevated cholesterol levels (**hyperlipidemia**). Cholesterol is a substance that is manufactured naturally in the body; however the body also receives cholesterol from dietary intake of food high in **lipids** or fats. Although there is a strong link between cholesterol and heart disease, not all people with high cholesterol level develop conditions of the cardiovascular system; likewise, some people develop cardiovascular conditions even though they do not have elevated cholesterol (Sherwood, 2007).

Symptoms of arteriosclerosis develop slowly and are generally nonexistent until blood flow becomes diminished to the extent that oxygen supply to a body part is hampered. At this point, individuals may experience pain, fatigue, or altered function in the body part affected.

Plaque can also contribute to **thrombus** (blood clot) formation within the narrowed vessel, blocking blood flow even more. Tissue death can occur if all blood flow to a body part stops. A thrombus can be dangerous even when blood flow isn't totally blocked. The thrombus can become an **embolus** if it becomes dislodged from the vessel wall and begins traveling in the bloodstream. (The term "embolus" can also refer to other substances traveling in the blood, such as an air bubble, fat globule, or other foreign matter.) The embolus can lodge in a blood vessel too small to allow its passage, occluding blood flow there. The effects of an *embolism* depend on the body part affected. For example, an embolism of the brain results in stroke, whereas embolism in a coronary artery causes **myocardial infarction** (heart attack). An embolus lodging in the lungs would be called a pulmonary embolus. In all instances, embolism can result in severe tissue damage and can be fatal.

Symptoms experienced by individuals with arteriosclerosis vary depending on the extent of stenosis of the vessels and the location of the impeded blood flow. For example, cognitive changes can result when blood flow to the brain is decreased, such as in carotid artery stenosis (narrowing of the vessels carrying blood directly to the brain).

Decreased blood flow to the kidneys may contribute to kidney damage, causing chronic renal failure. Decreased blood flow to the heart may cause **angina pectoris** (chest pain) or, if blood flow is severely restricted, heart attack.

Management of arteriosclerosis is directed toward preventing complications associated with the condition—namely, myocardial infarction, stroke (see Chapter 3), and kidney failure (see Chapter 15). A variety of medications are used to lower blood cholesterol levels. When the carotid artery leading to the brain is affected, a procedure called carotid endarectomy or a procedure called carotid artery stenting may be used to alleviate the problem (Furlan, 2006). These procedures seek to remove the obstruction or widen the passage of vessels leading to the brain, thereby increasing blood flow and oxygen supply to the brain. When narrowing of coronary arteries that supply blood and oxygen to the heart is identified prior to myocardial infarction (heart attack), surgical procedures to widen these vessels may also be used [coronary artery bypass graft (CABG) or percutaneous coronary intervention (PCI), both of which are discussed later in this chapter]. Because nicotine further constricts vessels already narrowed in arteriosclerosis, individuals with arteriosclerotic disease should avoid tobacco use.

Hypertension

Individuals with **hypertension** have a sustained elevation of pressure in the arteries. Both systolic and diastolic pressures may be elevated. This prolonged elevation of pressure can eventually damage other organs, such as the heart, kidneys, or brain. Hypertension in and of itself is not disabling, but it is a major health problem because of its associated high risk of myocardial infarction (heart attack), stroke, renal failure, and congestive heart failure, all of which cause significant disability (Oparil, 2000; August, 2003).

Blood pressure normally fluctuates with physical activity, becoming lower at rest and higher with changes in posture, exercise, or emotion. Individuals whose blood pressure remains high even at rest put increased strain on body organs and risk development of other complications such as heart attack, stroke, or end-stage renal disease.

The most common type of hypertension is primary (essential) hypertension, which has a gradual onset and few, if any, symptoms. The exact cause of primary hypertension is unknown.

Sometimes hypertension is a symptom of another medical condition, such as kidney disease, endocrine disorders, neurological disorders, or drug use or abuse. This type of hypertension is called secondary hypertension. A less common, but more severe type of hypertension is malignant hypertension, which has an abrupt onset, more severe symptoms, and more associated complications.

Often, primary hypertension is discovered for the first time during a routine physical examination. Because symptoms of hypertension are often vague or even nonexistent, hypertension may go undetected until complications such as heart attack, stroke, or visual problems arise (Glasser, 2001; Setness, 2001). Accurate measurement of blood pressure and verification of elevated blood pressure on several occasions are the chief way hypertension is diagnosed. Hypertension is most accurately diagnosed when blood pressure is measured under similar conditions over a period of time. Because blood pressure fluctuates throughout the day, and because it may be higher when measured in a healthcare setting than it would be at home, 24-hour blood pressure monitoring is gaining recognition as a more accurate appraisal of blood pressure throughout the day (White, 2003).

Management of Hypertension

The primary goal of treatment of hypertension is to lower blood pressure and reduce the risk of complications such as heart attack, stroke, or kidney failure. In mild cases of hypertension, lifestyle modifications—such as maintaining a proper body weight, exercising, cutting down on alcohol intake, ceasing to use tobacco, and limiting fats, calories, and sodium—may be sufficient to lower blood pressure (Victor, 2004; Appel et al., 1997; Sacks et al., 2001). Although stress itself may not directly cause primary hypertension, emotional stress does induce physiologic changes that may then raise the blood pressure. Learning how to reduce stress or avoid chronic stressful situations may also be important in the overall treatment of hypertension.

When lifestyle modifications are insufficient to control hypertension, or when blood pressure is too elevated to control with lifestyle modification alone, an important aspect of treatment is medication (Frohlich, 2007). A variety of medications, called *antihypertensives*, are prescribed to control high blood pressure. Antihypertensives can also cause numerous side effects, which can sometimes interfere with individuals' willingness to take medication as prescribed.

Psychosocial Issues in Hypertension

Although there usually are no symptoms associated with primary hypertension, the consequences of untreated hypertension can be severe, causing end-stage renal disease, myocardial infarction, or stroke. Consequently, treatment of hypertension is essential to prevent disability and/or death. Individuals with hypertension frequently experience few symptoms, so they may have less motivation to follow treatment. Treatment also often involves lifestyle changes that individuals may have difficulty accomplishing, such as weight loss, smoking cessation, or exercise. Consequently, individuals may be noncompliant with treatment and medical recommendations, which could help them prevent complications related to hypertension and prevent disability.

Adherence is defined as the degree to which individuals' behavior corresponds to the medical advice and instructions given. In treatment of hypertension, adherence includes not only taking medications prescribed, but also keeping scheduled medical appointments and making recommended lifestyle changes. Identifying potential problems that contribute to nonadherence, and working toward solutions to overcome them, can be beneficial in helping individuals prevent complications of hypertension and disability.

Vocational Issues in Hypertension

There are usually no specific limitations associated with hypertension per se; however, isometric activities such as pushing, lifting, or carrying heavy objects can increase blood pressure during the activity and may need to be avoided. Although some degree of emotional stress is inherent in many jobs, individuals need to recognize that chronic, sustained stress may have a detrimental effect on blood pressure. Individuals should be assisted in learning to manage the stress they experience on the job or should seek ways of modifying the work environment to make it less stressful. The major impact hypertension has on employment takes the form of disability, which can occur from uncontrolled hypertension and its complications. Consequently, reinforcement of adherence to medical recommendations is of major importance to ongoing employment.

Aneurysm

An **aneurysm** is the dilation or ballooning out of a weakened arterial wall. Although often associated with arteriosclerosis and hypertension, an aneurysm may also result from a congenital abnormality (Byrne & Darling, 2007). The weakened wall of the artery, if under increased pressure (e.g., because of hypertension), may burst and lead to hemorrhage. Common sites of aneurysms are in the brain and the aorta (the major trunk of the arterial system of the body). A dissecting aneurysm is a tear in the inner wall of the vessel so that blood leaks between the layers of the wall of the vessel, moving longitudinally to separate the layers along the length of the vessel rather than rupturing into an open body space.

Symptoms experienced as a result of an aneurysm vary according to its location. In some instances, there are no symptoms until the aneurysm becomes large enough to create pressure, causing pain at the site. In other instances, there are no symptoms until the aneurysm ruptures, which could result in sudden death.

Aneurysms may be treated surgically if they are diagnosed early or if surgery is not contraindicated because of associated medical problems. Surgical procedures to correct aneurysms involve removal of the weakened area of the artery, followed by connection of the two remaining ends (**anastomosis**). A graft to join the two remaining ends is used if a large portion of the vessel has been removed. Controlling hypertension, if present, is an important aspect of continuing treatment after surgery.

Coronary Artery Disease

Coronary artery disease is a condition in which the coronary arteries that supply blood and oxygen directly to the heart muscle (myocardium) become narrowed. The condition is usually caused by atherosclerosis in which plaques build up on the inner walls of blood vessels that supply the heart muscle. Buildup of plaques may narrow the coronary arteries to the extent that insufficient blood passes through the arteries to meet the oxygen demands of the heart muscle. In this situation, the heart muscle receives an inadequate supply of blood (**ischemia**). Depending on the extent of blockage of blood supply to the heart muscle, individuals may experience either angina pectoris or myocardial infarction.

Angina Pectoris

When there is a mismatch of the amount of oxygen a muscle needs and the amount of oxygen available, pain results. Insufficient supply of oxygen to the heart muscle results in chest pain, called **angina pectoris**. Because the heart muscle's need for oxygen is greatest when demands are placed on the heart, angina is often triggered by physical activity. Decreasing activity, and thus decreasing the workload of the heart, often causes chest pain to subside. This type of angina is called stable angina. When chest pain occurs at rest, with no precipitating activity, or when pain is more severe, more frequent, or more prolonged, individuals are said to have *unstable angina*. Diagnosis of angina is based on symptoms, laboratory evaluations, electrocardiogram (recording of electrical activity of the heart) or exercise electrocardiogram (stress test), or echocardiogram (discussed later in the chapter).

The system used for estimating functional capacity is expressed in *metabolic equivalents* (METs). The MET concept represents a procedure for determining energy cost (in terms of oxygen consumption) of certain physical activities. It provides a method for describing the functional capacity or exercise tolerance of individuals and for identifying physical activity in which individuals may safely participate without exceeding their capacity. The degree of activity individuals may participate in is determined with an exercise test, which focuses on the symptoms and signs individuals develop during exercise. Different types of activity have been classified in terms of how many METs are required. MET requirements range from 1 (the amount of oxygen an individual consumes at rest while awake) to 9 (for the heaviest tasks). Grading systems have been used to characterize the degree of limitation associated with angina pectoris. The most commonly used system was developed by the American Heart Association (see Table 13-1).

Management of angina pectoris is directed to reducing symptoms, increasing functional capacity, and preventing myocardial infarction, as well as including surgical measures to correct the cause. Treatment includes modification of ongoing risk factors, medication, and evaluation of need for surgical intervention. Cessation of tobacco use, treatment of hypertension, and weight loss, if obesity exists, are important ways to modify risk. Angina pectoris may also be helped by nitroglycerin, a medication that dilates the coronary arteries and enables the heart muscle to receive more oxygen, thereby relieving pain.

When angina pain occurs so frequently that limitation of activity becomes severely debilitating, or when occlusion of the coronary arteries becomes so pronounced that myocardial infarction is imminent, surgery such as

---

Table 13-1 Classification of Functional Capacity and Objective Assessment

Functional Capacity

Class I. Patients with cardiac disease but without resulting limitation of physical activity. Ordinary physical activity does not cause undue fatigue, palpitation, dispend or angina pain

Class II. Patients with cardiac disease resulting in slight limitation of physical activity. They are comfortable at rest. Ordinary physical activity results in fatigue, palpitation, dyspnea or anginal pain

Class III. Patients with cardiac disease resulting in marked limitation of physical activity. They are comfortable at rest. Less than ordinary activity causes fatigue, palpitation, dyspnea or anginal pain.

Class IV. Patients with cardiac disease resulting in inability to carry on any physical activity without discomfort. Symptoms of heart failure or the anginal syndrome may be present even at rest. If any physical activity is undertaken, discomfort increase.

Objective Assessment

1. No objective evidence of cardiovascular disease
2. Objective evidence of minimal cardiovascular disease
3. Objective evidence of moderately severe cardiovascular disease
4. Objective evidence of severe cardiovascular disease

PCI or CABG (both of which are discussed later in the chapter) may be indicated.

Myocardial Infarction

Like all other muscles, the heart muscle cannot live without oxygen. When the myocardium receives *no* oxygen (**anoxia**), **necrosis** (tissue death) of part of the heart muscle occurs. This situation is called myocardial infarction (heart attack), which means there has been death of part of the heart muscle. Myocardial infarction may occur anytime the blood supply to the heart muscle is insufficient. Not all individuals with angina go on to develop myocardial infarction, and not all people with myocardial infarction have first experienced angina, where there is only *diminished* blood supply and oxygen to the heart.

Total occlusion of a coronary vessel so that the heart muscle receives no blood supply can occur for the following reasons:

- Atherosclerosis, in which the coronary arteries become totally occluded
- Formation of a thrombus (blood clot) in a coronary artery, occluding blood flow
- Lodging of an embolus (a blood clot, a particle of vegetation from a diseased valve, or other foreign material that has traveled through the bloodstream) in a coronary artery, occluding blood flow

Once a portion of the heart muscle has been destroyed, it cannot regenerate. The ability of the heart to continue functioning as a pump is directly related to the amount of heart muscle damage that has occurred. Myocardial infarction can result in **arrhythmia** (irregular heartbeat), *heart failure*, or death. Individuals with myocardial infarction often experience chest pain that is not relieved by reducing activity as well as pressure in the chest. Myocardial infarction is a medical emergency and can be fatal. Consequently, immediate medical attention is required.

Myocardial infarction is diagnosed by the individual's symptoms, such as pain and pressure in the chest, and electrocardiogram and laboratory determinations, which helps physicians not only in making the diagnosis, but also in determining the most appropriate treatment.

Management of Myocardial Infarction

Myocardial infarction, as a potentially life-threatening condition, requires immediate medical attention. Individuals usually receive initial treatment in the emergency department, where the focus is on assessment, stabilizing their condition, relieving pain, and preventing sudden death. In the initial stages of myocardial infarction, pain may be treated with narcotics, thrombolytic drugs may be given to dissolve clots, anticoagulants may be given to decrease the likelihood of further clot formation, and oxygen is given to decrease **hypoxemia** (lowered oxygen in the blood).

After emergency room treatment, individuals are usually admitted to the coronary care unit (CCU), which specializes in critical care of individuals with cardiovascular conditions. The goal of treatment in the CCU is to limit the heart damage, promote electrical stability of the heart, promote comfort, and prevent additional damage to the heart muscle from occurring. Here individuals are monitored for life-threatening arrhythmias and receive continued pharmalogic and medical treatment directed toward these treatment goals. Some individuals also undergo surgical revascularization procedures (PTCA or CABG), as described later in this chapter.

After a cardiac event, the degree of disability and the types of activities in which individuals can engage are based on the energy expended to perform the activity. Energy is expressed in terms of calories per minute and based on the equivalent of one liter of oxygen equaling five calories. Cardiac rehabilitation (described later in this chapter) is crucial in the treatment of myocardial infarction so that individuals can improve exercise capacity, return to work, and reduce risk of mortality. Prior to exercise training, individuals undergo testing to assess their functional capacity so that the appropriate level of activity may be prescribed (see Table 13-1).

The functional capacity of individuals after myocardial infarction depends on the amount of damage the heart muscle sustained and the location of the damage. After experiencing myocardial infarction, individuals usually undergo cardiovascular risk factor assessment and are advised that steps to decrease risks— such as lowering blood pressure, increasing exercise, dietary modification, and smoking cessation—are fundamental to the risk reduction program. In addition, individuals are often placed on medication (aspirin or anticoagulants) to decrease the coagulability of blood. Individuals may also undergo surgical intervention, such as PCI or CABG.

Psychosocial Issues in Coronary Artery Disease

Depression and depressive symptoms are common after major cardiac events and are associated with higher mortality (Milani & Lavie, 2007). Pain associated with angina pectoris, as well as limited activity and anxiety caused by fear of potential heart attack, can limit the individual's ability to participate in a number of activities. As a result, individuals may experience low self-esteem and depression. In addition, symptoms associated with angina pectoris are indicative of the potential of a more serious consequence of obstruction to vessels supplying the heart muscle—the possibility of myocardial infarction and sudden death—causing anxiety and fear. Anxiety can become so extreme that individuals become increasingly fearful about engaging in activities. Alternatively, they may deny their symp-

toms, engaging in activities beyond their functional capacity.

Stresses experienced as a result of myocardial infarction are greatly influenced by individuals' psychological reactions to the heart attack. When individuals have a myocardial infarction, the realization that death could have occurred as well as the realization of the unpredictability and threat of sudden death can precipitate severe depression or anxiety, which can result in emotional disability. In the early stages of recovery from myocardial infarction, denial may have positive effects by helping individuals reduce the emotional distress associated with the knowledge that their condition is potentially life-threatening (Livneh, 1999). As individuals progress in recovery, however, denial may become detrimental if they deny the seriousness of the heart attack, failing to alter their lifestyle and refusing to follow other treatment recommendations.

The life-threatening nature of myocardial infarction may cause a variety of reactions in family members, which in turn affect individuals' adjustment to their condition. Overwhelming anxiety about the possibility that another myocardial infarction might occur can result in family members' overprotection of individuals, inhibiting their return to their full functional capacity. The extent to which family members believe individuals contributed to the development of their condition by engaging in activities viewed as precursors of heart disease, such as smoking, improper diet, or obesity, may further influence relationships. Family members may express anger, resentment, or frustration, placing blame on the individuals for their behavior. In turn, individuals who have had a myocardial infarction may experience guilt, low self-esteem, and self-blame.

Sexual readjustment after myocardial infarction may also be an issue. Depression and lowered self-esteem may both contribute to sexual dysfunction. In addition, some medications commonly prescribed after myocardial infarction may impair sexual function. Individuals and/or their partners may be especially anxious about engaging in sexual activity after a heart attack, fearing that sexual activity is too stressful and may precipitate another heart attack and possibly sudden death. Education and appropriate counseling, as well as reassurance, may be necessary to help the individuals and their partners alleviate these fears.

Vocational Issues in Coronary Artery Disease

After appropriate cardiac rehabilitation, most individuals are able to return to moderate levels of activity. Activity level is determined through appropriate medical evaluation of the energy cost of activities, as described previously. Work activity should not exceed individuals' limits. For the most part, isometric activities are avoided because of the additional stress they place on the heart. Likewise, because of the stress that extreme temperatures place on the heart, work environments with controlled temperature are preferable. Both the amount of stress experienced on the job and the individual's response to it should be considered as well.

Heart Failure

Heart failure is a common condition, affecting almost 5 million people in the United States (McMurray & Pfeffer, 2005). It can be disabling and significantly decrease quality of life (Neubauer, 2007).

When the heart muscle is weakened or damaged, and it cannot pump an adequate amount of blood to the rest of the body, a condition called heart failure occurs. Either one or both ventricles may be weakened in these circumstances. When the weakened ventricle cannot effectively pump all the blood it has collected, backup of blood and congestion occur.

The causes of heart failure include myocardial infarction (heart attack); damage from substances toxic to the heart muscle (such as alcohol or other chemicals); and hypertension, arteriosclerosis, valvular dysfunction, and lung diseases such as emphysema, all of which cause the heart to work harder (Sherwood, 2007). When the heart consistently must work harder to pump, over time it becomes enlarged (**hypertrophy**) and ineffective in its pumping action. As a result, fluid accumulates in the lungs, causing congestion, **dyspnea** (difficulty breathing), and difficulty breathing when lying down at night (**nocturnal dyspnea**). The decreased pumping action of the heart and congestion in the lungs result in inadequate supply of oxygen to the rest of the body, so individuals with heart failure may consequently experience fatigue and physical weakness. If oxygen supply to the brain is inadequate, cognitive changes may be present. Because of insufficient pumping and circulation of blood, fluid may also accumulate in the extremities, causing swelling (**edema**). Blood flow to the gastrointestinal system may be impaired, causing congestion with resulting **anorexia** (loss of appetite) or nausea and vomiting.

Management of Heart Failure

Management of heart failure depends on the type and causes of the condition. It is usually directed toward controlling or correcting the cause of heart failure and toward alleviating the symptoms. Often, medications to lower blood pressure (antihypertensives) are prescribed. These medications decrease the vascular resistance, thereby decreasing the amount of work that the heart must perform to circulate blood. Medications to help the heart muscle work more efficiently by increasing its pumping action (e.g., digitalis preparations) may also be prescribed. **Diuretics** (medications that help rid the body of excess fluid) and a low-salt diet to eliminate some of the excess fluid may be part of the treatment plan as well.

Severe heart failure can result in need for a heart transplant (discussed later in this chapter). When a donor heart isn't immediately available, a surgically implanted ventricular assistive device (VAD) can take over the function of the failing heart. This pump is used to sustain the individual until a donor for transplant can be found (Chapman, Parameshwar, Jenkins, Large, & Tsui, 2007; Baughman & Jarcho, 2007).

Psychosocial Issues in Heart Failure

Although some symptoms may be controlled, heart failure usually signifies the end stage of cardiovascular disease. Individuals with heart failure may experience depression and anxiety about their present and future situations. Symptoms of shortness of breath, fatigue, and edema of the extremities can severely limit activities and increase dependency on others, which may in turn lower self-esteem. Because heart failure is often the result of gradually deteriorating function of the heart, individuals also live with the knowledge that their condition can result in increasing disability and death. If individuals are candidates for cardiac transplant, uncertainty about whether a donor heart will be found before the condition deteriorates even more may be another source of continuing stress for individuals and their families.

If a ventricular assistive device is used, there may be body image disruption due to the incision and scarring from implantation of the device. In other instances, individuals may feel as if the device is an intrusion because of the noise and vibrations emitted from the device. Fear of potential device failure may be balanced with the hope the device brings for bridging the time to transplant (Miller et al., 2007; Barkley, Acosta, Starin, & Tan, 2004).

Caregiver stress may also be significant. Family members may feel overwhelmed with the training required and the need to be prepared for emergency in case of device failure. They may also experience guilt because of their feelings as well as anxiety at the realization of the severity of the situation (Casida, 2005).

Vocational Issues in Heart Failure

The extent to which individuals are able to continue to function in the work environment depends on the severity of symptoms experienced and the nature of the work. Individuals in sedentary occupations requiring limited activity will be able to function longer than individuals in occupations in which strenuous activity is required.

In general, emotional stress and physical demands on the job should be minimized as much as possible. Extremes in temperatures can put additional strain on the heart, so temperature-controlled environments are better tolerated.

Heart failure is often associated with gradual and progressive deterioration of cardiac function. Consequently, vocational goals may need to be short range to accommodate the potential for later functional decline.

Cardiac Arrhythmia

An arrhythmia is an abnormality of the heart rate or rhythm. A dysfunction in the heart's electrical conduction system may cause irregularities in its rhythm and/or rate. Arrhythmias decrease the heart's ability to work effectively and to supply adequate amounts of blood to any of the body's organs. The heart may beat too fast (**tachycardia**) or too slow (**bradycardia**), or it may beat irregularly (**dysrhythmia** or **arrhythmia**).

There are many different causes of arrhythmia and many different types. Types of arrythmias are usually named for the type of disorder or the part of the electrical impulse system that is affected. For example, a *sinus bradycardia* indicates that there is an abnormally slow rhythm arising in the SA node of the heart, whereas an atrioventricular *(AV) block* would be used to describe an arrhythmia in which electrical impulses are blocked at the atrioventricular junction. Some arrhythmias may be the cause of significant disability, some may be life-threatening (such as *ventricular fibrillation*), and others may be relatively minor and require little or no treatment. A common arrhythmia, *atrial fibrillation,* was once not treated, but it is now thought to increase the individual's risk of stroke (Saffitz, 2006). Consequently, treatment is important in preventing this complication (Fye, 2006). One of the treatment options used widely in atrial fibrillation is anticoagulant medications to prevent clots from forming in the atrium and traveling to the brain. Many people with atrial fibrillation have underlying cardiovascular disease; however, for many others no cause can be identified (Saffitz, 2006).

The symptoms experienced with arrhythmia depend on the type and extent of arrhythmia. Individuals may, for example, experience **palpitations** (feeling the heart beat), **exertional dyspnea** (shortness of breath with activity), fatigue, **vertigo** (dizziness), or **syncope** (fainting). Severe or prolonged arrhythmia can result in sudden death.

Management of Arrhythmia

Management depends on the underlying condition; it is directed toward correcting or controlling factors causing the arrhythmia. Some arrhythmias may be prevented by avoiding ingestion of stimulants such as caffeine or avoiding alcohol.

Medications

Medications called antiarrhythmics regulate the heartbeat and are often a central part of treatment. Other medications useful in the control of arrhythmia are digitalis preparations, beta blockers, and calcium-channel blockers. Because certain types of arrhythmia

(e.g., **atrial flutter**) can contribute to thrombus (blood clot) formation and possible embolus (traveling blood clot), some individuals may also need to be on anticoagulant medications (Hart, 2003).

In more severe arrhythmia, an electrical shock procedure called *cardioversion* may be indicated to return the heart to a normal rhythm. Individuals with a severe, recurrent arrhythmia, which could result in a life-threatening arrhythmia (e.g., ventricular tachycardia, which can become ventricular fibrillation), a device called an *implantable cardiovertor defibrillator* (ICD) may be surgically implanted. ICD placement involves creating a three-to four-inch incision into the left chest wall. The ICD produces visible scarring as well as a bulge around the implant site, which some people find objectionable because it shows under clothing (Sowell, Kuhl, Sears, Klodell, & Conti, 2006). The implanted defibrillator delivers an electric shock automatically to the heart when an arrhythmia occurs.

Pacemakers and Implantable Defibrillators

When the heart's ability to maintain an effective rate or rhythm is altered, an artificial cardiac pacemaker may be used to stimulate the electrical activity of the heart and to maintain function. Implantable pacemakers and defibrillators are undergoing rapid evolution (Cooper, Katcher, & Orlov, 2002) and can not only decrease the incidence of potentially fatal arrhythmias, but also enhance quality of life for those with problem arrhythmias (Newman et al., 2000). The pacemaker consists of a battery-operated pulse generator and a lead wire with an electrode tip. One end of the lead wire is inserted into a vessel and advanced into the individual's heart; the other end is connected to the generator. The generator then sends out an electrical stimulus to the heart muscle. The generator may be external if the need for pacing is only temporary. If the pacemaker is to be permanent, a small battery-operated generator is placed under the skin and fatty tissue of the upper chest or lower thoracic area.

A variety of pacemakers are available. Pacemakers are usually classified according to the chamber of the heart that is being stimulated, the chamber of the heart that is being monitored, and the response that the pacemaker is expected to deliver. The classification system uses a three-letter code to describe pacemaker function: The first letter of the code signifies the chamber being stimulated, the second letter indicates the chamber being monitored, and the third letter indicates the pacemaker response. For example, a code of VVI would indicate that a ventricle is being both stimulated and monitored. The "I" stands for "inhibited response," indicating that the pacemaker will not allow impulses from the atria to stimulate the ventricle.

Pacemakers may be designed to deliver any of several modes of pacing. The oldest type of pacing, fixed rate, is rarely used today. In this type of pacing, the pacemaker is set to fire at a fixed rate, usually about 70 beats per minute, and is unaffected by the heart's own rhythm. Another type of pacing, demand or standby, is accomplished with a pacemaker that has a special sensing circuit set at a specific rate. When the individual's own conduction system in the heart falls below that specific rate, the artificial pacemaker fires accordingly. Other types of pacing, called synchronous and bifocal, use pacemakers that are programmed in similar ways to monitor and deliver specific types of impulses.

The mode of pacing is determined on an individual basis according to the individual's specific arrhythmia. The physician chooses the type of pacemaker to be used and the amplitude of the stimulus based on the individual's condition. For most individuals, even permanent pacemakers may be inserted under local anesthesia with mild sedation.

Complications related to implantation of a pacemaker are rare, but can include **pneumothorax** (collapse of the lung), dislodgement, inflammation, or infection of the surrounding area (Morady, 2000). The level of activity in which individuals with a pacemaker can engage depends on the underlying disease process, the individual's age, and the degree of cardiac functional capacity. Normal daily activities can usually be resumed six weeks after the implantation of the pacemaker. Activities that could expose the internal pacemaker to a blow, such as contact sports, should be avoided. Although driving may be restricted for a short time after the pacemaker insertion, most individuals can begin driving in approximately one month, if the pacemaker is functioning well.

Individuals who have a pacemaker should at all times wear identification, such as Medic Alert, or should carry a card containing information about the type of pacemaker, the date of implant, and the pacemaker's programming. Because the pacemaker's generator is battery operated, failure of the battery means that the heart returns to beat at its previously abnormal rate or rhythm. Individuals with pacemakers should be aware of the signs of battery depletion such as a change in the cardiac rate or the appearance of symptoms similar to those experienced before the pacemaker was inserted. The length of time that a battery lasts depends on the model and can vary from one to several years. A physician should evaluate the pacemaker's function regularly. Periodic evaluations may be conducted with special telephone monitoring in which information about the pacemaker's function is transmitted over regular telephone lines to a special device in the physician's office.

Electromagnetic interference with permanent pacemakers and implantable defibrillators may have deleterious effects (Santucci, Haw, Trohman, & Pinski, 1998). Although the shielding around battery-operated generators has been improved significantly, individuals who wear these devices should be aware of possible interference from a variety of external electrical signals in the environment. Because implantable defibrillators are designed to be more sensitive to intracardiac electrical activity, they may demonstrate increased sensitivity to electromagnetic interference. Microwave ovens, radar installations, arc welding devices, antitheft devices, cellular phones, and other sources of electrical signals may all interfere with pacemaker signals. The pacemaker may also set off metal detection devices installed at airports.

Psychosocial Issues in Arrhythmia

The psychosocial impact of arrhythmia can be significant. Fearful of triggering a potentially fatal arrhythmia, individuals may curtail many activities related to both work and leisure in an effort to prevent such an occurrence. In many instances, the fear and anxiety experienced by individuals with arrhythmia may be more disabling than the arrhythmia itself.

Given that arrhythmias can be triggered by use of caffeine, alcohol, or tobacco, individuals may also need to modify their lifestyles to some extent. Commitment to lifestyle changes varies with the degree to which the individual accepts and understands the condition and the necessity for its treatment. Individuals who become extremely anxious about their condition may cope by employing denial as a way of decreasing the level of stress. If individuals engage in denial rather than making the necessary lifestyle changes, they may continue activities even though those activities could have a deleterious effect on their health.

Vocational Issues in Arrhythmia

Any activity that has been identified by the individual as triggering arrhythmia should be avoided. Avoiding excessive emotional stress as well as learning to manage stress may be an important component of the individual's ability to continue to perform adequately at work without danger of precipitating an arrhythmia. Individuals being treated with anticoagulants may need to be aware of the potential for excessive bleeding if injury should occur. Excessive anxiety about precipitating an arrhythmia can become disabling, immobilizing individuals and preventing them from carrying out normal tasks and activities. Individuals may develop chronic depression, which can further interfere with their ability to work.

Individuals with pacemakers may need to avoid activities that could potentially cause the pacemaker to become dislodged because of vibrations (such as use of an air hammer or shooting a rifle on the side of pacemaker placement). Individuals should avoid activities such as arc and resistance welding, use of power tools, or contact with radar transmitters, all of which could cause the pacemaker to malfunction. Consultation with a physician for clarification of level of activity as well as referral to a counselor may be indicated to help individuals deal with their fears and enhance their ability to perform work activities.

Other Conditions of the Heart

Congenital Heart Conditions

Congenital heart disease conditions include anatomic or physiologic abnormalities of the heart present at birth, such as the following common conditions:

- Ventricular septal defect
- Atrial septal defect
- Patent ductus arteriosus
- Coarctation of the aorta
- Tetralogy of Fallot
- Transposition of the great arteries

Many congenital heart conditions are identified in infancy or childhood; some, however, are not diagnosed until adulthood. Most congenital heart conditions are corrected surgically.

Ventricular septal defect is the most common congenital heart defect (McMahon, 2007). The degree of manifestations depends on the size of the defect. Adults with a small defect may have no significant manifestations aside from a heart murmur. Larger defects are generally identified and corrected in childhood.

The second most common congenital heart defect is atrial septal defect, which is also the most common congenital heart condition diagnosed in adulthood (McMahon, 2007). Manifestations are slight if the defect is small and may consist of slight heart murmur. In some instances, the defect closes spontaneously. If the defect is larger, there may be increasing symptoms such as arrhythmias and pulmonary hypertension in adulthood, requiring surgical repair.

Coarctation of the aorta may not be identified until later childhood, with the first symptom being hypertension. Although treatment consists of surgical repair, residual hypertension and long-term effects of surgical intervention require lifelong follow-up and periodic magnetic resonance imaging (McMahon, 2007).

Tetralogy of Fallot and transposition of the great arteries are congenital heart conditions known as cyanotic defects. **Cyanosis** (bluish discoloration of the skin caused by a lack of oxygen) is one of the primary manifestations of both conditions and, therefore, usually enables them to be identified shortly after birth and surgically corrected.

Valvular Conditions of the Heart

Damage to the valves of the heart is most often the result of **rheumatic fever** (a condition caused by the body's immune response against a streptococcal infection) (Liuzzo et al., 2005) or **endocarditis** (inflammation of the inner membrane of the heart), although valvular abnormalities may also be congenital. Two types of problems generally occur. Valves may become weakened or floppy, permitting a backflow (**regurgitation**) of blood from the ventricle to the atria, or valves may become scarred, narrowing the valvular opening (stenosis) and causing an obstruction of blood flow from a chamber of the heart. Although some valvular conditions are minimal and may require little intervention, more extensive valvular damage places an increased burden on the heart and can lead to dysfunction of the myocardium, congestive heart failure, and, in some cases, sudden death.

Types of Valvular Conditions

Valvular conditions are classified according to the nature of the abnormality and the valve affected. One type of valvular condition, *mitral prolapse*, consists of bulging of all or part of the mitral valve into the left atrium during ventricular contraction. Mitral regurgitation, mitral insufficiency, and mitral incompetence are terms that refer to the inadequate closing of the mitral valve, which allows blood to flow backward into the atria. *Mitral stenosis* refers to narrowing of the mitral valve, which obstructs the blood flow from the left atrium to the left ventricle. Tricuspid regurgitation and tricuspid stenosis are conditions similar to the regurgitation and stenosis conditions described earlier, but occur on the right side instead of the left side of the heart. The same process may affect the pulmonary or aortic valves.

Valvular defects of the aortic valve, such as aortic stenosis and aortic regurgitation, place additional loads on the left ventricle of the heart, possibly resulting in left ventricular heart failure. Symptoms of valvular disease vary in severity but often include fatigue, **dyspnea** (difficulty breathing), and **palpitations** (heartbeats that are perceptible to the individual).

Management of Valvular Conditions

Specific treatment for a valvular condition depends on the severity of the problem. Some conditions may require individuals to avoid strenuous activity. Others require no treatment or may not require individuals to take any precautions. Damaged valves are more susceptible to infection. Consequently, prophylactic antibiotics may be given to prevent endocarditis when there is the chance for a generalized bacterial infection, such as after a dental extraction.

Severe damage to a valve may require surgery to open or replace the valve. Surgical interventions for valvular abnormalities are intended either to widen a valve that is narrowed or constricted or, in the case of valvular insufficiency or regurgitation, to replace a diseased valve with an artificial valve. Individuals with stenosis of a valve may undergo a procedure known as **valvuloplasty** in which the stenosed (narrowed) valve is dilated with a balloon that is inserted through a peripheral vessel.

When valves are replaced, artificial valves (which are mechanical), or valves made of tissue may be used. Mechanical valves are made entirely from synthetic materials, while tissue valves may be made from a combination of synthetic and biological tissues. Mechanical valves require long-term anticoagulant therapy to prevent thrombus (blood clot) formation (Rey, 2005). Although tissue valves decrease the risk of clot development, they may not have the long-term durability of mechanical valves. Because prosthetic valves are more vulnerable to infection, individuals may need to take antibiotics before procedures in which infection is a risk (e.g., dental work) are performed.

Endocarditis

Endocarditis (inflammation of the membrane that covers the heart valves and chambers of the heart) is most often caused by an infection, but can also be the result of an immunological reaction. It is characterized by deposits of "vegetation" on the inner lining of the heart

(the endocardium) and, most frequently, on the valves. Damage to the valves can result.

Endocarditis may be associated with systemic infectious diseases or intravenous drug abuse, or it may be a complication of an invasive medical procedure. Sometimes even minor trauma can precipitate development of endocarditis. Most people have isolated incidents in which bacteria enter the bloodstream (**bacteremia**). In most instances, the body's own defenses overcome the organisms with no untoward results. At other times, because of the strength of the organisms or the reduced effectiveness of the body's defenses, the organisms settle on the inner lining of the heart, causing endocarditis.

Individuals with previous cardiac surgery, congenital heart disease, or conditions in which the heart valves have been damaged are more susceptible to development of endocarditis. Individuals with valve replacement, and especially those with prosthetic valves, are also at higher risk for endocarditis (Levinson, 2000).

Symptoms of endocarditis may be insidious at first, mimicking the flu. As the disease progresses, symptoms such as high fever, weight loss, and extreme fatigue become more pronounced. The condition is diagnosed based on history and symptoms, blood culture, and echocardiogram. Treatment consists of the administration of appropriate antibiotics to eradicate the infection before serious complications develop. When severe valvular dysfunction results, surgical replacement of the valve may be necessary.

Complications of endocarditis include embolism (obstruction of a blood vessel by a foreign substance), in which some of the vegetation from the affected valve breaks away and occludes a blood vessel in another part of the body. Any organ or part of the body can be affected. Depending on the part of the body affected and the extent of damage, embolism can sometimes result in death.

Pericarditis

Inflammation of the outer layer of the heart (pericardium) is known as **pericarditis.** Most commonly, it is caused by a virus (Manning, 2000). When inflamed, the pericardial layers can adhere to each other, creating friction as their surfaces rub together during cardiac contraction. The most common symptom of pericarditis is chest pain, which is aggravated by moving and breathing because of the rubbing together of the two inflamed surfaces. A low-grade fever may also be present.

Diagnosis is often based on symptoms, physical examination, and, at times, electrocardiogram (ECG). Treatment of pericarditis is directed toward alleviating pain caused by inflammation of the pericardium. Medications such as nonsteroidal anti-inflammatory drugs (NSAIDs) are commonly used for this purpose.

Severe inflammation of the pericardium can result in accumulation of excessive fluid within the pericardial sac, a condition known as **pericardial effusion**. Excess fluid in the sac surrounding the heart may constrict the myocardium, causing cardiac dysfunction. If constriction of the heart is severe because of increasing amounts of fluid, **cardiac tamponade** (severe constriction of the heart that prevents it from filling and emptying properly) may occur. A procedure called **pericardiocentesis** (puncturing of the pericardium to drain the fluid) may be performed to remove fluid and relieve the constriction. During this procedure, the physician inserts a needle into the pericardial sac to drain the fluid.

Although rare, after severe inflammation, the pericardium may become scarred, further constricting cardiac function (constrictive pericarditis). This condition may need to be treated surgically so that a portion of the pericardium is removed.

Rheumatic Heart Disease

Rheumatic heart disease is a type of heart condition caused by **rheumatic fever**. Rheumatic fever is an inflammatory condition that occurs as an inflammatory complication of infection with group A *Streptococcus* (Hahn, Knox, & Forman, 2005). Not everyone develops rheumatic fever after a streptococcal infection, and the reason for the allergic type of reactions in some individuals is unknown.

Recovery from rheumatic fever can be complete with no residual effects. Nevertheless, some individuals experience permanent cardiac damage as a result. Valves of the heart are most frequently affected, resulting in stenosis, insufficiency, or regurgitation.

Peripheral Vascular Conditions

Disorders of the peripheral blood vessels (i.e., those in the extremities) can lead to damage of the tissues supplied by those vessels. When oxygen supply is inadequate because of the diminished blood flow, extremities feel cold and appear pale or **cyanotic** (blue). Pain is also characteristically present when the oxygen supply is diminished.

Peripheral Vascular Disease

Peripheral vascular disease is a common manifestation of atherosclerosis and is associated with an increased risk of disability in combination with cigarette smoking (White, 2007). When arteriosclerotic changes have narrowed or occluded the larger peripheral vessels, an adequate blood supply cannot reach tissues in the extremities.

The symptoms experienced depend on the extent of the obstruction, the vessels involved, and the formation of any alternative blood supply routes, called **collateral circulation**.

Exercise requires increased demand for oxygen by muscles. Therefore, individuals who have deficient blood supply to the muscles because of peripheral vascular disease may, with activity such as walking, experience aching, cramping, or fatigue of the muscles in the legs—a condition known as **intermittent claudication**. Stopping to rest decreases muscles' need for oxygen and consequently relieves the pain. If the condition progresses, however, pain in the extremities may occur even at rest. In severe cases, the feet may become numb and cold, and ulcerations of the foot may appear.

Management is directed toward reducing risk factors, with recommendations including regular exercise and smoking cessation. Surgical procedures, such as a bypass graft of the severely affected vessel or a **percutaneous transluminal angioplasty (PTA)**, in which the vessel is widened, may restore vascularization to the extremity in selected cases (White, 2007). Aspirin may also be prescribed to reduce additional complications associated with vascular diseases, such as myocardial infarction and stroke.

Owing to the diminished blood supply in peripheral atherosclerotic disease, even tiny injuries in the extremities may become infected and not heal properly. If circulation becomes so severely impaired that **necrosis** (tissue death) results, amputation of the extremity may be necessary to prevent complications, such as the spread of infection throughout the body.

Thromboangiitis Obliterans (Burger's Disease)

Thromboangiitis obliterans is a rare condition of the small- and medium-sized arteries and superficial veins of the extremities that causes diminished blood flow to the affected part. In contrast to peripheral atherosclerotic disease, thromboangiitis obliterans occurs predominantly in individuals between the ages of 20 and 40 who do not have significant atherosclerosis. Symptoms include numbness, tingling, and pain in the upper or lower extremities. Although its exact cause is unknown, thromboangiitis obliterans occurs almost exclusively in individuals who smoke. Consequently, the major treatment of the condition is smoking cessation. If individuals continue to smoke, the disease continues to progress and can ultimately require the amputation of affected extremities.

Raynaud's Disease

Raynaud's disease is a condition in which spasms of the vessels in the fingers or toes impair the blood flow to those areas. Occasionally, this condition also affects the nose and the tongue. In most instances, the cause of the condition is unknown; however, it may be associated with other conditions, such as **rheumatoid arthritis** or **arteriosclerosis obliterans**. Attacks of vasospasm may last from minutes to hours, but rarely last long enough to cause tissue death. Attacks result in color changes in the fingers or toes, either *blanching* (white coloration) or **cyanosis** (blue coloration). Attacks may be precipitated by cold or emotional upsets.

If Raynaud's phenomenon is secondary to another condition, treatment is directed toward the underlying disorder. In the majority of cases in which the cause is unknown, treatment involves taking steps to prevent an attack from occurring, such as protection from the cold or avoidance of emotional upsets. Smoking constricts the blood vessels; consequently, tobacco use should be avoided. Treatment with biofeedback or the use of relaxation techniques may sometimes be helpful in reducing attacks.

Venous Thrombosis (Thrombophlebitis, Phlebitis)

A common and potentially lethal complication of bed rest or inactivity is thrombophlebitis. In chronic illness or disability in which activity is limited, thrombophlebitis can be a serious complication causing additional disability or potentially death. **Phlebitis** is the inflammation of a vein; **thrombophlebitis** is the inflammation of a vein with associated clot formation. Although phlebitis and thrombophlebitis can occur in any vein, they frequently occur in the veins of the lower extremities.

Individuals with thrombophlebitis may experience pain and tenderness in the affected area, especially if the lower extremity is affected. Individuals with loss of sensation as a result of spinal cord injury may be unaware of the condition, and consequently it may not be treated promptly. Other symptoms may include swelling and redness of the affected part or, at times, depending on the location of the inflammation, there may be no symptoms at all. If thrombophlebitis is unrecognized or inadequately treated, clots can break off, traveling to the heart, lungs, or to other parts of the body where they can lodge in a vessel, occluding blood supply to the body part. Depending on the location of the occlusion, individuals can experience stroke, myocardial infarction, or massive damage to whichever body part is affected.

Treatment of phlebitis and thrombophlebitis is directed toward decreasing inflammation and preventing or dissolving clots through use of anticoagulants, antithrombotic agents, or anti-inflammatory agents. Bed rest is usually prescribed during therapy, along with medications that decrease clotting.

Varicose Veins

When blood cannot be returned efficiently to the heart, backup of blood may cause distention and congestion of the veins, called **varicose veins**. Anything causing stricture or pressure on the veins—such as prolonged standing, obesity, or constriction of the leg by circular garters—can aggravate this condition.

Symptoms may include a sensation of heaviness in the legs, fatigue, and pain.

In mild cases, treatment may consist of application of compression hosiery. Surgery to tie and strip the veins may be indicated when the condition involves severe pain or recurrent phlebitis.

Vocational Issues in Peripheral Vascular Disease

Peripheral vascular disease can be significantly debilitating, causing vocational impairment and engendering psychological stress. Individuals with peripheral vascular conditions may be unable to stand for long periods of time or may be unable to walk without pain or muscle fatigue. Stamina in relation to these activities should be evaluated before the return to work. Environmental conditions, such as cold temperatures, or other factors that reduce blood supply to the extremities should be avoided. The potential for infection in the lower extremities because of inadequate blood supply necessitates avoidance of work environments containing hazards that could cause trauma to the feet or legs. Two thirds of all lower-extremity amputations performed are the result of peripheral vascular disease or diabetes (Jacobowitz, 2005). Consequently, not only should vocational concerns be related to functional capacity regarding the peripheral vascular condition itself, but concern must also be directed toward preventing injury and complications that could result in amputation and additional disability.

■ DIAGNOSTIC PROCEDURES IN CARDIOVASCULAR CONDITIONS

In addition to a physical examination and medical history, a variety of tests are used to diagnose cardiovascular conditions. These tests may also provide information that is used to make treatment determinations or to evaluate treatment effectiveness.

Chest Roentgenography (X-Ray)

A noninvasive radiographic procedure, **roentgenography** makes it possible to visualize organs in the chest cavity on x-ray film. Films may show evidence of congestion or fluid in the lungs, **hypertrophy** (enlargement) of any of the heart's chambers, or other abnormalities in the chest cavity.

Electrocardiography

An **electrocardiogram (ECG)**, a graphic representation of electrical currents within the heart, is helpful in identifying abnormalities of the heart's rhythm, assessing the amount and location of damage to the cardiac muscle, determining whether the cardiac muscle is receiving an adequate supply of oxygen, and obtaining information about the effects of certain medications. In this painless, noninvasive procedure, electrodes are placed externally on the skin and then connected to a special machine that transforms electrical impulses from the heart into a graphic printout that records the heart's activity. The ECG is usually performed in the physician's office, hospital, or other medical setting.

Holter Monitor

The *Holter monitor* is a form of ECG in which several electrodes attached externally to the chest are connected to a small portable device that records the heart's activity. The device is worn on the shoulder or waist so that the individual can go about his or her regular activities at home or work. The advantage of the Holter monitor is that the graphic reading of the heart's electrical impulses is continuous rather than a one-time reading in a laboratory situation. Readings from the Holter monitor enable physicians to assess the heart's functioning during various normal activities throughout a 24-hour period or longer.

Cardiac Stress Test

The *cardiac stress test* is a noninvasive exercise test that provides a graphic record of the heart's activity during forced exertion. It may be used diagnostically to determine the extent of cardiac disease. It can also be used as a basis for recommending either medical or surgical treatment, as well as for counseling individuals with cardiac disease about the type and amount of physical activity in which they may safely engage. The stress test is performed in a cardiology unit or clinic by a technician with a physician present.

In this test, electrodes are placed externally on the chest and connected to an ECG monitor. The individual is then asked to step on a motor-driven treadmill or to sit on a stationary bicycle with an ergometer. Activity is begun slowly, with a gradual increase of pace. During this time, the physician or technician monitors the individual's ECG reading, pulse, and blood pressure. The test is stopped if the individual is no longer able to keep up the pace or develops chest pain, or if the physician determines that blood pressure, pulse, or ECG readings indicate excessive strain on the heart.

The stress test is performed in a controlled, laboratory environment. In addition, consideration must be given to other stress—such as emotional stress, extremes in temperature, and physical terrain (such as steps or ramps)—that may be present in the individual's natural or work environment and that may increase the heart's workload beyond the workload experienced in the laboratory situation.

Angiography

When it is necessary to study one or more blood vessels, an invasive procedure called *angiography* (a series of x-ray pictures that define size and shapes of vessels and/or organs) is used. An angiogram of the heart enables physicians to identify abnormalities in the size or the shape of the vessels, the extent of narrowing or occlusion, and the sequence and time in which the vessel fills with blood.

Angiograms are named for the specific area of the body being studied. If arteries are being studied, the test is called an *arteriogram*. If veins are being studied, the test is called a *venogram*. If vessels of the heart are being studied, the test is called a *cardiac angiogram*.

A *radiologist* (a physician who specializes in x-ray procedures) performs an angiogram, usually in the radiology department. During the procedure, a special catheter is placed into a vein in the arm or leg and dye is injected. At this time, a rapid series of x-rays are taken, enabling the physician to visualize the vessels.

Echocardiography

Like the ECG, the *echocardiogram* is obtained by means of a noninvasive procedure. With this imaging technique, ultrasound is used to record the size, motion, and composition of the heart and large vessels. A transducer converts sound waves to electrical signals, which are then recorded as visual images and displayed on a type of television screen called an oscilloscope. Images can be photographed for further evaluation by a radiologist or cardiologist. Echocardiograms are helpful for identifying and evaluating valvular defects or other structural abnormalities of the heart.

Radionuclide Imaging

The procedure for radionuclide imaging begins with the intravenous injection of a radioactive substance that becomes localized in heart tissue. Multiple views of the heart are then taken with a special camera; additional views are repeated for comparison with the original images hours later. This procedure is most useful in evaluating the myocardium (heart muscle) or damage to the myocardial tissue. It may also be used to evaluate coronary artery disease or valvular disease. It can be performed with the individual either at rest or during exercise.

Cardiac Catheterization

An invasive procedure, *cardiac catheterization* is performed to study the chambers, valves, and blood supply to the heart. In this procedure, a catheter is passed into a vessel in an arm or a leg and then threaded into the heart. A special x-ray machine called a fluoroscope enables the physician to visualize the catheter advancing into the heart. When the catheter is in place, internal pressures in the heart are measured. Dye is then injected into the catheter, allowing the physician to visualize the pumping action of the heart and the blood flow through the coronary arteries.

Cardiac catheterization may be performed to determine the extent of coronary artery disease, valvular disease, congenital heart disease, or damage to the heart muscle. Information gained from this procedure may be used to determine whether cardiac surgery is indicated or to assess the function of the heart after cardiac surgery. The procedure may be performed in the radiology department, operating room, or special rooms within cardiac clinics.

■ GENERAL TREATMENT OF CARDIOVASCULAR CONDITIONS

Individuals with cardiovascular conditions may receive medical and/or surgical treatment. In any case, treatment requires regular medical follow-up to monitor the success of the treatment and the progression of the disease.

Medical Treatment

Although medical treatment of cardiovascular conditions varies with the type of disorder, treatment generally includes both medication and lifestyle changes. Hypertension is frequently associated with other cardiovascular disorders. Consequently, *antihypertensives* (medications that lower blood pressure) and/or medications that rid the body of excess fluid (*diuretics*) are often prescribed. When arrhythmias occur, *antiarrhythmic* medications may also be prescribed. *Nitroglycerin* may be taken to dilate the coronary vessels when there is chest pain from inadequate oxygen supply to heart muscle; it may also be taken prophylactically before any activity that may increase the heart's workload. *Anticoagulants* may be prescribed to reduce the coagulability of the blood, thereby diminishing the risk of clot formation. *Cardiotonic medications*, such as digitalis preparations, may be prescribed to change heart rhythm or rate and generally to strengthen the heart. Regardless of the type of medication prescribed, in all instances medications are taken under physicians' direction and supervision.

Physicians may also prescribe the degree and type of activity permissible for individuals with cardiovascular disease. Because the heart responds to different types of muscular activities in different ways, when prescribing activity physicians take into account the nature of the condition and the ability of the heart to function under various types of muscle actions. Exercise may also be prescribed to increase individuals' tolerance of activity.

Factors such as obesity, tobacco use, and stress, which may contribute to development of cardiovascular disease or place additional burdens on the heart, are also considered in planning treatment goals. Obesity increases strain on the heart, so individuals with cardiac disease are often placed on low-calorie diets.

Consumption of sodium, which contributes to water retention that increases the heart's workload, may also be restricted. Because high cholesterol levels have been associated with cardiovascular disease, individuals may be placed on a low-fat/low-cholesterol diet. Tobacco use is associated with an increased pulse rate, blood pressure changes, and blood vessel constriction. Consequently, individuals with cardiovascular conditions should avoid tobacco use.

Surgical Treatment

Surgical Interventions for Coronary Artery Disease

One of two **revascularization** procedures may be used in either angina pectoris or myocardial infarction to relieve obstruction in a coronary artery and restore blood flow: percutaneous coronary intervention (PCI) and coronary artery bypass graft (CABG) (Lambert, 2007; Théroux, 2004). PCI is used to widen narrowed vessels and, in some instances, to place a stent in the vessel to maintain blood flow. Some stents contain medication to further decrease the risk of blood clot formation (Curfman, Morrissey, Jarcho, & Drazen, 2007; Camenzind, 2006). CABG is also used to relieve narrowing or constriction of the coronary arteries, but rather than widening the vessel itself, a graft—usually a vein taken from the individual's leg—is used to bypass an obstructed coronary artery. Often, several coronary arteries are constricted, and more than one graft is needed. The bypass increases the myocardium's blood supply, potentially increasing individuals' ability to engage in activity.

Although PCI requires shorter hospital stays and lower initial cost, the effectiveness of this intervention may decrease over time, requiring additional surgical interventions at a later time. CABG requires longer hospitalization and is more expensive, but its effects appear to be more long lasting (Lytle, 2004).

One form of PCI, **percutaneous transluminal coronary angioplasty (PTCA)**, is performed to reopen a narrowed coronary artery. PTCA, which is also called balloon angioplasty, involves putting a special catheter (a thin, flexible tube) into the artery in the leg and then threading it under x-ray guidance into the blocked coronary vessel. Inflation of a balloon on the catheter's tip then stretches the vessel and flattens the arteriosclerotic plaque against the walls of the artery. The advantage of PTCA is that it is not an open heart procedure, so the recovery time from this procedure is shorter. It is, however, a temporary solution. Most individuals who undergo PTCA need to have the procedure repeated or need to have a coronary artery bypass at a later date. A coronary stent (a small mesh tube) may also be inserted and left in the artery to prop it open.

The CABG procedure, although not a cure, is intended to alleviate symptoms of arteriosclerotic heart disease, prevent myocardial infarction, or, if myocardial infarction has occurred, prevent additional damage from occurring. In addition, it has considerable impact on individuals' quality of life as well as ability to return to work (Charlson & Isom, 2003; McMurray, 1998). In the past, CABG involved open heart surgery, which also required use of a heart–lung machine. In recent years, less invasive procedures called *port-access coronary artery bypass surgery* and minimally invasive coronary bypass surgery have been developed that require much smaller incisions and use tiny cameras and video monitors to guide surgical procedures. These minimally invasive procedures do not require use of a heart–lung machine. Unless complications develop, the recovery time for the newer procedures is generally shorter than that for the regular CABG procedure.

Surgery for Valvular Conditions of the Heart

Individuals with valvular disease may have surgical treatment to widen a valve that is narrowed or to replace a valve that is diseased. All of these procedures are described elsewhere in the chapter. When the heart is severely impaired, cardiac transplantation may be performed.

Cardiac Transplantation

Cardiac transplantation is an accepted, established form of therapy when heart disease is so advanced (*end-stage heart disease*) that standard therapy is no longer effective and survival is severely threatened (House-Fancher & Foell, 2004). Individuals who undergo successful transplantation not only increase their chance for survival, but also increase their chance to return to a normal, productive life. In the United States, more than 2000 people undergo heart transplants each year, with year overall survival rate of 87.4 percent (Science Daily, 2008).

Pre-Transplant Considerations

Individuals selected for transplant often have end-stage cardiac disease with a life expectancy of less than one year without transplant (Rourke, Droogan, & Ohler, 1999). Prior to cardiac transplant, individuals undergo a complete physical and diagnostic workup. The individual and family also undergo a comprehensive psychological profile, assessing their coping skills, family support, and motivation to follow the rigorous medical regimen that is required. The evaluation period can be extremely stressful, with individuals becoming fearful they may be found unsuitable for transplant.

Not all individuals with heart disease are candidates for cardiac transplantation. Selection is based on factors such as general physical condition, absence of other systemic disease that would in itself limit survival, the ability to return to normal function after surgery, and the ability to comply with the complex medical regimen that necessarily follows transplantation. Usually a history of drug or alcohol abuse, mental illness, severe obesity, other systemic diseases, or end-stage renal disease or altered liver function are contraindications to cardiac transplant (House-Fancher & Foell, 2004).

To be eligible for transplant, an individual's physical condition must be strong enough to survive the transplant procedure, and he or she must be able to adhere to the complex medical regimen required after surgery. Individuals accepted for transplant are placed on a waiting list. A 24-hour national computer network links all organ procurement centers. When a donor organ is identified, the computer center searches the list of potential recipients for the best match. The donor–recipient match is based not only on blood type, but also on body and heart size.

The pre-transplant period may be extremely stressful for individuals and their families as they wait for a donor to be identified. Many individuals may put their lives on hold while waiting for a transplant. In addition, the pressure of uncertainty as to whether or when a heart will become available can cause severe stress in family relationships. Individuals and families have no control over when surgery will occur and, in the interim, the individual's condition may continue to deteriorate. Feelings of anxiety and depression are common. Individuals may also have feelings of guilt because they will receive a heart donated as a result of someone else's death. Organ preservation time is limited from the time of procurement to the time of implant (about four to six hours), so that individuals awaiting a transplant must be readily available for surgery at short notice.

Thus, if individuals do not live near a transplant center, they may need to relocate to be closer to the facility. Relocation can be an additional source of stress not only for the individual, but also for the family.

When a donor heart has been identified and the matching of donor–recipient blood types has been confirmed, the recipient is taken to surgery. His or her heart is removed and the donor heart transplanted. Immunosuppressant therapy to block the body's natural response to foreign objects begins immediately thereafter.

Post-Transplant Considerations

After cardiac transplant, individuals remain in the hospital for approximately five to ten days. After discharge from the hospital, they are required to have checkups by the transplant team biweekly and then every six to eight weeks for one to two years after transplant. Biopsies of the heart are often conducted weekly for the first four weeks, then every other week for the second and third months, and then monthly for the next eight months (Babruth, 2004). Monitoring of blood is also conducted frequently during the first six months to assess immune status; the frequency of this monitoring decreases over time if all is well. Individuals are evaluated for possible medicine toxicity or graft rejection as well as other complications of transplant, too. If signs of rejection are observed, additional medications are prescribed to augment immunosuppression.

Individuals undergoing cardiac transplantation must follow a complex medical regimen to prevent rejection of the donor organ and other complications. Because the body never really ceases its efforts to reject the donor heart, immunosuppressants must be taken indefinitely. These medications are a necessary part of treatment, but they have serious side effects, which must be monitored on a continuing basis. Too much or too little medication may cause the body to reject the transplant. Potential complications of immunosuppression include an increased susceptibility to infection and an increased rate of malignancy.

Individuals generally take approximately three to six months after surgery to become fully functional and adjust to the immunosuppressant medications. Survival rates after cardiac transplant increase as time after transplant increases. Transplant recipients have an 87% probability of surviving the first year after transplantation and longer with an expected increased quality of life (Hunt, 2006). When death does occur in the first year after transplant, the most common cause is tissue rejection or infection (Barkley et al., 2004; Rourke et al., 1999).

The costs associated with heart transplantation can be staggering. There are significant charges for the transplant surgery and hospitalization and the continuing immunosuppressant medication, of course, as well as costs associated with travel to and from the transplant center for checkups, food and lodging for family while the individual is hospitalized, and other support services that may be needed when the individual returns home.

Because the demand for cardiac transplantation far exceeds the supply of donor hearts available, mechanical support in the form of left ventricular assist devices (LVAD) or artificial hearts has emerged as a temporary measure to increase survival while waiting for a donor heart to become available (Casida, 2005; Mielniczuk et al., 2004). The mechanical devices have become a reliable bridge until cardiac transplant; they also have positive psychological and social benefits by enabling individuals to be more self-sufficient, possibly even going home (Morales, Argenziano, & Oz, 2000). These alternative devices do not require immunosuppression, but the extent to which they may be used over the long term remains unknown.

Psychosocial Issues in Heart Transplant

Heart transplant involves life-altering changes both for the individual and for the family (Brown, Launius, Mancini, & Cush, 2004). Individuals who had been in the terminal phase of heart failure and severely debilitated may, after heart transplant, progress to an active lifestyle. This process may cause the individual and family members to experience a number of emotional issues. Although individuals undergo psychological evaluation prior to transplant, some evidence suggests that individuals may experience grieving due to the loss of their own heart and take time to accept the donor heart on an emotional level (Kaba, Thompson, Burnard, Edwards, & Theodosopoulou, 2005).

Depression and anxiety are also issues in individuals after transplant. Individuals must learn to live with the possibility of rejection and infection, and in some instances they may develop a feeling of guilt or indebtedness to the donor. Some individuals may even experience post-traumatic stress disorder after transplant (Brown et al., 2004).

Vocational Issues in Heart Transplant

Although after transplant many individuals are able to be physically active and return to work, they may experience difficulty and require assistance in making the transition from their pre-transplant state to one in which they return to employment. One barrier to employment is prejudicial attitudes of employers who may have concerns about insurability and individuals' needs for continuing medical care and follow-up after transplant. Although functional limitations experienced by individuals after transplant are individually determined, some restrictions on heavy lifting or aggressive exercise are likely.

After transplant, individuals' immune status is compromised due to the continuing use of immunosuppressant therapy to prevent rejection of the transplanted heart. As a result, these individuals may be more prone to infection. Consequently, avoidance of situations in which they may be exposed to contagious infections should be avoided.

Psychological factors may also be a barrier to individuals' successful return to work. Prior to receiving the transplant, individuals may have been out of work for some time because of their condition. The adjustment to again being employed may be a difficult psychological transition. Individuals may also have difficulty with body image, or they may fear that work-related activity could interfere with their new heart's effective functioning. Fear of contracting an infection or anxiety about potential rejection of the transplant may also be psychologically debilitating, interfering with individuals' ability to work.

Cardiac Rehabilitation

Cardiac rehabilitation has been described by the U.S. Department of Health and Human Services (1995) as a program consisting of the following components:

- Medical evaluation
- Prescribed exercise
- Education
- Counseling

The goals of cardiac rehabilitation are to help individuals safely return to and maintain regular daily activities and to promote prevention measures, including healthy lifestyle practices (Bybee & Kopecky, 2007). Cardiac rehabilitation is a comprehensive and individualized program, the purpose of which is to reverse limitations developed following the adverse physical and psychological consequences of cardiac events. Specific aims are as follows:

- Curtail physical and psychological consequences of the cardiac event
- Limit the risk of future cardiac events
- Relieve symptoms
- Reintegrate individuals as functional beings in society and at work

Programs in cardiac rehabilitation use a multidisciplinary approach, incorporating exercise training, dietary consultation, smoking cessation (if needed), patient education, and counseling (Balady et al., 2000). Treatment programs are designed to maximize individuals' physical and psychosocial functioning. Education and increasing awareness of individuals and their family of the underlying condition and aspects of the prevention of future cardiac events are a cornerstone of cardiac rehabilitation programs. Because some individuals with cardiac conditions become disabled because of excessive fear, anxiety, or depression, interventions directed to helping individuals and their families deal with these feelings are also part of the total rehabilitation program.

Most cardiac rehabilitation programs include educational sessions to help individuals achieve necessary lifestyle changes, including dietary restrictions, smoking cessation, and graduated exercise training to help them achieve their maximum activity level and functional capacity. Psychological and vocational counseling are important components of cardiac rehabilitation programs as well.

■ PSYCHOSOCIAL ISSUES IN CARDIOVASCULAR CONDITIONS

Psychological Issues

The heart has been given symbolic significance for centuries. Consequently, individuals' reactions to conditions involving the heart can have far-reaching implications. Given the association between sudden death and cardiac malfunction, fear and anxiety are common reactions to cardiac conditions. Although many chronic illnesses trigger these reactions, because the heart is considered by many people as the most vital organ, any condition involving the heart can have significant emotional ramifications.

Most individuals come to accept their condition and its associated restrictions or treatment. In other instances, however, individuals' responses may adversely affect treatment and rehabilitation. Reactions of anger, anxiety, and depression can be the most debilitating factors in cardiac disease, as they can contribute to inactivity, social isolation, or withdrawal from the activities that were previously enjoyed. Consequently, it is necessary to consider how emotional reactions might affect an individual's ability to return to a comfortable, productive life.

Individuals with cardiovascular disease may be immobilized by fear, subsequently restricting their activities more than needed. Excessive concern that additional stress or exertion may lead to cardiac failure may cause individuals to dramatically alter job, recreational, and family activities. Depression may result from the concerns about work, family activities, sexual activities, and lifestyle changes that abound. In particular, when the cardiovascular condition requires significant modifications in lifestyle or employment, those changes may be associated with a sense of loss and bereavement.

Denial is part of a normal psychological defense that can be used to cope with a severe threat. Although denial can be an effective mechanism for reducing levels of anxiety, it can also have a detrimental effect on treatment. Symptoms may be ignored or trivialized, physical incapacity denied, or recommendations for treatment or lifestyle change ignored. As a result, care and treatment may be inadequate, leading to complications or hastening progression of the condition itself. Although the way in which individuals respond to cardiovascular conditions depends to some extent on personality, the magnitude of the response may reflect the individual's unique personal situation at the time. Financial, work, and family concerns, in addition to the diagnosis of a cardiac condition and its implications, can intensify the response expressed.

Lifestyle Issues

Although not all cardiovascular conditions require significant lifestyle changes, some changes are generally recommended. Modifications in diet, decrease in alcohol intake, or elimination of tobacco use may be required. Because smoking constricts blood vessels, persons with cardiovascular disease—particularly peripheral vascular disease—should not smoke so as to avoid diminishing blood flow to the heart or extremities further. Changes in exercise may also be recommended. For example, the physician may prescribe exercise, such as daily walks, as a therapeutic activity. Even when recommended changes are minimal, individuals may perceive the changes as having a negative effect on the quality of life; depression or anger may result.

The degree and the way in which stress contributes to the development of cardiovascular disease are unknown. Even if stress itself does not directly cause pathologic changes in the cardiovascular system, the behaviors used to cope with stress may have psychological components. Overuse of tobacco and alcohol as a reaction to stress are known to have adverse effects on cardiovascular function, so individuals who used tobacco and alcohol as a means to cope with stress in the past may need to learn different coping strategies after diagnosis with cardiovascular disease.

Stress is not always associated with overcommitment and activity. For some individuals, significantly cutting down on activity and involvement can be more stressful than continuing the activity itself. Therefore, helping individuals learn new ways to cope with stress may be more beneficial than insisting that potentially stress-producing activities be avoided altogether.

Many cardiovascular diseases require long-term treatment with medication. Often individuals' successful rehabilitation and subsequent progress depend on their willingness and ability to take medications accurately. Potential barriers to effective treatment with medication may be financial, attitudinal, or logistical. Appropriate strategies must be developed to maximize an individual's ability to comply with treatment as prescribed.

After diagnosis of a cardiac condition, sexual activity may be a special source of anxiety for both individuals and for their partners. In most instances, sexual activity can be resumed; however, associated fear and anxiety can hamper both enjoyment and performance, altering self-esteem and contributing to depression. Often, lack of information contributes to fear and misperceptions. Physicians should discuss specific recommendations regarding the resumption of sexual activity as well as any restrictions or modifications to such activities that should be heeded.

Social Issues

To some degree, the reactions of people in the environment influence the success with which individuals cope with any chronic condition. The quality of individuals' interpersonal relationships at the time of the cardiac event and the presence or absence of social supports can be major determinants of individuals' reaction to their condition.

Cardiovascular conditions can produce profound effects on family dynamics. Depending on the condition and extent of disability, there may be a shifting of family roles and role reversal. Owing to the invisible nature of many cardiac conditions, some family members may not understand that individuals may not be able to sustain the activity level they engaged in prior to their diagnosis. Lack of understanding may breed resentment or anger. Family members may, of course, be a source of support and consolation; however,

they may also contribute to individuals' fear and anxiety by being overly protective or showing anxiety out of proportion to the medical condition. Qualified professionals should discuss such reactions and their potential impact on individuals' return to function with family members.

Although individuals with cardiovascular disease may continue most forms of recreation, extremely rigorous activities may need to be curtailed. When recreational activities that were once a major social outlet must be restricted, social isolation and depression may result unless another recreational activity can be substituted.

Cardiac conditions often have few visible signs of disability. Although this may seem advantageous at first glance, the lack of visible cues may contribute to a misunderstanding of the activity restrictions that are part of the treatment protocol. As a result, individuals with such conditions may be pressured into participating in activities that are more strenuous than those at the prescribed level of activity. The absence of outward signs of disability may also foster individuals' denial of the condition and subsequent noncompliance with the medical treatment plan.

■ VOCATIONAL ISSUES IN CARDIOVASCULAR CONDITIONS

For most individuals, work is a source of pride as well as a financial necessity. The degree to which the cardiovascular condition inhibits the return to regular employment can influence individuals' reactions to the condition. In some instances, attitudes of employers represent formidable barriers to the successful return to work. Employers may be reluctant to employ or reemploy individuals with cardiovascular disease because of fear of liability or responsibility for medical costs if the condition should worsen.

Each job must be viewed in relation to the individual's physical and emotional abilities and the effect that the job has on the individual's health status. In some instances, a job change may be necessary, which can be an additional source of stress. In other instances, individuals can return to their former jobs with little or no modification.

Physicians generally prescribe the degree and type of activity in which individuals with cardiovascular disease may safely engage. Most individuals with heart conditions are able to engage in light to moderate activity.

Because of the effect on the cardiovascular system, environmental conditions such as excessive heat or cold should be avoided. Isometric exercise elevates blood pressure and places an extra burden on the heart; consequently, any exertion that involves muscular activity against a fixed, unmoving resistance should usually be avoided. Individuals with pacemakers should be aware that certain types of equipment may interfere with pacemaker function.

In most instances, once cardiovascular conditions are stabilized and appropriate treatment is instituted, functional decline is slow or minimal. The greatest barrier to productive vocational activity may be the individual's unwillingness or inability to make the recommended lifestyle changes or noncompliance with the medical treatment prescribed.

CASE STUDIES

Case 1

Mr. C., a 50-year-old high school teacher, has been employed in his current position since graduating from college. He teaches history and physical education. Mr. C. had a myocardial infarction at the age of 40; however, he went through intensive cardiac rehabilitation and has returned to most of his former functional capacity. Over the past year, however, he has had increasing fatigue and shortness of breath. Upon evaluation by his cardiologist, Mr. C. was found to be in the beginning stage of heart failure. Although his cardiologist is currently managing his symptoms with medication, he has told Mr. C. that if his cardiac condition continues to deteriorate within the next five years, he may need to have a heart transplant. Mr. C. is married and has three stepchildren.

1. How would you approach Mr. C. about his rehabilitation potential?
2. Is there additional medical information that would be helpful in establishing Mr. C.'s rehabilitation potential?
3. Which other factors should be considered in determining rehabilitation potential?
4. Is it feasible for Mr. C. to continue in his current job?
5. If Mr. C. would continue in his current job, which modifications might be considered?
6. What would Mr. C.'s rehabilitation potential be if he has a cardiac transplant?

Case 2

Ms. B., age 55, had rheumatic fever as a child and, as a result, experienced damage to her mitral valve. She is unmarried and lives alone. Ms. B. has supported herself by cleaning professional offices since she graduated from high school. Over the past year, she has noticed increasing fatigue and dyspnea. When evaluated by her physician, she was found to need valve replacement.

1. Which types of information would you find useful in helping Ms. B. develop a rehabilitation plan?
2. How will Ms. B.'s ability to perform in her current employment be affected by her surgery?

3. Which factors should you consider when helping Ms. B. develop a rehabilitation plan?

■ REFERENCES

Appel, L. J., Moore, T. J., Obarzanek, E., Vollmer, W., Svetkey, L., Sacks, F., et al. (1997). A clinical trial of the effects of dietary patterns on blood pressure. *New England Journal of Medicine, 336,* 1117–1124.

August, P. (2003). Initial treatment of hypertension. *New England Journal of Medicine, 348*(7), 610–616.

Babruth, A. J. (2004). What every patient should know: Pretransplantation and posttransplantation. *Critical Care Nursing, 27*(1), 31–60.

Balady, G. J., Ades, P. A., Comoss, P., Foody, J., Franklin, B., Sanderson, B., et al. (2000). Core components of cardiac rehabilitation/secondary prevention programs: A statement for health care professionals from the American Heart Association and the American Association of Cardiovascular and Pulmonary Rehabilitation Writing Group. *Circulation, 102,* 1069–1073.

Barkley, M. L., Acosta, J. D., Starin, E., & Tan, M. C. (2004). A ventricular assist device bridges the way to a new life. *Critical Care Nursing, 27*(1), 78–86.

Baughman, K. L., & Jarcho, J. A. (2007). Bridge to life: Cardiac mechanical support. *New England Journal of Medicine, 357*(9), 846–849.

Brown, P. A., Launius, B. K., Mancini, M. C., & Cush E. M. (2004). Depression and anxiety in the heart transplant patient: A case study. *Critical Care Nursing, 27*(1), 92–95.

Bybee, K. A., & Kopecky, S. L. (2007). In R. E. Rakel & E. T. Bope (Eds.), *Conn's current therapy* (pp. 417– 426). Philadelphia: W. B. Saunders.

Byrne, J., & Darling, R. C. III (2007). Acquired diseases of the aorta. In R. E. Rakel & E. T. Bope, (Eds.), *Conn's current therapy* (pp. 337–346). Philadelphia: W. B. Saunders.

Camenzind, E. (2006). Treatment of in-stent restenosis: Back to the future? *New England Journal of Medicine, 355*(20), 2149–2151.

Casida, J. (2005). The lived experience of spouses of patients with a left ventricular assist device before heart transplantation. *American Journal of Critical Care, 14*(2), 145–151.

Chapman, E., Parameshwar, J., Jenkins, D., Large, S., & Tsui, S. (2007). Psychosocial issues for patients with ventricular assist devices: A qualitative pilot study. *American Journal of Critical Care, 16*(1), 72–81.

Charlson, M. E., & Isom, O. W. (2003). Care after coronary-artery bypass surgery. *New England Journal of Medicine, 348*(15), 1456–1463.

Cooper, J. M., Katcher, M. S., & Orlov, M. Y. (2002). Implantable devices for the treatment of atrial fibrillation. *New England Journal of Medicine, 346*(26), 2062–2068.

Curfman, G. D., Morrissey, S. A., Jarcho, J. A., & Drazen, J. M. (2007). Drug-eluting coronary stents: Promise and uncertainty. *New England Journal of Medicine, 356*(10), 1059–1060.

Frohlich, E. D. (2007). Hypertension. In R. E. Rakel & B. T. Bope (Eds.), *Conn's current therapy* (p. 416). Philadelphia: W. B. Saunders.

Furlan, A. J. (2006). Carotid-artery stenting: Case open or closed? *New England Journal of Medicine, 355*(16), 1726–1729.

Fye, W. B. (2006). Tracing atrial fibrillation—100 years. *New England Journal of Medicine, 355*(14), 1412–1414.

Glasser, S. P. (2001). Hypertension syndrome and cardiovascular events. *Post Graduate Medicine, 110*(5), 29–36.

Hahn, R. G., Knox, L. M., & Forman, T. A. (2005). Evaluation of poststreptococcal illness. *American Family Physician, 71*(10), 1949–1954.

Hart, R. G. (2003). Atrial fibrillation and stroke prevention. *New England Journal of Medicine, 349*(11), 1015–1016.

House-Fancher, M. A., & Foell, H. Y. (2004). Heart failure and cardiomyopathy. In S. M. Lewis, S. McLean Heitkempei, & S. Ruff Dirksen (Eds.); P. Graber O'Brien, J. Foret Giddens, & L. Bucher (Section Eds.), *Medical surgical nursing* (6th ed., pp. 838–860). St. Louis: Mosby.

Hunt, S. A. (2006). Taking heart: Cardiac transplantation past, present, and future. *New England Journal of Medicine, 355*(3), 231–236.

Jacobowitz, G. R. (2005). Peripheral vascular disorders. In H. H. Zaretsky, E. F. Richter III, & M.

G. Eisenberg (Eds.), *Medical aspects of disability* (3rd ed., pp. 495–508). New York: Springer.

Kaba, E., Thompson, D. R., Burnard, P., Edwards, D., & Theodosopoulou, E. (2005). Somebody else's heart inside me: A descriptive study of psychological problems after a heart transplantation. *Issues in Mental Health Nursing, 26,* 611–625.

Lambert, C. R. (2007). Angina pectoris. In R. E. Rakel & E. T. Bope (Eds.), *Conn's current therapy* (pp. 342–346). Philadelphia: W. B. Saunders.

Levinson, M. E. (2000). Infective endocarditis. In L. Goldman & J. C. Bennett (Eds.), *Cecil's textbook of medicine* (21st ed., pp. 1631–1640). Philadelphia: W. B. Saunders.

Liuzzo, J. P., Shin, Y. T., Lucariello, R., Klapholz, M., Lang, S. J., Braff, R., et al. (2005). Triple valve repair for rheumatic heart disease. *Journal of Cardiac Surgery, 20,* 358–363.

Livneh, H. (1999). Psychosocial adaptation to heart diseases: The role of coping strategies. *Journal of Rehabilitation, 65,* 24–32.

Lytle, B., W. (2004). Surgical treatment of coronary artery disease. In L. Goldman & D. Ausiello (Eds.), *Cecil textbook of medicine* (22nd ed., pp. 428–431). Philadelphia: W. B. Saunders.

Manning, W. J. (2000). Pericardial disease. In L. Goldman & J. C. Bennett (Eds.), *Cecil's textbook of medicine* (21st ed., pp. 347–353). Philadelphia: W. B. Saunders.

McMahon, W. S. (2007). Congenital heart disease. In R. E. Rakel & E. T. Bope (Eds.), *Conn's current therapy* (pp. 378– 382). Philadelphia: W. B. Saunders.

McMurray, D. L. (1998). Psychological, social, and medical factors affecting rehabilitation following coronary bypass surgery. *Journal of Rehabilitation, 64,* 14–18.

McMurray, J. J., & Pfeffer, M. A. (2005). Heart failure. *Lancet, 365,* 1877–1899.

Mielniczuk, L., Mussivand, T., Davies, R., Mesana, T. G., Masters, R. G., Hendry, P. J., et al. (2004). Patient selection for left ventricular assist devices. *Artificial Organs, 28*(2), 152–157.

Milani, R. V., & Lavie, C. J. (2007). Impact of cardiac rehabilitation on depression and its associated mortality. *American Journal of Medicine, 120*(9), 799–806.

Miller, L. W., Pagani, F. D., Russell, S. D., John,

R., Boyle, A. J., Aaronson, K. D., et al. (2007). Use of a continuous-flow device in patients awaiting heart transplantation. *New England Journal of Medicine, 357*(9), 885–896.

Morady, F. (2000). Electrophysiologic interventional procedures and surgery. In L. Goldman & J. C. Bennett (Eds.), *Cecil's textbook of medicine* (21st ed., pp. 248–252). Philadelphia: W. B. Saunders.

Morales, D. L., Argenziano, M., & Oz, M. C. (2000). Output left ventricular assist device support: A safe and economical therapeutic option for heart failure. *Progress in Cardiovascular Disease, 43*(1), 55–66.

Nabel, E. G. (2003). Cardiovascular disease. *New England Journal of Medicine, 349,* 60–72.

Neubauer, S. (2007). The failing heart: An engine out of fuel. *New England Journal of Medicine, 356*(11), 1140–1150.

Newman, D., Dorian, P., Schwartzman, D., Paquette, M., Smith, J., Pitzer, P., et al. (2000). Effect of an implantable atrial defibrillator on health-related quality of life in patients with atrial tachyarrhythmias. *Circulation, 102*(suppl II), 715.

Oparil, S. (2000). Arterial hypertension. In L. Goldman & J. C. Bennett (Eds.), *Cecil's textbook of medicine* (21st ed., pp. 347–353). Philadelphia: W. B. Saunders.

Rey, M. (2005). Cardiovascular disorders. In H. H. Zaretsky, E. F. Richter III, & M. G. Eisenberg (Eds.), *Medical aspects of disability* (pp. 179–211). New York: Springer.

Rourke, T., Droogan, M. T., & Ohler, L. (1999). Heart transplantation: State of the art (advanced practice in acute and critical care). *Clinical Issues, 10*(2), 1–15.

Sacks, F. M., Svetkey, L. P., Vommer, W. M., Appel, L., Bray, G., Harsha, D., et al. (2001). Effects on blood pressure of reduced dietary sodium and the Dietary Approaches to Stop Hypertension (DASH) diet. *New England Journal of Medicine, 344,* 3–10.

Saffitz, J. E. (2006). Connexins, conduction, and atrial fibrillation. *New England Journal of Medicine, 354*(25), 2712–2714.

Santucci, P. A., Haw, J., Trohman, R. G., & Pinski, S. L. (1998). Interference with an implantable defibrillator by an electronic antitheft-surveillance device. *New England Journal of Medicine,*

339(19), 1371-1374.

Science Daily (February 1, 2008) Heart Transplants: Do More or Do None, study suggests. Science News. Retrieved March 2, 2008 from http://www.sciencedaily.com/releases/2008/01/080129125452.htm

Setness, P. A. (2001). Hypertension. *Postgraduate Medicine, 110*(5), 26.

Sherwood, L. (2007). Cardiac physiology. In Human physiology (6th ed., pp. 299-335). Belmont, CA: Thomson.

Sowell, L. V., Kuhl, E. A., Sears, S. F., Klodell, C. T., & Conti, J. B. (2006). Device implant techniques and consideration of body image: Specific procedures for implantable cardioverter defibrillators in female patients. *Journal of Women's Health, 15*(7), 830-835.

Théroux, P. (2004). Angina pectoris. In L. Goldman & D. Ausiello (Eds.), *Cecil's textbook of medi-*cine (22nd ed., pp. 389-400). Philadelphia: W. B. Saunders.

U.S. Department of Health and Human Services. (1995) Public Health Services AHCPR *Cardiac rehabilitation clinical practice guideline.* Rockville, MD: Author.

Victor, R. (2004). Arterial hypertension. In L. Goldman & D. Ausiello (Eds.), *Cecil's textbook of medicine* 22nd ed., (pp. 346-363). Philadelphia: W. B. Saunders.

White, C. (2007). Intermittent claudication. *New England Journal of Medicine, 356*(b12), 1241-1250.

White, W. B. (2003). Ambulatory blood-pressure monitoring in clinical practice. *New England Journal of Medicine, 348*(24), 2377-2378.

Chapter 14

Conditions of the Respiratory (Pulmonary) System

■ STRUCTURE AND FUNCTION OF THE RESPIRATORY SYSTEM

The respiratory system consists of air passages leading into the lungs, the lungs themselves, and the chest (**thorax**), which help move air in and out of the lungs (Sherwood, 2007). Functions of the respiratory system are to supply oxygen to the blood, where it can be distributed to body tissues. The respiratory system also removes carbon dioxide, a waste product of tissue metabolism, from the body. Abnormal functioning of the respiratory system affects every system of the body. A diminished supply of oxygen or an excess of carbon dioxide not only affects body function, but can also result in loss of consciousness and death.

Breathing is an involuntary activity that is under the control of the respiratory center in the brain. Changes in levels of carbon dioxide and oxygen in the blood bring about automatic changes in rate and depth of breathing. As the concentration of carbon dioxide in the blood increases, breathing rate increases to hasten elimination of the waste product.

Inspiration refers to the act of breathing in, whereas **ventilation** refers to the actual movement of gases (oxygen and carbon dioxide) into and out of the lungs. Air first enters the respiratory system through the nose during inspiration. Air entering the nostrils comes in contact with the mucous membranes, which warms and moistens it. Tiny hairs within the nostrils trap dust particles and organisms before they reach the **pharynx** (throat), which serves as a passageway for both air and food. At the bottom of the pharynx are two openings: one into the esophagus for the passage of food, and the other into the **larynx** (voice box) for the passage of air. The larynx contains the vocal cords, which are necessary for speech. A flap called the epiglottis, located on top of the larynx, closes over the larynx when food is ingested to prevent food from entering the respiratory system.

As air is taken in, it passes through the larynx into the main airway to the lungs, the **trachea** (windpipe). The trachea is a cartilaginous tube lined with special hair-like projections called cilia. The cilia are part of the body's defense against foreign objects, such as bacteria, or other particles that have not been filtered out by the upper part of the respiratory system. With a rhythmic motion, cilia project mucus or other particles up toward the pharynx, where they can be expectorated.

After entering the chest cavity, the trachea divides into two branches, called the right and left bronchi. Each bronchus, which also contains cilia, enters a lung and continues to branch into smaller segments called bronchioles. The bronchioles terminate in tiny sacs called alveolar sacs. Within the alveolar sacs are small balloon-like structures called alveoli, which make up most of the lung's substance. It is within the alveoli that the exchange of oxygen and carbon dioxide takes place through tiny blood vessels called **capillaries.**

External respiration is the process of exchanging oxygen and carbon dioxide in the lungs. The exchange of oxygen and carbon dioxide at the tissue level is called **internal respiration**. Oxygen diffuses through the alveolar walls into capillaries, allowing for it to be distributed by the blood to tissue cells throughout the body. Body cells release carbon dioxide into the blood, which then carries it to the alveoli. In turn, capillaries in the alveoli release carbon dioxide from the blood; the carbon dioxide then diffuses across the alveolar wall and is expelled from the lungs through **expiration** (the process of expelling air from the lungs).

The lungs are two sponge-like structures contained within the thoracic cavity (chest cavity) (see Figure 14-1). The thoracic cavity is lined with a thin membrane called the *pleura*, which secretes a thin layer of fluid to help minimize the friction created when the lungs expand and contract against the chest wall during respiration. The thorax cavity is surrounded by ribs. Muscles around the ribs (*intercostal muscles*) expand when air is inhaled and contract when air is exhaled. The thoracic cavity is separated from the abdominal cavity by the main respiratory muscle called the diaphragm.

The left lung contains two lobes: the upper and lower lobes. The right lung contains three lobes: the upper, middle, and lower lobes. The heart is located between the two lungs. Pulmonary vessels carry blood to and from the lungs from the heart. The **pulmonary artery** carries *deoxygenated blood* from the heart to the lungs, whereas the **pulmonary vein** carries *oxygenated blood* to the heart from the lungs.

After delivering oxygen to the body tissues, blood returns to the heart from the general circulation; at this point, it carries an excess of carbon dioxide. The blood is pumped from the right ventricle of the heart into the lungs. Here, the thin walls of the alveoli come in contact with capillaries. Carbon dioxide passes from the capillaries across the alveolar wall so that it can be expelled through expiration of the lungs. In turn, the oxygen that has been taken into the alveoli through inspiration passes across the alveolar wall into the capillaries. The red blood cells take up oxygen, and the blood returns to the heart, where it is pumped into the general circulation to supply body tissues with oxygen.

Air is able to move in and out of the lungs because of pressure changes, which occur because of the contraction and relaxation of the diaphragm and other breathing muscles. The pressure within the lungs and the thorax must be less than the pressure in the atmosphere for inspiration to occur. As air is taken into the lungs, the diaphragm contracts, moving downward, increasing the size of the thoracic cavity, and lowering the pressure within the thoracic cavity. The lungs expand. Atmospheric air, which is at higher pressure, then flows into the lungs, bringing in oxygen as inhalation occurs. Next the diaphragm moves in the opposite direction, relaxing and moving upward, causing the thoracic cavity to become smaller, and thereby increasing intrathoracic pressure. As the lungs are squeezed, air is forced out and carbon dioxide is exhaled.

■ CONDITIONS OF THE RESPIRATORY SYSTEM

Infections of the Respiratory System

Upper Airway Infections (Pharyngitis, Laryngitis)

The upper respiratory tract consists of the nose, the pharynx, and the larynx. **Pharyngitis** (sore throat) is a condition of the upper airway

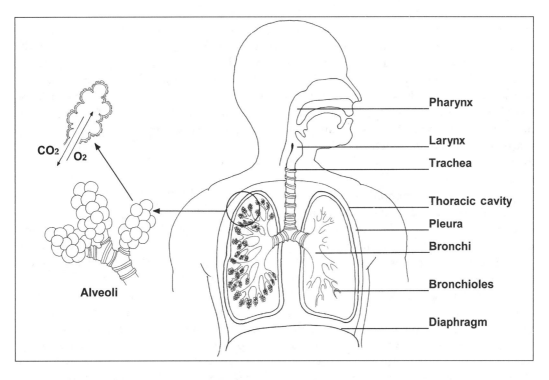

Figure 14-1   The respiratory system

that may be caused by infection with viruses or bacteria. In this condition, the mucous membrane lining the throat becomes inflamed, which may cause symptoms such as sore throat, fever, or difficulty in swallowing. **Laryngitis** (inflammation of the larynx) is usually caused by a virus and can produce hoarseness, loss of voice, cough, and sore throat. Both pharyngitis and laryngitis are relatively minor and tend to be self-limiting.

Pneumonia

Pneumonia is an acute illness caused by inflammation and infection, which affect the bronchioles and alveolar tissue in the lung. It is characterized by cough, chest pain, fever, and breathlessness. Although not in and of itself a disability, pneumonia can be a major problem and is often a life-threatening condition when it is superimposed on other chronic illnesses and disabilities. Individuals with conditions such as heart conditions, alcoholism,

neuromuscular conditions (such as multiple sclerosis), chronic obstructive lung disease, spinal cord injury (especially quadriplegia), dementia, altered immune status, or swallowing abnormalities are at particular high risk for developing pneumonia.

The term "pneumonia" is usually further qualified to describe the cause or location. For example, lobar pneumonia refers to pneumonia that affects one lobe of the lung, whereas bronchopneumonia refers to patchy and diffuse inflammation and infection of one or both lungs. Pneumonia can be caused by a number of organisms, including viruses, bacteria, fungus, yeasts, or other pathogens. Pneumonia caused by a virus would be called viral pneumonia, whereas pneumonia caused by a bacterium would be called bacterial pneumonia.

Usually the defenses of the respiratory system are sufficient to ward off infection. However, when the body is weakened or when the causative agent is overwhelming, defenses in the respiratory system cannot withstand the organism and pneumonia develops. Individuals with chronic illness or disability, and particularly those who have limited mobility or who are subject to prolonged inactivity owing to bed rest, have an increased susceptibility for developing pneumonia. Pneumonia caused by inactivity or immobility such that the lungs do not expand sufficiently is known as *hypostatic* pneumonia.

Another type of pneumonia can occur in individuals who have difficulty swallowing or who are unconscious. In these situations, the epiglottis may not close adequately, allowing food, liquid, or other substances to enter the lungs. The consequent accumulation of foreign material in the lung contributes to development of aspiration pneumonia. Persons who are especially vulnerable to aspiration pneumonia include individuals with altered mental status, neuromuscular conditions, or abnormalities of the esophagus. Aspiration of toxic materials such as oils, bile, gastric acid, or alcohol causes additional complications because of direct damage to the alveolar membrane, leading to chemical pneumonitis.

Inflammation and infection of the alveoli interfere with oxygen and carbon dioxide exchange in the lungs. The greater the extent of inflammation and infection, the greater the interference with respiration. Infection triggers changes in the capillary walls in the alveoli, causing fluid to flow into the alveoli and accumulate there. The accumulation of fluid serves as an excellent growth medium for organisms, so that the infection becomes worse. Accumulation of fluid in the lungs further interferes with the exchange of carbon dioxide and oxygen. When the infection becomes widespread, there is danger of the organisms invading the bloodstream, which is a potentially life-threatening complication of pneumonia.

Diagnostic Testing for Pneumonia

Diagnosis of pneumonia is usually made by assessment of symptoms as well as chest x-ray, which helps to identify the location and degree of lung involvement. Culture of sputum specimens may be done to identify the precise organism responsible for the infection so that appropriate medication can be prescribed. If the sputum culture is inconclusive or if the individual's condition deteriorates rapidly, *bronchoscopy* (insertion of a special tube through the mouth and into the trachea to examine the bronchi) may be indicated.

Management and Prevention of Pneumonia

Once the cause of pneumonia is identified, treatment with medication is directed toward eradicating the specific organism. Medications that facilitate removal of secretions from the lungs (**expectorant**s) may also be administered. Because individuals with pneumonia may have lowered oxygen content in the blood (**hypoxia**) owing to poor gas exchange, oxygen may be administered. Manual chest physiotherapy may also be conducted to facilitate drainage from the lungs.

Individuals at high risk for developing pneumonia should be especially vigilant to prevent infection that opens the door to subsequent pneumonia. Good nutrition, adequate hydration, and adequate sleep are all measures that help bolster immunity. Individuals should attempt to minimize situations in which they are exposed to infection, especially during cold and flu season. Exposure to others with cold or flu should be avoided as well. The position of individuals with limited mobility should be changed frequently to facilitate lung expansion and drainage. In addition, flu and pneumococcal vaccinations may be important to prevent pneumonia from occurring. Respiratory irritants such as secondhand cigarette smoke or other pollutants can make individuals more susceptible to infection and consequently should be avoided.

Vocational Issues in Pneumonia

Pneumonia can cause significant morbidity and consequent loss of workdays, not to mention threat to life itself. Because individuals with chronic illness or disability often have increased susceptibility to pneumonia, the steps mentioned previously to minimize development of pulmonary complications are especially important. The presence in the workplace of conditions that can induce or aggravate lung conditions may require job modification or complete avoidance or exposure to the risk. Although risk of exposure may be present in a number of work situations, specific exposure to respiratory irritants or to large numbers of people who may have respiratory symptoms should be avoided as much as possible.

Tuberculosis

Tuberculosis (TB) is an infectious condition that is curable and preventable, but can also potentially be fatal (Lahart, 2007). It is caused by an organism called the tubercle bacillus. Although it most frequently affects the lungs, tuberculosis can occur in almost any part of the body. Tuberculosis of the lung is called *pulmonary* tuberculosis. Infection occurs primarily through inhalation of infectious droplets that an infected individual has released through coughing. As a result of the infection, nodules form in the lung.

Exposure to the tubercle bacillus may or may not lead to infection or to an active form of the condition. Whether infection or active tuberculosis develops depends on individual's general physical condition and intensity of the exposure. Ordinarily, tuberculosis is not contracted from brief exposure to a person with TB.

Many factors predispose individuals to develop tuberculosis. Lowered body resistance owing to inadequate rest and poor nutrition may be one predisposing factor. Persons with other chronic conditions—for example, diabetes, alcoholism, HIV infection, and conditions that affect the lungs (e.g., silicosis)—are more likely to develop tuberculosis if they should come in contact with the infectious agent (Poss, 2000).

Individuals infected with tuberculosis for the first time are said to have a *primary infection*. Primary infections may or may not become active. The infection may remain dormant for years until the person's physical resistance is lowered. The most common form of tuberculosis is reinfection, also called *secondary tuberculosis*. Individuals with active pulmonary tuberculosis may have few symptoms until nodules in the lung are large enough to be seen on x-ray. Initial symptoms may include weight loss, **anorexia** (loss of appetite), and a slight elevation of temperature. Symptoms may then progress to cough, overproduction of sputum, and **hemoptysis** (blood-streaked sputum).

Diagnosis of Tuberculosis

Infection with the tubercle bacillus is diagnosed through cultures of sputum, chest x-rays, and tuberculin skin tests. Skin tests can be a valuable screening tool to determine if the individual has been infected with the tubercle bacillus. After being infected by the tubercle bacilli, the body develops an allergic response over time, resulting in tissue sensitivity. This sensitivity can be identified through the tuberculin skin test, which involves injection of a small amount of filtrate from dead tubercle bacilli under the skin. If an individual has been exposed to and infected by the tubercle bacillus, a local skin reaction will occur at the injection site. Skin tests are interpreted for reaction at 24 hours and again at 48 to 72 hours after injection.

A positive reaction to a skin test indicates that the individual has been exposed to and infected with the tubercle bacillus, but it does not indicate whether the condition is active. Individuals who have a positive skin test, but who do not have any symptoms or other evidence of the active form of the condition on x-ray or sputum specimens, do not have the active form of tuberculosis and are not contagious to others. It is now recommended that individuals with positive skin tests be treated even though they have no active signs of the tuberculosis, so as to prevent the possibility of tuberculosis becoming active at a later date, when their resistance may be diminished due to other causes such as chronic conditions or aging (Horsburgh, 2004).

To determine whether the individual with a positive skin test has active TB, physicians obtain chest x-rays and sputum specimens from the individual to check for signs of active tuberculosis. Identification of nodular changes in the lung and/or the finding of tubercle bacillus in the sputum or other body secretions confirms the diagnosis of active tuberculosis. Individuals with active TB are infectious and, theoretically, would be able to transmit the condition to others.

Management of Tuberculosis

Individuals with active tuberculosis should undergo prompt treatment, not just for their own well-being, but also for the protection of others. Treatment consists of taking medication from 6 to 24 months. The average length of treatment with medication ranges from 9 to 12 months. Usually, after 2 to 4 weeks of intensive treatment with medication, individuals are no longer a public health threat in terms of being contagious, and they can return to normal activities.

It is of the utmost importance that individuals being treated for tuberculosis take the medication accurately as prescribed and consistently if treatment is to be effective. Because individuals have not always been compliant with the drug regimen prescribed, there are more cases in which the tubercle bacillus has become resistant to the regular medications, which had once been effective. *Multidrug-resistant (MDR) tuberculosis* and *extensively drug-resistant (XDR) tuberculosis* have become a global health problem (Raviglione & Smith, 2007).

Case identification and consistent treatment are crucial in the control of tuberculosis (Lahart, 2007). Compulsory isolation (which refers to individuals who have been infected) and quarantine (which refers to individuals who have been exposed but are not yet infected) have been suggested as ways to protect public health. In most instances, individuals are willing to participate in voluntary directly observed therapy so that compulsory detention isn't necessary (Parmet, 2007).

Tuberculosis that occurs outside the lungs is called *extrapulmonary tuberculosis*. Possible sites of infection include the lining of the brain and spinal cord, the kidney, bones, or the abdomen. Tuberculosis that is widespread throughout the body is called *miliary tuberculosis*. Treatment of extrapulmonary tuberculosis is similar to that of pulmonary tuberculosis, although treatment may continue for a longer period.

Psychosocial Issues in Tuberculosis

Although anyone of any social class or educational level can be infected by the tubercle bacillus, development of tuberculosis is often associated with crowded conditions, poverty, alcoholism, substance abuse, and homelessness (Campion, 1999). In many cultures, social stigma of tuberculosis may contribute to individuals' denial that they have the condition and abandonment of treatment. Individuals with tuberculosis who remember the social stigma once associated with the condition may feel ashamed and embarrassed. They may try to hide their diagnosis from others, ignore the physician's recommendations, or discontinue treatment. Such reactions have serious consequences for both individuals with tuberculosis and those in close contact with them.

Vocational Issues in Tuberculosis

When tubercle bacilli are no longer present in the sputum after patients begin treatment, individuals are no longer considered infectious to others and are able to return to work (usually within 2 to 4 weeks). Once an individual has undergone treatment, providing there have been no associated complications, the ability to return to work or to perform tasks performed previously should not be affected. Because of this stigma attached to this condition and misinformation employers or co-workers may have about it, however, one of the major barriers to employment for person with TB may be the attitudes of employers and fellow employees.

Chronic Lung Conditions

Asthma

Asthma is a condition characterized by airway hyperresponsiveness (Ho, 2007) and contraction of the smooth muscles of the airway, leading to constriction of the bronchi (Cox et al., 2007; Doherty, 2004). It is associated with episodic attacks of wheezing, **dyspnea** (difficulty breathing), chest tightness, and cough triggered by a variety of stimuli. Triggers of asthma exacerbations appear to involve complex interactions with factors within the environment (Holgate & Polosa, 2006).

The prevalence of asthma has increased dramatically over the last 25 years, as air quality has declined in industrialized Western countries (Moorman, Rudd, Johnson, King, Minor, Bailey et al., 2007). Exposure to air pollutants increases the risk of developing asthma (Gilmour, Jaakola, London, Nei, & Rogers, 2006). Other factors such as exercise, emotional stress, inhalation of cold air, and exposure to respiratory irritants such as fumes from paint or gasoline, cigarette smoke, or perfumes may also precipitate an asthma attack. For some people, attacks are triggered by food preservatives or substances found in some medications, such as aspirin. Most triggers set off an allergic response, which causes the immune system to initiate an inflammatory response in which the airway swells and secretes excess mucus that clogs the passages. At the same time, muscles that control air passages constrict and go into spasm, causing the airways to narrow. As a result, individuals have difficulty breathing and the lungs work less efficiently.

The severity of symptoms and the frequency of asthma attacks vary with the individual. Some people may have a slight cough and shortness of breath during an attack, whereas others may be so restricted by cough and shortness of breath that they are unable to speak more than a few words at a time. Chronic bronchitis or emphysema may coexist with asthma, especially in older adults.

Asthma may be classified as mild, moderate, or severe. Individuals with mild asthma may have intermittent brief symptoms several times per month, but have no symptoms in between attacks, so that medication is required only during an attack. Individuals with moderate asthma may have an attack several times per week and require medication almost daily. Individuals are classified as having severe asthma when symptoms are almost continuous and physical activities are limited due to symptoms. Severe asthma requires daily medication, and it may be accompanied by frequent hospitalizations and potentially life-threatening exacerbations.

Atelectasis (collapse of the lung) is a possible complication of asthma. A severe, prolonged attack (**status asthmaticus**) is a severe exacerbation of asthma that is unresponsive to treatment methods and can be fatal. Status asthmaticus requires emergency medical intervention.

Management of Asthma

Management of asthma is directed toward the identification and avoidance of precipitating factors, the symptomatic relief of attacks, and the prevention of future attacks. Identification and management of factors causing exacerbations, rather than simply obtaining more medications to treat symptoms, are crucial (Harrison, 2005).

If asthma is caused by allergy, individuals should attempt to rid the environment the substance causing the allergic response (**allergen**) to the maximum extent possible. Common allergens include dust mites, mold, pollen, and animal dander.

When individuals know what triggers a response, whether allergic or not, precipitating factors should be eliminated as much as possible. Common precipitating factors that can aggravate asthma and possibly bring on an attack include irritants such as dust, smoke, exhaust fumes, chemicals, and perfumes. Some food preservatives, such as sulfites, can also bring on an attack. In some instances, attacks may be brought on by stress or fatigue.

Several medications are commonly used to treat asthma. Although medications can help individuals manage symptoms, they do not cure the condition (Selgrade et al., 2006). Individuals may take medications daily, or they may use medications for relief of symptoms during an asthma attack. *Corticosteroids* are substances produced naturally in the body by the adrenal glands that perform a number of vital functions, including regulating metabolism, maintaining proper water balance, and fighting against inflammation. The corticosteroids prescribed by a physician for treatment of asthma are *anti-inflammatory* medications, meaning that they reduce inflammation and swelling of the lining of the bronchial tubes. They are usually taken on a regular basis to prevent asthma attacks. These agents may be inhaled, taken orally, or administered by injection.

Cromolyn sodium may be prescribed as an alternative to inhaled steroids or to help reduce the amount of steroids needed. It helps to prevent asthma attacks by blocking the release of substances that narrow airways during an asthmatic reaction. Cromolyn sodium may be especially helpful when taken prior to exercise or prior to exposure to triggering factors.

Medications called *bronchodilators*, which dilate the narrowed and constricted bronchioles, are commonly used in the treatment of acute asthma attacks. These medications dilate the bronchioles by relaxing the muscles of their walls, thereby creating a larger opening for the passage of air.

Bronchodilators may be taken orally, or they may be administered with inhalers or nebulizers. A *nebulizer* is a device that converts liquid medication into tiny droplets that individuals then inhale. Nebulizers and inhalers deliver medication directly to the lungs so that the medication begins to act immediately. Individuals with asthma may also use special instruments called *metered-dose* or *aerosol inhalers*. When inhalers are used correctly, medication is delivered directly into the lungs for quick relief of symptoms. Metered-dose inhalers dispense aerosol medication in measured doses, but to receive the full effect individuals must learn and remember to use the proper technique with the inhalers. *Spacer devices* may also be used. A spacer device is a tube or bag that is attached to the metered-dose inhaler at one end and has a mouthpiece for the individual to inhale through the other end. The spacer acts as a holding chamber, slowing down the delivery of the medication so the individual can inhale it more efficiently. A peak-flow meter is a device that determines changes in the size of the individual's airways. Individuals are able to measure and record their peak flow rate to help determine the severity of their asthma and identify how well they are responding to treatment.

Individuals with asthma require periodic medical assessment to ensure that the goals of treatment have been achieved and to monitor their condition. The severity of the condition and the appropriate therapy vary widely among individuals, and an individual's condition can change over time, with new allergies developing or the severity of the asthma increasing or decreasing.

One of the most important aspects of treatment of asthma is patient education and monitoring (Naureckas & Solway, 2001). Individuals should be aware of how to recognize and manage exacerbations of the condition; they should also be able to identify and, if possible, avoid environmental triggers. Asthma self-management education should be tailored to the need of the individual, with the provider exhibiting sensitivity to the person's cultural beliefs and practices. In addition, annual influenza vaccination may be indicated for individuals with persistent asthma.

Psychosocial Issues in Asthma

Effective management of asthma requires adherence to the medical recommendations to control attacks. However, psychological or behavioral responses may prevent or limit individuals' compliance with recommendations. Individuals may experience a variety of obstacles that impede their ability to adhere to medical interventions. Resistance to the treatment plan may be one of the greatest barriers to successful asthma control. Asthma, unlike many other chronic conditions, has associated symptoms that are usually reversible when treated with medications. Consequently, with proper treatment, the condition should only minimally affect daily living. Unfortunately, individuals may feel that the level of adherence to treatment necessary to control the symptoms draws attention to them. Consequently, they may feel stigmatized and avoid implementing treatment as needed. Individuals with asthma may view daily medications as a negative, constant reminder of their condition. Social opportunities may also be affected by asthma if, depending on the factors that appear to precipitate an attack, there are limitations on physical activities or exposure to environmental factors because they trigger attacks. Fear and panic may also be experienced during acute asthma attacks.

Individuals who have had asthma since childhood may be especially vulnerable to social adjustment problems because of stressors experienced due to hospitalizations and restrictions, which may have impeded their social development. Obstacles such as lack of medical insurance coverage may encourage episodic care and inadequate follow-up and monitoring. Out-of-pocket expenditures for health care and prescription costs may impose an undue hardship on affected individuals and their families, making it difficult to obtain necessary medication and medical care. Transportation obstacles, if they prevent individuals from obtaining access to health care for follow-up, may also pose a challenge.

In other instances, individuals may not understand the importance of certain recommendations, such as taking medication daily even when they are not having an asthma attack, reducing exposure to allergens, or modifying the home or work environment to reduce irritants that can trigger attacks.

Individuals with asthma may experience feelings of anger and low self-esteem, which in turn may cause difficulty in acceptance of their condition. They may have difficulty coming to terms with the limitations imposed by their condition and have a sense of loss of control over themselves and their life.

Vocational Issues in Asthma

Asthma is a common cause of morbidity and mortality in the United States (Marik, Varon, & Fromm, 2002) and a major cause of missed school or work days (Eisner, Yelin, Katz, Lactao, Iribarren, & Blanc, 2006; Li, 2001). It imposes some limitations on individuals regardless of the level of severity. Because exposure to irritants and allergens can increase asthma exacerbations in individuals who are sensitive to these factors, the individual should avoid environmental pollutants or allergens to which he or she is particularly sensitive. Environmental factors that can contribute to asthma include chemicals such as cleaning solutions, craft supplies, industrial and vehicle emissions, tobacco smoke or wood-stove emissions, pollens, and animal dander. Exertion should be avoided in situations where air pollution is high. Individuals with asthma should also avoid exposure to individuals with respiratory infections.

Chronic Obstructive Pulmonary Disease (COPD, Chronic Bronchitis, and Emphysema)

Chronic obstructive pulmonary disease has a major impact on both physical and psychological well-being (Goldberg, Hillberg, Reinecker, & Goldstein, 2004). The term *chronic obstructive pulmonary disease* (COPD) is a diagnostic term used to describe a group of conditions that are characterized by respiratory symptoms such as **dyspnea** (shortness of breath), cough, sputum production, limitation of air flow, and chronic inflammation of the lungs (Rabe, 2007). COPD involves chronic inflammation of the airways, which subsequently causes enlargement of the mucous glands in the lungs, with increased mucus secretion. As the inflammation continues, airways become narrowed so that airflow is obstructed. The structure of alveolar walls is destroyed so that there is permanent enlargement of the airspaces. Eventually alveolar units become less functional, such that the amount of lung area available for gas exchange becomes reduced (Dewar & Curry, 2006).

COPD, in addition to affecting the lungs, has far-reaching effects on other body systems. It attacks the cardiovascular system, increases risk of lung cancer, is associated with

osteoporosis and other metabolic syndromes, and can lead to depression (Sin, Anthonisen, Soriano, & Agusti, 2006). COPD is generally progressive and can lead to increasing disability and death (Mannino et al., 2002). Risk factors include exposure to a wide variety of inhaled particles and gases (Rabe, 2007). Cigarette smoking is the major risk factor for developing COPD (Barnes, 2004; Petty, 2001), although not everyone who has COPD has a history of smoking (Rennard, 2004). Environmental pollutants, occupational chemicals, passive smoke, and a genetic predisposition to COPD are also risk factors (Garcia & Jenkinson, 2007; Hogg, Chu, Utokaparch, Woods, Elliott et al., 2004; Barnes, 2000). While there is no universally accepted definition of COPD (Snider, 2003), the primary criteria these conditions share is air flow limitation that is not fully reversible, that is progressive, and that is associated with exposure to noxious particles or gases (Pauwels, Buist, Calverley, Jenkins, & Hurd, 2001). Included in this definition are *chronic bronchitis* and *emphysema*.

Acute bronchitis should be distinguished from chronic bronchitis. *Acute bronchitis* is a self-limited inflammation of the airways of the lung that is associated with viral infections (Wenzel & Fowler, 2006). *Chronic bronchitis* is a chronic condition associated with coughs and linked with another chronic condition, emphysema.

Although, chronic bronchitis and emphysema are two distinct conditions, they frequently coexist. Both share similar symptoms including **dyspnea** (shortness of breath), especially on exertion; intermittent cough; and fatigue. This combination of symptoms is a major contributor to disability, with dyspnea in particular significantly altering quality of life (Luce & Luce, 2001). Fatigue is a common symptom in most individuals with COPD. The dyspnea of COPD can affect individuals' ability to exercise or perform tasks of daily living. Individuals with early COPD may experience dyspnea after walking for short distances, while those in later stages of the condition may experience significant dyspnea with even minimal activity such as brushing their teeth.

Chronic bronchitis is clinically defined as a chronic productive cough on most days for a minimum of three months in the year, for not less than two consecutive years. Symptoms consist of a persistent cough, especially in the early morning, accompanied by an excessive volume of mucus and expectoration. The lining of the air passages becomes irritated, swollen, and clogged with mucus. Mucus obstructs airflow into and out of the **alveoli** (the small air sacs in the lung where oxygen–carbon dioxide exchange takes place). Sometimes the small muscles around the air passages tighten—a phenomenon called *bronchospasm*—which makes breathing even more difficult. Chronic bronchitis often leads to emphysema. Although bronchitis may predispose individuals to develop emphysema, it can also result from other conditions of the lung, such as occupational lung diseases and cystic fibrosis.

Emphysema is defined as a permanent enlargement of the alveoli caused by the over-inflation of and destructive changes in the alveolar walls (Kerstjens, 1999). As a result, the alveoli have less surface area available for the exchange of oxygen and carbon dioxide, and the bronchioles close before exhalation is complete. As more and more alveoli are affected, the lungs lose some of their natural ability to stretch and relax, diminishing the efficiency of expiration. Airways become obstructed; stale air, which is high in carbon dioxide and low in oxygen, becomes trapped in the alveoli; and the lungs become over-inflated because all of the air cannot be expelled.

Cigarette smoking is the most important risk factor for developing COPD, and smoking and air pollution in combination may facilitate development and progression of the condition. Nevertheless, COPD may also develop in individuals who have had chronic asthma for years and do not smoke. The course of COPD varies. In most cases, the condition develops slowly, with respiratory function remaining relatively stable for years. In other cases, respiratory function deteriorates rapidly. Many people have COPD for years before it is diagnosed. Individuals usually seek medical advice when they note shortness of breath with exercise or at rest. At this point, more than 50% of their lung function may already have been lost.

Because of the airway obstruction that accompanies COPD, **hypoxemia** (decreased levels of oxygen in the blood) may occur. As COPD becomes more advanced and hypoxemia increases, oxygen supply to the brain may become inadequate, resulting in impaired judgment, confusion, or motor incoordination. A buildup of carbon dioxide (**hypercapnia**) may also occur because of inadequate gas exchange in the lungs, resulting in drowsiness or apathy. To counteract the low concentration of oxygen, the body's production of red blood cells increases, resulting in a condition called *polycythemia*. The increased number of red cells in the blood increases blood viscosity, which in turn can impede blood flow. When polycythemia is severe, periodic **phlebotomy** (removal of blood) may be performed to reduce the number of red blood cells, thereby decreasing the viscosity of the blood. As COPD advances, individuals may experience increased difficulty expectorating secretions; increased shortness of breath, especially upon exertion; and increased vulnerability to respiratory infections. For individuals with COPD, respiratory infections can be life threatening because they may further compromise an already-diminished gas exchange.

Failure of the right ventricle of the heart (**cor pulmonale**) may develop as a complication of COPD. As a result of the obstruction of air flow in the lungs and the subsequent breakdown of the alveolar walls, many capillaries in the lungs are destroyed. The surrounding capillaries become constricted, as a compensatory mechanism in response to lower concentrations of oxygen. Constriction of the capillaries channels additional blood flow to areas of the lungs that are better oxygenated; however, constriction of capillaries also creates a resistance to the blood being pumped into the lungs by the right ventricle of the heart. As a consequence, the right ventricle must pump against resistance and becomes hypertrophied (enlarged), losing its ability to pump effectively (see Chapter 13). Because of the inefficient pumping action of the enlarged right ventricle, blood returning to the right side of the heart from the general circulation begins to back up, causing **edema** (swelling) in other parts of the body. Organs of the digestive system may become engorged with fluid, causing nausea and vomiting. There may also be edema of the lower extremities, predisposing individuals to skin ulcerations.

Diagnosis of COPD

Despite the many detrimental effects of COPD, this condition is grossly underdiagnosed in many individuals (Mannino, Gagnon,

Petty, & Lydick, 2000). Although history of smoking, smoker's cough, and excess mucus secretion may be indicative of COPD, spirometric measurements are required to diagnose COPD and document the degree of loss of lung function. Measurements of air flow limitation during forced expiration are measured through spirometry (Hurd & Pauwels, 2002). Spirometry is discussed in detail later in this chapter.

In an effort to increase awareness of COPD and to develop a consensus on the criteria necessary for diagnosis of COPD, the Global Initiative for Chronic Obstructive Lung Disease (GOLD) has introduced a five-stage classification for the severity of COPD based on the degree of air flow as measured by spirometry and presence of symptoms (Garcia & Jenkinson, 2007). These stages are outlined in Table 14-1.

Management of COPD

COPD is irreversible and incurable. The major goals of treatment include smoking cessation, symptom relief, improvement in functional capacity, and limitation of complications

---

Table 14-1   Classification of COPD

Stage	Manifestations
Stage 0: at risk	Chronic cough and sputum production. Lung function as measured by spirometry normal. No functional limitations.
Stage I: mild	Potential chronic cough and sputum production. Mild limitation of airflow as measured by spirometry. Individual may still be unaware of declining lung function.
Stage II: moderate	Progression of symptoms with shortness of breath on exertion. Abnormalities found in spirometry.
Stage III: severe	Increased shortness of breath. Significant changes in spirometry. Quality of life affected.
Stage IV: very severe	Quality of life and activity severely affected, with potentially life-threatening consequences.

Adapted from Global Initiative for Chronic Obstructive Lung Disease. (2005). Global strategy for the diagnosis, management, and prevention of chronic obstructive pulmonary disease [executive summary]. Accessed January 17, 2006, at http://www.goldcopd.com/Guidelineitem.asp?l1=2&l2=1&intid=996

(Sutherland & Cherniack, 2004). Individuals with COPD may be referred to a **pulmonologist** (a physician who specializes in evaluation and treatment of lung conditions) for evaluation and treatment.

Pulmonary rehabilitation is an important nonpharmacologic treatment of COPD and is directed toward increasing the ability to compensate for and live with the condition, rather than attempting to cure it (Rochester, 2000). Pulmonary rehabilitation consists of a structured program of education, exercise conditioning, energy conservation, physiotherapy, and psychosocial and vocational counseling. Goals are to provide symptomatic relief, decrease functional consequences, and enhance lifestyle. For individuals who smoke, the most important intervention to alter the clinical course of the condition is smoking cessation (Barnett, 2006; American Thoracic Society, 1995; Petty, 1999).

A variety of medications may be used in the treatment of COPD. Bronchodilators, which help to reduce hyperinflation and thus dyspnea, are a mainstay of treatment for COPD (Barnes, 2000). Most individuals with COPD have chronic inhaled bronchodilator therapy prescribed. Some individuals with COPD may have features of asthma; during exacerbation of their symptoms, systemic steroids may be prescribed for their anti-inflammatory effect (Irwin & Madison, 2003). Individuals with COPD are susceptible to respiratory infections and pneumonia, which, because of their already-reduced lung function, may be fatal. For bacterial lung infections, antibiotics are usually prescribed. In addition, individuals with COPD should have annual vaccines for both flu and pneumonia.

In addition to medication, other forms of therapy may include *postural drainage* or *chest physiotherapy*, (to remove secretions from the lungs) or *resistive breathing devices* (to increase breathing capacity). Avoidance of pulmonary irritants, especially smoking, is of primary importance. Many individuals with COPD benefit from learning new breathing techniques that stress abdominal, diaphragmatic breathing (to reduce use of accessory muscles for breathing and to conserve energy,) or *pursed-lip breathing* (to slow breathing rate and help remove trapped air from the lungs). Others find it helpful to use a simple resistive breathing device in the home daily to "exercise" muscles of respiration. Physicians may advise individuals with COPD to engage in a daily walking or exercise program to keep in shape, to build strength and endurance, and to maintain their physical condition and improve work capacity. Physicians may also recommend that individuals with COPD consume a series of small meals throughout the day rather than a few large meals because a distended stomach or abdomen can push against the lungs, further interfering with breathing. Foods that cause gas and bloating should be avoided. Adequate fluid intake is important to facilitate clearance of respiratory secretions.

Supplemental home oxygen therapy may be required, depending on the amount of lung damage and the oxygen level in the blood. Often individuals with COPD have right ventricular failure, **polycythemia** (elevated level of red blood cells), severe dyspnea, and sleep-associated hypoxemia. Oxygen administration during ambulation can reduce the effects of dyspnea and increase endurance and the ability to carry out daily activities. Physicians may prescribe home oxygen therapy for individuals with advanced COPD as well. The prescription for oxygen therapy usually depends on the degree of hypoxemia experienced at rest or during exercise, and the amount of oxygen needed for each person will vary. Some people need oxygen only at night and during exercise, whereas others will require supplemental oxygen 24 hours a day. Supplemental oxygen provides the additional oxygen that the lungs cannot deliver.

Oxygen may be supplied from several different sources. Weight, portability, ease of refilling, availability, and cost are taken into account when choosing a system. Compressed gas usually comes in large cylinders, which can weigh as much as 200 pounds. These cylinders are stationary and may be mounted near the bed to be used at night during sleep. Small portable devices that contain oxygen and that can be carried and used by the individual throughout the day are also available. Portable systems generally consist of canisters containing liquid oxygen, each of which weighs 6 to 9 pounds. Larger units are available, but the difficulty of carrying these devices may make it necessary for them to be wheeled around. Therefore, the larger device may limit mobility; in addition, there is the possibility of tripping over the device or becoming entangled in the tubing.

Supplemental oxygen reduces dyspnea and can improve quality of life. Nevertheless, it is a medicine and should be prescribed and used as such. Although oxygen can improve an individual's functional capacity and quality of life, use of portable oxygen machines may also cause others to perceive the individual as an invalid, hampering social interaction because of false perceptions. Because the body's ability to respond to different concentrations of oxygen diminishes in some respiratory conditions, oxygen should be used only as prescribed, and its use should be carefully monitored. Individuals should never increase or decrease the amount of oxygen prescribed without first checking with their physician. Individuals using oxygen should not smoke or allow smoking around them because of the danger of combustion. Likewise, oxygen equipment and tubing should be kept away from open flames. Combustible material such as aerosol sprays, paint thinners, or petroleum-based products should also be removed from the area.

Surgical Intervention for COPD

Surgical interventions may be used in severe cases of COPD. The goal of surgical therapy for individuals with advanced disease is to prolong life by preventing complications, relieving dyspnea, and enhancing quality of life through improving functional status. Until recently, lung transplantation was the last surgical option available for individuals who faced limited life expectancy because of emphysema. Lung transplantation may involve one or both lungs. Selection of an individual as being an appropriate candidate for lung transplant is generally based on the individual's inability to survive without it as well as specific selection criteria (Gunes, Aboyoun, Morton, Plit, Malouf, & Glanville, 2006; O'Brien & Criner 1998).

More recently, lung volume reduction surgery has been proposed as a palliative treatment for individuals with severe emphysema (Twedell, 2007; Geddes et al., 2000; Pompeo, Marino, Nofroni, Matteucci & Mineo, 2000). Emphysema causes the lungs to become overinflated and lose much of their elastic recoil, such that the remaining functional part of the lung essentially becomes compressed within the chest wall. Removal of some of the nonfunctioning area of the lung, allows lung capacity to decrease, so that a more normal physiologic state is restored (Twedell, 2007). A major requirement for lung reduction surgery is manifestations so severe that individuals without the surgery are not expected to live longer than 18 to 24 months. Individuals must be within normal body weight, abstain from cigarette smoking for at least 6 months, and have no coexisting medical problems or severe psychological problems. Although lung volume reduction surgery has been found to increase the chance of improved exercise capacity and quality of life (Geddes et al., 2000), it has not been found to increase survival rates any more than medical therapy. (National Emphysema Treatment Trial Research Group, 2001).

Prior to undergoing the surgery, individuals are expected to attend pulmonary rehabilitation for at least 6 weeks. This program includes exercises with the treadmill, exercise bike, stair climbing, and the like under medical supervision. During exercise, the oxygen saturation of the individual's blood is measured. To qualify for surgery, individuals must build their exercise tolerance to 30 minutes while maintaining a predetermined oxygen level in the blood, using supplemental oxygen as necessary.

After lung reduction surgery, individuals undergo pulmonary rehabilitation; in this respiratory muscle retraining, they learn how to use the diaphragm and accessory muscles of respiration to assist in breathing. Pulmonary rehabilitation is also directed toward helping individuals increase their overall fitness and endurance.

Psychosocial Issues in COPD

Psychosocial issues can be manifested as anxiety, depression, fatigue, and withdrawal from family and social life. Individuals may require extensive psychosocial support to deal with these issues. Many of the psychosocial issues individuals experience are related to dyspnea. Shortness of breath can lead to anxiety and panic, whether or not it is associated with a physical condition. For individuals with COPD, dyspnea may produce severe anxiety, accompanied by fear of death, avoidance of all activities that cause dyspnea, and preoccupation with bodily complaints. Because strong emotions naturally raise the respiratory rate, fear of becoming short of breath may in itself increase dyspnea, causing a vicious cycle that can prove totally incapacitating. Because shortness of breath is anxiety provoking, individuals may adopt an abnormally and poten-

tially unnecessarily restricted lifestyle even though they are physically capable of being more active. Maladaptive avoidant responses may result, severely limiting interpersonal activities and causing individuals to become isolated. Individuals may be unable to work and may feel less interested in participating in social and family events.

Individuals with COPD may experience intense emotions such as anger and depression related to coping with their illness. Suppression of emotions can further compromise individuals' physical condition, increasing their functional decline and restricting individuals' activity and involvement with others even more.

Sexual difficulties may be a particular problem for individuals with COPD. Problems may stem from a fear of becoming short of breath rather than from any physical limitation attributable to the condition. Although it is physically safe for most people with COPD to engage in sexual activity, sexual inhibition may be present if individuals interpret the dyspnea that can occur during sexual activity as an exacerbation of their condition or as a life-threatening symptom. These concerns can inhibit further sexual activity and can affect intimate relationships with others. In other instances, sexual function may be negatively affected by depression.

Individuals with COPD may also confront a number of losses. Employment, physical independence, self-esteem, and social interactions may be lost or limited because of their condition. Some individuals may be reluctant to use portable oxygen in public because of embarrassment, whereas others may become psychologically dependent on it and be reluctant to venture out without the oxygen source, even when they do not need it. Some people with COPD insist on using oxygen even though their difficulty in breathing is not the result of lowered oxygen content of the blood. In such instances, the psychological dependency on the oxygen may be more debilitating than the respiratory condition itself.

Individuals may find themselves excluded from activities of their families and friends because of their limited functional capacity. In some instances, coughing and expectoration of foul-smelling mucus may interfere with the ability to interact socially. Counseling and support groups can help to increase self-esteem and help family members cope with the individual's illness. Education of both individuals with emphysema and their family members is important. In addition, both the individual with COPD and family members should develop reasonable expectations of what can be accomplished with treatment and be helped to understand the importance of adhering to medical recommendations.

Vocational Issues in COPD

The most limiting factor related to COPD is dyspnea. Chronic hypoxemia may cause neuropsychological deficits that diminish individuals' ability to perform a number of mental functions, which can further contribute to difficulties in the work setting.

In later stages of COPD, dyspnea may become so severe that walking and communicating become difficult. Individuals may need to learn energy conservation techniques so that activities are planned and paced to improve performance within the limitations of their condition. They may need to change their methods of performing more energy-consuming activities so as to improve their energy efficiency. Proper attitude, breathing techniques, body mechanics, pacing, and relaxation can all increase work tolerance.

Although stress is a part of every job, when demands are too challenging muscles tense, heartbeat increases, and breathing becomes more difficult; as a conquence, more oxygen is required. Working in a relaxed atmosphere

can reduce the emotional strain that may contribute to dyspnea.

Sitting to do work (rather than standing) as much as possible requires less energy. Proper height of stools or chairs in relation to tables or desks and arrangement of equipment, tools, or supplies so that they are placed within easy reach can minimize strain on breathing. Unnecessary motion or movements should be eliminated. Arranging work to make tasks simpler can increase functional ability. For example, pushing or sliding objects is easier than lifting them. Placing casters on items can facilitate movement. Pushing a wheelbarrow or cart with a light load of items is less strenuous than carrying items.

Individuals may also need to prioritize tasks. Distributing more difficult tasks throughout the day and breaking up activities into constituent parts, with periods of rest in between, can enable individuals to accomplish tasks more easily. Individuals with COPD may be limited in how much they can use their arms and upper body because of the additional stress placed on accessory muscles of respiration. For this reason, they may need to avoid activities that involve lifting or reaching. Using special long-handled tools to access materials can also help individuals avoid stooping, bending, and reaching. With such accommodations, individuals may be able to continue in sedentary lines of work even in the later stages of the condition.

Transportation to and from work is another issue that should be considered. Although many people with COPD continue to drive, driving in crowded conditions in which fumes and pollutants are present may be a detriment to their health. Planning to drive via alternative routes that are less congested, or driving earlier or later in the day can help to conserve energy and decrease exposure to pollutants.

The work environment should also be relatively free of allergens as well as dust, fumes, or chemicals that are irritating to the airways. Generally, extremes such as heat, cold, wind, distance, and duration should be avoided. The work environment should be well ventilated and climate controlled so that the temperature is not too hot or too cold.

Occupational Lung Conditions (Pneumoconiosis, Asbestosis, Silicosis, Occupational Lung Disease)

Some lung conditions, collectively known as occupational lung disease, are directly related to matter inhaled from the occupational environment. Occupational lung conditions are preventable and are classified by the type of material particles inhaled. The term **pneumoconiosis** refers to a group of lung conditions in which there has been inhalation of dusts. Examples of types of pneumoconiosis are silicosis, coal miner's pneumoconiosis, asbestosis, byssinosis, and berylliosis.

Silicosis is an occupational lung condition caused by exposure to silica dust, usually in the form of quartz. It may occur in people who work in quarries, metal mining, foundries, pottery making, sandblasting, or other occupations in which there is exposure to silica. Development of silicosis generally takes 15 to 20 years of exposure. When particles of silica enter the alveoli, special cells within the lungs engulf the foreign material and then die. In response, a special substance is released in the lung, and **fibrosis** (fibrous tissue within the lung) results. There may be no respiratory consequences initially, although initial damage in the form of nodules may be identified by x-ray.

In the early stages of the condition, individuals may show no symptoms. As damage continues, however, there is a progressive restriction of lung function with associated hypoxemia (decreased oxygen in the blood), shortness of breath on exertion, cough, and expectoration. Symptoms are worse when the person engages in tobacco use. If the condition progresses further, complications such as right ventricular failure may result.

There is no effective treatment for silicosis, other than removing the individual from the environment in which silica is present. The condition can continue to progress without additional exposure, however. Some individuals are able to continue to work in the environment with the use of an air stream helmet that offers dust protection. Silicosis also predisposes individuals to the development of tuberculosis (Sood & Beckett, 2007). Diagnosis is based on an occupational history of silica exposure as well as demonstration of nodule filtration on x-ray. Persons with airway obstruction as a result of silicosis are treated similarly to individuals with COPD.

Coal miner's pneumoconiosis, also known as black lung disease, is an occupational lung condition in which there has been excessive exposure to coal dust. It is characterized by a wide distribution of coal dust throughout the lungs, leading to a mild dilation of the bronchioles and the development of abnormalities surrounding the bronchioles. Although not all cases of coal miner's pneumoconiosis progress, a small percentage of individuals develop progressive scarring of the lung, which in turn interferes with air exchange. There is no specific treatment for coal miner's pneumoconiosis; treatment is similar to that for COPD.

Asbestosis is an occupational lung condition resulting from long-term inhalation of asbestos fibers. Asbestos is now restricted or banned in many Western countries (Sood & Beckett, 2007), but exposure to it may occur through the mining, milling, or manufacturing processes involved in the production of items such as cement, shingles, or siding, or through asbestos products such as insulation. The inhalation of asbestos fibers can cause fibrinous changes within the lung. Individuals usually notice dyspnea (difficulty breathing) on exertion. Treatment of asbestosis is symptomatic. Because asbestosis increases the risk of lung cancer, it is recommended that individuals with this condition abstain from smoking.

Inhalation of dust or fumes that contain beryllium compounds may cause another type of occupational lung condition called *berylliosis*. Exposure to beryllium is common in many chemical plants, in factories (e.g., those that manufacture fluorescent light bulbs), and in the aerospace industry. Symptoms of this condition may not appear for as long as 10 to 20 years after the exposure. Inhaled beryllium creates an inflammatory process in the lungs that alters the lung tissue. Symptoms may include progressive difficulty with breathing on exertion, with progressive loss of respiratory function. The treatment of berylliosis is largely symptomatic.

The occupational lung condition called *byssinosis* occurs primarily in textile workers. It is caused by inhalation of dust from fibers such as cotton, flax, and hemp. The resulting bronchoconstriction causes chest tightness. Unlike persons with other occupational lung conditions, which become worse with increased exposure, individuals with byssinosis experience symptoms after they return to work from days off; as the week goes on, however, symptoms gradually lessen. With prolonged exposure over a number of years, chest tightness may extend for longer periods.

Occupational asthma is a condition characterized by airway restriction and hyperresponsiveness induced by exposure to sensitizing agents in the work environment (Bernstein, Bernstein, Chan-Yeung, & Malo, 1999). The term "occupational asthma" is not used to describe instances in which environmental factors provoke an attack in someone who already has asthma but, rather, is applied to individuals who become asthmatic because of exposure to environmental agents in the workplace.

This process may take from days to years. The list of agents considered potential causes of occupational asthma is growing daily. If a person's asthma is proven to be occupational, in origin, exposure must be reduced or avoided completely, depending on the severity of the condition. The treatment and management of occupational asthma must be tailored to the individual. In some instances, even those who leave the work environment continue to have symptoms for a number of years.

■ OTHER CONDITIONS AFFECTING RESPIRATORY FUNCTION

Restrictive Pulmonary Conditions

Restrictive pulmonary conditions prevent affected individuals from receiving an adequate supply of air; that is, the volume of air is diminished during inspiration. Conditions that cause restrictive pulmonary conditions may include skeletal problems such as **scoliosis** (lateral curvature of the spine) and **kyphosis** (forward curvature of the spine; see Chapter 4) in which chest expansion is decreased. Other conditions that may cause pulmonary restriction include nervous system conditions such as polio, spinal cord injury, and Parkinson's disease (see Chapter 4), in which the muscles that assist in respiration are hindered. Obesity also restricts lung expansion.

Bronchiectasis

Bronchiectasis is a chronic condition characterized by chronic respiratory tract infection and increased inflammatory response of the bronchi and bronchioles; the latter structures become dilated and inflamed, leaving them permanently vulnerable to recurrent infection. Bronchiectasis is caused by repeated respiratory tract infections associated with conditions such as chronic sinusitis, bacterial infections, cystic fibrosis, or rheumatic conditions, or it may result from a genetic or immune deficiency (Barker, 2002). In this condition, **purulent** (pus-containing) material collects in the dilated airways. Individuals with bronchiectasis experience cough and chronic sputum production. They may also complain of fatigue, weight loss, or loss of appetite or experience hemoptysis (expectoration of blood).

Bronchiectasis is usually diagnosed based on the person's symptoms, chest x-ray, and, in some instances, a computed tomography (CT) scan to pinpoint the location and extent of damage. Treatment includes the administration of antibiotics to control the infection, bronchodilators to clear the airways, maintenance of general health through rest and nutrition, and avoidance of further infections. Individuals may also learn special techniques (bronchopulmonary hygiene) or receive treatment (postural drainage and chest physiotherapy) to remove respiratory secretions.

Damaged bronchi do not return to normal. If the inflammatory and destructive process continues, surgical removal of the affected part of the lung may be necessary, although the role of surgery in treatment of bronchiectasis has declined in recent years.

Cystic Fibrosis

Cystic fibrosis is a genetic condition in which there is faulty regulation of salt and water movement across cell membranes (Esmond, Butler, & McCormack, 2006). This multisystem condition affects the respiratory, digestive, skin, and reproductive systems (Dickinson-Herbst, 2001). The defective regulation of salt and water causes abnormally concentrated and thick mucus, which then blocks ducts primarily in the lungs and pancreas (Esmond, 2000). As a result, there is degeneration and scarring of the organs involved.

Individuals with cystic fibrosis once rarely lived beyond childhood. However, with recent improvements in the management of complications, many individuals with this disease now survive well into adulthood (Cystic Fibrosis Foundation, 2003). While survival rates have improved significantly, morbidity continues to be high, especially when individuals experience progressive deterioration of respiratory function (Burker, Sedway, Carone, Trombley, & Yeatts, 2005).

Lung involvement is one of the most frequent causes of functional limitations in cystic fibrosis and, when complications occur, can result in death. Respiratory involvement occurs because of formation of thick mucus in the small bronchi, which can lead to severe bronchitis and emphysema. **Atelectasis** (collapse of the lung) is not uncommon. Individuals may have intermittent episodes of acute respiratory infections, which persist for long periods. Coughing may be pronounced and accompanied by thick and purulent sputum. As the condition progresses, there is usually a gradual decline in pulmonary function.

Although the lungs are involved, other organs, such as the pancreas, are also affected. In particular, the pancreas may become inflamed so that individuals develop **pancreatitis.** Because ducts of the pancreas are plugged by the thick mucus production, enzymes produced by the pancreas that aid in digestion are unable to function in this capacity, leading to poor digestion of protein and fat. As a result, individuals experience chronic malnutrition and delayed growth.

Individuals with cystic fibrosis also have poorly functioning sweat glands, so that excessive loss of salt occurs. This phenomenon may result in **hyponatremia** (decreased concentration of salt in the blood).

Fertility problems are also common. Males with cystic fibrosis have high rates of infertility (Knowles & Durie, 2002), with an almost 99% rate of sterility. Women have lower rates of infertility but higher rates of complications, such as progression of the condition with pregnancy (Hamlett, Murphy, Hayes & Doershuk, 1996).

Diagnosis of Cystic Fibrosis

Because of the increased concentrations of sodium and chloride in the sweat of individuals with cystic fibrosis, a *sweat electrolyte* test is an important diagnostic tool in identifying individuals with this condition. This noninvasive test involves collecting and analyzing sweat from a small area of the individual's arm. When the test is positive, additional genetic testing may be instituted.

Management of Cystic Fibrosis

Individuals with cystic fibrosis have grown up learning to manage their condition through chest physiotherapy, nebulizer therapy, and nutritional supplementation (Esmond, Butler, & McCormack, 2006). Because mucus production is increased, individuals with cystic fibrosis may have difficulty clearing secretions. The clearance of secretions is important so that organisms do not have an environment in which they can grow and thrive. Pulmonary symptoms require the administration of antibiotics to prevent or treat infection.

To help clear secretions, individuals learn specific procedures to assist coughing, and they are encouraged to increase their fluid intake to liquefy the secretions. *Positive expiratory pressure (PEP) therapy* is a method of airway clearance that may be used (Newbold, Tullis, Corey, Ross, & Brooks, 2005). In this technique, the individual places the PEP mask over the mouth and nose and breathes out through resistance created by the system. The resistance helps to stabilize the airway and prevent it from closing. Other measures to clear resistance include breathing warm, humidified air or inhaling steam several times a day. Individuals may also be instructed in various forms of postural drainage to be used at home to drain mucus. For example, they may be instructed to lie over the side of the bed with their head lower than the rest of the body several times a day to facilitate drainage of mucus. In some instances, individuals may be referred for chest physiotherapy in which procedures such as percussion are used. Percussion is a form of massage in which the chest is repeatedly tapped or vibrated to loosen mucus and allow it to drain. This procedure may be done by a physical therapist, or it may be done at home, either with an electric percussor or manually by a family member. Supplemental oxygen may also be used on an as-needed basis to maintain lifestyle and work activities.

Diet plays a direct role in treatment of pancreatitis. If pancreatic ducts become blocked, supplemental enzymes may be taken at mealtimes to aid in digestion and prevent malnutrition. Despite use of supplemental enzymes, individuals with cystic fibrosis often experience delayed growth and malnutrition, and they are typically underweight. Owing to the increased salt loss characteristic of cystic fibrosis, dietary prescription is necessary to assure adequate salt intake. Adequate hydration is necessary to liquefy secretions, and other dietary prescriptions may be needed to prevent nutritional deficiencies.

When progression of the lung changes associated with cystic fibrosis reaches a magnitude in which manifestations result in severe functional limitations, double-lung transplantation may be performed to halt progression of the condition and restore function (Dickinson-Herbst, 2001; Lanunza, Lefaiver, & Farcas, 2000).

Psychosocial Issues in Cystic Fibrosis

Because cystic fibrosis is a genetic condition, with symptoms usually present in childhood, issues of growing up with a chronic and potentially fatal condition can affect individuals' successful passage through normal growth and development. Attitudes of family, teachers, and peers are instrumental in helping children develop their self-concept, their view of their condition, and its impact on future function.

Psychological impact of cystic fibrosis in adulthood varies (Burker, Carels, Thompson, Rodgers, & Egan, 2000; Crews, Jefferson, Broshek, Barth, & Robbins, 2000). Management of cystic fibrosis requires time, energy, and resources to perform many of the home therapy treatments such as chest physical therapy, dietary adjustment, monitoring for respiratory infection, enzyme administration to aid in digestion, and routine use of other mediations such as bronchodilators and antibiotics. Special skills are required for monitoring symptoms, interpreting changes, and making decisions about need for alteration of treatment. Children who have been encouraged to assume more responsibility for their self-care will be more likely to grow into gradual independence (Esmond, 2000).

During adolescence, behavioral responses to a chronic condition may be made more difficult by the "need to fit in" or by the attitudes of rebellion and defiance characteristic of that age. These factors may potentially result in health-compromising behaviors. Without appropriate support, individuals may be less able to adapt and cope with chronic illness, resulting in isolation and altered relationships.

Individuals with any chronic condition may find adherence to treatment difficult because of its long-term and complex nature. Adhering to treatment is a daily reminder of the condition. Some individuals may feel that, given the likelihood of increasing deterioration and potential mortality, adherence is not worthwhile.

Fertility problems in individuals with cystic fibrosis may bring an emotional toll. In addition to coping with the challenges of daily management of the condition, these persons must incorporate issues of infertility into their relationships with significant others.

Vocational Issues in Cystic Fibrosis

Cystic fibrosis is an incurable chronic condition, which may lead to increasing functional consequences over time. The rate of progression of the condition varies significantly from individual to individual. Owing to the incurable and progressive nature of cystic fibrosis, employment of adults with the condition has not been considered feasible until recently (Mungle, Burker, & Yankaskas, 2002).

Individuals with cystic fibrosis have heightened susceptibility to respiratory infections; consequently, they should avoid environments in which exposure to respiratory infections is likely. Flu and pneumonia vaccinations are important to prevent respiratory complications from occurring. Individuals should also avoid exposure to dust or toxic fumes. They may demonstrate intolerance if placed in an environment in which they are exposed to sudden temperature changes or air pollutants. If supplemental oxygen is needed for maintaining work activities, oxygen precautions (as discussed previously in this chapter) should be instituted.

Because excessive loss of salt through sweat occurs in cystic fibrosis, and because adequate hydration is necessary to avoid excessive viscosity of mucus that can clog airways, individuals should avoid hot, humid environmental conditions. Although many individuals with cystic fibrosis are able to be employed full-time, the time and energy required to carry out daily treatment routines needed for management of cystic fibrosis as well as the potential for disruptions because of periodic hospitalizations must be incorporated into individual's vocational plans.

Apnea

The term **apnea** refers to cessation of breathing. Apnea is associated with a variety of conditions. One of the more common conditions associated with apnea is sleep apnea, in which repeated episodes of the cessation of breathing occur during sleep. This condition is more common in middle age. Individuals with sleep apnea may be unaware that they stop breathing during sleep, but may experience excessive daytime drowsiness, difficulty with attention or concentration, and irritability because of the disruption of their sleep. Individuals with sleep apnea may be unaware of periods of apnea during sleep, but sleep partners may complain of being awakened by the individual's loud snoring or sudden body movements during an attack of apnea.

Several types of sleep apnea are distinguished. The least common type is *central sleep apnea*, which is caused by a disruption of the signals from the central nervous system that stimulate respiration. This condition may be due to a variety of conditions affecting the central nervous system (see Chapter 3). *Peripheral sleep apnea*, also called obstructive sleep apnea, is the most common type; it is caused by an upper airway obstruction. The obstruction can be caused by narrowing of the airways due to obesity, *hypertrophy* (enlargement) of the tonsils, or structural abnormalities that predispose the airway to narrowing or closure during sleep (Flemons, 2002). Mixed-type sleep apnea is a combination of central and peripheral sleep apnea. Individuals with sleep apnea, regardless of the type, experience **hypoxia** (decrease of oxygen), resulting in **hypoxemia** (decreased oxygen in the blood) and **hypercapnia** (buildup of carbon dioxide in the blood).

The consequences of sleep apnea go beyond sleep disruption and daytime drowsiness. Individuals with sleep apnea have an increased risk of **hypertension** (high blood pressure), heart failure, **myocardial infarction** (heart attack), and stroke. Because of sleep deprivation, people with sleep apnea are also at increased risk of accidents.

The evaluation of sleep apnea often takes place in a sleep laboratory, where breathing during sleep is monitored and recorded. Portable monitoring systems can also be used outside the hospital, but readings may not be as accurate.

Treatment of Sleep Apnea

Sleep apnea may be treated behaviorally, medically, or surgically. The type of treatment chosen depends on the individual's symptoms and the function of his or her cardiopulmonary system. Treatment goals are directed toward establishing normal breathing and oxygenation of the blood and toward eliminating disruption of sleep. Because alcohol consumption reduces muscle tone of the upper airway and increases the frequency of abnormal breathing during sleep, treatment recommendations often include limiting alcohol use. Individuals who are obese are encouraged to lose weight to reduce obstruction. Some individuals have more difficulty with sleep apnea when lying on their back; in these instances, they are trained to sleep on their side.

The treatment of choice for some individuals with sleep apnea is *continuous positive airway pressure (C-pap)* delivered through a mask. Machines used for this purpose weigh only about 5 pounds. These devices are used at night and fit on a bedside table. Individuals may use a mask that covers only the nose, nasal prongs, or a mask that covers both the nose and the mouth. The amount of continuous positive pressure applied is determined through evaluation in a sleep laboratory. Rather than using the positive airway pressure machine, some individuals choose oral appliances, which are worn during sleep to help keep the airway open.

Surgical treatment can range from **tracheostomy** (in which a surgical opening is made through the neck into the trachea to enable the individual to breathe) to surgical correction of structural abnormalities of the palate or the facial structure, that contribute to obstruction. Insufficient awareness of sleep apnea among physicians and the public in general may result in sleep apnea going undiagnosed and consequently untreated.

Vocational Issues in Sleep Apnea

Sleep apnea can cause significant vocational impairment. Individuals with sleep apnea, in addition to daytime sleepiness, may experience irritability, impatience, or even depressive manifestations, which can affect their relationships with others at work. Individuals with sleep apnea may also experience cognitive consequences including difficulty with attention and concentration, visual/motor abilities, and difficulties with memory. Tasks involving planning, verbal fluency, or general intellectual performance may be impaired. As mentioned earlier, because of sleep deprivation, individuals with sleep apnea may be more accident prone.

If sleep apnea is diagnosed and treated, symptoms can be reversed. Unfortunately, in many cases the condition is not diagnosed and a decrease in job performance is attributed to other causes.

Chest Injuries

Fractured ribs are a common chest injury. Although painful, they are usually treated relatively easily by wrapping a strap or binder around the chest for support. In some instances, however, a fractured rib punctures other organs, such as the lungs or heart, and the consequences are more serious.

An open wound to the chest, such as a puncture wound, may allow air to enter the thoracic cavity. This condition, called **pneumothorax**, may cause the lung on the affected side to collapse. Pneumothorax unrelated to trauma can occur secondary to a number of pulmonary conditions, such as COPD, asthma, or cystic fibrosis. Such a *spontaneous* pneumothorax is caused by a tear or rupture of air sacs in the lung, causing air to escape into the thoracic cavity. Pneumothorax is generally treated by insertion of a tube through the chest wall to facilitate expansion of the lung. Individuals who have experienced pneumothorax should avoid smoking, high diving, or flying in unpressurized aircraft all of which can cause recurrence of the condition.

Escape of blood into the thoracic cavity because of an injury to the chest that damages vessels in the thoracic cavity is called **hemothorax**. It may also cause collapse of a lung. In the case of pneumothorax or hemothorax, the lung is compressed, hampering breathing. A large pneumothorax or hemothorax requires emergency treatment to remove air or blood in the chest and repair the injury. The removal of fluid from the thoracic cavity is called **thoracentesis.** In this procedure, a needle is inserted into the thoracic cavity and fluid is then aspirated through the needle.

■ DIAGNOSTIC PROCEDURES FOR RESPIRATORY CONDITIONS

Chest Roentgenography (X-Ray)

Roentgenography (x-ray) of the chest is a radiographic procedure that allows bony structures (e.g., the ribs), the lungs, and other organs in the thoracic cavity to be viewed as a still image on x-ray film. It may be useful in diagnosing tuberculosis, in noting changes in the lungs caused by COPD, and identifying structural abnormalities or tumors.

Bronchoscopy

Visual examination of the bronchial tubes through a long hollow tube inserted through the mouth and into the bronchus is called **bronchoscopy.** With the bronchoscope, the physician can view the walls of the bronchus and note any abnormalities. A *pulmonologist* (a physician who specializes in evaluation and treatment of conditions of the lung) usually performs the procedure, although other physicians with special training in the procedure may also do so. Individuals undergoing bronchoscopy are usually given a sedative, but they remain awake during the procedure.

Laryngoscopy

Laryngoscopy is a visual examination carried out through a hollow tube called a laryngoscope. The procedure enables the physician to inspect the structures of the larynx and to assess the function of the vocal cords. The procedure is usually performed under a local anesthetic, although the individual may be sedated for the procedure.

Pulmonary Angiography

In a procedure called pulmonary angiography, a catheter is inserted into a vessel and a *contrast agent* (a special dye that enhances visualization of a structure) is injected into the catheter to enable the physician to visualize the pulmonary vessels. X-ray films are then taken and the circulation of the lungs studied. Pulmonary angiography may be used to assess the extent to which emphysema has destroyed lung tissue. Alternatively, it may be used prior to surgery for lung cancer to assess the potential benefits of surgery.

Pulmonary Function Tests

Pulmonary function tests are used to detect abnormalities in respiratory function and to determine the degree of impairment of respiratory function. Physicians use these tests to assess the volume of air that an individual can take in and expel from the lungs, as well as the individual's ability to move air into and out of the lungs. Pulmonary function tests may be used to determine the cause of dyspenea, the extent to which the lung is affected, or the effectiveness of treatment for lung conditions. Generally done in a pulmonary laboratory, the tests involve breathing into a special machine called a spirometer, which measures several

types of pulmonary function. The results are then printed out in a graphic representation called a *spirogram*. Types of pulmonary function that are measured in terms of lung capacity are listed below and illustrated in Figure 14-2:

- *Vital capacity*: the maximum volume of air that can be inspired and expired.
- *Forced expiratory volume (FEV)*: the volume of air that the individual can forcibly exhale at 1-, 2-, and 3-second intervals. Readings of the FEV are reported as FEV_1, FEV_2, and FEV_3.
- *Residual lung volume*: the amount of air left in the lungs after maximum expiration.
- *Maximum voluntary ventilation (MVV)*: the maximum volume that an individual can breathe in 12 seconds, breathing in and out as rapidly and forcefully as possible.
- *Tidal volume*: the amount of air breathed in and out at rest.
- *Inspiratory capacity*: the volume of air taken in by maximal inspiration after normal expiration.
- *Functional residual capacity*: the volume of air remaining in the lungs after normal expiration.

Ventilation/Perfusion Scan (Lung Scan)

Ventilation is the process by which gases are transported between the atmosphere and the alveoli. **Perfusion** is the process by which blood or other fluid passes to a body part through a vascular bed. The *ventilation/ perfusion scan* is a radiographic procedure that makes it possible to measure the ventilation and/or perfusion of the lung. The test may be performed to determine whether a blood clot has traveled to the lung and lodged there or to diagnose other conditions, such as emphysema. For the *ventilation scan*, the individual inhales radioactive gas; the image taken shows where ventilation is occurring in the lung. For a *perfusion scan*, a radioactive dye is injected

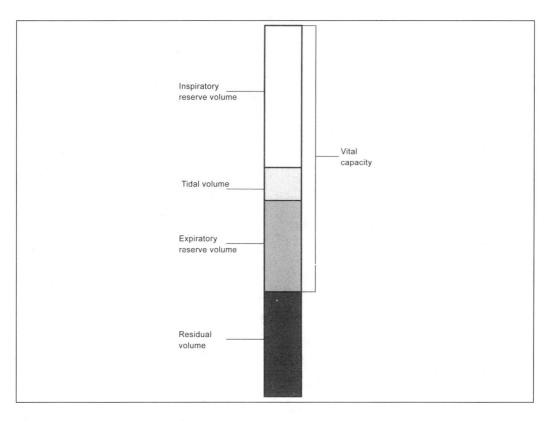

Figure 14-2   Pulmonary volumes

intravenously, enabling the radiologist to visualize blood flow to the lung.

■ GENERAL TREATMENT FOR RESPIRATORY CONDITIONS

Because many conditions of the respiratory system are irreversible, treatment may be directed toward the control of symptoms and the prevention of complications or further deterioration. Pollutants and other irritants—especially cigarette smoke—should be avoided, as they can aggravate respiratory conditions. In areas where pollution is severe or if allergies complicate the condition, special air filters or purifiers may be needed. Even when pulmonary function is compromised, physicians often advise individuals with pulmonary conditions to engage in a daily walking and exercise program to keep in shape and build strength and endurance.

A number of medications may be used for respiratory conditions, depending on the nature of the respiratory dysfunction.

- *Bronchodilators* help to open the airway so that more air can move in and out. Bronchodilators come in several forms, including pills, liquids, and sprays.
- *Antibiotics* may be taken for infections. They may be taken orally (by mouth) or injected.
- *Diuretics*, sometimes called *water pills*, rid the body of extra fluid, such as fluid buildup because of right ventricular failure.
- *Expectorants* are oral medications that make mucus thinner and easier to clear.

- *Steroid*s are hormonal preparations that help reduce swelling in the airway, consequently easing breathing. Steroids are usually taken orally, but may also be injected. Because of their serious side effects, they are usually prescribed only for temporary relief of severe symptoms rather than for long-term use.

A variety of breathing aids may be used in the treatment of respiratory conditions. Many devices are designed to deliver medicines, oxygen, or moist air deep into the lungs and to help individuals clear their lungs of mucus. An *intermittent positive-pressure breathing (IPPB) machine* is a device used to deliver air under pressure to the lungs. It may have a nebulizer attached so that it delivers medication and humidity to the lungs as well. Individuals with cancer or severe chest injuries may require surgery. At times, the removal of the lung (**pneumonectomy**) or a portion of the lung is indicated. Most people are able to function normally even with a portion of the lung removed.

■ PSYCHOSOCIAL ISSUES IN RESPIRATORY CONDITIONS

Psychological Issues

Difficulty breathing can be a frightening and distressing experience. Associated fear and anxiety may lead to inactivity, which in turn may result in additional physical problems. Prolonged breathing difficulty often causes feelings of helplessness and despair. For those individuals who have been active and self-sufficient, the inability to engage in even simple activities without breathing difficulty can be devastating. Depression is common in such cases. Individuals may focus on the activities in which they can no longer participate, at least not as vigorously, rather than attempting to attain their highest level of functional capacity.

When a respiratory condition reduces the oxygen concentration in the blood and the amount of oxygen available to the brain is insufficient, associated cognitive changes may result. Clouding of consciousness or changes in cognitive function can be frightening both for individuals who experience these changes, and for the family members who observe them. Close monitoring of oxygen and carbon dioxide concentrations is important in the care of individuals with respiratory conditions so that low oxygen or high carbon dioxide concentrations can be identified and appropriate measures instituted to reestablish normal concentrations.

Emotional factors can compound the effects of physical symptoms of respiratory conditions. Anxiety or emotional upset may increase the difficulty in breathing, causing more anxiety and leading to yet more difficulty in breathing. When it is possible to identify situations that increase anxiety or stress, it is important to institute interventions to decrease anxiety so that the difficulty in breathing does not escalate.

Responses of family and friends to respiratory conditions may affect an individual's ability to cope with his or her condition. Family members may unintentionally place individuals in an invalid role, reducing expectations of them in the family structure or removing responsibility from them, even though individuals may be capable of engaging in a number of activities. Individuals may respond by using breathing difficulty to escape from life's demands, to receive emotional rewards, or to manipulate or control the behavior of others. In other instances, family members may overestimate individuals' abilities, not fully understanding the seriousness of the condition and its implications for function. Such reactions may push individuals to go beyond their functional capacity or to ignore physicians' specific recommendations for controlling the condition.

The circumstances that surround the development of a respiratory condition may elicit guilt on the part of the individual with the condition or anger on the part of family members. Because smoking is linked to a variety of respiratory conditions, individuals who have smoked heavily may feel guilty for having contributed to the condition. Family members may express anger, blaming the individual for smoking and possibly contributing to the development of the condition. When respiratory conditions are related to occupational factors, individuals and the family members may be angry because of individual's exposure to unrecognized hazards or, if hazards were identified, because of the employer's failure to take proper precautions to protect employees from them.

Unless the individuals have severe respiratory distress or use some type of breathing aid, respiratory conditions are not usually recognizable as easily as are conditions associated with visual cues, such as crutches or a wheelchair. Consequently, the expectations of employers, co-workers, or casual acquaintances regarding individuals' ability to perform various activities may not be consistent with the individuals' functional capacity. Similarly, the lack of visual cues may enable individuals to deny their condition and avoid treatment, which can prove hazardous not only for the individual but also, in the case of infectious conditions (e.g., tuberculosis), for others with whom the individual comes in contact.

Activities and Participation

As with other chronic conditions, the lifestyle changes required by respiratory conditions depend on the seriousness and on the individual's previous state of health and functional capacity. In general, it is important for individuals with respiratory conditions to maintain good nutritional status and normal weight. Because of the increased burden that obesity or overeating can place on breathing capacity, individuals with respiratory conditions should be urged to avoid both.

Cessation of smoking is a necessary component of treatment, regardless of the type of respiratory condition. Many individuals consider this requirement to be the most difficult part of their treatment. Even when they are aware that smoking exacerbates their respiratory condition, they may find it difficult to alter their behavior. Enrollment in specially designed smoking cessation programs may be necessary to help individuals stop smoking. Some individuals resist participation even in these interventions, however.

Although exertion can cause difficulty breathing, individuals with respiratory conditions are generally able to maintain some level of activity unless they have associated cardiac complications. Exercise programs can both improve self-esteem and reduce symptoms to some extent. If individuals experience dyspenea partly due to ineffective breathing patterns and partly from lack of conditioning, it is crucial that they work to increase exercise tolerance through daily breathing or conditioning exercises, in addition to participating in other exercise routines.

Unless the cause of dyspenea can be corrected, individuals with respiratory conditions need to become accustomed to feeling short of breath and to adapt to the sensation so that they can maintain their maximum level of activity without undue fear or anxiety. Finally, they may need extra time to accomplish tasks so that they can take rest periods. They may need to divide some activities into smaller tasks rather than trying to accomplish the entire task at one time.

Although an environment near sea level with a mild climate and minimal air pollution is ideal for individuals with chronic respiratory conditions; it is not always possible to live in this type of setting. Individuals living in less moderate climates should avoid extremes in temperatures. Home and work temperatures should be kept cool. Radiant or baseboard heaters may be better than forced-air heating systems, as the latter have filters that need to be cleaned or changed regularly. If a humidifier is used, it should be cleaned regularly to forestall mold growth. Fireplaces and wood burning or coal-burning stoves should be avoided, as they are potential sources of air pollution in the home.

Maintaining adequate hydration is important in respiratory conditions characterized by an overproduction of mucus. The environment should be well humidified, and a nebulizer or aerosol may be used periodically throughout the day to deliver humidity directly to the lungs. High levels of humidity may make breathing more difficult, however. For this reason, individuals living in hot, humid environments should have air conditioning to maintain the temperature and the humidity at acceptable levels. Filters on air conditioners should be changed on a regular basis.

If factors in the home contribute to the respiratory condition, environmental modifications—such as removing the cause of the allergic reaction—may be required. This change may be especially distressing if the offending factor is a pet. The environment should also be kept dust free. It may be necessary to install special filters to cut down on molds and household dust.

Individuals with respiratory conditions may become very anxious about participating in any type of physical activity that increases respiratory difficulty. Because both the rate and the depth of respiration are increased during sexual excitement, the fear of suffocation may cause some individuals to be reluctant or restrained when engaging in sexual activity. Although dyspnea may be uncomfortable, those who have respiratory conditions with no complications can generally maintain sexual activity. They can often increase their tolerance for sexual activity through conditioning, or their partners may assume a more active role.

Individuals with respiratory conditions may avoid social contacts and social situations that they once enjoyed if dyspnea, especially on exertion, is pronounced. The resulting social isolation can contribute to depression and lowered self-esteem. As much as possible, individuals should continue to participate in social activates, albeit modifying the circumstances as necessary. For example, use of a golf cart may reduce the exertion required in golf to the extent that those with respiratory conditions can still enjoy the game as a form of recreation and time to be spent with friends. Outdoor activities should be avoided, when temperatures are very hot or very cold, or when pollution levels are especially high.

Even though crowded, polluted environments aggravate respiratory conditions; individuals with respiratory conditions need not refrain from participating in activities in urban areas. It may be necessary to plan travel time to and from such events so that traveling does not take place during the time of heaviest traffic. Arriving early at events can help cut down on crowding and the potentially anxiety-provoking rush.

Establishments that do not prohibit smoking altogether usually provide nonsmoking areas. Individuals should check on smoking rules ahead of time and request seating in nosmoking sections.

Some respiratory conditions cause pronounced coughing, which may be accompanied by excessive, foul-smelling mucus production. Both the cough and excessive mucus can be embarrassing and interfere with communication and social interactions. Individuals with respiratory conditions should be open and honest about their condition with others, not making excuses or excessive apologies. Frequent mouth care can help to alleviate foul-smelling breath.

Because of the potential seriousness of respiratory infections in individuals with lung conditions, they should avoid contact with persons who have upper respiratory infections or flu to the greatest extent feasible. Although not always possible without severely limiting social contacts, exposure to large groups of people in confined environments at the height of the flu season, for example, should be discouraged.

■ VOCATIONAL ISSUES IN RESPIRATORY CONDITIONS

The extent to which individuals with respiratory conditions can continue regular employment depends on the type of work, the work environment, and the severity of the respiratory condition. Individuals with severe respiratory incapacity may continue to function in the workplace if their job requires little physical exertion. Conversely, individuals with a small degree of respiratory incapacity may be unable to maintain employment in an environment that requires strenuous activity. Work that requires extensive use of the body's upper extremities requires higher levels of ventilation than does work that mostly involves use of the lower extremities.

If factors in the work environment have contributed to or aggravated the respiratory condition, a change may be needed. A mounting body of evidence indicates that exposure to high levels of air pollution not only is associated with respiratory conditions, but also has potential cardiovascular consequences (Mittleman, 2007). In some instances, individuals may transfer to another location in the facility where the offending factors are not present. Compensation and litigation may also be an issue for individuals who experience respiratory conditions after exposure to occupational contaminants (Samet, Geyh, & Utell, 2007).

The extent of activity that individuals with respiratory conditions can tolerate should be evaluated. If, for example, they can walk the length of the hall but cannot walk up one flight of stairs without severe dyspnea, using an elevator may be indicated or the individual's workstation may need to be moved to a different floor. The degree to which upper body movements are used in work and the effects of these movements on dyspnea should be considered. If the work demands lifting and carrying that increase dyspnea, alternative strategies may be devised so that the work can be performed with less exertion. Individuals, their employers, and their co-workers should be helped to understand that moderate dyspnea, although uncomfortable, is not in itself life-threatening. Because cough and sputum production can be cosmetically displeasing, they may interfere with individuals' effectiveness in jobs that require close personal contact or continued conversation. The degree to which the workplace demands this type of interaction and the impact of these symptoms on job effectiveness should be assessed.

If any type of breathing device or aid is used, the extent to which the aid will be a hazard in the work environment must be considered. The tubing in some portable devices may become caught in machinery, for example, or cause falls. Oxygen, because of the danger of fire or explosion, should not be used in close proximity to an open flame.

In addition to stress in the work setting that could increase anxiety and subsequently exacerbate breathing difficulty, stressors such as those involved in transportation to and from work should be noted. If commuting necessitates travel in polluted, congested areas, it may be possible to modify the work schedule to allow travel at less busy times. Flexibility of the work schedule may also be important if specific treatments or rest periods are required during the day.

The legal implications of many lung conditions, especially if they appear to be occupationally related, may be barriers to continued employment (Samet, Geyh, & Utell, 2007). For individuals who are eligible for worker's compensation or other benefits, financial considerations may influence their motivation and cooperation with treatment. In other instances, the employer's fear of liability may limit job opportunities for individuals with respiratory conditions. Medical rehabilitation programs for individuals with respiratory conditions can be important to helping them increase their activity level to their optimal capacity.

CASE STUDIES

Case 1

Mr. L., a 55-year-old bartender in a large metropolitan area, has been a heavy smoker for 40 years. He was diagnosed as having COPD 7 years ago. Mr. L. lives in the city and takes the city bus to work, although he still has to walk about three blocks to the bar where he works. He has found it increasingly difficult to walk the three blocks without stopping to rest at frequent intervals. At work, his manager has also expressed concern about the effect Mr. L.'s continuous coughing has on customers.

1. Is it feasible for Mr. L. to continue working as a bartender?
2. Which factors would you consider when discussing with Mr. L. whether he can remain in his current line of employment?
3. What is the general prognosis for Mr. L.'s condition?
4. Which lifestyle factors need to be considered in working with Mr. L. on his rehabilitation plan?

Case 2

Ms. Q., a 32-year-old female, was diagnosed with HIV infection 5 years ago. She has continued to work as a receptionist at an insurance agency. Ms. Q. recently had a tuberculin skin test, which was interpreted as positive. She has shared this information with the office manager out of concern for its implications for her employment as well as concern for her co-workers and customers of the agency.

1. What vocational implications does a positive tuberculin skin test have for Ms Q.?
2. What, if any, additional information is needed prior to making decisions regarding Ms. Q.'s employment?
3. What are the vocational implications of a positive TB test alone for for Ms. Q.?

■ REFERENCES

American Thoracic Society. (1995). Standards for the diagnosis and care of patients with chronic obstructive pulmonary disease. *American Journal of Respiratory Critical Care Medicine*, 152(5 suppl), S77–S120.

Barker, A. F. (2002). Bronchiectasis. *New England Journal of Medicine*, 346(18), 1383–1393.

Barnes, P. J. (2000). Chronic obstructive pulmonary disease. New England Journal of Medicine, 343(5), 269–280.

Barnes, P. J. (2004), Small airways in COPD. *New England Journal of Medicine*, 350(26), 2635–2640.

Barnett, M. (2006). COPD: The role of the nurse. *Journal of Community Nursing*, 20(2), 18–22.

Bernstein, I. L., Bernstein, D. I., Chan-Yeung, M., & Malo, J. L. (1999). Definition and classification of asthma. In: Asthma in the workplace I. L. Bernstein, M. Chan-Yeung, J. L. Malo, & D. I. Bernstein, (Eds.), (pp. 1–3). New York, Marcel Dekker.

Burker, E. J., Carels, R. A., Thompson, L. F., Rodgers, L., & Egan, T. (2000). Quality of life in patients awaiting lung transplant: Cystic fibrosis versus other end-stage lung diseases. *Pediatric Pulmonology*, 30, 453–460.

Burker, E. J., Sedway, J., Carone, S., Trombley, C., & Yeatts, B. P. (2005). Vocational attainment of adults with CF: Success in the face of adversity. *Journal of Rehabilitation, 71*(2), 2, 22–27.

Campion, E. W. (1999). Liberty and the control of tuberculosis. *New England Journal of Medicine, 340*(5), 385–386.

Cox, G., Thomson, N. C., Rubin, A. S., et al. (2007). Asthma control during the year after bronchial thermoplasty. *New England Journal of Medicine, 356*(13), 1327–1337.

Crews, W., Jefferson, A., Broshek, D., Barth, J., & Robbins, M. (2000). Neuropsychological sequelae in a series of patients with end-stage cystic fibrosis: Lung transplant evaluation. *Archives of Clinical Neuropsychology, 15,* 59–70.

Cystic Fibrosis Foundation. (2003). Cystic Fibrosis Foundation, patient registery, 2002 annual data report. Bethesda, MD: Author

Dewar, M., & Curry, R. W. (2006). Chronic obstructive pulmonary disease: Diagnostic considerations. *American Family Physician, 73*(4), 669–676.

Dickinson-Herbst, D. (2001). Cystic fibrosis and lung transplantation: Ethical concerns. *Pediatric Nursing, 27*(1), 87–94.

Doherty, D. E. (2004). The pathophysiology of airway dysfunction. *American Journal of Medicine, 117* (Suppl 12A) 11S–23S.

Eisner, M. D., Yelin, E. H., Katz, P. P., Lactao, G., Iribarren, C., & Blanc, P. D. (2006). Risk factors for work disability in severe adult asthma. *American Journal of Medicine, 119*(10), 884–891.

Esmond, G. (2000). Cystic fibrosis: Adolescent care. *Nursing Standard: Harrow-on-the-Hill, 14*(52), 47–59.

Esmond, G., Butler, M., & McCormack, A. M. (2006). Comparison of hospital and home intravenous antibiotic therapy in adults with cystic fibrosis. *Journal of Clinical Nursing, 15,* 52–60.

Flemons, W. W. (2002). Obstructive sleep apnea. *New England Journal of Medicine, 347*(7), 498–504.

Garcia, J. A. & Jenkinson, S.G. (2007). Management of chronic obstructive pulmonary disease. In R. E. Rakel & E. T. Bope (Eds.), *Conn's current therapy* (pp. 264–274). Philadelphia: W. B. Saunders.

Geddes, D., Davies, M., Koyama, H. et al. (2000). Effect of lung-volume-reduction surgery in patients with severe emphysema. *New England Journal of Medicine, 343*(4), 239–245.

Gilmour, M. I., Jaakola, M. S., London, S. J., Nei, A. E., & Rogers, C. A. (2006). How exposure to environmental tobacco smoke, outdoor air pollutants, and increased pollen burdens influence the incidence of asthma. *Enviromental Health Perspectives, 114,* 627–633.

Global Initiative for Chronic Obstructive Lung Disease. (2005). Global strategy for the diagnosis, management, and prevention of chronic obstructive pulmonary disease [executive summary]. Retrieved January 17, 2006, from http://www.goldcopd.com/Guidelineitem.asp?I1=2&I2=1&intid=996

Goldberg, R. T., Hillberg, R., Reinecker, L., & Goldstein, R. (2004). Evaluation of patients with severe pulmonary disease before and after pulmonary rehabilitation. *Disability and Rehabilitation, 26*(11), 641–648.

Gunes, A., Aboyoun, C. L., Morton, M., Plit, M., Malouf, M. A., & Glanville, A. R. (2006). Lung transplantation for chronic obstructive pulmonary disease at St. Vincent's Hospital. *Internal Medicine Journal, 36,* 5–11.

Hamlett, K. W., Murphy, M., Hayes, R., & Doershuk, C. F. (1996). Health independence and developmental tasks of adulthood in cystic fibrosis. *Rehabilitation Psychology, 41*(2), 149–160.

Harrison, B. D. W (2005). Difficult asthma in adults: Recognition and approaches to management. *Internal Medicine Journal, 35,* 543–547.

Hogg, J. C., Chu, F., Utokaparch, S., et al. (2004). The nature of small-airway obstruction in chronic obstructive pulmonary disease. *New England Journal of Medicine, 350*(26), 2645–2653.

Holgate, S. T., & Polosa, R. (2006). The mechanisms, diagnosis, and management of severe asthma in adults. *Lancet, 368,* 780–793.

Horsburgh, C. R. (2004). Priorities for the treatment of latent tuberculosis infection in the United States. *New England Journal of Medicine, 350*(20), 2060–2067.

Hurd, S., & Pauwels, R. (2002). Global Initiative for Chronic Obstructive Lung Diseases (GOLD). *Pulmonary Pharmacoly and Therapeutics, 15*(4), 353–355.

Irwin, R. S., & Madison, J. M. (2003). Systemic corticosteroids for acute exacerbations of chronic obstructive pulmonary disease. *New England Journal of Medicine, 348*(26), 2679–2680.

Kerstjens, H. A. M. (1999). Stable chronic obstructive pulmonary disease. *British Medical Journal, 319,* 495–500.

Knowles, M. R. & Durie, P. R. (2002). What is cystic fibrosis? *New England Journal of Medicine, 347*(6), 439–442.

Lahart, C. J. (2007). Tuberculosis and other myobacterial diseases. In R.E. Rakel & E. T. Bope (Eds.), *Conn's current therapy.* (pp. 330–336). Philadelphia. Saunders.

Lanunza, D. M., Lefaiver, C. A., & Farcas, G. A. (2000). Research on the quality of life of lung transplant candidates and recipients: An integrative review. *Heart & Lung, 27*(3), 180–195.

Li, J. T. (2001). Asthma and allergy. *Postgraduate Medicine, 109*(5), 43.

Luce, J. M., & Luce, J. A. (2001). Management of dyspnea in patients with far-advanced lung disease: "Once I lose it, it's kind of hard to catch it." *Journal of the American Medical Association, 285*(10), 1331–1337.

Mannino, D. M., Gagnon, R. C., Peatty, T. L., & Lydick, E. (2000). Obstructive lung disease and low lung function in adults in the United States; Data from the National Health and Nutrition Examination Survey, 1988-1994. *Archives of Internal Medicine 160*(11), 1683–1689.

Marik, P. E., Varon J., & Fromm, R. (2002). The management of acute severe asthma. *Journal of Emergency Medicine, 23*(3), 257–268.

Mittleman, M.A. (2007) Air pollution, exercise, and cardiovascular risk. *New England Journal of Medicine, 357*(11), 1147–1149.

Moorman, J. E., Rudd, R. A., Johnson, C. A., King, M., Minor, P., Bailey, C. et al. (2007). National Surveillance For Asthma—United States, 1980–2004. *MMWR Surveillance Summaries, 56(5508);* 1–14; 18-54.

Mungle, J., Burker, E. J., & Yankaskas, J. R., (2002). Vocational rehabilitation counseling for adolescents and adults with cystic fibrosis. *Journal of Applied Rehabilitation Counseling, 33*(4), 15–21.

National Emphysema Treatment Trial Research Group. (2001). Patients at high risk of death after lung-volume-reduction surgery. *New England Journal of Medicine, 345,* 1075–1083.

Naureckas, E. T., & Solway, J. (2001). Mild asthma. *New England Journal of Medicine, 345*(17), 1257–1262.

Newbold, M. E., Tullis, E., Corey, M., Ross, B., & Brooks, D. (2005). The flutter device versus the PEP mask in the treatment of adults with cystic fibrosis. *Physiotherapy Canada, 57,* 199–207.

O'Brien, G. M. & Criner, G. J. (1998). Surgery for severe COPD: Lung volume reduction and lung transplantation. *Post Graduate Medicine, 103*(4), 179–202.

Parmet, W. E. (2007). Legal power and legal rights: Isolation and quarantine in the case of drug-resistant tuberculosis. *New England Journal of Medicine, 357*(5), 433–435.

Pauwels, R. A., Buist, A. S., Calverley, P. M., Jenkins, C. R., & Hurd, S. S. (2001). Global strategy for the diagnosis, management, and prevention of chronic obstructive pulmonary disease: NHLBI/WHO Global Initiative for Chronic Obstructive Lung Disease (GOLD) Workshop summary. *American Respiratory Critical Care Medicine, 163,* 1256-7126.

Petty, T. (1999). Rehabilitation options for chronic obstructive pulmonary disease. *Annals of Long-Term Care, 7*(5), 200–205.

Petty, T. (2001, April 15). Early diagnosis of COPD. *Hospital Practice,* 7–8.

Pompeo, E., Marino, M., Nofroni, I., Matteucci, G., & Mineo, T. C. (2000). Reduction pneumoplasty versus respiratory rehabilitation in severe emphysema: A randomized study. *Annals of Thoracic Surgery, 70,* 948–953.

Poss, J. E. (2000). Factors associated with participation by Mexican migrant farm workers in a tuberculosis screening program. *Nursing Research, 49,* 20–28.

Rabe, K. F. (2007). Treating COPD: The TORCH Trial, *p* values, and the dodo. *New England Journal of Medicine, 356*(8), 851–854.

Raviglione, M. M. C., & Smith, I. M. (2007). XDR tuberculosis: Implications for global public health. *New England Journal of Medicine, 356*(7), 656–658.

Rennard, S. I. (2004). Looking at the patient: Approaching the problem of COPD. *New England Journal of Medicine, 350*(10), 965–966.

Rochester, C. L. (2000). Which pulmonary rehabilitation program is best for your patient? . *Journal of Respiratory Diseases, 21*(9), 539-550.

Samet, J. M., Geyh, A. S., & Utell, M. J., (2007). The legacy of World Trade Center dust. *New England Journal of Medicine, 356*(22), 2233-2236.

Selgrade, M. J. K., Lemanske, R. F., Gilmour, M. I., Neas, L. M., Ward, M. D., Henneberger, P. K. et al. (2006). Induction of asthma and the environment: What we know and need to know. *Environmental Health Perspectives, 114*(4), 615-619.

Sherwood, L. (2007). The respiratory system. In L. Sherwood (Ed.), *Human physiology* (pp. 451-499). Belmont, CA: Thomson Brooks/Cole.

Sin, D. D., Anthonisen, N. R., Soriano, J. B., & Agusti, A. G. (2006). Mortality in COPD: Role of comorbities. *European Respiratory Journal, 28,* 1245-1257.

Snider, G.L. (2003). Nosology for our day: Its application to chronic obstructive pulmonary disease. *American Respiratory Critical Care Medicine, 167,* 678-683.

Sood, A., & Beckett, W. S. (2007). Silicosis and asbestosis. In R. E. Rakel & E. T. Bope (Eds.), *Conn's current therapy* (pp. 324-327). Philadelphia. Saunders.

Sutherland, E. R., & Cherniack, R. M. (2004). Management of chronic obstructive pulmonary disease. *New England Journal of Medicine, 350*(26), 2689-2697.

Twedell, D. (2007). Emphysema and lung volume reduction surgery. *Journal of Continuing Education in Nursing, 38*(4), 150-151.

Wenzel, R. P., & Fowler, A. A. III. (2006). Acute bronchitis. *New England Journal of Medicine, 355*(20), 2125-2130.

Chapter 15

Kidney and Urinary Tract Conditions

■ STRUCTURE AND FUNCTION OF THE URINARY TRACT

The urinary system enables the body to eliminate by-products of metabolism and regulate body fluids and electrolyte content. The urinary system consists of two kidneys which are bean-shaped organs about the size of a fist lying behind the abdominal cavity (*retroperitoneal*) on either side of the vertebral column, and the urinary tract, consisting of two **ureters** (tubes, one from each kidney, leading from the kidneys to the bladder), the bladder (a storage place for urine until it is eliminated), and the **urethra** (a single tube leading from the bladder to the outside opening—urinary meatus—through which urine is eliminated. (See Figure 15-1.) The term **renal** refers to the kidney, while the term urinary refers to the collecting system for urine (i.e., the ureters, bladder, and urethra).

The kidneys have multiple functions:

- They maintain the body's internal chemical balance (**homeostasis**) by regulating the water content and **electrolyte** (electrically charged particles of substances that are important to many of the body's internal functions) concentrations.
- They rid the body of metabolic waste products (**urea,** *uric acid,* **and creatinine**).

- They remove foreign chemicals from the body (drugs, pesticides).

They secrete hormones:

1. *Renin* that influences blood pressure and sodium and potassium balance in the body. It stimulates a hormone (*angiotensin*) that in turn stimulates an endocrine gland, the adrenal cortex (see Chapter 11), to secrete a hormone called *aldosterone,* which influences how the kidney regulates potassium and sodium levels in the body.
2. *Erythropoietin,* controls production of red blood cells
3. *Vitamin D* regulates calcium absorption from the intestine and influences the calcium balance in the body.

A thin layer of white fibrous tissue called the renal capsule surrounds the kidney. The outer layer of the kidney is called the *cortex*; the inner portion is called the *medulla*. The *renal pelvis* is a funnel-shaped structure through which urine passes into the ureters. The medulla contains 10 to 15 triangular structures called *renal pyramids*, which serve as a portion of the renal drainage system. The cortex and medulla contain units called *nephrons,* which are the functional units of the kidney. There are approximately 1 million nephrons in each

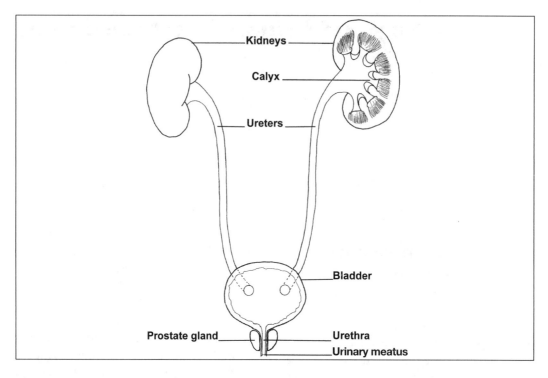

Figure 15-1   The urinary tract

kidney. Each nephron contains an initial filtering systems (**glomerulus**), each of which is surrounded by a *Bowman's capsule*. Glomeruli are loops of capillaries (*glomerular capillaries*). Extending from the glomerulus are the renal tubules, which end in a collecting duct. Collecting ducts from each nephron merge to empty into the renal pelvis. (See Figure 15-2.)

The kidney filters a large volume of blood each day. Approximately 20% of the body's blood flow passes to the kidney through the renal arteries, at a rate averaging about one liter of arterial blood per minute. The remaining 80% of blood remains in the general body circulation. Blood enters the kidney through the renal artery and leaves from the kidney to enter the general body circulation through the renal vein.

Blood entering the kidney flows first to the glomerular capillaries, where it is filtered, and then to a second capillary bed surrounding the tubules (peritubular capillaries), which form the veins through which blood leaves the kidney. The process by which the kidney removes waste products from the blood is called *glomerular filtration*. The level of kidney function is measured by the **glomerular filtration rate** (**GFR**), which is the rate at which a given compound passes through the glomerulus in a given time (usually measured in milliliters per minute), or the filtration rate of blood through the renal glomerular capillaries into Bowman's capsule per unit of time.

Initial filtration, which occurs as the blood enters the glomerulus, removes some waste products. As the glomerular filtrate continues to move through the tubules of the nephrons, substances are either reabsorbed into the bloodstream, continue through the tubules, or are added back to the filtrate. As the filtrate moves into the collecting system, it eventually drains into the calyx at the mouth of each

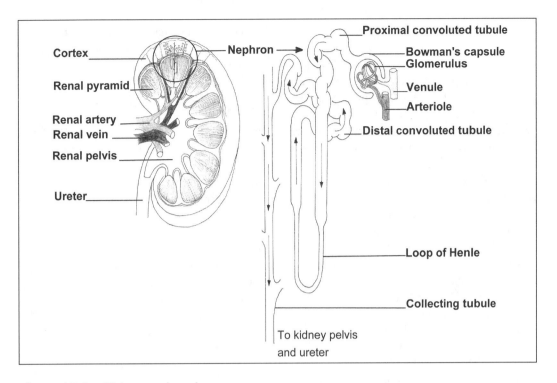

Cortex

Renal pyramid

Renal artery

Renal vein

Renal pelvis

Ureter

Nephron

Proximal convoluted tubule

Bowman's capsule

Glomerulus

Venule

Arteriole

Distal convoluted tubule

Loop of Henle

Collecting tubule

To kidney pelvis
and ureter

Figure 15-2   Kidney and nephron

pyramid and empties into the renal pelvis as urine. From the renal pelvis, urine drains into the ureters to the bladder, where it is stored until it is ready to be excreted through the urethra and urinary meatus.

Metabolic end products and toxic substances are removed from the blood through the filtration process, and are then subsequently eliminated from the body as urine. Conversely, other substances such as sugar and amino acids (the building blocks of protein) are reabsorbed into the bloodstream. Consequently, in healthy individuals, sugar and protein should not be found in the urine. Electrolytes (e.g., sodium and potassium) are also returned to the bloodstream along with 99% of the water in the filtrate. *Potassium* is important to muscle contraction, nerve function, and heart function, whereas *sodium* is important to heart and nerve function as well as water balance. The amounts of water and electrolytes reabsorbed are variable, being regulated according to the body's specific needs; however, this internal chemical balance is crucial for the general function of most other organs. Because of the kidneys' many functions, disorders of the kidney affect many body systems.

■ URINARY TRACT AND KIDNEY CONDITIONS

Cystitis (Lower Urinary Tract Infection)

The bladder and the urine contained within it are usually sterile. **Cystitis** is a condition in which bacteria enter the bladder, causing it to become infected and inflamed. Bacteria can invade the bladder through the external urinary meatus, or infection of the bladder can occur secondary to an infection in another location of the urinary tract. Although cystitis itself is generally not a disabling condition, it can be a serious complication for individuals with chronic illness or disability.

Symptoms of cystitis may include *frequency* (frequent urination), even though the bladder may not be full; **dysuria** (painful urination); *urgency* (a need to urinate immediately); pain in the lower abdomen or lower back; or **hematuria** (blood in the urine). Recurrent or inadequately treated cystitis can produce more serious consequences if the infection travels up the urinary tract and leads to infection of the kidney (**pyelonephritis**). If bacteria enter the blood, a (**septicemia**), potentially life-threatening systemic infection can result.

Cystitis is diagnosed by symptoms reported and by examination of the urine for evidence of bacteria, white blood cells, or other indications of infection or inflammation. Treatment of uncomplicated infections includes the administration of medications, such as antibiotics (Norrby, 2004). If cystitis is recurrent, treatment may include identifying and removing or correcting factors that contribute to the development of urinary tract infections. Examples include structural conditions such as stricture (narrowing) of part of the lower urinary tract that prevents adequate emptying of the bladder, thus predisposing individuals to infection.

Immobility, use of external catheter, poor perineal hygiene, or generally weakened physical condition can predispose individuals to develop cystitis. Because of the potentially serious nature of this complication in individuals with chronic illness or disability, symptoms suggestive of the presence of urinary tract infection should be treated promptly. Prevention of cystitis is important to reduce the risk of serious complications. Proper bladder care (i.e., wiping from front to back; avoiding contamination with fecal matter), adequate fluid intake, maintaining acidity of urine (e.g., drinking cranberry juice), or periodic urine analysis and cultures for presence of bacteria to ensure early detection of unsuspected infection may help individuals prone to cystitis prevent or lessen the chance of its occurrence.

Pyelonephritis

Pyelonephritis (infection of the kidney) can be a complication of cystitis when bacteria progress to the kidneys from an infection of the lower urinary tract, or it can be caused by spread of infection from elsewhere in the body to the kidney (McCammon & McCammon, 2007). This condition can also be caused by obstruction or narrowing of a portion of the urinary tract that leads to **stasis** (stagnation) of urine, which provides an environment amenable to growth of bacteria.

Pyelonephritis may be acute or chronic. No long-term debilitation is usually associated with acute pyelonephritis, although individuals may be acutely ill with fever and chills, flank or abdominal pain, nausea, and vomiting. Prompt treatment with appropriate antibiotics can eradicate the infection or, in the case of an obstruction or stricture, surgical intervention to remove any obstruction or stricture can prevent acute pyelonephritis from recurring. If acute pyelonephritis is not adequately treated or if treatment is not permanently successful owing to urinary tract obstruction or stricture, chronic pyelonephritis can develop. Chronic pyelonephritis can cause irreversible degenerative changes in kidney structure and function, leading to kidney failure, described later in the chapter.

Diagnosis of pyelonephritis is based on symptoms and an examination of urine for the presence of bacteria and white blood cells.

Urinary or Renal Calculi (Kidney Stones, Nephrolithiasis, Urolithiasis)

Ranging in size from a stone as tiny as a grain of sand to a stone large enough to fill the inner portion of the kidney, kidney stones (*renal cal-*

culi) may occur anywhere in the urinary tract. They cause very severe pain (renal colic) and can be a source of obstruction and secondary infection. Some individuals appear to be more prone to developing kidney stones than others. In addition to structural or metabolic abnormalities, prolonged immobility or bed rest, inadequate fluid intake, and a variety of chronic illnesses and disabilities can predispose individuals to develop kidney stones.

Kidney stones may produce no symptoms, or they may produce excruciating pain in the flank or kidney area, nausea and vomiting, **hematuria** (blood in the urine), or frequency of urination. Diagnosis is based on the symptoms, together with an examination of the urine for hematuria or bacteria.

The presence of stones may also be identified with ultrasound and confirmed with computerized tomography (CT). A radiologic examination called an intravenous pyelogram (IVP; described later in the chapter) may also be performed to detect the presence of stones and, if they are present, to evaluate the extent of the obstruction. Because IVPs are time-consuming and require exposure to x-ray and injection of contrast media, noncontrast CT is often used instead to visualize kidney stones (Hegarty & Streem, 2007).

If a stone severely obstructs its flow, urine may back up to the kidney (**hydronephrosis**), causing kidney damage. Most calculi are passed through the urinary meatus spontaneously. If a stone does not pass spontaneously, it may have to be removed surgically. The type of surgery depends on the size and location of the stone. A procedure called *lithotripsy* (described next) may be used to break up the stone through the use of ultrasound.

Shock-wave lithrotripsy (SWL), which is also known as *extracorporeal shock-wave lithrotripsy (ESWL)* is a noninvasive procedure in which high-frequency sound waves from an external source are used to fragment the kidney stone. It is usually performed on an outpatient basis;

if it is performed in the hospital, it requires only a minimal stay.

If the stone is lodged in the ureter, an attempt may be made to remove it using a special instrument called a *cystoscope* that is inserted into the bladder. The surgeon may directly remove the stone, break it up with a laser, or push it back into the renal pelvis via ESWL. Individuals undergoing this procedure may be positioned in a padded chair that is lifted into a stainless-steel tub of warm water, or a fluid bag may be placed between the individual and the source of the high-frequency sound waves to serve as a buffer against the sound waves. Once the individual is positioned to receive the maximal effect, sound waves from a machine called a *lithotriptor* are directed to the stones, which are visualized radiographically. The stones are broken apart by the sound waves, and the fragments can then be passed in the urine.

In some instances, if lithotripsy fails or cannot be performed, a procedure called *percutaneous nephrolithotomy* may be performed. In this procedure, an incision is made into the kidney and the stone is then removed surgically (Juknevicius & Hruska, 2004).

Hydronephrosis

An obstruction can occur anywhere in the urinary tract for a variety of reasons: a stone; a narrowing caused by an infection; an injury; a congenital abnormality; a tumor; or enlargement of the prostate gland (known as **benign prostatic hypertrophy**) (**BPH**), a condition seen in older men. Obstructions prevent urine from flowing through the urinary tract so that urine backflows into the kidneys. Because the kidneys continue to produce urine even though there is backup of urine from the urinary tract, the kidney pelvis eventually becomes swollen and distended. This distention is called **hydronephrosis.** Obstruction of the urinary tract and backflow of urine also predisposes individuals to infection of the kidney (**pyelonephritis**).

The symptoms experienced by individuals with hydronephrosis depend on the location of the obstruction, the degree of blockage, and the duration of the blockage (Klahr, 2004). Individuals with hydronephrosis may experience pain, or they may feel little discomfort. Diagnosis of hydronephrosis is usually made through ultrasound.

To prevent permanent damage to the kidney, whatever is causing the obstruction must be removed. The degree of disability experienced because of hydronephrosis depends on the degree of permanent damage to the kidney. In severe cases, hydronephrosis can result in kidney failure.

Glomerulonephritis

Nephritis is an inflammation of the kidney. **Glomerulonephritis** is a type of nephritis characterized by inflammation of the glomeruli of the kidney (Appel, 2004). Glomerulonephritis results from an immunologic response to bacteria or viruses or, in some cases, as part of an autoimmune process found in conditions such as lupus (see Chapter 16). The immunologic response can follow an infection elsewhere in the body, such as streptococcal pharyngitis ("strep throat") or bacterial endocarditis (see Chapter 13).

Glomerulonephritis may be acute or chronic (Cattran & Turner, 2007). Symptoms often include **hematuria** (blood in the urine); **proteinuria** (protein in the urine); some impairment in kidney function, with the retention of salt and water, possibly leading to elevated blood pressure (**hypertension**); and **edema** (swelling), especially in the legs and around the eyes. Generalized edema (**anasarca**) may also occur and may be accompanied by other symptoms, such as **dyspnea** (difficulty breathing) on exertion, visual disturbances, and headache.

Although some individuals recover completely, glomerulonephritis can result in irreversible, permanent structural changes in the kidney leading to chronic kidney disease. The extent of kidney damage depends on the cause of the glomerulonephritis and the speed and the effectiveness with which the process can be stopped through appropriate treatment. Treatment of glomerulonephritis focuses on relieving the symptoms and eliminating the underlying cause.

Nephrosis (Nephrotic Syndrome)

Nephrosis is a general term used to describe conditions in which a kidney has been damaged by conditions other than direct infection of the kidney itself. It may be a manifestation of glomerulonephritis, or it may occur secondary to conditions such as systemic lupus erythematosus or diabetes mellitus. In some cases no cause is found.

In *nephritic syndrome*, the glomerular filter allows excessive proteins (especially albumin) to pass into the filtrate and urine. This leads to *albuminuria* (albumin in the urine). Eventually, the albumin level in the blood falls, with accompanying high levels of lipids. Individuals with nephritic syndrome often have severe edema. Other manifestations include proteinuria (protein in the urine). When the kidneys are damaged, substances such as protein, which normally would be reabsorbed into the bloodstream during the filtering process, are passed through the membranes of the glomerular capillaries and excreted in the urine. Thus an important complication of nephritic syndrome is severe protein malnutrition, which may require nutritional supplementation. Prognosis depends on the cause of nephritic syndrome.

Polycystic Kidney Disease

Polycystic kidney disease (PKD) is a hereditary disease characterized by the presence of many cysts in the kidneys. The most common form of PKD is called *autosomal dominant PKD*, which means that a person with this condition has a 50% chance of transmitting the condition to his or her children. The cysts become enlarged in PKD, compressing and exerting pressure on functioning kidney tissue. The disease progresses slowly over many years, so individuals may be unaware that they have it. Physicians may discover the condition by accident during a routine examination, or as cysts enlarge, individuals may begin to experience symptoms such as low back pain, hematuria (blood in the urine), or frequent urinary tract infections.

PKD often progresses to chronic kidney disease, though this progression sometimes takes as long as 20 years. Treatment of chronic kidney disease may include dialysis and/or kidney transplantation (both of which are discussed later in this chapter). Although transplantation is feasible for those individuals with PKD, close family members may not be appropriate donors because of the hereditary nature of this condition.

Nephrectomy

If trauma has severely injured the kidney, if stones have caused severe damage or are too large to remove, or if the kidney is chronically infected or nonfunctional, the entire kidney may be removed. This surgical procedure is called *nephrectomy*. Individuals can live normal lives with one functioning kidney, but should guard against infection or injury that could compromise the function of the remaining kidney.

Acute Renal Failure

Acute renal failure (**ARF**) has a sudden onset and can occur within hours or days as a complication of other medical conditions, surgery, or trauma (Mitch, 2004). Diminished blood volume (**hypovolemia**) due to hemorrhage or

severe dehydration, extremely low blood pressure (*hypotension*), **septicemia** (bacteria in the blood), urinary tract obstruction, and **nephrotoxins** (substances harmful to the kidneys such as certain drugs, solvents, or metals) are all potential causes of acute renal failure.

Treatment of ARF is directed toward removing the cause of the kidney failure when possible, preventing permanent damage to the kidney and complications, and restoring the body chemistry to its normal state (Barrett & Parfrey, 2006). If the causative factor can be corrected before irreversible structural changes occur in the kidney, this condition may be temporary. Depending on the cause, ARF can often be reversed with no permanent damage to the kidney. To prevent permanent kidney damage, treatment must begin immediately. Dialysis may be instituted temporarily to take over kidney function until the cause of the kidney failure can be corrected (Weisbord & Palevsky, 2007). Dialysis may also be used to remove toxic substances from the body, such as in drug overdose.

Chronic Kidney Diease

Chronic kidney disease (CKD) also called *chronic renal failure (CRF)* refers to conditions in which the kidney has become damaged. There are many causes of CKD. Unfortunately, in most cases CKD is progressive and can eventually lead to kidney failure in which the kidney is unable to maintain adequate function (Barsoum, 2006). The course of CKD may span many years. Individuals with such CKD have impaired kidney function and should receive ongoing evaluation to detect any change in kidney function so that progression of kidney impairment may be slowed, if possible.

When the kidneys become so damaged or the functional capacity of the kidneys declines to the extent that it is insufficient to meet the body's demands, individuals are said to be in *kidney failure*. Kidney failure can be acute or chronic, temporary or permanent. Signs and symptoms of kidney failure, whether acute or chronic, depend on three factors:

- The cause of the kidney failure
- The degree of dysfunction of the kidney
- The rate of development of kidney failure

In some cases, kidney function may no longer be sufficient to support life. Symptoms experienced by individuals whose kidneys have failed depend on the stage of the condition. Individuals may lose a significant amount of kidney function before any symptoms are noted. Both acute and chronic kidney disease diminish the kidneys' ability to filter blood adequately and remove water and wastes. As a result, wastes, which once would have been excreted by the kidneys through the urine, continue to circulate in the body. This decreased function affects the body's delicate internal chemical balance. Because the kidneys have many functions important to the body, kidney dysfunction has effects on all other organ systems.

The presence of chronic kidney disease is established by evidence of kidney damage and level of kidney function. Estimate of kidney function is made from the *glomerular filtration rate* (GFR), which was discussed earlier in the chapter (Stevens, Coresh, Greene, & Levey, 2006). CKD is defined as either kidney damage leading to a GFR of less than 60 mL/min (in relationship to body mass) or the presence of albumin in the urine for more than 3 months (Jafar, 2006). Kidney damage is determined by abnormalities in blood or urine tests or abnormalities or evidence of damage found in imaging studies (National Kidney Foundation, 2002).

CKD can result from acute renal failure in which irreversible damage occurs before the cause of the ARF can be corrected, or it can result from complications of a number of other conditions related to the kidney, such as glomerulonephritis, pyleonephritis, and polycystic kidney disease. In addition, CKD can result from complications of systemic conditions such as hypertension (see Chapter 13), diabetes (see Chapter 11), autoimmune diseases such as lupus erythematosus (see Chapter 16), vascular disease resulting in **nephrosclerosis** (a condition in which the arteries of the kidney become thickened), or exposure to nephrotoxins, drug toxicity, or drug overdose. Nearly two thirds of cases of chronic kidney failure are caused by diabetes and hypertension (Luke, 2004).

Symptoms of Chronic Kidney Disease

Whereas acute renal failure occurs rapidly, chronic kidney disease may progress gradually over time. Its severity can be classified according to the level of the GFR, regardless of the cause of this disease (Stevens & Levey, 2005). Staging of CKD assists physicians in the evaluation, monitoring, and treatment of individuals with kidney disease (Kraut, 2007). The stage of the CKD is based on the level of kidney function in terms of the GFR in the context of the individual's body mass. Individuals are diagnosed with chronic kidney disease when there is kidney damage and the GFR falls below the level considered normal. Stages are defined as follows (National Kidney Foundation, 2000):

- Stage 1: evidence of kidney damage with normal GFR or GFR greater than 90 mL/min
- Stage 2: kidney damage with a mild decrease in GFR (60–89 mL/min)
- Stage 3: moderate decrease in GFR (30–59 mL/min)
- Stage 4: severe decrease in GFR (15–29 mL/min)
- Stage 5: kidney failure (GFR of less than 15 or dialysis)

In the early stages of CKD, symptoms may be barely perceptible. Fatigue may be one of the first noticeable symptoms. It may result from anemia that accompanies kidney failure. The kidneys normally produce a substance called *erythopoietin* (EPO) that stimulates the bone marrow to produce blood cells. With CKD, EPO production is too low and so anemia occurs.

In the early stages, CKD may be accompanied by increased urine production (**polyuria**). Examination of the urine (**urinalysis**) may reveal protein in the urine as an early sign. Because protein is usually reabsorbed into the regular body circulation after being filtered through the kidney, presence of protein in the urine is an indication of failure of this mechanism.

As kidney function declines, waste products of metabolism (urea and creatinine) build up in the blood, a condition called **uremia**. As waste products continue to increase and circulate in the general circulation, individuals may experience overall itching (**pruritus**). Fatigue, anemia, and buildup of waste products in the blood may also contribute to manifestations of disease including difficulty with concentration or development of shortened attention span.

Individuals with advanced CKD must be treated through dialysis; alternatively, they may receive a kidney transplant to survive. Individuals with severe CKD are unable to regulate water balance in their body. Urine production is severely diminished (**oliguria**) or nonexistent (**anuria**). Consequently, water that would have been excreted as urine remains in the body, creating fluid overload. Although some water is excreted through the gastrointestinal and respiratory systems, as well as through perspiration, the kidneys are the main source of fluid excretion. Overload of fluid in the body puts stress on the circulatory system, and especially on the heart, potentially causing cardiac dysfunction and failure. Outward symptoms of fluid overload consist of weight gain, edema, and difficulty breathing (**dyspnea**).

The problem of fluid overload is compounded if there is also increased sodium in the blood. Sodium, an electrolyte, helps regulate fluid content of the body's tissues and, along with potassium and another electrolyte (chloride), regulates the body's internal chemistry. In CKD, the kidneys are unable to excrete sodium. Too much sodium in the body causes retention of fluid and swelling (**edema**) and high blood pressure (**hypertension**). As a result, individuals may experience sudden weight gain, as well as puffiness or swelling of the face, feet, ankles, legs, and, at times arms and abdomen. Individuals may complain of feeling uncomfortable and bloated; they may also experience difficulty breathing due to fluid overload on the heart and lungs.

Potassium is important in regulating contraction and relaxation of muscles, including the heart and muscles used for respiration. When there is too little potassium, muscle weakness can occur along with dangerous disturbances in heart and respiratory function. Normally most potassium taken in through the diet is excreted by the kidney; however, in CKD the kidney is unable to secrete potassium, so it is retained, leading to subsequent high blood levels of potassium (**hyperkalemia**). Excessive amounts of potassium in the blood can adversely affect the heart, potentially causing cardiac arrest and death.

Calcium in the blood is decreased below normal levels in CKD, partially because the kidney is unable to produce sufficient amounts of the active form of vitamin D, which is necessary for calcium absorption, and because calcium absorption in the intestine is decreased. Low calcium in the blood due to CKD also causes overactivity of the parathyroid glands (see Chapter 11), causing calcium loss from the bone (**osteoporosis**), and contributing to bone pain and fractures.

Individuals with CKD may become malnourished because of **anorexia** (loss of appetite), nausea and vomiting, or lack of appetite due to depression. **Anemia** (reduction of circulating red blood cells), accompanied by iron deficiency, is characteristically seen in kidney failure not only because of poor diet, but also because of the kidneys' inability to produce EPO, the hormone responsible for initiating red blood cell production, and because of individuals decreased ability to absorb iron from the intestine (Drueke et al., 2006). As a result, individuals with CKD tend to experience weakness and have low exercise tolerance. It may be difficult for many individuals with CKD to walk very far without resting.

Uremia has toxic effects on nerves, especially the peripheral nerves of the hands and feet. It may, therefore, result in **peripheral neuropathy**, a disabling symptom leading to weakness and loss of sensation in the upper and/or lower extremities. Peripheral neuropathy is a symptom commonly observed in individuals with chronic kidney disease (U.S. Renal Data System, 2006). As a result of peripheral neuropathy, individuals may have both difficulty manipulating objects with their hands and difficulty walking.

The central nervous system may also be affected by CKD. Intellectual impairment may coincide with worsening uremia, so that individuals have increased difficulty concentrating or demonstrate a shortened attention span. In addition, the incidence of **dementia** (see Chapter 8) is increased in individuals with CKD. Individuals on hemodialyis have a three times greater incidence of dementia than do members of the general population (U.S. Renal Data System, 2006).

Individuals with CKD are not restricted from engaging in sexual activity. Nevertheless, because of both physical and emotional changes present in CKD, individuals may experience impaired sexual function (Neelakantappa & Lowenstein, 2005; Ifudu, 1998). Hormonal changes, circulatory problems, changes in the nervous system, lack of energy, or side effects of medication may all contribute to diminished sexual desire or performance. Likewise, changes in self concept and body image may hamper sexual interest and activity.

Management of Chronic Kidney Disease

Physicians who specialize in the treatment of kidney disease are called **nephrologists**. Because there is no cure for CKD, except by transplantation, treatment is directed at controlling and delaying disease progression. Progression can be delayed by control of high blood pressure, control of diabetes, and control of other primary processes involved in CKD. In very early stages of CKD, treatment may include restricting water to an amount equal to urine output, carefully monitoring body weight, and managing the diet to provide adequate nutrition without overtaxing the kidney with metabolic waste products. This effort may require a low-sodium diet, with restrictions on excessive protein and on the intake of potassium, water, or phosphorus.

Medications may also be administered to slow the progression of kidney disease (Herbert, 2006; Hou et al., 2006). The kidneys can usually continue to function with as little as 10% of normal kidney function. Loss of function beyond this point requires renal replacement therapy (RRT) to survive (Luke, 2004). RRT consists of hemodialysis, peritoneal dialysis, or kidney transplant (all of which are discussed later in this chapter). In 2004, nearly 95,000 people were on hemodialysis and 6686 on peritoneal dialysis. More than 2000 people received kidney transplants (U.S. Renal Data System, 2006).

Diet

When kidney function is significantly reduced, individuals' diet and fluid intake must be regulated to accomodate the limited or absent function of the kidneys. Intake of protein, sodium, potassium, fluid, and calories must be carefully regulated and monitored to achieve the following goals:

- Minimize waste products in the body
- Maintain electrolyte levels in the body within normal limits
- Avoid either too much or too little fluid in the body.

Diets are tailored to the individual; there is no single diet prescription that is appropriate for all individuals with kidney failure. Individuals with chronic kidney failure work closely with *dietitians* (individuals who specialize in the science of applying nutritional information to the regulation of diet to maximize health) to develop a diet plan right for them. The type of dietary prescription is based on individual needs and the type of kidney disease. In CKD, the kidney is no longer able to filter out waste products of protein metabolism, so dietary intake of protein must be controlled. Consequently, dietary intake of foods especially high in protein—meat, fish, eggs, poultry, and dairy products—is restricted to 8 to 10 ounces per day (National Kidney Foundation, 2007).

Because in CRF the kidneys are unable to excrete potassium, and because of the adverse and potentially fatal effects of high levels of potassium on heart and other muscles in the body, potassium buildup in the blood (**hyperkalemia**) must be avoided. Dietary intake of foods rich in potassium must, therefore, be restricted. Examples of foods with high potassium content are listed in Table 15-1. The more severe the loss of kidney function, the more carefully potassium levels must be regulated.

Because sodium is important in the regulation of fluid in the body as well as in maintaining the body's internal chemical balance, and because the kidneys in CRF cannot excrete sodium effectively, individuals with CKD must also regulate dietary intake of sodium. Sodium restrictions affect not only intake of salt, but also intake of a number of other foods high in sodium. Foods containing high levels of sodium must, therefore, be restricted. (See Table 15-2.)

Individuals with CKD are unable to regulate fluid balance so the amount of fluid taken orally may need to be restricted. Included in this measure of fluid intake are ice cubes, gelatin desserts, sherbet, or any other food that liquefies at room temperature. Physicians calculate the amount of fluid individuals may consume based on the amount fluid lost through perspiration and respiration. The amount of fluid intake permitted is based on

---

Table 15-1   Restricted Foods in Chronic Kidney Disease: Foods High in Potassium

Oranges and orange juice	Strawberries
Grapefruit, grapefruit juice	Raisins
Bananas	Beets
Apricots	Cabbage
Cantaloupe	Carrots
Kidney beans	Celery
Pears	Many breakfast cereals
Potatoes	Many breads
Spinach	Many nuts
Tomatoes	Salt substitutes
Peaches	

(continues)

Table 15-2 Restricted Foods in Chronic Kidney Disease: Foods High in Sodium	
(continued)	
Corned and chipped beef	Hot dogs
Bacon	Cheddar and swiss cheese
Ham	Snack foods such as pretzels, popcorn,
Cold cuts such as bologna	potato chips, some crackers
Pork sausage	Most canned vegetables
Canned tuna, salmon, sardines	Olives
Pork sausage	Soft drinks

the individual's weight gain at specific intervals, and may be severely restricted.

Due to food restrictions, individuals may have difficulty maintaining sufficient caloric intake. Foods low in sodium, potassium, and protein may be needed throughout the day as supplements to provide additional calories. For snacks in between meals, the dietitian may recommend specialized products that are high in calories but low in protein and electrolyte.

Medications

Due to dietary restrictions on their intake of dairy products and other foods high in calcium, individuals with CKD may experience calcium depletion. Consequently, calcium supplements as well as supplements of vitamin D derivatives normally produced in the kidney are given by mouth to these persons. The physician may also prescribe supplementary vitamins and certain minerals.

Vitamin D is essential for proper bone health and it stimulates calcium absorption from the intestine. The body normally produces vitamin D when the skin is exposed to the sunlight or the person consumes vitamin D in fortified foods such as milk. Vitamin D normally goes to the liver and then to the kidney for chemical conversion to its active form. In case of kidney disease, this chemical conversion does not occur. Consequently, individuals with CKD do not have sufficient amounts of

active vitamin D and must take supplements to avoid a deficiency.

Oral iron supplements are frequently given as apart of the medical treatment of CRF. In addition, *erythropoietin* (a substance normally produced in the kidney that stimulates production of red blood cells) may be given **subcutaneously** (into the fatty tissue under the skin) three times a week after each dialysis treatment. Individuals with CKD are often placed on antihypertensive medications to help control blood pressure. Medications may also be given to limit the intestinal absorption of phosphorus.

Dialysis

Individuals with kidney failure, whether acute or chronic, cannot survive unless they have a way of compensating for their absent kidney function. Dialysis artificially performs the function of the kidney—that is, removal of waste and fluid from the body. It may be used temporarily, as in the case of acute renal failure, or it may be used to sustain life when kidney damage is irreversible and permanent, as in CKD. For individuals with acute renal failure, dialysis is a life-saving procedure until kidney function can be restored. When individuals develop CKD and kidney function cannot be restored, either dialysis or transplant is necessary for survival.

If individuals with CKD are suitable candidates for kidney transplantation, dialysis may be used until an appropriate donor kidney is available. Not all individuals with chronic kidney failure are suitable candidates for kidney transplant, however. If a transplant is not feasible, individuals with CRF must remain on dialysis for the rest of their lives.

Two types of dialysis are possible: *peritoneal dialysis* and *hemodialysis*. Both types simulate kidney function to achieve the following goals:

- Waste products of metabolism are removed from the blood.
- An appropriate balance in the body chemistry is maintained.
- Excess fluid is removed from the blood (Tolkoff-Rubin & Goes, 2004).

Both types of dialysis involve use of a *semi permeable* membrane, a porous material that allows some substances to pass through the membrane while keeping other substances in the blood. The blood of individuals undergoing dialysis is on one side of the membrane, and a specially prepared solution called a *dialysate* is on the other side of the membrane. Differences in concentrations of the blood and dialysate allow certain particles—but not others—to pass from the blood through the membrane and into the dialysate, where they can then be removed through dialysis.

The development of dialysis for CKD has enabled many people who otherwise might have died from their condition to live useful and productive lives (Himmelfarb, 2002). Nevertheless, dialysis is not without risk (Bonventre, 2002). Individuals with CKD who are receiving dialysis have a first-year mortality rate of approximately 25% (U.S. Renal Data System, 2001). Pneumonia and other pulmonary infections, stroke, and cardiovascular complications are all more prevalent in individuals having hemodialysis (U.S. Renal Data System, 2006). Given that people with CKD frequently have other medical conditions that have caused or contributed to their kidney failure, achieving a better outcome with dialysis depends on medical care in the early stages of chronic kidney disease (Kinchen et al., 2002).

Peritoneal Dialysis

In peritoneal dialysis the semipermeable membrane needed for dialysis consists of the **peritoneum** (the thin membrane that lines the abdominal cavity). A tube or catheter is surgically placed within the abdominal cavity. During peritoneal dialysis, dialysate from a bag is drained through the catheter into the abdominal cavity (see Figure 15-3). The catheter is clamped, and the dialysate is left in the abdominal cavity for a specified amount of time. During this time, waste products and excess fluid pass from the blood through the peritoneal membrane and into the dialysate. At the end of the specified period, the catheter is unclamped and the dialysate, which now contains the waste products and excess fluid, is drained from the body through the catheter. The tube is again clamped and remains in place for the next dialysis treatment.

Peritoneal dialysis is performed at home, manually or with a machine. There are several methods of peritoneal dialysis:

- Continuous ambulatory peritoneal dialysis
- Intermittent peritoneal dialysis
- Continuous cycling peritoneal dialysis

Regardless of the method used for peritoneal dialysis, the principles remain the same. With *continuous ambulatory peritoneal dialysis (CAPD)*, dialysate is instilled into the abdominal cavity manually, using gravity. A bag of dialysate solution is connected to the catheter. The individual then elevates the bag, causing the dialysate to flow into the abdominal cavity. The catheter is clamped, and the dialysate is left in place for 4 to 8 hours. The catheter is then unclamped and the bag lowered so that the dialysate drains from the abdominal cavity by gravity. When the bag is full, the individual

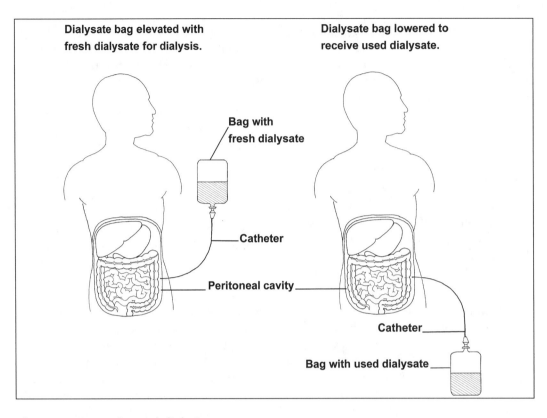

Dialysate bag elevated with fresh dialysate for dialysis.

Dialysate bag lowered to receive used dialysate.

Bag with fresh dialysate

Catheter

Peritoneal cavity

Catheter

Bag with used dialysate

Figure 15-3   Peritoneal dialysis

detaches the bag from the catheter, attaches a new bag of dialysate, and begins the process again. Individuals change the dialysate manually four to five times per day. Each exchange takes about 30 to 40 minutes. Individuals using this type of peritoneal dialysis are able to continue their regular daily activities, stopping only for periodic intervals to drain the dialysate and attach a fresh bag.

Intermittent peritoneal dialysis (IPD) and *continuous cycling peritoneal dialysis (CCPD)* both use a machine. IPD is now infrequently used as a form of periotoneal dialysis, but when it is used it is performed three or more times a week, with each exchange lasting for 10 or more hours. With IPD, the catheter is connected to the cycling machine at night. The exchange takes place while the person sleeps;

consequently, individuals are free to engage in their regular activities during the day.

CCPD also uses a cycling machine but is performed daily. In CCPD, the catheter is connected to the cycling machine, which performs multiple solution exchanges while the individual sleeps. In the morning, the individual disconnects the catheter from the machine, sometimes leaving the last solution in the abdomen all day, while engaging in his or her regular activities.

Peritoneal dialysis may be chosen as the dialysis method for individuals who have, in addition to kidney disease, other medical conditions that increase the risk of complications associated with hemodialysis. In other instances, it may be chosen because of its relative ease and the limited use of sophisticated equipment—both factors that enable individuals to use peritoneal dialysis in the home. Depending on the type of procedure used, individuals may enjoy more mobility with peritoneal dialysis than with hemodialysis. If severe vascular disease interferes with the blood supply to the peritoneum or there is an increased vulnerability to infection, however, peritoneal dialysis may be contraindicated.

Although generally a safe procedure, peritoneal dialysis can have a number of associated complications. The most common is **peritonitis** (inflammation of the peritoneum), which occurs when the peritoneum is contaminated with bacteria. If peritonitis develops, antibiotics may be used to treat the infection, or peritoneal dialysis may be discontinued and hemodialysis begun. Other complications that may occur as a result of peritoneal dialysis include plugging or displacement of the catheter, development of hernias, and pain during dialysis. Over time, infection or the dialysate concentration itself may damage the peritoneum. Peritoneal dialysis is usually a limited procedure because of the loss of membrane function.

Hemodialysis

The most common type of dialysis used for individuals with CKD is *hemodialysis*, in which an artificial kidney machine (**dialyzer**) circulates and filters the blood outside the body to remove waste products and excess fluid. Hemodialysis requires access to the individual's circulation. Access routes through which blood is removed from the individual to be circulated through the dialysis machine and then returned to the individual's circulation may be surgically created through a graft, an external arteriovenous shunt (less commonly used today), an internal arteriovenous fistula (Figure 15-4), or an internal jugular cannula (Figure 15-5).

Access routes are created surgically, most often in the forearm. The internal arteriovenous fistula is the most widely used venous access because it is more durable and has fewer complications, such as clotting or infection.

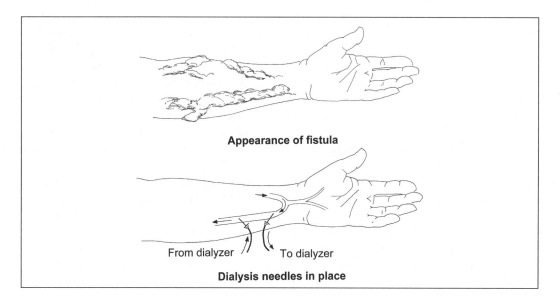

Appearance of fistula

From dialyzer   To dialyzer

Dialysis needles in place

Figure 15-4   Access for hemodialysis through a fistula

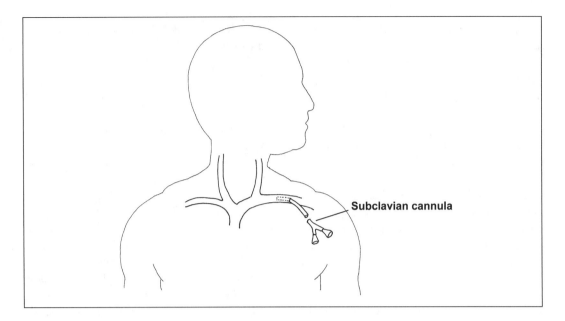

Figure 15-5 Access for hemodialysis through a subclavian cannula

In this procedure, an artery is surgically joined to a vein underneath the skin, establishing an opening called a **fistula** between the two. Shunting arterial blood into the vein causes the vein to become thickened and enlarged, allowing it to be used repeatedly as a point of access to the circulation for dialysis. It may take from 2 to 6 weeks for the fistula to become thickened and enlarged enough so that it can be used for dialysis. In the meantime, temporary access may be maintained through the internal jugular vein.

Grafts, which are used less commonly, connect an artery and a vein. The graft may be made by surgical placement of either synthetic material or a vein that has been removed from another part of the individual's body. The external arteriovenous shunt is rarely used, unless immediate and temporary access is needed, such as in the case of acute renal failure. This procedure consists of surgical placement of a tube (*cannula*) under the skin to connect an artery to a vein.

For hemodialysis purposes, a large needle is placed into the artery side of the access route; another large needle is placed in the vein side of the access. Tubes are then attached to the needles and connected to the dialysis machine. Blood moves from the first tube to the dialysis machine, where it is cleansed and filtered. The cleansed blood is then returned to the individual through the second needle in the vein (see Figure 15-6). Blood flow typically is 8 to 14 ounces of blood per minute.

The artificial kidney includes two compartments: one for the individual's blood and one for the dialysate solution. A synthetic semipermeable membrane separates these compartments within the artificial kidney. Blood cells and other important substances are too large to pass through the pores of the membrane, so they remain in their compartment. Most waste products are small enough to pass through the membrane into the dialysate, however, so they are washed away. The cleansed blood then returns through the tube to the individual.

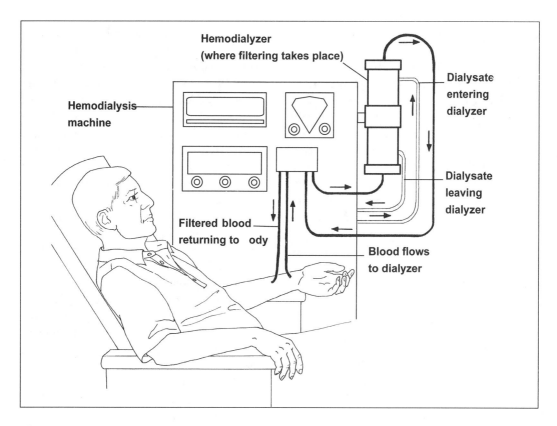

Figure 15-6   Hemodialysis machine

Hemodialysis is usually performed from 3 to 4 hours per day, three times per week (Owen, Pereira, & Savegh, 2000). It has also been performed successfully on a daily basis for 2 hours per day (Schiffle, Lang, & Fischer, 2002).

Hemodialysis can be performed at a kidney dialysis center or, in some instances (albeit rarely), at home. Because home hemodialysis requires a high degree of individual control, self-destructive tendencies in individuals or unwillingness of family members or caregivers to participate in the procedure is a contraindication for home hemodialysis. Home dialysis requires someone (a family member, or someone who has been hired) who has been trained to assist with the procedure. The level of responsibility as well as the need to be always present at specified times of dialysis can cause considerable stress for the helper, especially if he or she is a family member. Stress levels associated with home hemodialysis are usually evaluated and monitored before the implementation of such a home dialysis program.

The success of hemodialysis depends on individuals' level of motivation, the presence of other medical conditions that may cause complications, and development of complications from the hemodialysis itself. The numerous potential complications related to hemodialysis range from technical problems with the access route to more generalized complications that could result in death. Arteriovenous grafts and central venous catheters are especially prone to infection that can result in **septicemia** (bacteria in the blood), a potentially life-threatening complication.

Cardiac-related complications, such as **pericarditis** (inflammation of the outer layer of membrane surrounding the heart), **myocardial infarction** (heart attack), **arrhythmias** (irregular heartbeat), or **hypertension** (high blood pressure), may also occur (Ifudu, 1998). Another possible complication of hemodialysis is stroke or some other thrombolytic event. Because of the risk of clot formation in the access route, individuals on hemodialysis may receive anticoagulant medication during the procedure. Administration of this medication, however, may also increase the risk of bleeding. Hemodialysis itself is painless, although some minor discomfort may occur when needles are inserted for dialysis. During dialysis individuals are confined to the dialysis unit, but they can still read, use a computer, watch television, or sleep.

Rapid changes that occur in fluid and chemical balances in the body during dialysis cause some individuals to experience nausea, vomiting, headaches, or muscle cramps in association with hemodialysis. Some individuals may become anemic, and some experience sleep disturbances or mental cloudiness. Individuals on prolonged hemodialysis may develop changes in nerves of the extremities resulting in **peripheral neuropathy** (loss of sensation and weakness in the arms and legs).

Hemodialysis can relieve many of the symptoms of kidney disease, but not all of them. Individuals on hemodialysis may develop secondary conditions that increase the risk of bone fractures, or the procedure may not adequately clear all wastes, leading to a feeling of weakness. The degree of functional capacity varies from individual to individual. Many continue to lead near-normal lives, except for their dialysis treatments.

Kidney Transplantation

Kidney transplantation involves surgically placing a kidney from a donor into the body of an individual with kidney disease. Individuals who receive transplants usually have Stage 5 chronic kidney disease. The diseased kidney is usually not removed from the individual receiving the kidney transplant, unless there is uncontrolled infection, uncontrolled hypertension, or a limitation of space. Transplants may be received from a family member (living-related donor), an individual who is not related to the individual (living-unrelated donor), or an individual who has recently died (deceased donor). Regardless of the status of the donor, the donor's blood must be the same type as that of the recipient and tissues must closely match those of the recipient to decrease the chances of the body rejecting of the transplant (Soulillou & Giral, 2006; El Nahas, Harris, & Anderson, 2000). In addition, donors must undergo in-depth psychological evaluation and verification that they have not been coerced into donation. Donation must be altruistic and totally voluntary.

Kidney transplant frees individuals from restrictions associated with dialysis, diminishes many symptoms of chronic kidney failure, and improves overall quality of life (Tolkoff-Rubin & Goes, 2004). Before being considered for kidney transplant, recipients undergo careful and thorough medical evaluation to see if they are suitable candidates. It is essential prior to transplant that the individual knows that transplantation is a treatment, not a cure. Transplantation is simply a form of renal replacement therapy. Individuals having the transplant may still have the chronic condition that caused the initial kidney damage.

When being considered for transplant, the recipient's general health—including presence of other diseases that may potentially affect the success of the transplant or make it impossible—is evaluated. Pre-transplant evaluation also includes a thorough psychological evaluation. Discussion of risk of rejection and infection and the lifelong need to use immunosuppressants with their corresponding risk is a part of the pre-transplant protocol. In some instances, the ability to finance the procedure and the cost of medications needed after transplant may be assessed before someone is evaluated for eligibility for transplantation.

Expectations for the transplant are discussed with both the recipient and the living donor. Also evaluated is the recipient's ability to adjust to the transplant as well as his or her ability to adjust should the transplant fail. The degree of family and social support is assessed as well. Besides the cost of the kidney transplant itself the costs associated with travel to the transplant center, lodging for family members, and lifelong medication needed after the transplant can be staggering. Consequently, the social service evaluation includes the financial status of the candidate for transplant and identification of resources that can help to cover costs.

Scarcity of donors is the major factor that limits kidney transplantation. In 2004, 60,393 people were waiting for a transplant (U.S. Renal Data System, 2006). Whether the donor is living or deceased, compatibility of tissue type and blood type and a variety of other factors determine of the success of the transplantation (Soulillou & Giral, 2006). Tissue typing is most important in decreasing the possibility of rejection. The most desirable sources of kidneys for transplantation are closely related, living donors, but unrelated donors are now acceptable and new protocols are being developed so that blood type–incompatible donors. may be used (Delmonico, 2004).

At the time of transplant, both donor and recipient are hospitalized. The individual with CKD has dialysis the day before the transplant. The donor has renal angiography to determine which kidney will be used for the transplant. The surgical procedure for the kidney transplant consists of removing the kidney from the donor and placing it in a surgically con-structed pocket in the lower abdomen of the recipient.

Once the donor kidney has been transplanted, it may begin to function immediately. Early functioning of the transplanted kidney is a good prognostic sign for success of the transplant. When the recipient is discharged from the hospital, he or she must be careful to avoid infection owing to use of immunosuppressant drugs (medications prescribed to prevent rejection of the new kidney). The risk of infection is greatest in the first 6 months after surgery (Soulillou, 2001). During this time, the individual needs to be particularly careful to avoid contact with persons with communicable disease. After transplant, prophylactic antibiotics should be administered prior to any dental work.

After transplant, the individual receiving the kidney may return to work within 6 to 8 weeks. Because of the extensive surgical procedure necessary for removing the kidney from the donor, the recovery time for the donor had traditionally been considerably longer. The donor surgical procedure is now frequently done with a laparoscopic approach, which has greatly decreased recovery time; even so, the donor should expect to be away from work for at least 4 to 6 weeks. Donors who undergo traditional flank incisions will have a longer recovery time than the recipient and should expect to be absent from work for 8 to 12 weeks.

The major complication of kidney transplantation is rejection, which can destroy the transplanted kidney (Pascual, Theruvath, Kawai, Tolkoff-Rubin, & Cosimi, 2002). Rejection most commonly occurs within the first 6 weeks after the transplantation; however, chronic rejection may occur months or even years later. Although the rejection rate in the first year after kidney transplant has dramatically decreased over the last decade (Hariharan, Johnson, Bresnahan, Taranto, McIntosh & Stablein, 2000), long-term success has been elusive. Ultimately, failure occurs after 10 years in about half of individuals who receive a deceased-donor kidney (Marsden, 2003).

The body's defense system, or immune system, naturally attacks foreign substances in the body. Unfortunately, the immune system does not distinguish between a life-saving transplanted kidney and harmful substances. The immunosuppressants that are prescribed after transplant block the body's normal immune response. Unfortunately, immuno-suppressants can cause a number of complications—namely, increased susceptibility to infection, formation of cataracts, degeneration of bone (**avascular necrosis**), and an increased rate of **malignancy** (cancer), especially skin cancer. If rejection takes place immediately, it may be necessary to remove the transplanted kidney to avoid a generalized body reaction that could prove fatal.

Psychosocial Issues in Chronic Kidney Disease

Chronic kidney disease has a significant impact on quality of life (Hicks, Cleary, Epstein, & Ayanian, 2004; Franke, Reimer, Philipp, & Heemann, 2003). The initial shock and real-ization of kidney failure and its ramifications may be immobilizing. Reactions vary in degree from severe depression to total denial. Denial can be helpful in reducing stress levels, but it can be life-threatening if it leads to noncom-pliance with the recommended treatment.

Individuals who begin dialysis may also have a period of adjustment. When first begin-ning dialysis, individuals may be hopeful and confident because of the immediate physical improvements they experience after dialysis. In the early sessions of dialysis, individuals may experience apprehension or uneasiness about the possibility that the machine may malfunc-tion. As they become more comfortable with dialysis, these fears generally subside.

As the individuals continue in dialysis, they may become discouraged and disenchanted when they come to the realization that there is no hope that the kidneys will miraculously begin to function again. They may experience loss of self-esteem and feelings of helplessness and inadequacy as they come to recognize that they are dependent on the dialysis machine for their existence. Fears of death may then conflict with fears of continuing to live a life sustained by dialysis with its subsequent restrictions. Many individuals reach a stage of acceptance in which limitations and complica-tions of dialysis are incorporated into their daily lives. Even when individuals reach this stage of adjustment, however, they may experi-ence alternating periods of depression.

Anger and hostility are frequent manifes-tations of conflicts between dependency and independence—even conflicts between liv-ing and dying. Feelings of hostility may be expressed openly, but they may also be inter-nalized as individuals on dialysis realize the degree of their dependence not only on a machine, but also on those who provide their care. These internalized feelings can be self-destructive if individuals rebel against the necessary care and treatment. Feelings of sad-ness, hopelessness, and despair may become so severe that individuals with chronic kidney disease consider suicide as a way to resolve the problems surrounding the condition. Sui-cide attempts may be subtle and overt, such as nonadherence to diet, taking in too much fluid, skipping dialysis treatment, or in other ways failing to cooperate with treatment.

Transplantation involves a number of psy-chological issues as well. Individuals identi-fied as eligible recipients of a transplanted kidney are often elated about the anticipated improvement in their quality of life after the transplantation. Consequently, rejection of the transplanted kidney can be devastating. Even if rejection does not occur and quality of life is significantly improved, individuals with a transplanted kidney may express disappoint-ment that long-term care and evaluation are still necessary. In addition, they may be disappointed if transplantation has not restored the state of health that was theirs prior to the onset of chronic kidney disease. Even after the initial postoperative period, the chance of later rejection or the risk that infection will damage the transplanted kidney may be a source of anxiety.

Individuals having transplantation may have unmet expectations after surgery. Infection, rejection, or other complications may affect their energy level, their ability to work, and their sense of well-being. Loss of work time, side effects of medications, and the high cost of medications and medical care may be surprising and disappointing to both individuals and their families. If complications prevent a return to what they perceive as "normalcy" they may feel they have simply traded one set of problems for another. Individuals may also go through several stages of adjustment after transplantation.

Despite the significant psychological preparation that usually is implemented prior to transplantation, postsurgical psychological reactions may still occur. If the donor is a family member or friend of the recipient, the relationship may be altered. At times the relationship is strengthened, but it may also become weakened. Recipients may experience guilt, anxiety, or depression because of the donation of the kidney they received. If potential donors felt pressure, either real or imagined, to donate a kidney, they may experience stress, conflict, or guilt, especially if they decided to decline, or resentment if they donated their kidney under duress (Hanto, 2007). If the kidney was received from a deceased donor, recipients may have fantasies about embodying the spirit of someone who is dead. Whether the transplant was from a living or deceased donor, recipients may still feel that the kidney is foreign to them.

Individuals with kidney failure face profound changes in their daily activities. When kidney function is impaired or nonexistent, intake of foods and fluids must be carefully monitored. Such restrictions are necessary to minimize the amount of waste products and to avoid the presence of too much or too little fluid in the body. In chronic renal failure or chronic kidney disease, the kidney is no longer able to excrete wastes adequately, so total fluid intake between dialysis sessions must also be monitored. Fluid intake includes not only beverages, but also water contained in foods. Individuals are weighed before and after each dialysis treatment to monitor fluid gain so that the dialysis procedure may be adjusted accordingly.

Although there are no limitations or restrictions regarding sexual activity, sexual dysfunction is common in many individuals on dialysis (Stewart, 2006). Some men with chronic kidney disease experience impotence or have a diminished interest in sexual activities. Women with chronic kidney disease often report general disinterest or diminished interest in sexual activities, or a decreased response to sexual stimulation. Sexual dysfunction among individuals on dialysis probably results from a combination of generally poor health and emotional reactions to a life-threatening illness. Reproductive capacity of both men and women on dialysis is severely diminished. Sexual function may improve after kidney transplant, however, and conception is possible. If the transplant is rejected or the individual is heavily medicated, sexual function may be impaired.

Kidney conditions may not affect individuals' social activities until the kidneys become dysfunctional, causing restrictions or alterations in regular activities. Although family, friends, and associates play an important supportive role in individuals' adjustment to kidney failure, an overindulgent attitude can impede individuals' return to the earlier level of independence. Individuals on dialysis may have to alter activities, both because of their physical condition and because of the dialysis schedule. Those with shunts should avoid any activity that could expose the shunt area to potential injury. Because heat intolerance is often associated with chronic kidney disease, activities requiring exposure to heat should be avoided.

Previously existing relationship problems may be amplified after a diagnosis of chronic kidney disease. The additional stress brought on by dialysis or the wait for transplantation may intensify discord if it exists. If dialysis is conducted at home, the family member assisting with dialysis may feel burdened and strained by the added responsibility and regimen of the dialysis program, given that activities must be programmed around the schedule. Individuals' physical complaints, fatigue, and loss of interest in sexual activities may compound the problem. Although financial assistance for dialysis is usually available through government or private agencies, the overall financial burden imposed by medical bills, dialysis, and lost income if the individual with kidney disease is not able to continue working may put additional stress on relationships.

Even if individuals feel well enough to participate in social activities, many activities may need to be altered because of dietary and fluid restrictions. Individuals may be reluctant to accept the dinner invitations of friends because of dietary restrictions, for example, or they may themselves give up entertaining because of limitations associated with their condition. Increasing social isolation can exacerbate loss of self-esteem, feelings of depression, and hopelessness.

Vacations are still possible, but require careful planning for individuals who are on hemodialysis. Dialysis units near the vacation spot must be located, and arrangements must be made for dialysis at the center prior to departure. Peritoneal dialysis, although offering more flexibility, also requires that individuals plan for travel. Depending on the amount of time away and the method of travel, they may need to prearrange shipment of dialysate or a cycling machine to their destination.

Although transplantation can free individuals from some limitations, other issues may arise. If the donor is a family member or friend, a strong bond may develop between the donor and the recipient; in some cases, however, problems may arise in the relationship. The donor may resent the attention paid to the recipient after the transplant or may feel abandoned. The recipient, by contrast, may have feelings of guilt because of the potential jeopardy to the donor, who is left with only one kidney.

Vocational Issues in Chronic Kidney Disease

As chronic kidney disease progresses and symptoms become more pronounced, the impact on vocational function increases. Fatigue may necessitate a shortened workday or rest periods during the day. In addition, problems of impaired judgment, difficulty with memory, or irritability may interfere with adequate job performance. Peripheral neuropathy may make it difficult or impossible to perform tasks such as lifting or to complete tasks that require manual dexterity.

Individuals on dialysis may need a flexible work schedule to accommodate the dialysis schedule. Many dialysis centers operate 24 hours each day, enabling individuals to arrange dialysis in off-hours. Blood access routes, such as fistulas, require protection, so occupations that pose a potential threat of damage to the fistula should be avoided. Fatigue or the decreased ability to walk caused by peripheral neuropathy may necessitate a change to a more sedentary line of work. Environmental issues should also be considered. Specifically, work that requires exposure to high temperatures should be avoided because of the heat intolerance associated with kidney diseases.

After transplant, many individuals are able to return to work. In other instances, complications related to immunosuppressant drugs, such as infection or fatigue, may make returning to work more difficult. Sometimes, because of the cost of the medications that are an inevitable part of the post-transplant protocol, individuals may be reluctant to return to work if it means they might lose benefits as a result of having a higher income.

■ DIAGNOSTIC PROCEDURES FOR CONDITIONS OF THE KIDNEY AND URINARY TRACT

Urinalysis

Urine may be examined by direct visualization, under a microscope, or through other laboratory tests. The urinalysis report contains information about the concentration, acidity, and appearance of the urine, as well as the presence of any other components such as protein, sugar, blood, bacteria, or various types of cells. A urinalysis not only provides a gross estimate of kidney function, but also permits identification of other potential problems (e.g., infection) or systemic conditions (e.g., diabetes) that may exist.

A urinalysis is often a screening test to help determine what, if any, other tests are needed. Collection of urine can be external or, if a sterile specimen (one that is uncontaminated by organisms outside the urinary tract) is needed, can occur through a tube or catheter passed through the external opening (urinary meatus) into the bladder.

Urine Culture

Laboratory examination of a sterile urine specimen—a urine culture, helps to determine whether there is an infection within the urinary tract and, if so, which organisms are causing the infection. Specimens for a urine culture are usually obtained through catheterization.

Blood Urea Nitrogen (BUN)

Measuring the level of urea nitrogen (a waste product of protein metabolism) in the blood can be helpful in evaluation of kidney function. The kidneys normally excrete urea nitrogen, so elevated urea nitrogen in the blood indicates potential kidney impairment. The urea level may also be elevated in conditions other than kidney disease. For example, elevated urea nitrogen levels may be apparent in starvation, dehydration, or conditions in which the blood supply to the kidneys is poor.

Serum Creatinine

Creatinine is a waste product of a high-energy compound (creatine phosphate) found in skeletal muscle tissue. It is usually filtered out of the blood through the kidney, so elevation in creatinine levels in the blood indicates damage to a large number of nephrons. Determination of the creatinine level is a more sensitive test than BUN level and is a better reflection of kidney function.

Creatinine Clearance Test

The creatinine clearance test is used to determine the kidneys' glomerular filtration rate. It involves a comparison of the amount of creatinine in the blood serum (serum creatinine) with the amount of creatinine excreted in the urine over a specified period of time. For this test, individuals collect and save all of their urine during a specified period of time. Blood tests are performed at various points during that period, and the amounts of creatinine in the blood serum and in the urine are compared. A decreased creatinine clearance rate indicates decreased glomerular function and, therefore, kidney dysfunction. This rate is a better indicator of kidney function than is the measurement of serum creatinine alone. Creatinine clearance tests may be used to diagnose kidney dysfunction or to evaluate the progress of kidney disease.

Cystoscopy

A **urologist** (a physician who specializes in diagnosis and the treatment of conditions of the urinary tract) may visualize the urethra and bladder directly through a special tube, called a cystoscope, inserted through the urinary meatus and urethra into the bladder. This procedure, which is called **cystoscopy**, can be used either as a diagnostic procedure or as a part of treatment. It may be performed on an outpatient or inpatient basis and may be performed under local or general anesthesia. The cystoscopic examination makes it possible to identify any abnormalities in the internal structure of the bladder, to remove foreign objects or calculi from the bladder, to remove tumors or other abnormal tissue from the bladder, or to perform a retrograde pyelogram.

Intravenous Pyelogram

Radiologic examination of the kidneys, ureters, and bladder through an intravenous pyelogram may be done on an outpatient basis. During this test, a special dye is injected into a vein in the individual's arm. The dye is filtered by the kidney and excreted through the urinary tract, during which time x-ray films are taken at intervals for approximately one hour. The intravenous pyelogram helps to identify not only any structural abnormalities of the kidney, but also any problems with passage of the dye through the urinary system. Because some individuals are hypersensitive to components of the dye and may have severe allergic reactions to it, questions about known allergies and skin tests are usually routine prior to testing.

Kidney, Ureters, and Bladder Roentgenography (KUB)

A simple x-ray of the kidney, ureters, and bladder is called a KUB. The x-ray film outlines the size, shape, and location of these structures, but does not indicate kidney function.

Renal Angiography

To examine the vascular function of the kidney, a diagnostic procedure called renal angiography may be done. This procedure is performed by inserting a needle into the femoral artery (located in the groin). A small catheter is passed through the needle into the artery and advanced until it reaches the renal arteries. Dye is then injected through the catheter, and x-ray films are taken at 2- to 3-second intervals to examine the functioning of the renal artery.

Noncontrast Computed Tomography

Noncontrast computed tomography is a radiographic procedure, that uses no contrast media to visualize a body part or organ—in this case, the kidney. It produces three-dimensional pictures of cross sections of the organ.

Renal Biopsy

In some cases, it is necessary to remove a small piece of kidney tissue for the diagnosis of kidney disease. This procedure, which is called a renal biopsy, may be done in several ways. One method involves a surgical incision over the kidney so that the physician can directly view the kidney and remove the specimen. Because this procedure is done under general anesthesia in a hospital setting, it has a prolonged recuperation period. The second, more commonly used method involves the insertion of a specially designed needle through the skin over the kidney. The needle is then inserted into the kidney, and a small amount of kidney tissue is removed. This technique, which is called percutaneous renal biopsy, is generally performed under a local anesthetic in a hospital setting. Because it requires no incision or general anesthesia, only limited recuperation time is needed.

Retrograde Pyelography

Retrograde pyelograms are performed to assess function of the kidneys and ureters, and to detect possible abnormalities or obstructions in the collecting system. During a retrograde pyelogram, a small catheter is inserted through a tube (cystoscope), which is then directed into the ureters to the pelvis of the kidney. A special dye is injected through the catheter, and x-ray films are taken to visualize the collecting system. This procedure may be done on an outpatient or inpatient basis.

▨ PSYCHOSOCIAL ISSUES IN KIDNEY AND URINARY TRACT CONDITIONS

Not all kidney conditions are life-threatening, and not all impose major changes in functional capacity. Although they may cause some pain and discomfort, conditions such as cystitis frequently have no functional or psychological sequelae. Chronic kidney disease, however, has profound effects on all areas of individuals' lives, causing significant psychological stress.

Psychological changes are associated both with the emotional reactions to a life-threatening disease and with the physiological changes that occur with chronic kidney disease. Emotional reactions to chronic kidney disease vary. Mourning loss of part of body function, loss of control, feelings of disconnectedness, and anger are all emotional reactions commonly

reported (Moua, 2000). Elevated levels of toxic waste in the blood can produce cognitive changes, such as impaired judgment, drowsiness, and difficulty with concentration. Other possible cognitive changes include memory loss, speech impairments, and irritability. The physical discomfort associated with dialysis—such as interrupted sleep patterns, nausea, lethargy, and shortness of breath—may increase the individual's psychological distress. Individuals eligible for kidney transplant may also experience stress while waiting for a transplant as well as fear of rejection if the transplant actually takes place.

Uncertainty is also an issue in chronic kidney disease. Treatment choices are not always final. Individuals who choose peritoneal dialysis rather than hemodialysis may need to switch if complications from peritoneal dialysis occur. Individuals using hemodialysis may later consider a kidney transplant should an organ become available. Even after individuals receive a kidney transplant, uncertainty remains because there is always the chance that rejection of the transplant may occur.

Many kidney and urinary tract conditions require lifestyle changes during the acute phase of the condition; however, after treatment, few limitations may exist. The exception is those individuals with chronic kidney disease for whom lifestyle implications are profound. Not only are there stringent dietary restrictions, but the requirement of regular dialysis treatments restricts individuals' freedom of time. Even if an individual receives a transplant that succeeds, the medical regimen is demanding both before and after the transplant,

Exercise can increase strength and endurance and reduce stress. Although individuals with chronic kidney disease may be unable to tolerate as much physical activity as before the disease struck them, exercise programs individually tailored to and prescribed for individuals' specific needs and abilities may be possible. Although many of individuals' daily activities can be continued, individuals should approach activities with flexibility, given that their physical tolerance for various activities may be unpredictable from day to day.

Desire for sexual activity may change for individuals with chronic kidney disease both because of side effects of medications or because of physical manifestations of the disease itself. Sexual desire may also change for emotional reasons. If individuals experience depression or anxiety, or if relationship problems exist, sexual desire and/or function may also be altered.

Traveling is possible whether individuals are using hemodialysis or peritoneal dialysis if arrangements are made well in advance. Individuals on hemodialysis must locate a dialysis unit in the area to be visited so that dialysis sessions can be scheduled prior to their arrival. Individuals with peritoneal dialysis need to make plans for backup medical care as well as arrange for availability of dialysate and a cycling machine, if used.

Many conditions of the kidney and urinary tract have few implications for social functioning. There may be significant effects, however, for individuals with chronic kidney disease. Chronic kidney disease is a serious condition whose severity fluctuates but that requires lifelong management and treatment for survival. Dialysis regimens, dietary restrictions, and medications may limit activities and socialization to some degree. For these reasons, pre-existing social or relationship problems are frequently made worse by the problems associated with chronic kidney disease.

Physiologic changes, treatment demands, and the chronic nature of chronic kidney disease affects not just individuals with the condition, but the whole family unit. Family members' reactions and stability can either help or hinder individuals' acceptance of their condition. Family members can be over-solici-

tous or rejecting, making it more difficult for individuals to reestablish their own emotional balance and their role within the family. Individuals and their families may focus on the chronic kidney disease as the center of family functioning. They may require assistance in developing a life that incorporates the disease into the family structure, rather than overwhelming it.

Individuals with chronic kidney disease may withdraw from family and friends owing to feelings of inadequacy. They may struggle to resolve qualms about their dependence on dialysis and on others for assistance with their treatment. Individuals with unresolved dependency conflicts may become uncooperative and ill tempered. Rather than confronting the individual, family and friends may excuse his or her behavior, reinforcing the sick role.

■ VOCATIONAL ISSUES IN KIDNEY AND URINARY TRACT CONDITIONS

Many kidney and urinary tract disorders have no long-term impact on individuals' ability to work. Kidney failure, however, affects psychological, social, and vocational function, such that, a variety of alterations in individuals' daily life may become necessary. The impact of treatment or other stressors associated with the condition may contribute to disruption of job performance (Murphy, 2006). The degree to which kidney disease affects employment depends on individuals' occupation, previous work history, medical condition and treatment, and status of any secondary disabilities. Individuals with early-stage kidney failure can generally continue their previous jobs, especially if the job is sedentary and does not require strenuous activity. Individuals with chronic kidney disease may experience reduced work tolerance owing to impaired concentration and fatigue. If they are no longer capable of performing the physical activity that the work requires, a job modification or change may be necessary.

Work schedule flexibility may be necessary to accommodate recurring medical problems, periods of hospitalizations, dialysis treatment, and time away due to normal medical check-ups. At times financial disincentives or employer concerns about lost work time may also be barriers to employment.

Individuals with chronic kidney disease who experience a decreased attention span or an inability to concentrate may require jobs that accommodate these limitations. Excess heat in the work environment should be avoided, as individuals with chronic kidney disease are unable to adequately regulate body heat. Individuals with peripheral neuropathy as a result of kidney failure may have difficulty with manual dexterity or walking. In addition, individuals with a fistula for hemodialysis may need to limit the use of the arm containing the access route.

CASE STUDIES

Case 1

Mrs. M. is a 29-year-old female who has worked as a certified nursing assistant for the last 9 years. She was diagnosed with Type I diabetes when she was 10 years old and also has hypertension. Her kidney function has continued to decline over the last few years, and recently Mrs. M. has been told that she is in Stage 3 renal failure. It is recommended that she begin hemodialysis.

1. Given Mrs. M's type of work, which specific factors related to her medical condition would you consider when establishing a rehabilitation plan?

2. Which factors regarding hemodialysis would you consider?

3. Are there special accommodations that will need to be made if Mrs. M. is to continue in her current line of employment while still on dialysis?

Case 2

Mr. B. is a 48-year-old male who had been in dialysis for the past five years, and who recently had a kidney transplant. He continued to work as a high school history teacher throughout his period of dialysis and is looking forward to returning to his job on a full-time basis.

1. Which specific factors might you consider in evaluating Mr. B.'s rehabilitation potential?

2. Is his goal of returning to work full-time realistic? Why or why not?

3. Which specific issues related to his transplant would you consider when helping Mr. B. establish a rehabilitation plan?

■ REFERENCES

Appel, G. B. (2004). Glomerular disorders. In L. Goldman & D. Ausiello (Eds.), *Cecil textbook of medicine* (pp. 726–733). Philadelphia: W. B. Saunders.

Barrett, B. J., & Parfrey, P. S. (2006). Preventing nephropathy induced by contrast medium. *New England Journal of Medicine, 354*(4), 379–386.

Barsoum, R. S. (2006). Chronic kidney disease in the developing world. *New England Journal of Medicine, 354*(10), 997–999.

Bonventre, J. V. (2002). Daily hemodialysis: Will treatment each day improve the outcome in patients with acute renal failure. *New England Journal of Medicine, 346*(5), 362–364.

Cattran, D., & Turner, P. (2007). Primary glomerular disease. In R. E. Rakel & E. T. Bope (Eds.), *Conn's current therapy* (pp. 808–813). Philadelphia: W. B. Saunders.

Delmonico, F. L. (2004). Exchanging kidneys: Advances in living-donor transplantation. *New England Journal of Medicine, 350*(18), 1812–1814.

Drueke, T. B., Locatelli, F., Clyne, N., Eckardt, K. U., Macdougall, I. C., Tsakiris, D., et al. (2006). Normalization of hemoglobin level in patients with chronic kidney disease and anemia. *New England Journal of Medicine, 355*(20), 2071–2084.

El Nahas, A. M., Harris, K., & Anderson, S. (Eds.). (2000). *Mechanisms and clinical management of chronic renal failure* (2nd ed.). New York: Oxford University.

Franke, G. H., Reimer, J., Philipp, T., & Heemann, U. (2003). Aspects of quality of life through end-stage renal disease. *Quality of Life Research 12,* 103–115.

Hanto, D. W. (2007). Ethical challenges posed by the solicitation of deceased and living organ donors. *New England Journal of Medicine, 356*(10), 1062–1066.

Hariharan, S., Johnson, C. P., Bresnahan, B. A., Taranto, S. E., McIntosh, M. J., & Stablein, D. (2000). Improved graft survival after renal transplantation in the United States, 1988–1996. *New England Journal of Medicine, 342,* 605–612.

Hegarty, N. J., & Streem, S. B. (2007). Renal calculi. In R. E. Rakel & E. T. Bope (Eds.), *Conn's current therapy* (pp. 1062–1066). Philadelphia: W. B. Saunders.

Herbert, L. A. (2006). Optimizing ACE-inhibitor therapy for chronic kidney disease. *New England Journal of Medicine, 354*(2), 189–191.

Hicks, L. S., Cleary, P. D., Epstein, A. M., & Ayanian, J. Z. (2004). Differences in health-related quality of life and treatment preferences among black and white patients with end-stage renal disease. *Quality of Life Research, 13,* 1129–1137.

Himmelfarb, J. (2002). Success and challenge in dialysis therapy. *New England Journal of Medicine, 347*(25), 2068–2070.

Hou, F. F., Zhang, X., Zhang, G. H., Xie, D., Chen, P. Y., Zhang, W. R., et al. (2006). Efficacy and safety of benazepril for advanced chronic renal insufficiency. *New England Journal of Medicine, 354*(2), 131–140.

Ifudu, O. (1998). Care of patients undergoing hemodialysis. *New England Journal of Medicine, 339*(15), 1054–1062.

Jafar, T. H. (2006). The growing burden of chronic kidney disease in Pakistan. *New England Journal of Medicine, 354*(10), 995–997.

Juknevicius, I., & Hruska, K. A. (2004). Renal calculi (nephrolithiasis). In L. Goldman & D. Ausiello (Eds.), *Cecil textbook of medicine* (22nd ed., pp. 761–767). Philadelphia: W. B. Saunders.

Kinchen, K. S., Sadler, J., Fink, N., Brookmeyer, R., Klag, M. J., Levey, A. S., et al. (2002). The timing of specialist evaluation in chronic kidney disease and mortality. *Anuals of Internal Medicine, 137,* 479–486.

Klahr, S. (2004). Obstructive uropathy. In L. Goldman & D. Ausiello (Eds.), *Cecil textbook of medicine* (pp. 740–744). Philadelphia: W. B. Saunders.

Kraut, J. A. (2007). Chronic renal failure. In R. E. Rakel & E. T. Bope (Eds.), *Conn's Current Therapy* (pp. 845–852). Philadelphia: W. B. Saunders.

Luke, R. G. (2004). Chronic renal failure. In L. Goldman & D. Ausiello (Eds.) *Cecil Textbook of Medicine* (22nd ed., pp. 708–716). Philadelphia: W. B. Saunders.

Marsden, P. A. (2003). Predicting outcomes after renal transplantation: New tools and old tools. *New England Journal of Medicine, 349*(2), 182–184.

McCammon , K. A., & McCammon, C. F. (2007). Acute pyelonephritis. In R. E. Rakel & E. T. Bope (Eds.), *Conn's current therapy* (pp. 813–816). Philadelphia: W. B. Saunders.

Mitch, W. E. (2004). Acute renal failure. In L. Goldman & D. Ausiello (Eds.), *Cecil textbook of medicine* (pp. 703–708). Philadelphia: W. B. Saunders.

Moua, M. N. (2000). End-stage. *Rehabilitation Counseling Bulletin, 45*(1), 53–55.

Murphy, F. (2006). A care study exploring a patient's non-compliance to haemodialysis. *British Journal of Nursing, 15*(14), 773–776.

National Kidney Foundation. (2002). K/DOQI clinical practice guidelines for chronic kidney disease: evaluation, classification and stratification. *American Journal of Kidney Disease, 39* (suppl), S1–S266.

National Kidney Foundation. (2007). http://www.kidney.org/atoz/atoz/tem.cfm?id=95

Neelakantappa, K., & Lowenstein, J. (2005). Chronic kidney disease. In H. H. Zaretsky, E. F. Richter, & M. G. Eisenberg (Eds.), *Medical aspects of disability* (3rd ed., pp. 563–582). New York: Springer.

Norrby, R. (2004). Urinary tract infections. In L. Goldman & D. Ausiello (Eds). *Cecil textbook of medicine* (22nd ed., pp. 1909–1913). Philadelphia: W. B. Saunders.

Owen, W. F., Pereira, B. J. G., & Savegh, M. H. (Eds). (2000). Dialysis and transplantation: A companion to Brenner and Rector's *The kidney*. Philadelphia: W. B. Saunders.

Pascual, M., Theruvath, T., Kawai, T., Tolkoff-Rubin, N., & Cosimi, A. B. (2002). Strategies to improve long-term outcomes after renal transplantation. *New England Journal of Medicine, 346*(8), 580–588.

Schiffle, H., Lang, S. M., & Fischer, R. (2002). Daily hemodialysis and the outcome of acute renal failure. *New England Journal of Medicine, 346*(5), 305–310.

Soulillou, J. P. (2001). Immune monitoring for rejection of kidney transplants. *New England Journal of Medicine, 344*(13), 1006–1007.

Soulillou, J. .P., & Giral, M. (2006), Influence of graft characteristics on the outcome of kidney transplantation. *New England Journal of Medicine, 354*(19), 2060–2062.

Stevens, L. A., Coresh, J., Greene, T., & Levey, A. S. (2006). Assessing kidney function: Measured and estimated glomerular filtration rate. *New England Journal of Medicine, 354*(23), 2473–2483.

Stevens, L. A., & Levey, A. S. (2005). Chronic kidney disease in the elderly: How to assess risk. *New England Journal of Medicine, 352*(20), 2122–2124.

Stewart, M. (2006). Narrative literature review: Sexual dysfunction in the patient on hemodialyis. *Nephrology Nursing Journal, 33*(6), 631–641.

Tolkoff-Rubin, N. S., & Goes, N. (2004). In L. Goldman & D. Ausiello (Eds.), *Cecil textbook of medicine* (22nd ed., pp. 716–726). Philadelphia: W. B. Saunders.

U.S. Renal Data System. (2006). *USRDS 2006 Annual data report: Atlas of end-stage renal disease in the United States*. Bethesda, MD: National Institutes of Health, National Institute of Diabetes and Digestive and Kidney Diseases.

Weisbord, S. D., & Palevsky, P. M. (2007). Acute renal failure. In R. E. Rakel & E. T. Bope, (Eds.), *Conn's current therapy* (pp. 837–845). Philadelphia: W. B. Saunders.

Chapter 16

Conditions of the Musculoskeletal System

■ STRUCTURE AND FUNCTION OF THE MUSCULOSKELETAL SYSTEM

The Skeletal System

Bones make up the general framework of the body. The skeletal system, which consists of 206 bones, supports the surrounding tissues and assists in movement by providing leverage and attachment for muscles (see Figure 16-1). It also protects vital organs, such as the heart and brain. The tough outer covering of bone is called the **periosteum**. Bones also have a network of sensory nerves and a network of tiny vessels to supply blood. They serve many functions other than support, movement, and protection.

Red blood cells are manufactured in the red bone marrow by means of *hematopoiesis.* Bone also stores calcium and other mineral salts. New bone is constantly being produced and old bone replaced, creating a dynamic relationship between calcium in the bone and calcium in the blood.

Types of Bone

Bones are classified according to shape. Long bones are found in the arms and legs (e.g., the humerus and the femur). Short bones are found in the hands and feet (e.g., the carpals

and the tarsal). Flat bones are those like the skull (**cranium**) and ribs, while irregular bones have differing shapes, such as the vertebrae and **mandible** (jaw bone).

The **vertebrae** (irregular bones that surround the spinal cord) support the head and trunk of the body, protect the spinal cord, and enable bending and flexing. The seven vertebrae at the neck and upper back are called *cervical vertebrae.* The 12 vertebrae that extend from the upper to lower back are called **thoracic vertebrae**. In the lower back there are five **lumbar vertebrae**; a bony prominence called the *sacrum*, which consists of fused bone; and the **coccyx**, or small residual "tail bone," which extends from the end of the sacrum.

Connective Tissue

Connective tissue supports and (as its name implies) connects other tissues and tissue parts. In addition to bones, ligaments, tendons, and cartilage serve as connective tissue. **Ligaments** are tough bands of fiber that connect bones at the joint site and provide stability during movement. **Tendons** are bands of tissue that connect muscle to bone, enabling muscle movement. *Cartilage* is a dense type of connective tissue that creates form, maintains

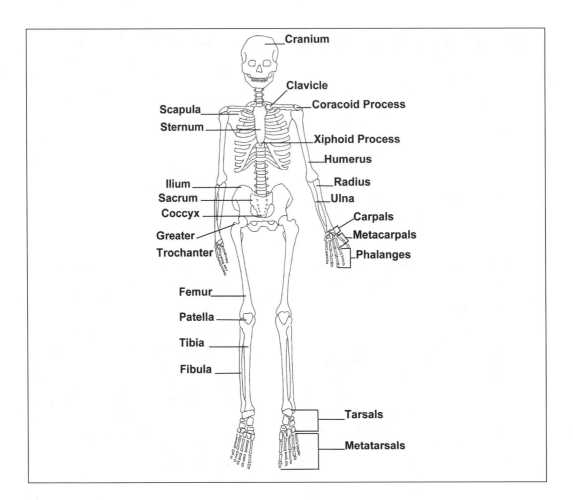

Figure 16-1 The skeleton

structure, and can withstand considerable tension. Several different types of cartilage exist. For example, cartilage is found between the vertebral disks of the spine and in the joint of the knee to absorb shock and prevent friction. In addition, the cartilage in the external ear and nose provide form to these structures.

Between each two vertebrae, which surround the spinal cord, are disks of cartilage called *intervertebral disks* that act as cushions against shock. The tough, fibrous outer portion of the disk is called the *annulus*, and the spongy inner portion is called the *nucleus pulposus*. Vertebrae are connected by ligaments

and are surrounded in part by a joint capsule containing synovial fluid like other synovial joints.

Joints

A **joint** is the place where two or more bones are bound together. The coming together of two bones at a joint is called **articulation**. Some joints, such as those in the skull, are fibrous (fixed), meaning that they provide no movement. Other joints, such as the *pubis symphysis* (pubic bone) in the pelvis, are *cartilaginous* (contain cartilage) and provide slight movement.

Synovial joints are freely movable, enabling both motion and change of position (Figure 16-2). They are enclosed in a sac called the **bursa**, which is lined with a *synovial membrane*. This membrane secretes **synovial fluid**, which aids joint movement by acting as a lubricant. Synovial fluid also helps cushion the joint against the shock produced by joint movement. *Articular cartilage* lines the end of each bone, helping to absorb shock; it receives its nourishment from the synovial fluid.

Synovial joints are capable of many types of movements (see Figure 16-3):

- **Circumduction**: circular movement
- **Eversion**: movement in which a body part is turned outward
- **Inversion**: movement in which a body part is turned inward
- **Flexion**: bending movement
- **Extension**: straightening movement
- **Abduction**: movement of a body part away from the midline of the body
- **Adduction**: movement of a body part toward the midline of the body
- **Ulnar deviation**: lateral movement of the hand away from the body
- **Radial deviation**: lateral movement of the hand inward, toward the body

- **Pronation**: turning movement of a body part downward
- **Supination**: turning movement of a body part upward
- **Dorsiflexion**: backward movement of a body part

The type of motion of a particular synovial joint depends on the type of joint:

- *Circular motion* is provided by ball-and-socket joints, such as those found in the hip and shoulder.
- *Back-and-forth motion* is provided by hinge joints, such as those in the elbow and knee.
- *Gliding motion* is provided by joints of the vertebrae.
- *Pivotal motion* is provided by vertebrae that connect the head and the spine.

The Muscular System

Several types of muscles are found in the body. Involuntary muscles work automatically, such as the cardiac muscle (myocardium) of the heart and the smooth muscle found in the digestive tract. In contrast, *striated* (skeletal muscle), which makes up 40% to 50% of an individual's body weight, is under voluntary control.

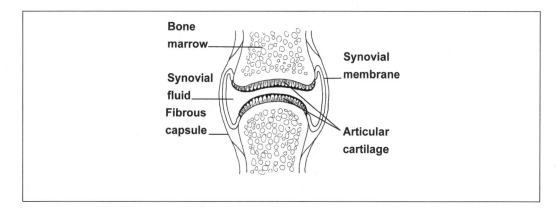

Figure 16-2   A synovial joint

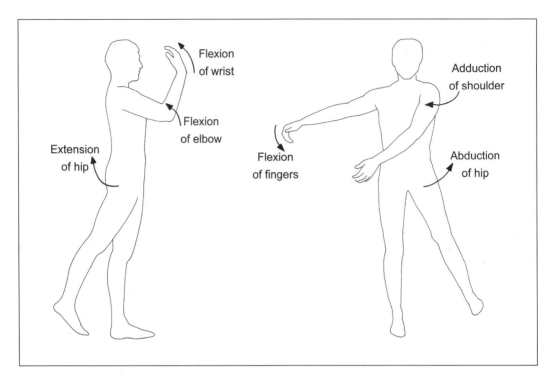

Figure 16-3   Movement of synovial joints

A *muscle sheath* (a hard band of connective tissue) contains blood vessels and nerve fibers and surrounds every muscle. Each of the two ends of the muscle is attached to a different bone. The muscle attachment closer to the midline of the body is called the *origin* of the muscle, while the attachment of the end farther from the midline of the body is called the **insertion.**

Muscles produce movement by the contraction of opposite muscle groups. Muscles are classified by their function. Muscles that bend a limb are called **flexors**; those that straighten a limb are **extensors**. Muscles that move a limb laterally, away from the body, are called **abductors**, while muscles that move a limb closer to the body are called **adductors**. Muscles that bend a body part backward are called **dorsiflexors**. Because of continuous nerve stimulation to muscle, muscles main-

tain a partial state of contraction (tone) even at rest, when they aren't being used.

■ CONDITIONS OF THE MUSCULOSKELETAL SYSTEM

Trauma

Fractures

Fractures of bone result in pain and immobility. Depending on which bone is fractured and what type of fracture occurs, the functional consequences may be either temporary or, in some cases, permanent. Individuals with chronic conditions may be especially vulnerable to fractures if immobility associated with their condition increases demineralization of bone or because of physiological processes involved in the condition itself (such as in osteoporosis or certain types of cancer) (Kyle & Rajkumar, 2007).

Any break or disruption in the continuity of bone is termed a *fracture*. Several types of fractures are distinguished, with varying levels of severity (see Figure 16-4):

- *Closed (simple) fracture* is an uncomplicated break in a bone with no breaking of skin.
- *Open (compound) fracture* is a break in a bone in which the skin is broken so that the bone protrudes through it.
- *Complete fracture* is a break in a bone that extends through the bone from one side to the other, including the periosteum, or outer cover.
- *Incomplete (partial) fracture* is a break that does not extend all the way through the bone.
- *Transverse fracture* is a fracture that extends straight across the bone.
- *Oblique fracture* is a fracture across the bone at a slant angle.
- *Spiral fracture* occurs in a spiral around the bone and is usually caused by a twisting injury.
- *Impacted fracture* is a break in which one portion of the bone is impacted, or forcibly driven, into another portion of the bone.
- *Comminuted fracture* is a break in which the bone has been shattered, leaving fragments of bone at the site of the break.
- *Displaced fracture* refers to a break in a bone in which the two ends of the bone are separated.
- *Complicated fracture* refers to a break in a bone in which the tissue surrounding the bone, such as blood vessels and nerves, has also been injured.
- *Compression fracture* refers to a break in which the ends of the bones are pressed against each other. Compression fractures often occur in the vertebrae.

- *Pathologic fracture* refers to a break in a bone owing to changes in the bone that are associated with another condition.
- *Colles' fracture* refers to a break in a bone near the wrist.
- *Stress fracture* is a small break in a bone that occurs as the result of prolonged or unaccustomed activity.

Some fractures may be treated by *closed reduction*, a procedure in which bone fragments are realigned manually, without surgery, and immobilized with a plaster cast. Other fractures must be treated by **open reduction**, a procedure in which bone fragments are realigned and stabilized surgically. Traction may be used in combination with either closed or open reduction.

Many fractures heal well and result in no permanent functional consequence. In other instances, complications can occur, leading to significant functional consequences. For example, bone edges or fragments of a compound, displaced, or comminuted fracture may injure tissue or nerves in the surrounding area, causing permanent damage. In fractures of large bones, such as the femur, blood loss can be significant. Open or compound fractures can become infected, leading to **osteomyelitis** (infection of the bone). In addition, when individuals with other chronic conditions fracture a bone, additional complications related to the fracture as well as the subsequent immobility imposed by the fracture can develop, posing a significant threat not only to function, but also to general health and well-being.

Dislocation

Displacement or separation of a bone from its regular joint position is called a **dislocation**. If the bone is not totally separated from the joint, the condition is called a **subluxation**. In addition to causing extreme pain, a dislocation causes a partial loss of movement at the

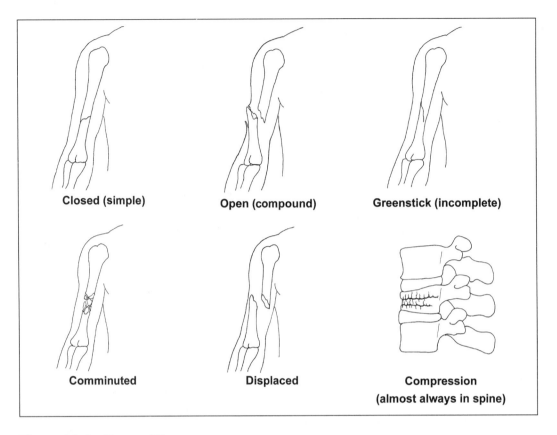

Figure 16-4 Types of fractures

joint and can impede the blood supply to the surrounding tissue.

Dislocations can result either from trauma or from a congenital weakness or irregularity of joint predisposing individuals to dislocation when a joint is moved a certain way. The shoulder and the hip are common sites of dislocation, although any joint can become dislocated.

Prompt intervention to correct joint dislocation is important to prevent complications, such as nerve damage or injury due to the decreased blood supply. The bones can usually be slipped back into place manually. If no damage has occurred to the nerves, blood vessels, or surrounding tissue, there are usually no permanent functional consequences. If

dislocations recur in the same joint, however, individuals may need to avoid movements that appear to contribute to the dislocation. When dislocation recurs frequently, surgical fixation of the joint may be necessary.

Contusions

Musculoskeletal injuries may not always involve bone; sometimes the injury involves underlying structures, such as the soft tissue under the skin. A **contusion** is a soft-tissue injury that results from a blunt, diffuse blow. Although the skin is not usually broken and no bones are broken, local hemorrhage with associated bruising, swelling, and damage to the deep soft tissue under the skin occurs. Bleeding under the skin is responsible for the purplish discoloration at the site of injury—the bruise (**ecchymosis**). When a major vessel or a muscle is injured, a **hematoma** (a sac filled with accumulated blood) may develop under the skin.

Strains and Sprains

Although the terms "strain" and "sprain" are often used interchangeably, they refer to two different types of injuries. A **strain** is an overstretching or overuse of tendons and muscles, while a **sprain** is an injury or overstress of a ligament and its attachment site.

Strains may be acute, resulting from a sudden twisting or wrenching movement, or they may occur with unaccustomed vigorous exercise. Chronic strain may be the result of repetitive muscle overuse. Individuals with strains may be treated with analgesics, muscle relaxants, or anti-inflammatory drugs. One goal of therapy is to increase muscle strengthening. Consequently, immobilization is usually not recommended.

Sprains are categorized as mild, moderate, or severe (first-, second-, or third-degree sprains). First- and second-degree sprains are usually treated with analgesics, anti-inflammatory agents, or muscle relaxants. Treatment of second-degree sprains may also include immobilization of the injured joint and therapeutic exercises and physical therapy to promote an early return to motion. A severe sprain can tear a ligament completely from its attachment and may require surgical repair. Most sprains heal spontaneously with rest and support of the body part affected (Chuan & Taylor, 2007).

Lacerations

An injury that has torn or cut the skin and underlying tissues is referred to as a **laceration**. Puncture and penetration injuries generally have a small entrance wound but cause extensive damage to tissues under the skin. Stabbing wounds and gunshot wounds are puncture wounds and penetration wounds, respectively.

The degree of functional consequence experienced with lacerations, puncture wounds, or penetration wounds depends on the injury's location; the amount of damage to the underlying tissues, such as nerves, blood vessels, and internal organs; and any associated complications, such as infection. The risk of infection depends on the source and circumstances of the injury.

Overuse and Repetitive-Motion Injuries
Bursitis, Tendonitis, and Tenosynovitis

Bursitis is associated with persistent mild injury and overuse of a joint (Colburn, 2007). The term **bursitis** refers to inflammation of the bursa (the sac that contains the synovial fluid in the synovial joints). It may be acute or chronic. Although bursitis may affect any synovial joint, it commonly occurs in the shoulder, elbow, wrist or hand, hip, or knee (Boulware, 2004).

Bursitis is characterized by pain and tenderness over the joint and by limitation of joint motion. Acute attacks may last for days to weeks, and they may recur. Splinting and rest of the joint are generally recommended. Bursitis may become chronic, causing varying degrees of functional consequence.

The term *tendonitis* describes a condition in which there is an inflammation of a tendon. The term **tenosynovitis** describes a condition in which there is an inflammation of the sheath of tissue that surrounds the tendon. The two conditions usually occur simultaneously. Although the exact cause is unknown, tendonitis may be associated with trauma, strain, or unaccustomed exercise. Its primary manifestation is pain on motion at the site of inflammation. Tendonitis usually subsides with appropriate management, although surgery may be indicated on rare occasions.

Carpal Tunnel Syndrome

Nerves (including the median, ulnar, and radial nerves) travel from the spinal cord to innervate the hands (Maher, 2007). These nerves are contained in small "tunnels" that may become narrowed, compressing the nerves. **Carpal tunnel syndrome** is a condition in which there is compression of the median nerve in the wrist, causing pain and **paresthesia** (a tingling, pricking sensation) in the hand. This condition is classified as a *compression* or *entrapment neuropathy*.

Carpal tunnel syndrome can be associated with various autoimmune conditions, such as rheumatoid arthritis (discussed later in this chapter); metabolic conditions, such as diabetes (see Chapter 11); heredity; or obesity. Activities involving rapid repetitive movement of the hands with few rest periods, or awkward or forceful movements, may contribute to the development of carpal tunnel syndrome (Simmons & Borsch, 2006). In most instances, they do not: Instead, individuals engaging in these activities may experience a condition called *repetitive-strain injury* (Steinmehl, 2006). Confirmation of carpal tunnel syndrome is made through evaluation based on case definition guidelines established by the National Institute of Occupational Safety and Health (NIOSH). These guidelines include positive findings on physical examination and nerve conduction studies that indicate median nerve damage irregularities (Werner, 2006).

With carpal tunnel syndrome, muscle strength in the hand may be weakened to the extent that individuals have difficulty opening jars or twisting lids. They may experience pain that can be dull and aching or that may radiate into the forearm. Individuals may complain of waking at night because the affected hand is numb. They may also complain of numbness in the hands in the morning, feeling they have to shake their hands to get the circulation back. Manifestations may be mild and of short duration or may become chronic.

Management of Carpal Tunnel Syndrome

Irreparable nerve damage may occur if carpal tunnel syndrome is left untreated. In mild cases, a wrist splint at night may be sufficient to relieve manifestations, along with medications such as nonsteroidal anti-inflammatory drugs (Colburn, 2007). If the splint does not interfere with activity, individuals may also wear it or another type of wrist support during the day. Corticosteroids are sometimes injected into the area if the splint is unsuccessful at relieving manifestations; however, any improvement may be only temporary. When the hand becomes weakened, or when manifestations become intolerable, surgery to relieve pressure on the nerve may be indicated (Griffin, 2004).

Vocational Issues in Carpal Tunnel Syndrome

Repetition, force, and posture are risk factors that can contribute to the development of carpal tunnel syndrome. Other risk factors—including conditions such as diabetes, arthritis, and obesity—may be more prevelant, however (Steinmehl, 2006). Because carpal tunnel syndrome is a compensable condition in most worker's compensation systems in the United States (Werner, 2006), evaluation is important to establish this diagnosis.

Carpal tunnel syndrome can become severe enough to limit individuals' ability to work. It can be of particular concern to individuals who rely on sign language as a major form of communication (Smith, Kress, & William, 2000). With continued exposure to risk factors without adequate care or rest, permanent damage to the soft tissue and nerves can result.

When carpal tunnel syndrome is related to activity, both the nature of the work and the amount of time spent on a task contribute to the potential for injury. If carpal tunnel syndrome is related to a specific activity, ergonomic modifications such as forearm support when typing, adjusting the height of the keyboard or work area, or positioning the hands differently may be indicated. For individuals with carpal tunnel syndrome that is aggravated by work-related activity, the factors in the work environment may need to be modified. Office workers and those using computer keyboards may need to take periodic rest breaks throughout the day. When using a desk and chair, different body positions may help reduce muscle fatigue and prevent exacerbation of manifestations of carpal tunnel syndrome. Individuals should avoid bent, extended, or twisted hand positions for long periods. When possible, they should alternate hands for work tasks and avoid awkward hand positions.

Degenerative Conditions

Osteoporosis

Osteoporosis is a metabolic condition in which the bone mass (the amount of bone) is reduced, causing bones to become weakened, fragile, and easily broken (Barzel, 2007; Prestwood & Raisz, 2002). In some instances, although there has been no bone fracture, individuals may experience aching in various bones and often have chronic backache. Vertebral fractures—a serious consequence of osteoporosis—can lead to acute and chronic back pain as well as structural irregularity of the spine (Meunier et al., 2004).

Individuals with osteoporosis commonly have no manifestations until a bone is broken as a result of minimal or no trauma. Frequent sites of bone fractures include the hips, especially in older or frail individuals, and the wrist (**Colles' fracture**). Crush or compression fractures may occur in the vertebrae (see Figure 16-4).

Risks for Osteoporosis

Osteoporosis commonly occurs in individuals after middle age. Nevertheless, secondary osteoporosis may occur as a result of other conditions, such as rheumatoid arthritis or multiple myeloma (see chapter 18) or as a side effect of the overuse or long-term use of alcohol, steroids, or other medications such as anticonvulsants. Individuals with chronic conditions in which they are nonambulatory or with conditions that require immobilization are also at higher risk of developing osteoporosis (Finkelstein, 2004). Women with physical and cognitive disabilities are at especially high risk for osteoporosis and osteoporosis-related fractures (Schrager, 2004).

Management of Osteoporosis

Osteoporosis is a progressive condition, but appropriate interventions may slow this deterioration process. Fractures related to osteoporosis can result in substantial morbidity and mortality (Solomon, Finkelstein, Katz, Mogun, & Avorn, 2003). Consequently, prevention is a key component of any plan to prevent functional consequences. The best intervention for osteoporosis is prevention through the daily intake of adequate amounts of dietary calcium; weight-bearing exercise throughout life; avoidance of long-term use of steroid medications, which promote bone loss; and prevention of falls (Boskey, 2001; Marcus, 2000).

When osteoporosis does occur, analgesics, heat, or rest may relieve the pain. In some instances, braces or splints may be indicated. Exercise that strengthens muscles, thereby providing additional support, may be beneficial. Although general activity is encouraged, heavy lifting or any activity that increases the risk of falls should be avoided.

Calcium supplements are usually prescribed for both men and women with osteoporosis. Women with osteoporosis may be given hormones to decrease bone loss and to increase absorption of calcium. When calcium absorption is impaired, supplemental vitamin D may also be given.

Osteoarthritis (Degenerative Joint Disease)

Osteoarthritis is a local joint condition, *not* a systemic condition. Although the term implies inflammation of a joint, inflammation is not present in all cases (Ehrlich, 2007). This condition was formerly called "degenerative joint disease," a term that has now largely been discarded.

Osteoarthritis is the culmination of all life events at the joints and, to some degree, occurs in almost all individuals past middle age. Not everyone affected has manifestations, however (Ehrlich, 2007). Although any joint may be involved, joints in the knees are the most frequently affected. Risk factors for osteoarthritis of the knee include previous surgery or injury of the knee, occupational kneeling and squatting, and obesity (Rajan & Kerr, 2000). Obesity is the most significant independent factor in development of osteoarthritis and its progression (Schnitzer & Lane, 2004).

Because osteoarthritis is not systemic, manifestations occur around the affected joint. Bone spurs (**osteophytes**) may develop on the surface of the joints, eroding the cartilage so that it can no longer serve as a cushion or shock absorber. Consequently, ends of the bones at the joint rub against each other, causing pain and inflammation. Weight-bearing joints, such as the knees, hips, and spine, are frequently affected. In addition, finger joints are often involved. When osteoarthritis affects the knees or hips, it may be considerably disabling, interfering with mobility.

Joints affected by osteoarthritis may have been previously injured or exposed to long-term strain. Obesity places extra strain on joints and is thought to be a predisposing factor for osteoarthritis. The reason why some individuals who have no known predisposing factor develop osteoarthritis is unknown, although the condition may be associated with the aging process.

Osteoarthritis is generally unremitting. Overuse of the affected joints, exposure to cold and damp weather, or other factors may intensify manifestations. The functional consequences experienced depend on the type and magnitude of joint damage, the number of joints involved, the particular joints involved, and the daily activity of the individual.

Management of Osteoarthritis

Management of osteoarthritis is directed toward increasing function and preventing further functional consequences. Specific exercises, including range-of-motion and strengthening exercises, are often part of the management plan to meet this goal. It may be necessary to balance rest of the joint with its use.

The use of assistive devices, such as canes or crutches, may prevent undue weight bearing on joints. If individuals with osteoarthritis are obese, weight reduction may be advisable to remove undue pressure on the joints. Oral administration of aspirin or nonsteroidal anti-inflammatory drugs (NSAIDs), as well as injection of steroids into the joint, may also be helpful. In cases of severe joint damage, total joint **arthroplasty** (surgery to replace damaged joints with artificial joints) can restore many individuals to pain-free functional independence (Ritz & Mann, 2000).

Vocational Issues in Osteoarthritis

Osteoarthritis can have long-term functional consequences (Hawker et al., 2000), though the precise consequences experienced depend on the specific joints affected. Individuals with osteoarthritis of the knees, for instance, may be unable to walk long distances or stand for long periods of time. They may also have difficulty with bending or stooping. Individuals with osteoarthritis of the upper extremities or vertebrae of the spine may have difficulty lifting, turning, and reaching. When fingers are affected, individuals may be unable to perform tasks that require significant finger motion.

Back Pain

Back pain can be caused by a variety of conditions (Aminoff, 2004). (See Table 16-1.) It can produce a number of manifestations in addition to pain, depending on its location. Because of the subjective nature of pain and the different meaning of pain to different individuals, identification of the cause of back pain and its management may be difficult. Although muscle strain is frequently identified as a cause of back pain, underlying conditions of the spine may also be responsible (McCann, 2007). It is important that the cause

of back pain be established so that appropriate interventions can be implemented.

Back pain is classified as mild, moderate, or severe. Given that pain is a subjective measure, the extent of impaired function associated with back pain is often an indicator of the severity.

Types of Back Pain

Low Back Pain

Low back pain is one of the most common health-related conditions experienced. It is defined as pain in the lumbar or sacral region of the lower back. It may be experienced in the erect, nonmoving spine (**static pain**) or during movement (**kinetic pain**). Low back pain may result from any of the following causes:

- Mechanical problems due to poor posture, such as **lordosis** (swayback posture)
- Poor body mechanics at work, causing sprain or strain
- Injury due to falls, motor vehicle accidents, or sports

Table 16-1 Causes of Back Pain	
Cause	**Example**
Degenerative conditions	Osteoarthritis
Congenital conditions	Spinal stenosis
Structural irregularitiy	Scoliosis
Muscle condition	Spasm
Metabolic conditions	Osteoporosis
Injury	Compression fracture of vertebrae, muscle trauma
Cancer	Tumor, multiple myeloma, metastasis
Inflammatory conditions	Ankylosis spondylitis, rheumatoid arthritis
Infection	Meningitis
Referred pain (pain experienced in the back, but caused by another source)	Aneurysm of the aorta, conditions involving abdominal organs
Psychological causes	Anxiety, malingering

- **Spondylolisthesis** (forward slippage of a vertebrae)
- **Spondylolysis** (breakdown or degeneration of a vertebrae)
- Arthritis or osteoporosis
- Infection of the bones of the spine or tissue between vertebrae
- Tumors in the spine, or metastasis of cancer from another part of the body
- Herniation of an intervertebral disk
- **Referred pain** from other organs of the body, such as kidneys or uterus

Back pain may be accompanied by sciatica, or it may occur alone. **Sciatica** is a syndrome of pain that radiates from the lower back into the hip and down the leg. It may be accompanied by numbness, tingling, and muscle weakness. Sciatica can accompany a number of conditions of the lower back, with herniated disk being the most common.

Herniated or Ruptured Disk (Herniated Nucleus Pulposus)

Rupture of the soft, inner portion of the intervertebral disk (*nucleus pulposus*) through a tear in the tougher outer portion of the disk (*annulus*) is called a herniation (see Figure 16-5). A sprain or strain of the back or any condition that weakens the annulus may cause herniation of a disk. It results in back pain, often accompanied by spasms of the back muscles. Protrusion of the herniated disk exerts pressure on the nerves that surround the area. Pressure on the nerves can cause a partial loss of sensation and/or weakness in lower extremities. In severe cases, pressure on the nerves can cause problems with bowel or bladder function.

Pain experienced with a herniated disk is frequently exacerbated by straining, coughing, or lifting. Manifestations may be intermittent

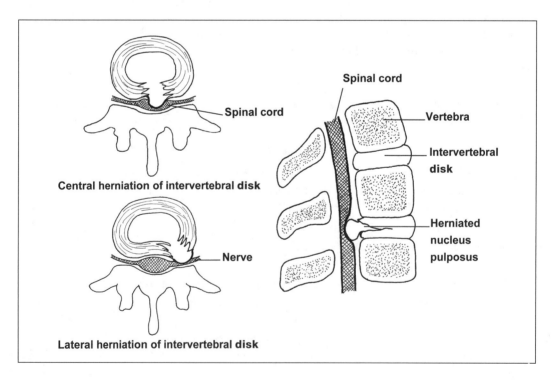

Central herniation of intervertebral disk

Lateral herniation of intervertebral disk

Spinal cord

Nerve

Spinal cord

Vertebra

Intervertebral disk

Herniated nucleus pulposus

Figure 16-5   Vertebral herniation

at first, but later progress to continuous pain or loss of sensation. Interventions, consisting of physical therapy and the use of anti-inflammatory medication, usually eliminate pain. Even so, herniated disk is the most common reason for back surgery (Deyo, 1998). When surgical intervention for herniated disk is necessary, **diskectomy** (removal of the disk) may be performed (Deyo, Nachemson, & Mirza, 2004).

Degenerative Disk Disease

Degenerative spondylolisthesis is characterized by slippage of the vertebral body into the one below. It is associated with degeneration and narrowing of the involved disk. The major manifestation is back pain, especially with bending, lifting, or twisting. Individuals may also complain of leg pain or may have neurologic signs.

One intervention that may be part of the management plan is flexion exercises. Some individuals find corset support to be helpful. In addition, NSAIDs may be utilized as part of the management plan. The most important measures are life-style changes such as avoidance of repetitive bending, heavy lifting, or twisting of the trunk of the body. *Spinal fusion surgery* (**spinal arthrodesis**), in which two disks are fused, may also be necessary for management of instability and structural irregularity of the disk.

Scoliosis

Scoliosis is a lateral, S-shaped curvature of the spine, which can be either **congenital** (present at birth) or a complication of amputation or another condition that alters posture, such as poliomyelitis or cerebral palsy. Scoliosis can be corrected with early recognition and proper intervention. If the spinal irregularity becomes fixed, however, the condition is difficult to reverse. In severe cases, scoliosis can interfere with respiratory capacity and can cause pressure on organs in the thoracic or abdominal cavity, thereby interfering with organ function.

Diagnosis of Back Pain

Back pain can sometimes be diagnosed by taking a history of manifestations, observation of individuals in various body postures and activities, and physical examination. Although x-rays can be helpful in identifying bony irregularities of the spine, other conditions—such as ruptured disk, for example—may not be seen on a regular x-ray. Other diagnostic tests may involve electromyography (EMG), which provides information about nerve function and nerve damage. Computerized tomography (CT) scan or magnetic resonance imaging (MRI) may also be used for identification of disk degeneration or ruptured disk.

Management of Back Pain

Exercise is an important part of both prevention and management of either acute or chronic back pain. In the past, bed rest was thought to be the intervention of choice; more recent studies have shown that individuals who maintain bed rest do not have any different outcomes than those who maintain regular activities during the acute period of back pain (Deyo, 1998; Deyo & Weinstein, 2001). Maintaining activity is, of course, dependent on the demands of the individual's regular activities, such as the need for heavy lifting.

Back pain may be treated with muscle relaxants, or antidepressants may be used for some individuals if they experience depression (Deyo & Weinstein, 2001). Physical therapy or acupuncture may be used to provide relief of the physical manifestations they may be experiencing.

Preventive measures, such as conditioning of the muscles of the back or the use of proper body mechanics, are helpful in avoiding recurrences. Unfortunately, maintaining adherence to specific exercise routines after manifestations have subsided may be difficult. Although most back pain subsides spontaneously, over-reaction to the condition can result in drug-seeking behavior, which can precipitate a more serious consequence of substance dependency.

Low back pain persisting for 6 months or longer is considered *chronic back pain*. Chronic back pain may be an extension of manifestations due to injury or may result from osteoporosis, degenerative spondylolisthesis, or a narrowing (**stenosis**) of the spinal canal. It may be more difficult to resolve chronic back pain, depending on the cause, and extensive, long-term therapy may be necessary. Chronic back pain may be treated either non-surgically or surgically. Management may consist of exercise, biofeedback, stress management, and medications such as muscle relaxants or steroids to reduce inflammation and non-narcotic analgesics to reduce pain. Spinal surgery has a limited role in alleviating chronic back pain and is usually reserved for those individuals who also have neurologic manifestations such as loss of urinary or bowel control or foot drop. The surgical intervention employed varies, depending on the cause of the pain. Some surgical interventions include simple diskectomy.

Vocational Issues in Back Pain

Acute back pain caused by strain or sprain may significantly impair function for a period lasting from days to weeks. Pain is precipitated by repeated twisting or lifting, prolonged sitting, or operating vibrating equipment. Individuals may have difficulty standing erect and may need to change position frequently. Most individuals with acute back pain return to work within six weeks. Recurrences are common, however, and the functional consequences of back pain have steadily increased across the population (Deyo, 1998). Although low back pain is rarely permanently disabling, return to work after an episode of low back pain is influenced by clinical, social, and economic factors (Deyo & Weinstein, 2001).

Prevention is the best way to reduce back injury. Education about good body mechanics and conditioning can help to reduce the chance of further injury. Individuals who are the least physically active are more likely to have acute lower back injury; consequently, exercises that increase strength and muscle tone can help prevent injury. Modification of the workplace to reduce mechanical stresses may also be important to decrease both the frequency and the cost of lower back injuries.

Individuals whose jobs require lifting or heavy physical work may need mechanical assistance devices or tables to allow lifting from the waist. Regular rest breaks may be needed as well as instruction regarding good lifting techniques. Ergonomics review of the workstation and equipment can help to assure that individuals are sitting and moving in ways that reduce the risk of strain. As much as possible, any equipment that causes whole-body vibration should be modified to reduce the amount of vibration. Individuals using equipment with significant vibration should schedule frequent rest periods or should rotate among workstations so that they also perform less strenuous tasks.

Chronic Pain

Approximately one in six Americans experiences chronic or recurrent pain (Schedler, 2006). Pain is a complex human experience that can dramatically affect quality of life (Molton, Jensen, Ehde, & Smith, 2007). This multidimensional concept includes physical, psychological, spiritual, and social functioning (Glajchen, 2001). The purpose of pain is mainly protective: It serves as a signal or warning that an area of the body needs attention. Pain and pain-related problems may be associated with a number of body systems and with a number of conditions. Chronic pain can be experienced because of a number of conditions, ranging from cancer to chronic headaches. It may also be associated with a number of conditions of the musculoskeletal system, ranging from trauma to rheumatoid arthritis.

Pain is subjective, difficult to quantify, and has different meanings to different individuals (Max, 2004). *Pain perception* may be influenced by anxiety, fear, and depression as well as cultural, ethnic, and other life influences (Adams, Poole, & Richardson, 2006). Individuals have different **pain thresholds** (the point at which sensation is perceived as pain) as well as different levels of **pain tolerance** (the point at which the individual finds the pain unbearable). Individuals with heightened pain tolerance may minimize the importance of manifestations and delay seeking attention for the pain until the pain is severe. Individuals with low pain tolerance may tend to have an exaggerated reaction to pain. **Pain intensity**, as demonstrated by the reaction of the individual, is not always a reliable index of the seriousness of the condition.

Individuals' response to pain (**pain expression**) is influenced by a number of cognitive, emotional, behavioral, and cultural factors. Some cultures encourage a stoic response to pain, whereas other cultures permit free expression of feelings in response to pain. Different individuals may not respond to the same pain stimuli in the same way, and the same person may react differently to pain in different circumstances. Anxiety and fear tend to enhance the perception of pain and the intensity of the pain response, whereas distractions tend to lessen the perception of and response to pain (Carr, 2007).

Acute Versus Chronic Pain

Pain can be classified as acute or chronic. *Acute pain* is defined as pain that occurs with the onset of illness or injury and is generally of short duration. It usually has an identifiable cause. As healing occurs or the cause of pain is corrected or removed, pain usually decreases within an established course of time.

The control of most acute pain is based on management of the underlying cause. When the underlying cause cannot be eradicated, or when interventions are not effective in relieving or controlling the source of pain, pain becomes chronic. Four basic factors determine the transition from acute pain to chronic pain (Rowbotham, 2004):

- On-going tissue damage
- Irregular function of the nervous system
- Nervous system damage
- Psychological factors

When pain becomes chronic, it is often treated as a condition in itself. *Chronic pain* is defined as pain that continues for longer than 3 months. As it persists over time, chronic pain loses its biologic function of signaling injury and imposes psychological and physical stress on individuals who experience it. Individuals experiencing chronic pain may develop *chronic pain syndrome*, a condition characterized by physical, social, and behavioral consequences. Individuals with chronic pain syndrome often have marked alteration of behavior, as shown by depression or anxiety, restriction in daily activities, excessive use of medications, and frequent use of medical services. Pain becomes a central issue in their lives.

Types of Chronic Pain

Chronic pain may be of three types:

- Pain that persists beyond the regular healing time (e.g., pain at the site of a fractured bone after the bone has healed; phantom pain in an amputated limb)
- Pain related to a chronic, degenerative, or malignant condition (e.g., rheumatoid arthritis, osteoporosis, cancer)
- Pain that persists for months or years but has no readily identifiable organic cause (psychogenic pain), such as back pain or headache with no identifiable physical reason for the pain

For some people, pain is unrelenting and persists at intolerable levels despite analgesic medication and futile attempts for other cures. Some individuals with chronic pain engage in cycles of false hope, frustration, and guilt. They may be unable to work and begin to withdraw from family and social activities. Personal relationships may deteriorate. They may believe no one else has ever endured the type of pain they are enduring and, consequently, may become demoralized, depressed, and angry.

Management of Chronic Pain

Management of chronic pain includes pharmacologic, physical, and psychological interventions (Douglass, 2007). Pain that cannot be controlled or eradicated is managed by helping individuals learn to cope with the pain. Physicians may find management of chronic pain difficult because of concern over the ineffectiveness of various interventions for chronic pain or concern that individuals may become addicted to medications used in management (Foley, 2003). Consequently, physicians may refer individuals with chronic pain to a clinic that uses multiple, simultaneous therapeutic approaches to chronic pain. Alternative forms of pain control may be used alone or in combination with analgesic medication.

Medications

Generally, medications are used more often in the management of acute pain rather than in the management of chronic pain. When medications are used as a part of pain management, the type chosen depends on the cause and the type of pain. Muscle relaxants may be prescribed to relax tight muscles or calm muscle spasms. Analgesics, which range from over-the-counter medications such as aspirin to narcotics such as Demerol or morphine, may also be used. In many instances, professionals tend to under-utilize narcotic analgesics for the long-term management of chronic

pain (unless pain is part of a terminal condition) because of their fear of physical and/or psychological dependence or addiction, even though studies have shown that there is little risk of addiction in individuals who have had no history of substance abuse (Portenoy, 1994). Because individuals with chronic pain frequently experience depression, antidepressant medications may occasionally be prescribed as well.

Noninvasive Procedures

Physical Therapy

Physical therapy may be prescribed to help individuals with chronic pain gradually increase their exercise tolerance and activity level. It is directed toward stretching and strengthening specific muscles and joints. Physical therapy may also be used to improve functional activity and reduce muscle spasms. Splints or braces may be used to support painful body parts or may be prescribed to help individuals increase their activity level.

Transcutaneous Electrical Nerve Stimulation

Transcutaneous electrical nerve stimulation (TENS) may help to relieve pain. In this technique, electrodes of a small, battery-operated device are placed over the painful area. When the unit is on, it stimulates nerve fibers electrically, providing a counter-irritation that in turn blocks pain impulses. The intervention itself is painless. The length of time for which individuals wear the unit varies, ranging from all day to only 1 or 2 hours per day.

The success of TENS depends to some extent on individuals' understanding of the technique and their motivation to use it. The degree and duration of pain relief with TENS units are variable. For some individuals, the effects wear off after a few months. Others may use the TENS unit successfully for a longer period of time. Owing to the expense of using a TENS unit, long-term or permanent use of the unit is rarely feasible.

Stress Management

Other specific techniques may be used to help individuals reduce their stress response. When individuals are tense, the heart beats faster, blood pressure rises, and muscles tighten. These responses can make pain more intense. Stress management includes specific procedures designed to reduce stress and promote relaxation.

Stress management may be useful in the management of a variety of conditions, but especially in the management of chronic pain. Because tension and anxiety tend to accentuate pain perception, removal of tension and anxiety can also serve to reduce the perception of pain. Many types of stress management programs are available. Some individuals may be helped to identify the sources of stress and learn ways to control their reaction to it. Other individuals may learn specific relaxation techniques.

Guided Imagery

Guided imagery uses instruction or descriptive narrative provided by a trained professional, to help individuals direct their thoughts to a relaxed, focused state. Guided imagery uses the individual's imagination to help the body respond to what he or she is imagining. Guided imagery can be used to promote relaxation, manage pain, promote healing, or to help individuals reach goals, such as weight loss.

Relaxation Therapy

Relaxation therapy is a technique aimed at assisting individuals to learn the relaxation response, which decreases blood pressure, heart rate, oxygen consumption, and alpha wave (a type of brain wave) activity on EEG. This technique, which can be learned through practice, may include both breathing techniques and progressive relaxation.

Individuals who undergo progressive relaxation training are taught to tighten and relax different muscle groups gradually. This procedure promotes relaxation, decreases anxiety, and lessens muscle tension. When such techniques are used on a daily basis, they can help the individual cope with stress.

Cognitive-Behavioral Therapy

Cognitive-behavioral therapy (CBT) has become recognized as an important intervention in pain management (Richardson, Adams, & Poole, 2006). CBT incorporates a number of interventions—such as education, cognitive restructuring, coping strategies training, problem solving, and goal setting—that influence the individual's cognition and behavior. This approach combines a biopsychosocial and holistic approach to pain management and seeks to help individuals change their pain-related behaviors.

Meditation

Meditation is a technique that helps individuals achieve a relaxed state by pinpointing attention on a repetitious event, usually a word or phrase recited repeatedly. Thus this technique removes individuals' focus from the painful sensation. Individuals concentrate on a variety of other processes, such as breathing, chanting, or forming a visual image.

Hypnosis

Hypnosis is a procedure by which individuals are induced into a trance-like state, during which suggestion is used to alter attitudes, perceptions, or behaviors. The hypnotic state is attained through focusing on a soothing image or situation, purposeful relaxation of voluntary muscles, and controlled breathing. For individuals with chronic pain, hypnosis may be used to alter the reaction to painful stimuli or the perception of pain. Skilled hypnotherapists may help individuals distract their thinking about pain through post-hypnotic suggestion.

Hypnosis should be conducted only by trained, certified individuals. It has varying degrees of success in the management of chronic pain.

Biofeedback

Some individuals find biofeedback helpful in controlling pain, especially if the pain is due in part to muscle tension. Biofeedback is a technique based on operant conditioning and feedback learning of a physiologic response. In principle, it involves measuring a naturally occurring body function and amplifying it so that individuals can acquire the ability to voluntarily control that function. Through biofeedback, individuals learn to elicit the relaxation response and control physiologic mechanisms that produce stress-related manifestations.

During a biofeedback session, individuals receive feedback from a specific physiologic measurement such as heart rate, muscle tension, or skin temperature. Electrical equipment produces real-time information about physical function, such as muscle tension or heart rate. Electrodes are placed on the skin over localized muscles; wires from the electrodes are then attached to an electromyogram machine, which measures electrical activity of the muscles. Information is delivered to the individual through a tone or lights.

After learning different methods to reduce the amount of muscle tension, individuals can monitor the effectiveness of these methods in controlling muscular activity through the feedback system. With practice, they can learn to reduce the stress response at will without the benefit of physiologic monitoring.

Operant Conditioning

As a behavioral technique designed to decrease the functional consequences associated with chronic pain, operant conditioning does not cure or reduce the pain itself, but rather, alters the individual's behavioral response to the pain. This technique is based on theories of learning and conditioning. The pain experience often results in a series of behaviors that communicate discomfort (e.g., grimacing, guarding, limping) and usually elicit responses from others in the form of sympathy, decreased expectations for performance or success, or even monetary compensation. Behavioral responses to pain may also be reinforced by the fact that they may help individuals avoid activities that they find unpleasant. Such reinforcement of pain behaviors may condition individuals to display them and, as a result, may increase the functional consequences associated with the pain behaviors. Operant conditioning involves withdrawing reinforcement for "pain" behaviors and reinforcing "well" behaviors.

Pain Groups

Chronic Pain Anonymous (CPA) groups may help individuals learn to live with their pain when no other technique or intervention has done so. The CPA model borrows from Alcoholics Anonymous (AA) and is based on the concept that there are similar psychological and emotional disturbances seen in alcoholism and intractable benign pain: Both disrupt personal and work relationships; both cause loss of control, obsession, and isolation; and both are chronic conditions. CPA uses the same 12 steps as AA, substituting the word "pain" for the word "alcohol."

Invasive Procedures

Acupuncture

Acupuncture has gained increased acceptance in management of chronic pain (Vas, Aguilar, Perea-Milla, & Méndez, 2007). In this ancient Chinese form of analgesia, long, fine needles are inserted into selected points (trigger points) of an individual's body to eliminate the pain sensation.

There is no simple explanation for the mechanisms that underlie the analgesic effects of acupuncture. Although it is considered an invasive technique, it has few, if any, complications when it is done under sterile conditions by those who have been trained and certified in acupuncture techniques.

Nerve Blocks

Nerve blocks eliminate pain locally. They are commonly used during surgical procedures as well as in the management of chronic pain. In this technique, local anesthetics are injected close to nerves, blocking their ability to conduct the painful stimuli. Generally, nerve blocks are given for the temporary relief of pain. However, in cases of severe pain, such as in terminal cancer, nerve blocks may be performed so that the effects are irreversible.

Neurosurgical Procedures

Neurosurgical procedures in which surgeons sever sensory nerves supplying the painful area may be used when severe pain cannot be ameliorated or controlled by other means. Cutting the nerves removes not only the sensation of pain, but also the sensations of pressure, heat, and cold. Consequently, individuals who have undergone these procedures must be aware of the necessity of protecting the area from injury.

The type of neurosurgical procedure used depends on the type and location of the pain. For example, *sympathectomy* involves the autonomic nervous system; *neurectomy*, either the cranial or the peripheral nerves; and *rhizotomy* and *chordotomy*, the nerves close to the spinal cord (see Chapter 4).

Amputation

The general term used to describe loss of all or a portion of a body part is **amputation**. Amputation can occur for several reasons. *Traumatic amputation* due to injury is most common in younger, predominately male adults (Herbert & Ashworth, 2006). Common causes of traumatic amputation include explosions and

motor vehicle accidents (Proehl, 2004; Blank-Reid, 2003). Amputation may be performed surgically as an intervention to manage a condition, such as amputation of a breast (**mastectomy**) because of cancer or amputation of a leg because of gangrene. Amputation may also be congenital, as when individuals are born without a limb.

Upper extremity amputations are often associated with accidents, burns, explosions, or other types of traumatic injury. Lower extremity amputations are more frequently associated with chronic conditions, such as conditions of the peripheral vascular system (see Chapter 13).

Levels of Extremity Amputation

Amputation of an extremity may be performed at different levels. To provide for maximal length of the stump of the extremity and, thereby, maximal function with a prosthesis, surgeons usually perform an amputation as **distal** (farthest from the center of the body) as possible. The following levels of upper extremity amputation are possible:

- *Forequarter or interscapular–thoracic amputation*: the most severe upper extremity amputation, in which the entire arm, clavicle, and scapula are removed
- *Shoulder disarticulation (S/D)*: removal of the arm at the shoulder joint
- *Above the elbow (A/E)*: removal of the arm anywhere between the shoulder and the elbow joints
- *Elbow disarticulation (E/D)*: removal of the arm at the elbow joint
- *Below elbow (B/E)*: removal of the arm anywhere between the elbow and the wrist
- *Wrist disarticulation (W/D)*: removal of the hand at the wrist
- *Partial hand*: amputation of one or more fingers or the loss of a portion of the hand

The following levels of lower extremity amputation are distinguished:

- *Hemipelvectomy* or *hindquarter amputation*: the most severe lower extremity amputation, in which the entire lower limb and half of the pelvis are removed
- *Hip disarticulation (H/D)*: removal of the leg at the hip joint
- *Above the knee (A/K)*: removal of the leg anywhere between the hip and the knee joints
- *Knee disarticulation (K/D)*: the removal of the lower leg at the knee
- *Below the knee (B/K)*: the removal of the lower leg anywhere between the knee and the ankle
- *Syme's amputation*: the removal of the foot at the ankle
- *Transmetatarsal* or *partial foot*: the removal of a portion of the foot

It is especially important to retain the maximal length of the stump in lower extremity amputations, where the amount of energy required to use an artificial limb increases with the height of the amputation. Individuals with a below-the-knee amputation, for example, require approximately 10% to 37% more energy for movement than do individuals without an amputation (Wilson, 1998).

Management of Amputation

Surgery

When underlying conditions such as cancer or artierosclerosis necessitate amputation, the type of surgical amputation performed, the postoperative course, and type of rehabilitation depend to a great extent on the circumstances surrounding the amputation and the individual's general condition. Individuals who undergo amputation because of an underlying condition may be at risk for additional amputations because of the condition itself or because of complications that result from the condition.

Reimplantation

An extremity or a portion of an extremity that has been totally severed by an injury can sometimes be surgically reattached to the body with partial restoration of function. This process is called *reimplantation*. Reimplantation may be especially important after amputation of an upper extremity, because upper limb prostheses provide only limited function (Daigeler, Fansa, & Schneider, 2003).

With the evolution of surgical techniques and scientific technology, reimplantation procedures have resulted in better outcomes. The degree of success of surgical reimplantation depends on the general condition of the individual, the availability of rapid transportation to a reimplantation center, and appropriate care of the severed body part prior to reimplantation. The goal of reimplantation is to preserve quality of life by improving function and appearance (Brown & Wu, 2003). Studies have demonstrated that reimplantation can, in many cases, achieve 50% function and 50% sensation of the replanted part (Wilhelmi, Lee, Pagensteert, & May, 2003), although in some cases return of motor function is greater than return of sensory function (Wiberg et al., 2003). Nevertheless, the success of this kind of surgery in achieving increased quality of life and function is partly determined on individuals' appropriate and realistic expectations of appearance and function of the body part after reimplantation (Wilhelmi et al., 2003).

Prostheses

A **prosthesis** is a fabricated substitute for a missing body part, such as an artificial limb that replaces an amputated limb. Prosthetic devices may enable individuals to regain independent function, or they may be prescribed only for cosmetic purposes. The type of prosthesis, its purpose, and maximal use depend on the reason for the amputation, the type and level of the amputation, the presence of any underlying conditions, the development of any complications, and, most importantly, the needs of the individual and his or her motivation to use the prosthesis (Bussell, 2000).

The physician, usually the *orthopedic surgeon* (a physician who specializes in surgical treatment of bones) who performed the surgery, prescribes the prosthesis on the basis of the individual's daily activities, occupation, and cosmetic needs. A *certified prosthetician* (an individual who specializes in making prosthetic devices) then fabricates the prosthesis.

In some instances, the surgeon may place a temporary prosthesis on the stump of a lower extremity immediately after surgery. In this case, a rigid total-contact dressing is applied to the stump in the operating room, and a pylon or adjustable rigid support structure is attached. An ankle-foot assembly is then attached to the lower end of the pylon. The immediate placement of a temporary prosthesis may have a psychological benefit for individuals, fostering a sense of independence and optimism as soon as they wake from surgery. It also promotes ambulation, reducing the risk of complications associated with immobility. Immediate placement of a temporary prosthesis is contraindicated when there is a severe underlying condition, such as diabetes or infection, or if there has been extensive damage as a result of injury. It is also contraindicated for individuals with limited mental capabilities, who may unable to understand instructions or to regulate the weight placed on the stump in the early postoperative period.

When immediate prosthetic fitting is not advisable, individuals receive a temporary prosthesis 2 to 3 weeks after their surgery. Placement of a temporary prosthesis is necessary, whether the fitting is immediate or delayed, so that **edema** (swelling) can subside and the stump can shrink before the permanent prosthesis is fitted. A permanent prosthesis can usually be placed within 3 months.

As much as possible, lower extremity prostheses are designed to enable ambulation. The individual's walking ability after lower limb amputation is determined by many factors, including the presence of other conditions that may affect general health and the person's physical capacity (van Velzen, van Bennekom, van der Woude, & Houdijk, 2006). Generally, the lower the level of amputation, the easier the use of the lower extremity prosthesis. The ankle-foot attachment may be either immovable or movable. A commonly used ankle-foot mechanism is the solid ankle–cushion heel foot (SACH). In above-the-knee amputations, the prosthesis must also replace knee function, providing a joint that is stable for both standing and walking. Good alignment and fit of the socket of the prosthetic device are crucial for optimal balance and support. Because proper alignment varies with the heel heights of shoes, individuals who wish to wear shoes with different heel heights on occasion may need several removable prosthetic feet designed to accommodate the varying heel heights.

Prosthetic devices for use after hemipelvectomy are more difficult to use. The increased energy needed for ambulation often makes use of a prosthesis after hemipelvectomy unrealistic for other than cosmetic use, although such a prosthesis can be functional. For example, a prosthesis may be worn after hemipelvectomy to help individuals maintain proper posture while sitting in a wheelchair. When using the prosthesis for ambulation, individuals with hemipelvectomy can usually walk only at a slow pace and only on level ground. Most individuals who have undergone hemipelvectomy choose to use crutches or a wheelchair for their daily activities, reserving the prosthesis for special events when cosmetic appearance is more important than ambulation (Amputee Coalition of American, 2000).

Upper extremity prostheses vary in type and purpose and are custom made according to individual need. Complex function of the hand cannot be replaced, but functions such as lifting, grasping, and pinching can often be restored with a prosthesis. A *terminal device* is a prosthesis that substitutes for a hand. The level of amputation and the individual's needs determine the type of terminal device used. In general, the better the cosmetic appearance of the device, the less its functional capacity. Individuals who need grasping, holding, or lifting actions may find a hook more beneficial as a prosthesis. For others, prosthetic hands that have grasp or pinch function for light objects may be most useful. The cosmetic appearance of the prosthetic hand may be more important to some individuals than the prosthetic hand's functional capacity.

Activation of the function of a prosthesis is obtained by using the muscles in the remaining portion of the limb. For this reason, a prosthesis for a high upper extremity amputation may have limited function. A prosthesis placed after a shoulder disarticulation or an interscapular–thoracic amputation, for example, may be mostly cosmetic with little, if any, functional capacity.

Myoelectrical prostheses, the function of which is activated by electrical potentials produced by muscles, may be considered in some instances. In this type of prosthetic device, electrodes are placed over the skin of the muscles to be used. The electrodes pick up electrical impulses from the muscles, transferring them to a motor in the prosthesis, which then stimulates the hand to open and close. Function of the electric prosthesis does not, however, approximate function of regular hand movement and dexterity. Myoelectrical

prostheses are best suited for individuals with below-the-elbow prostheses. They are heavier because of the battery and motor that they contain, and they are more expensive than regular prosthetic devices.

Complications of Amputation

Complications may develop after either upper or lower extremity amputation. It is extremely important that the prosthesis fit well and that there be no undue pressure or rubbing that could lead to ulceration. All individuals—but especially those whose amputation was made necessary by underlying peripheral vascular disease—must be careful to avoid skin ulceration that could become infected and necessitate a higher-level amputation.

Swelling (edema) of the stump after the permanent prosthesis has been placed can not only interfere with the proper fit of the prosthesis, but also increase pressure and restrict the blood flow to the stump, contributing to the likelihood of ulceration. An improper fit of the prosthesis, rubbing, or swelling of the stump should be immediately brought to the attention of the physician and prosthetist so that the prosthesis can be adjusted appropriately.

Individuals undergoing amputation must also concentrate on preserving the range of motion in the remaining joints of the amputated limb. **Contractures** (deformities in which permanent contraction of a muscle makes a joint immobile) may occur because of improper positioning or limited activity of remaining joints. Contractures may impede or prevent effective use of the prosthetic device. These complications are easier to prevent through regular range-of-motion exercises of joints than they are to cure. When contractures develop, they may be corrected with extensive physical therapy and, occasionally, surgery.

Other complications of amputation may include bone spurs, scoliosis, and phantom pain. Bone spurs or bone overgrowth may develop at the end of the stump, changing its shape and causing pain. Scoliosis (an S-shaped lateral curvature of the spine) may occur after a lower extremity amputation because of the improper alignment of the body or because of improper use of the prosthesis. Whether or not scoliosis occurs, lower back pain may also be experienced with lower extremity prosthesis use (Friel, Domhold, & Smith, 2005). After a higher upper extremity amputation, scoliosis may develop if the prosthetic device unbalances the trunk. In both instances, scoliosis can be prevented by making sure that the prosthesis is in good alignment. Individuals who have had an upper extremity amputation may also perform exercises to strengthen the muscles that support the prosthesis.

Although all individuals who have had an amputation experience some degree of **phantom sensation** (a sensation that the amputated extremity is still present), this sensation usually diminishes over time. Some individuals, however, experience chronic, severe pain sensation in the amputated extremity called **phantom limb pain** (Hanley, Jensen, Ehde, Hoffman, Patterson, & Robinson, 2004; Kooijman, Dijkstra, Geertzen, Elzinga, & van der Schans, 2000). Phantom limb pain may gradually diminish over time, but it sometimes becomes disabling. In some instances, interventions to block the nerves that serve the amputated extremity may alleviate the pain. At times, **neuromas** (bundles of nerve fibers) embedded in the scar tissue of the stump may cause pain and can be removed; however, this measure may not totally alleviate phantom limb pain. Individuals with chronic phantom pain may need chronic pain management.

Psychosocial Issues in Amputation

Individuals with amputation must make permanent behavioral, social, and emotional adjustments to cope with the multiple problems that can exist with amputation (Gallagher & MacLachlan, 1999). Amputation forces individuals to make a major adjustment not only to a change in body image, but also to a change in functional capacity. When individuals are fitted with a prosthetic limb, they are confronted head-on with the irrevocable fact that they have lost a limb as well as the need to learn how to incorporate the prosthesis into daily function (Gallagher, 2004).

Traumatic amputation produces psychological and social effects that can be overwhelming if not addressed openly and candidly. The earlier that psychosocial intervention can be implemented, the more likely that psychological factors will not impede functional outcome (Meyer, 2003). Individuals whose amputation was due to chronic condition may find it less difficult to adjust, especially if the body part amputated had been a source of pain or immobility prior to the amputation. Individuals who have who lost a body part suddenly—such as amputation of the breast because of breast cancer or loss of a limb because of traumatic injury—may have more difficulty with adjustment because they have had inadequate time to prepare for the loss.

Regardless of the reason for the amputation, it is important to understand individuals' interpretation of the loss. Individuals' ability to adapt to amputation depends on the circumstances surrounding the amputation, the usefulness of the prosthetic device, and individuals' perception of their condition. Some individuals who have lost a limb no longer consider themselves whole. They may fear that they will never again be able to function as they did prior to the amputation. For these individuals, a prosthesis is a reminder of perceived inadequacy rather than restoration of function. In some instances, loss of a limb is comparable to the loss of a loved one. Individuals may need sufficient time to grieve and adjust to their loss.

Individuals who have undergone amputation, especially loss of a lower extremity because of a chronic condition, such as diabetes must guard against injury and infection to the stump. Consequently, skin care is a vital part of rehabilitation. Bathing in the evening rather than in the morning is advisable, as damp skin may swell and stick to a prosthesis, causing irritation and rubbing.

The extent of activity in which individuals can participate depends to some extent on the level of the amputation. Most individuals with lower extremity amputation can bicycle, swim, dance, and participate in many athletic activities with adaptive equipment. Driving a car is usually not a problem, although automatic transmissions may allow individuals to drive more easily. Activities such as climbing, squatting, and kneeling may be more difficult; however, even these tasks are mastered by some individuals. Individuals with upper extremity amputation may require other assistive devices in addition to the prosthesis to perform a number of activities of daily living.

Although the amputation of an extremity has no direct effect on sexual activity, psychological factors and/or the reaction of sexual partners to the amputation may alter sexual function (Ide, 2004). Reaction of individuals' partners to amputation may be either supportive or nonsupportive. The stability of the relationship prior to amputation as well as communication and understanding are important components to adjustment, and, consequently to the quality of the relationship.

Vocational Issues in Amputation

Individuals with amputation who wear a prosthesis may need to avoid hot, humid environments that can cause skin breakdown or contribute to the deterioration of the prosthesis. Dust or grit can be abrasive to the skin, exacerbating skin problems, and can interfere with the functioning of the movable parts of the prosthesis.

In the case of lower extremity amputation, physical demands of a job, such as the need for walking, climbing, or pushing, should be eval-

uated and altered, if necessary. The increased energy expenditure required for the use of a prosthesis should also be considered part of the physical demands of the job. Individuals in professional or managerial careers may have fewer functional consequences following the amputation of either an upper extremity or a lower extremity. Those with upper extremity amputation may have a greater need for a cosmetic-oriented prosthesis, however, than do those workers whose jobs require the prosthesis for tasks such as lifting.

Rheumatoid and Autoimmune Conditions

More than 105 conditions are classified as rheumatic conditions. Many rheumatoid conditions are also considered *autoimmune conditions*. Autoimmune conditions are thought to be mediated by an autoimmune response in which the body's immune system fails to recognize body tissue and attacks the tissues as if they were foreign objects. The reason for this autoimmune response is unknown.

The term **rheumatic disease** describes conditions that produce manifestations that affect the joints, connective tissues, and muscle. Rheumatoid conditions are characterized by pain, inflammation, fatigue, and loss of motion in joints. **Arthritis** is a general term used to describe a musculoskeletal condition of the joints (Heesch, Miller, & Brown, 2007). **Myositis** refers to inflammation of the muscle.

The effects of rheumatoid conditions are diverse, with manifestations ranging from mild to severe. Manifestations are often unpredictable, so individuals with rheumatoid conditions can never predict when pain, stiffness, or structural irregularity may occur.

Rheumatoid Arthritis

Rheumatoid arthritis is a chronic, progressive, systemic condition that causes signification pain, joint destruction, and functional consequence (Kvien, 2004). It is characterized by inflammation and swelling of the synovial joints, resulting in pain, stiffness, and structural irregularity of the joints. One of the most common of the rheumatoid conditions, rheumatoid arthritis has an unpredictable and fluctuating course.

Rheumatoid arthritis is thought to result, in part, from an autoimmune response in which the body's regular mechanisms of defense produce an inflammatory type of reaction against itself, leading to cell destruction. Although much of the focus of rheumatoid arthritis is on the joints, rheumatoid arthritis is a systemic condition affecting other body systems. Affected individuals may experience a range of manifestations, such as fatigue, weight loss, fever, joint pain, and structural irregularity of the joints. The inflammatory process may also affect other body organs (e.g., the eyes, heart, lungs, or spleen), causing changes that alter organ function.

Rheumatoid arthritis is a progressive condition, but not all individuals are affected to the same degree. The condition may be severe in some individuals, causing moderate structural irregularity of the joint in a relatively short amount of time. In others, it may progress more slowly or may never become severely debilitating.

Rheumatoid arthritis may be characterized by a series of remissions, in which manifestations subside for a period of weeks to years, and exacerbations, in which manifestations become worse. During an exacerbation, joints may sustain increased damage so that they never return to their regular state, even during remissions.

During the exacerbations of rheumatoid arthritis, the synovial membrane becomes inflamed and thickens, and the joints become warm, swollen, and painful. As the condition progresses, a layer of scar tissue forms over the synovial membrane. This tissue, called *pannus*, interferes with provision of nutrients to the cartilage of the joint, thereby leading to erosion and joint destruction. Scar tissue may become so tough and fibrous that **ankylosis** (stiffness and fixation of the joint) occurs, impeding movement.

Rheumatoid arthritis may not affect all joints, or it may affect different joints at different times. The joints that are most commonly involved include these:

- Wrists
- Ankles
- Knees
- Elbows
- Fingers and toes

Occasionally, shoulders, hip, and neck joints are also involved.

Joints are usually affected symmetrically. For example, both knees—rather than just one knee—will be affected. Joint pain and stiffness are generally worse in the morning, subside somewhat during the day, and again become painful at night.

The prognosis for individuals with rheumatoid arthritis varies. Some individuals may experience rapid progression of manifestations with functional consequences, whereas others remain in a state of remission for years, continuing their regular employment and full activity.

Nonsurgical Management of Rheumatoid Arthritis

Rheumatoid arthritis is a lifelong condition with no known cure (O'Dell, 2004a). A physician, who specializes in the treatment of rheumatoid conditions, including rheumatoid arthritis, is called a *rheumatologist*. Its management is directed toward suppressing the condition, reducing pain, restoring function, and preventing additional joint damage (Shanahan & St. Clair, 2007; Oliver, 2007). There is no cure for rheumatoid arthritis, so goals of management are remission, including decreasing joint destruction, maintaining joint function, preventing structural irregularity of the joint, and maintaining remission (O'Dell, 2004b). Cornerstones of therapy are rest and exercise.

Exercise

Exercise is almost always directed toward strengthening and increasing the flexibility of muscles without placing additional wear and tear on the joints. Although activity alone is not necessarily therapeutic, prescribed exercise is important in the management of rheumatoid arthritis to restore muscle strength, maintain joint mobility, and prevent contractures. Individuals should follow the specific exercise plan recommended by their physician.

Exercises usually consist of specific range-of-motion exercises for joints. They should be performed regularly and daily to prevent structural irregularity. Other exercises are used to help strengthen muscles to prevent structural irregularities of the joints.

Rest

Complete bed rest may be recommended for short periods during the acute phases of rheumatoid arthritis. In other instances, rest periods throughout the day may be prescribed. Splinting of specific joints may occasionally be prescribed to reduce local inflammation. When acute inflammation is present, active exercises may not be possible and splints may be prescribed for various joints. Splints, if used, are typically used only at night and at rest and are designed to maintain the joints in extension. Splints are prescribed as a temporary measure and always under the direction of a physician. Long-term use of splints can cause structural irregularities because they immobilize affected joints.

Thermal Intervention

Thermal intervention (applications of either hot or cold) may be used to relieve pain. Interventions may include hydrotherapy, such as a whirlpool bath, or paraffin baths, in which the affected body part is placed in a bath of hot paraffin and then removed. As the paraffin cools externally, warmth to the body part is held in, reducing both pain and inflammation.

Occupational and Physical Therapy

Occupational therapists and physical therapists may be consulted to assist individuals in increasing their functional capacity. Occupational therapists generally focus on tasks of daily living, whereas physical therapists focus on mobility issues.

Medications

Medications are a mainstay of management in rheumatoid arthritis (Olsen & Stein, 2004). They are used to reduce inflammation, thereby also reducing pain. Medications used for rheumatoid arthritis are characterized into three main classes: NSAIDs, corticosteroids, and disease-modifying antirheumatic drugs (DMARDs) (O'Dell, 2004b). Often these medications are used in combination.

NSAIDs provide partial relief of pain and stiffness. Because they do not slow progression of rheumatoid arthritis, they are typically used in combination with DMARDs (American College of Rheumatology Subcommittee on Rheumatoid Arthritis Guidelines, 2002). Long-term administration of these medications can, however, result in stomach irritation, gastrointestinal ulcer, and, in some instances, perforation and hemorrhage (O'Dell, 2004b).

In some instances, salicylates (e.g., aspirin) may be prescribed in large doses, to nearly the toxic level, to obtain the desired therapeutic effect. This high concentration of salicylate in the blood may exceed the liver's ability to metabolize it, causing toxic effects such as ringing in the ears (**tinnitus**). Because of the large doses required, individuals may experience other side effects from the medication, such as stomach discomfort and/or bleeding caused by irritation of the stomach lining.

Corticosteroids are added to the management plan to suppress the inflammatory response. When and how they are used in the management of rheumatoid arthritis remains controversial (Moreland & O'Dell, 2002). Corticosteroids can have serious side effects, such as thinning of skin, cataracts, osteoporosis, and hypertension. Given this potential for serious side effects, these drugs are rarely used on a long-term basis, but are more commonly used when individuals are having a major exacerbation of the condition. To prevent serious complications, individuals taking steroids must not stop medication suddenly, but rather should gradually withdraw from the medication under a physician's supervision.

DMARDs are used to retard or halt progression of rheumatoid arthritis by suppressing inflammation. One example of a DMARD is methotrexate, which is often selected as the initial therapy for rheumatoid arthritis (Mikulus & O'Dell, 2000).

Complementary and Alternative Therapies

Complementary and alternative medicine (CAM) is a term that describes a diverse range of products and practices outside the mainstream of Western medical practice for promoting health and preventing or treating conditions (Harpham, 2001). Several studies have found that more than 40% of individuals with rheumatoid conditions use some form of complementary or alternative therapy (Vecchio, 1994; Boisset & Fitzcharles, 1994; Resch, Hill, & Ernst, 1997).

The types of alternative therapies used in the United States vary. Some individuals use topical ointments, ranging from silicon lubricant to alcohol extract from marijuana leaves; others use copper bracelets or other special jewelry to relieve manifestations; others take dietary supplements such as glucosamine, vitamins,

or herb preparations; still others undergo acupuncture (Kolasinski, 2001). Alternative therapies such as massage, tai chi, yoga, and hypnosis are also used in the management of rheumatoid arthritis (Swann, 2007b).

Many complementary and alternative therapies have few side effects. Nevertheless, because individuals with rheumatoid arthritis often continue to receive traditional interventions, interactions of traditional therapies and alternative therapies may be of concern. Consequently individuals should make both traditional healthcare providers and alternative healthcare providers aware of all types of interventions they are currently using.

Surgical Management of Rheumatoid Arthritis

Most individuals with rheumatoid arthritis manage their condition with a combination of medication, exercise, and rest. At times, because of severe joint inflammation or structural irregularity of the joint, surgical procedures are necessary. The following surgical procedures are performed in cases of rheumatoid arthritis (Swann, 2007a):

- **Arthroscopy** is a procedure in which a needle is inserted into the joint space. It may be done for diagnostic purposes, to inspect the joint, or it may be done to repair damage.
- **Synovectomy** is the surgical removal of the synovial membrane surrounding a joint. It prevents recurrent inflammation, thereby reducing joint pain and further joint destruction.
- **Arthroplasty** (surgical replacement, formation, or reformation of a joint) may be necessary when the joint has become nonfunctional because of destruction, or when movement of the joint becomes so painful that activity is severely hampered.
- **Osteotomy** involves partial removal of a damaged bone.

Psychosocial Issues in Rheumatoid Arthritis

The consequences of rheumatoid arthritis and its associated pain can affect individuals' ability to work or fulfill responsibilities at home as well as curtail their social life and ability to engage in recreational activities (Stucki et al., 2004; Walsh, Blanchard, Kremer, & Blanchard, 1999). Living with pain is a factor to which individuals with rheumatoid arthritis must adjust. Awareness of the lack of a cure and the progressive nature of the condition may lead to feelings of hopelessness. Individuals with rheumatoid arthritis may also experience sleep disturbances, which may increase fatigue and contribute to depression and irritability (Martens et al., 2006).

In its early stages, before structural irregularities of joints occur, rheumatoid arthritis may be essentially an invisible condition. It hidden nature may lead to misunderstandings on the part of family and friends, who may perceive individuals as merely seeking attention with their complaints of pain or attempting to avoid work or other activities, rather than acknowledging the manifestations as real. The unpredictable nature of rheumatoid arthritis not only contributes to this misunderstanding, but can also cause stress for individuals who are unsure on a day-to-day basis whether they will be able to participate in various activities.

Individuals may develop learned helplessness as a result of the unpredictable, chronic, and incurable nature of the condition. Helping individuals gain a feeling of control by increasing their self-management of arthritic pain and their ability to cope with the vagueness of the condition can improve both social functioning and overall quality of life.

Independence is a critical issue for individuals with rheumatoid arthritis. Loss of the ability to perform certain tasks or associated role changes may require significant adjustment. For homemakers with rheumatoid arthritis whose partners must now assume some of the housekeeping duties, adjustment may be difficult for both parties. Conversely, individuals with rheumatoid arthritis who once prided themselves on being self-sufficient and strong may view having someone else perform what they consider simple tasks as a sign of weakness.

If individuals have to leave their jobs because of rheumatoid arthritis, their social identity may be threatened. Family roles may also be changed, with other family members taking over tasks once performed by the individual. As rheumatoid arthritis progresses and individuals become more dependent on others or on assistive devices, they may feel a loss of control, which can lead to poor self-esteem.

Also contributing to poor self-esteem is altered body image, resulting from structural irregularities of joints or the need for assistive devices that accompanies joint changes. Use of devices can, however, help individuals to gain independence and overcome feelings of helplessness. For grooming needs, individuals may use devices such as adaptive handles for combs and brushes or toothbrushes. They may use a long-handled sponge that has a compartment to hold a bar of soap. Devices such as a zipper-pull or button aid may be of help with dressing.

Some individuals may be resistant to using an assistive device, viewing it as "giving up" or fearing that if they use the device rather than their joint, they will lose their ability to perform the task. Others may be concerned about appearances or fear that using the assistive device will call attention to their condition. Thus the use of assistive devices can be an emotionally charged issue. The degree of support from family and friends can make a difference in the individual's willingness to use such a device.

Vocational Issues in Rheumatoid Arthritis

Individuals with rheumatoid arthritis experience a number of work barriers, ranging from physical barriers (such as the need to handle items, writing, and energy-related barriers) to psychosocial barriers (such as hostility of others in the workplace) (Allaire, Li, & LaValley, 2003). Because not all individuals with rheumatoid arthritis are affected in the same way, vocational implications will vary with the severity of the condition and its progression. Not all individuals with rheumatoid arthritis will become totally disabled, but most individuals will experience reductions across a broad spectrum of activities.

A major limitation associated with this condition is its unpredictability—that is, not knowing when the condition will change and if additional functional loss will occur. Occupations characterized by significant physical demands may be more difficult for individuals to maintain than those that are sedentary or require light activity. Even when individuals are still able to perform moderate physical function in their work, the progressive nature of the condition and its potential for affecting mobility should be considered. Pain on motion, limited motion, and muscle weakness may all affect individuals' ability to perform tasks. Tasks requiring manual dexterity or pinch grip may also be difficult, if not impossible, if structural irregularity of the hands has occurred. Work that places stress or strain on joints may exacerbate the condition and should be avoided.

If joints in the lower extremities are involved, standing for long periods of time or walking for long distances may be affected. Individuals may have difficulty with climbing, stooping, bending, reaching, and kneeling. They may find it uncomfortable or difficult to remain in one position for long periods of time and may need to change position frequently, as arthritic joints should not stay immobile for long periods. If they spend long periods of time traveling in a car, they should take frequent stops; if the travel on trains or planes, they should walk around frequently.

Individuals should attempt to organize and plan tasks as much as possible to conserve energy, protect joints, and minimize fatigue. They may attempt to do as much as they can while seated. If cervical joints are affected, individuals should avoid working with their neck bent over. They may use a slanted or elevated table or desk to avoid neck flexion.

Individuals should set priorities, giving up those activities of least importance. They may consider alternating more difficult tasks with those requiring less energy. In all cases, they should learn to pace themselves, stopping to rest occasionally, rather than persisting with the task until they are exhausted.

If individual manifestations are increased by temperature and humidity, an indoor, climate-controlled environment may be preferable. In most instances, sudden, frequent changes in environmental conditions will prove more bothersome than the exact level of temperature or humidity itself. Consequently, going in and out of excessively cold or warm environments should be avoided.

Effects of rheumatoid arthritis are more far-reaching than simply affecting one aspect of the person's life: All activities of daily living are affected. Consequently, individuals may require extra time to get ready for work or perform tasks at home, which can in turn affect their work schedule. The need for prescribed periods of rest and exercise must also be considered, both at home and in the work environment. A variety of environmental alterations may assist individuals with rheumatoid arthritis maximize their functional capacity, whether at work or at home. The need for reaching and bending can be reduced with modifications such as storing heavy objects on lower shelves and using pullout shelving or baskets to retrieve them. Pullout shelves can also be used to minimize bending and stretching for hard-to-reach items. Counters can be raised or lowered, permanently or with adjustable components.

Assistive devices can help individuals manage their work environment as well as essential daily activities more easily and should be used as appropriate. Devices may enhance muscle strength, endurance, range of motion, manual dexterity, and mobility. Assistive devices such as long-handled reachers may be used to open cabinets. Knobs can be replaced by levers so that the whole hand can be used. This may be helpful if manual dexterity or hand strength is affected. Individuals with moderate to severe rheumatoid arthritis may use a motorized wheelchair to increase mobility and to conserve energy.

Although intellectual functioning or cognitive ability remains intact with rheumatoid arthritis, the effect of pain on individuals' ability to concentrate should be considered. The combination of pain and the disabling consequences of rheumatoid arthritis may be associated with depression, which in turn can affect functional capacity. Management of depression, when identified, as well as interventions to enable individuals to decrease their pain and cope more effectively, may be beneficial in increasing their capacity for maintaining their vocational status.

Systemic Lupus Erythematosus

The potential variety and severity of manifestations and unpredictable course of systemic lupus erythematosus present significant challenges for individuals who are living with this condition (Sohng, 2003). An autoimmune condition of unknown cause, **systemic lupus erythematosus** can affect the skin, joints, kidney, heart, lungs, nervous system, blood, and other organs of the body (Giffords, 2003). It is most common in young women and does not usually develop in individuals past middle age (Trethewey, 2004). This condition produces inflammation and structural changes in many body organs and may cause neurological and psychiatric manifestations, including cerebrovascular conditions, movement and/or cognitive consequences, seizures, and anxiety disorder (ACR Ad Hoc Committee on Neuropsychiatric Lupus Nomenclature, 1999). It may progress rapidly or slowly, or it can become chronic with associated remissions and exacerbation.

Manifestations vary from individual to individual, but may include a characteristic "butterfly rash" on the face, increased sensitivity to sunlight, loss of appetite, and weight loss. As the condition progresses, it may have more serious effects, such as kidney damage, accumulation of fluid around the heart or lungs, and mental changes, including forgetfulness, confusion, and, in some instances, seizures.

The prognosis for individuals with systemic lupus erythematosus depends on the organs that are involved and the degree of autoimmune reaction experienced. This condition is not curable and requires long-term management. For many individuals, appropriate management interventions can control or suppress the manifestations; however, the disease may also result in death (Ruiz-Irastorza, Khamashta, Castellino, & Hughes, 1999). Some individuals experience years of remission in which they are almost free of manifestations, whereas others rapidly develop kidney damage. Women may experience flare-ups of the condition at certain times of the menstrual cycle and during or after pregnancy. Complications such as cardiac manifestations or renal damage are treated as appropriate. Persons with severe kidney involvement may require dialysis (see Chapter 15).

Management of Systemic

Lupus Erythematosus

Systemic lupus erythematosus requires individualized lifelong management. The goal is to improve or maintain organ function and to prevent permanent organ damage (Schur, 2004). Mild cases may require few or no interventions. When interventions are necessary, the type and location of the condition determine the type of intervention prescribed. If major organs such as the heart or kidney are involved, management is directed toward preserving function and preventing organ failure that could result in functional consequences or death. In mild cases, salicylates or NSAIDs may be used. In more severe cases, steroids may be indicated (Schur, 2004).

Individuals with systemic lupus erythematosus may need more than the regular amount of rest. Exercise to the point of exhaustion and stressful situations should be avoided, as both can cause exacerbation of the condition.

Psychosocial Issues in Systemic Lupus Erythematosus

Although the identification of systemic lupus erythematous may cause emotional reactions and psychological issues, some psychological manifestations may be manifestations of the condition itself. Individuals may need considerable emotional support. Not only is systemic lupus erythematosus a potentially fatal condition, but most individuals affected are in young adulthood, when the psychosocial and vocational impact of the condition can have a profound effect.

Individuals with systemic lupus erythematosus may need considerable rest, which may be difficult due to other responsibilities. The stress of pregnancy and childbirth may exacerbate manifestations; consequently, the decision of whether to have children may be a difficult one for women with this condition.

The degree of psychosocial distress resulting from the condition depends, to some degree, on the severity of the manifestations.

Vocational Issues in Systemic Lupus Erythematosus

Fatigue is a challenge for many individuals with systemic lupus erythematosus (Varga, Manzi, & Lakos, 2007), such that individuals may need more than the regular amount of rest. Exercise to the point of exhaustion and stressful situations should be avoided, as both can cause exacerbation of the condition. For this reason, adequate rest periods and appropriate scheduling are important.

Individuals with systemic lupus erythematosus are often sensitive to sunlight, which may trigger manifestations. Individuals should avoid excessive exposure to the sun, wear protective clothing, and use sunscreen routinely (Varga et al., 2007). Other musculoskeletal conditions may become worse in cold, damp environments.

While in remission, and if there is no associated permanent organ damage, individuals with systemic lupus erythematosus may have few physical or emotional disabilities.

Gout

Gout is a condition that results from hyperuricemia—that is, buildup in the body of uric acid (Terkeltaub, 2004). Uric acid is a waste product of the metabolism of purines, which are found in a variety of foods. It is usually carried in the blood until it is excreted by the kidneys. With gout, uric acid levels in the blood increase, either because the kidneys are not excreting uric acid fast enough or because the body is making too much uric acid. Excess uric acid changes into crystals, called urate crystals, which settle in the joints, causing swelling and excruciating pain. Individuals with gout are more likely than are others to develop kidney stones (*urolithiasis*; see Chapter 15), which occasionally cause obstruction and severe kidney damage (Terkeltaub, 2003).

Manifestations of Gout

Gout can be inherited, or it can be a complication of another condition. Manifestations, which appear suddenly, may be precipitated by the intake of foods and beverages rich in purines, such as organ meats (e.g., liver, sweetbreads), gravies, and alcohol. Manifestations may also be precipitated by minor injury, stress, or fatigue. Attacks may last for only a few days at first, but, if the condition is not adequately controlled, later attacks may last for weeks.

If left untreated, gout may result in chronic joint manifestations with permanent joint damage and restriction of motion. Although gout cannot be cured, prophylactic interventions can control its manifestations.

Management of Gout

The objectives in the management of gout are to terminate the acute attack, to prevent recurrent attacks, and to prevent or reverse complications that result from uric acid crystals being deposited in the joints, kidneys, or other sites (Wortmann, 2002). Management involves not only reducing acute inflammation and urinary tract stones (*urolithiasis*), but also lowering urate crystal levels in an attempt to prevent recurrent attacks and progression of the condition (Wortmann, 2002; Schlesinger & Schumacher, 2001).

During acute attacks, the affected joint is placed at rest and anti-inflammatory agents are prescribed. Prevention of further attacks may require daily use of medications for lowering the level of uric acid in the blood or for increasing its excretion by the kidneys. Occasionally, surgery is necessary to remove **tophi** (deposits of crystals in the joints).

Individuals with gout should increase their fluid intake so as to decrease the risk of kidney stones; follow a diet that excludes foods high in purines and fats, such as sardines, anchovies, organ meats, veal, and bacon; and avoid excessive alcohol intake.

Vocational Issues in Gout

Because gout can cause significant pain in affected joints, individuals may be unable to work during a gout attack. The extent of absences from work depends on the frequency and severity of the attacks. Not all joints are affected. Consequently, the degree of functional consequences that occur if there is resulting joint damage or loss of motion is dependent on the joint involved and the degree to which that joint is crucial to job performance. Because stress can precipitate gout attacks, individuals should avoid stressful situations or should be helped with stress management.

Ankylosing Spondylitis

Ankylosing spondylitis comprises a group of inflammatory rheumatic conditions also referred to as *spondyloarthropathies* (SpA). There appears to be a strong genetic predisposition to developing this condition, and, although once thought to occur mainly in males, cases in females are also common (Breban, 2007). Ankylosing spondylitis primarily affects the spinal and pelvic skeleton, although skin and gastrointestinal manifestations may be present as well (Breban, 2007). It is a progressive condition that frequently leads to deterioration in spinal posture (Swinkels & Dolan, 2004).

Manifestations most often involve persistent back pain, beginning in the lumbar area and moving upward (Inman, 2004). Individuals may also experience *uveitis* (inflammation of the iris, ciliary body, and choroid layer of the eye; see Chapter 5), psoriasis (see Chapter 17), and inflammatory bowel disease (Breban, 2007).

The inflammatory process around these joints causes pain and can result in a fusing of the joints, with subsequent loss and/or restriction of motion. Back pain, of varying intensity, is the most common initial complaint. It is often worse at night. Other complaints may include morning stiffness, which is relieved by activity, and systemic manifestations, such as fatigue, weight loss, loss of appetite, and anemia. Postural irregularities may develop with resulting spinal deformities. If the condition is untreated, a permanent postural manifestation called **kyphosis** (humpback) may occur.

The course of ankylosing spondylitis and its severity is highly variable (Inman, 2004). With proper management, many individuals have little permanent functional consequence. There may be occasional flare-ups when the manifestations become worse, but there may also be long periods with no manifestations (Cornell, 2004).

Management of Ankylosing Spondylitis

Management of ankylosing spondylitis involves relieving pain and inflammation and maximizing function through physical therapy and exercise. NSAIDs may be administered to decrease inflammation and pain, thereby facilitating exercise.

Exercises prescribed are designed to strengthen supporting muscles and to maintain good posture and function. Good posture is essential to prevent spinal irregularity. Physical therapy should begin early to keep the spine as straight as possible, thereby preserving the chest's ability to expand. In the case of severe spinal irregularity, surgical intervention may be indicated.

Vocational Issues in Ankylosing Spondylitis

Individuals with ankylosing spondylitis experience no limitation with regard to their cognitive skills, vision, or motor coordination. Because of the stiffness and potential fusing of

joints of the spine, however, twisting and turning motions as well as lifting may be limited. If individuals develop kyphosis, the altered self-image may be accompanied by embarrassment and a reluctance to work in situations in which the public is encountered.

Other Conditions of the Musculoskeletal System

Osteomyelitis

Osteomyelitis (infection of the bone) can be acute or chronic, can occur at any age, and can have significant functional consequences with a long course of management interventions (Brause, 2004; Calhoun, Laughlin, Mader, & Maher, 1998). This disease can occur in several hours. For example, pathologic organisms can enter the bone directly through an injury, such as an open or compound fracture in which the broken bone fragment has penetrated through the skin, allowing pathologic organisms to enter and invade the bone. Osteomyelitis may also result from infection of surrounding tissue, with the infection then extending to the bone. For example, ulceration of tissue in a lower extremity that occurs due to **vascular insufficiency** (inadequate supply of blood and oxygen to a body part) in conditions such as arteriosclerosis or diabetes may cause the tissue to become infected, and infection may then extend to the bone. In other instances, pathologic organisms present in the blood may settle and localize in the bone.

Management of Osteomyelitis

Osteomyelitis is often difficult to cure. Interventions for management of osteomyelitis may be either nonsurgical or surgical. Nonsurgical interventions consist of the administration of antibiotics and bed rest until the infection has been eradicated. Surgical interventions may be indicated to remove infected tissue, replace a portion of bone with a graft, or replace an infected prosthetic joint (Lazzarini, 2007).

Fibromyalgia

Fibromyalgia is a chronic pain syndrome characterized by aching, stiffness in muscles and/or joints, and exaggerated tenderness at 18 specific tender points on the body (Abeles, Pillinger, Solitar, & Abeles, 2007). It is also frequently associated with sleep disturbance and fatigue (Millea & Holloway, 2000). Manifestations may range from mild to moderate to severe.

The pain and discomfort associated with fibromyalgia are diffuse, involving the neck, shoulders, lower back, and hips, as well as other sites. Fibromyalgia is not a progressively degenerative condition and does not cause damage to bones or joints; consequently, there are no objective findings or definitive diagnostic tests available that can legitimize the condition (Bennett, 2004). As a result, the condition can be quite perplexing both for the individuals with manifestations and for their physicians, who are often unable to establish a clear-cut diagnosis (Clauw, 2000).

Given that there are no definitive laboratory or radiographic tests available to identify fibromyalgia, diagnosis is based on individuals' self-reports of history and types of manifestations, with the identifiable tender points being a prime diagnostic marker. Individuals with fibromyalgia can also experience manifestations other than musculoskeletal pain, including headache and irritable bowel syndrome (see Chapter 12). Complaints of sleep disturbances and fatigue are common. Any significant life stress can exacerbate manifestations.

Psychological manifestations of anxiety and depression frequently accompany this condition (Longley, 2006). Adjustment to manifestations may be more difficult due to the uncertainty associated with the condition (Johnson, Zautra, & Davis, 2006). Fibromyalgia can interfere with individuals' quality of life and may cause interpersonal difficulties when manifestations occur. Individuals often find it helpful to be reassured that the condition is "real." Legitimizing individuals' experience of manifestations can help reestablish self-control and self-esteem, enabling them to cope with their condition.

Management of Fibromyalgia

Fibromyalgia is a chronic condition in which only relative improvement can be expected. Management may include medications such as NSAIDs and antidepressants, as well as exercise, nutrition, acupuncture, and stress reduction (Massey, 2007). No one intervention seems to be universally effective (Adams & Sim, 2005). Recent studies have suggested that hyperbaric oxygen therapy (discussed later in this chapter) may also be useful in management of fibromyalgia (Yildiz et al., 2004).

Although simple analgesics such as acetaminophen or NSAIDs may be prescribed by physicians for their patients with fibromyalgia, medications such as systemic corticosteroids or stronger pain relievers are not recommended. Low-dose tricyclic antidepressants (see Chapter 8) may also be beneficial to assist individuals with sleep. If individuals are experiencing stress or have other underlying psychological factors that exacerbate sleep disturbances or pain perception, then stress management, relaxation, or counseling may be needed to help them cope with the condition. Some individuals also find support groups useful. It is important that individuals remain physically and socially active, and efforts should be made to identify and eliminate stresses or environmental disturbances that may exacerbate manifestations.

Vocational Issues in Fibromyalgia

Individuals with fibromyalgia may have repeated absenteeism at work because of pain, fatigue, or both. The direct effect on individuals' ability to work depends on a number of factors, including the nature of the job, the person's motivation to follow suggested lifestyle changes, and the presence of any underlying psychological factors.

Many individuals with fibromyalgia must learn how to pace themselves, as certain physical activities may take longer than before the condition arose. Very active individuals may have to cut back on activities. Individuals should be encouraged to remain active but not to push themselves beyond their limit.

Flexibility in scheduling may be beneficial. Some job modification and restructuring may be necessary to prevent overuse or over-exertion of muscle groups. Any physical stressors identified should also be avoided. Because sleep disturbance is an accompanying manifestation, individuals may have difficulty concentrating while at work. Because of the vague nature of manifestations and the fact that there is presently no definitive test with which to diagnose fibromyalgia, individuals may be subject to the scrutiny of co-workers or employers, who may question the legitimacy of their condition and its manifestations. Individuals may be labeled as malingerers, and resentment from co-workers may result. Education of employers and co-workers can help to dispel myths and misinformation.

■ DIAGNOSTIC PROCEDURES FOR CONDITIONS OF THE MUSCULOSKELETAL SYSTEM

Roentgenography (Radiography, X-Rays)

The most widely used diagnostic tool for musculoskeletal conditions is x-ray. This painless procedure involves positioning the body part to be studied against photographic film and exposing the film by irradiation. A radiographic technician generally takes the x-ray films, and a **radiologist** (a physician who specializes in radiation and the use of radioactive materials for the diagnosis and management

of conditions) interprets them. For musculoskeletal conditions, x-ray is useful for identifying irregularity or injury of bones.

Arthrography

To perform an **arthrogram** (a radiographic study of a joint), the radiologist first injects the joint to be examined with a local anesthetic and then injects a special material or contrast medium and/or air into the joint cavity. The joint is then moved through its range of motion, and a series of x-ray films is taken. This diagnostic procedure is done to identify injury to the joint or supporting ligaments.

Discography and Myelography

Although discography and myelography are similar to arthrography, they involve the study of different areas of the body. **Discography** is a radiographic study of the cervical or lumbar disks, while *myelography* is a radiographic study of the spinal cord.

Arthroscopy

Arthroscopy is the visualization of a joint through a small instrument, called an *arthroscope* that is inserted into the joint to be studied. Videotaped pictures may be taken of the internal joint structures.

Arthrocentesis

Arthrocentesis is a procedure in which the physician aspirates synovial fluid via a needle that has been inserted into the joint cavity. The synovial fluid is then examined for irregularities, such as blood, crystals, or infection. In some instances, arthrocentesis may be used to remove fluid from the joint to relieve pain. If the joint has been injured or is infected, examination of blood or pus in the synovial fluid can help in determining the type or degree of injury or infection.

Bone Scan

A bone scan is a procedure in which radioactive substances, called radioisotopes, are injected intravenously. The radioisotopes concentrate in the bone, and the amount of concentration is measured by a special machine called a scanner. The scanner produces a picture of the bone (scan), enabling physicians to identify any irregularities.

Magnetic Resonance Imaging

A painless, noninvasive procedure, magnetic resonance imaging (MRI) produces rapid, detailed pictures of body tissue. It is widely used to assist in the identification of musculoskeletal conditions as well as conditions affecting other body systems. The MRI procedure requires no radiation. It may be performed without contrast (a substance that is injected and enables visualization) or with contrast (i.e., individuals are injected with a contrast substance intravenously).

For MRI studies, individuals are placed in a horizontal cylinder, where they are exposed to a magnetic field much greater than the earth's normal magnetic field. During this procedure, hydrogen atoms within the body line up parallel to the magnetic field. Low-energy radio waves are then directed into the individual's body, causing protons in the body to move out of alignment, a process is called resonance. When the radio waves are discontinued, the protons realign. The machine picks up the amount of energy released by the protons as they swing back into alignment and converts it to produce an image of the body part being studied.

Because of the strength of the magnetic field used for the procedure, individuals with metal in their body should not undergo MRI. Thus this imaging technique is contraindicated for individuals with a cardiac pacemaker, metal clips that have been placed in the body as part of a prior surgical procedure, or small pieces of metal embedded by injury (e.g., shrapnel).

MRI is used for diagnosing conditions of many body systems. In the musculoskeletal system, it is helpful in diagnosing conditions of the joints, confirming infection of the bone (**osteomyelitis**), discovering small fractures of the bone that may not be detectable by other means, and identifying soft-tissue and bone tumors.

Computed Tomography (Computed Axial Tomography, CAT Scan, CT Scan)

Computed tomography (CT scan) is a noninvasive radiographic procedure that may be performed either with or without contrast. It may be used to diagnose a number of conditions affecting many different body systems. In the musculoskeletal system, this imaging technique may be helpful in identifying fractures, tumors, bone deformities, or soft-tissue damage.

During the imaging procedure, individuals are placed within a hollow tube, and then x-rays are passed through the body part at many different angles. Because each tissue has a different density, each density is given a numerical value, which is computed and displayed on a screen. The resulting image is then recorded on film. The CT scan is performed by the radiologist.

Blood Tests

In and of themselves, blood tests are not diagnostic for specific conditions of the musculoskeletal system. Nevertheless, some blood tests indicate inflammation or tissue injury and, therefore, may be used as part of the diagnostic process. For example, a determination of the *erythrocyte sedimentation rate* may be part of the diagnostic workup for conditions such as rheumatoid arthritis. Another test, *C-reactive protein*, may also be used to identify inflammatory processes or tissue destruction.

A blood test commonly used in identification of rheumatoid arthritis is the *rheumatoid factor (RF)*. The *latex fixation* or *agglutination tests* for RF are not definitive tests for rheumatoid arthritis but merely provide supportive evidence when individuals have corresponding manifestations. The blood test determines whether abnormal protein is present in the serum. Many individuals with rheumatoid arthritis have such protein, although individuals with many other conditions (e.g., tuberculosis, bacterial endocarditis) may also have the factor in their serum.

Another blood test that may be used, especially in identification of systemic lupus erythematosus, is the *antinuclear antibodies (ANA) test*. Antinuclear antibodies are proteins found in the blood of some individuals with autoimmune conditions; the ANA tests identify the presence of these proteins. However, because the test may be positive in many different autoimmune conditions or may be positive as a result of some medications, it is not definitive proof of a particular condition.

■ GENERAL MANAGEMENT OF CONDITIONS OF THE MUSCULOSKELETAL SYSTEM

Medications

Pain and inflammation are manifestations of many musculoskeletal and connective tissue conditions. *Salicylates* (e.g., aspirin) are commonly the first choice of medication to reduce pain and inflammation. For some conditions, such as rheumatoid arthritis, it may be necessary to prescribe as many as 15 or more tablets of salicylate per day to reach a therapeutic dos-

age. This high concentration of aspirin in the blood may exceed the liver's ability to metabolize it. The side effects of such a high salicylate dosage include gastric irritation and ringing or noise in the ears (**tinnitus**).

NSAIDs may also be used to reduce the pain and inflammation associated with musculoskeletal conditions. Like salicylates, these drugs can irritate the stomach lining, causing pain and, in some instances, bleeding.

Corticosteroids can produce dramatic short-term anti-inflammatory effects, but they do not prevent progression of joint destruction and, because of their potency and subsequent side effects, can be used only on a short-term basis. Side effects of prolonged use may include cataracts, demineralization of bone, delayed wound healing, poor resistance to infection, and manifestations similar to those of Cushing's syndrome (see Chapter 11). More serious systemic effects may involve severe adrenal insufficiency following withdrawal (see Chapter 11). Steroid use should always be carefully monitored by a physician, and steroids should never be discontinued suddenly. Although steroids for musculoskeletal conditions are generally taken orally, they are sometimes injected directly into an inflamed joint for the temporary suppression of the inflammation.

Hyperbaric Oxygen Therapy

Hyperbaric oxygen therapy is an intervention in which 100% oxygen is given at two to three times the atmospheric pressure at sea level. It is used for a number of conditions in addition to musculoskeletal conditions—for example, carbon monoxide poisoning, decompression sickness, radiation-induced tissue injury, and severe skin injury. Specific conditions of the musculoskeletal system for which hyperbaric oxygen therapy is used include chronic osteomyelitis (Sugihara et al., 2004), crush injuries or other severe trauma to the extremities that results in insufficient blood flow to the extremity resulting in **necrosis** (tissue death) (Chen, Ko, Fu, & Wang, 2004), thermal burns and skin grafts or flaps (see Chapter 17) that have inadequate blood flow or oxygen and are not healing properly, and foot and leg ulcers associated with diabetes (see Chapter 11) (Kranke, Bennett, Roeckl-Wiedmann, & Debus, 2004).

Hyperbaric oxygen therapy works by restoring the body's defenses against infection and increasing the rate at which the body is able to kill common bacteria. Individuals inhale hyperbaric oxygen in the atmosphere of a special cylindrical single-occupant chamber in which they have been placed, or through masks, hoods, or special tubes that are inserted into the individual's **trachea** (windpipe).

The length and amount of intervention depend on the reason for the intervention. Single interventions can range from 45 minutes of hyperbaric oxygen for carbon monoxide poisoning to almost 5 hours for conditions involving severe decompression. For musculoskeletal conditions, the individual may undergo 20 to 30 interventions, averaging approximately 90 minutes each. Although hyperbaric interventions can be costly, when comparing the cost with hospitalization for conditions that are not successfully managed, the savings can be extensive.

Physical Therapy

Many types of musculoskeletal conditions can be improved through physical therapy techniques. These techniques are usually performed by a physical therapist or a physical therapy assistant. A *physical therapist* is an individual with a bachelor's degree in physical therapy who provides services that help develop, restore, or preserve physical function. A physical therapy assistant is generally an individual with an associate's degree who works under the direction of a physical therapist.

The type of physical therapy administered depends on the particular musculoskeletal condition. Physical therapy may be directed toward increasing or maintaining a joint's range of motion, increasing muscle strength, relieving pain or muscle spasms, or teaching techniques for ambulation.

Some techniques used in physical therapy involve therapeutic exercise, which may be passive or active. In **passive exercise**, the therapist or a mechanical device exercises the body part. In **active exercise**, the individual independently performs a specified exercise regimen under the direction or supervision of the physical therapist or physical therapy assistant. Exercise may be designed to increase or maintain range of motion, prevent **atrophy** (shrinking of the muscles), prevent irregularity due to contractures, or increase muscle strength.

Other physical therapy techniques may involve application of heat or cold or the massage of muscles for relaxation or relief of pain. Heat may be applied through hot packs, hot soaks, infrared radiation, or whirlpool baths. Another procedure for applying heat is *diathermy*, a process in which the temperature of the body part is raised through high-frequency ultrasonic waves. Because cold has a numbing effect, it may also be used to relieve pain; that is, cold packs or chemical packs may be applied to the painful area. *Massage*—the manipulation of muscles through rubbing or kneading—may be used to relax muscles, improve muscle tone, relieve muscle spasm, or increase blood flow to the area.

Casts

Another intervention used in the management of a variety of musculoskeletal conditions is casting. Although casts may be synthetic, they are more commonly made of plaster of Paris.

Casts provide immobilization and support for a body part while it is healing. They may also be used to prevent or correct various musculoskeletal deformities. The type and size of cast depend on the condition and the purpose of the casting. In addition to casts used on extremities, *spica casts*, which extend the entire length of the lower extremity from the middle of the trunk of the body, may be used. In some instances, a full body cast is necessary.

Assistive Devices

Individuals with musculoskeletal conditions may use assistive devices to aid in ambulation, prevent undue strain on a body part, or restore or enhance functional capacity. Assistive devices may be used therapeutically in the healing period after musculoskeletal injury, or they may be used on a continuing basis. Examples of assistive devices that aid in ambulation or prevent excessive weight bearing on a lower extremity include canes, crutches, and walkers. Other examples of assistive devices include the special devices used by individuals with upper extremity irregularities that assist the individual in performing activities of daily living, such as long-handled grippers, zipper pulls, or jar-opening devices (see Chapter 19 for a fuller discussion of assistive devices).

Orthosis

Devices used to straighten or correct an irregularity of a body part (**orthosis**) are applied to the body to control the motion of joints and the force or weight distribution to a body part. A brace, for example, is an orthotic device used to provide support or to prevent or correct an irregularity. The type of device used depends on the purpose of the bracing and the condition itself. An **orthotist** is an individual who constructs orthotic devices to meet individual needs.

Orthoses may be prescribed for any musculoskeletal area, depending on the nature of the problem. For example, lower limb orthoses include orthopedic shoes and orthoses for the foot, ankle, knee, or hip. Spinal orthoses may be used to relieve compression forces on the spine, restrict movement of the spine, or modify the alignment of the spine.

At least 50 types of spinal orthoses are distinguished based on the level of application. Cervical orthoses may be prescribed for a wide variety of problems, ranging from whiplash to fracture of the cervical spine. *The Taylor, Jewett Hyperextension TLSO*, and *C.A.S.H.* spinal orthoses are prescribed to restrict trunk flexion and rotation or to provide hyperextension and reduce flexion in the thoraciclumbar spine. *Lumbar–sacral spinal* orthoses, such as the *Knight Chairback* and *Williams,* are prescribed primarily for low back pain and may consist of flexible or semi-rigid corsets that provide support and protection. The *Milwaukee brace* is an orthotic device used as an intervention for **scoliosis** (lateral S-shaped curvature of the spine).

Orthotic devices may also be used for the upper extremities. In these instances, they are most frequently prescribed because of injury. Upper-extremity orthoses may be applied to the shoulder, elbow, or wrist/hand. Newer orthotic devices, called *fracture orthoses*, are designed to allow early ambulation on fractures of the lower extremity. These devices permit functional use of the extremity much earlier than does conventional casting. Recently, fracture orthoses have also been used as interventions for some upper- extremity fractures.

Traction

Individuals with a variety of musculoskeletal conditions may benefit from **traction**, a therapeutic method in which a mechanical or manual pull is used to restore or maintain the alignment of bones or to relieve pain and muscle spasm (see Figure 16-6). It may be applied in several ways. When traction exerts a constant pull, it is said to be *continuous*. If the pull is relieved periodically, the traction is said to be *intermittent*. Traction may be applied externally or internally.

Skin traction is applied by fastening straps, belts, or other external devices around the body and then to a source of counter-traction. In contrast, skeletal traction is applied internally; metal wires (*Kirschner wires*), pins (*Steinmann pins*), or tongs (*Crutchfield tongs*) are inserted through the bone surgically and attached to a source of counter-traction outside the body. Kirschner wires and Steinmann pins are typically used to reduce (align) fractures of the long bones of the extremities so as to promote bone healing or to stabilize the fracture until surgical intervention can be undertaken to correct the fracture. Crutchfield tongs are inserted into the skull for injuries of the cervical spine.

The use of traction may prevent surgical intervention in some cases, and it offers more freedom of movement than does a cast. However, it usually requires prolonged hospitalization. Furthermore, in the case of skeletal traction, there is a risk of complications, such as osteomyelitis, that can contribute to permanent functional consequences.

Surgical Management

Individuals with musculoskeletal conditions may require surgical interventions to correct, remove, or replace injured or damaged structures. Surgery may be performed on an emergency basis in the case of traumatic injury or on an elective basis in the case of damage experienced due to a chronic condition or an old traumatic injury. Several types of surgical interventions are possible:

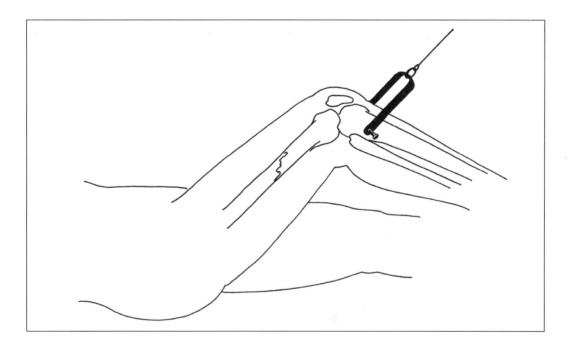

Figure 16-6 Skeletal traction

- **Open reduction**: surgical alignment of the fractured bone.
- **Internal fixation**: placement of screws, pins, wires, rods, or other devices through the bone to hold the bone fragments together.
- **Arthroplasty**: replacement of all or part of a joint with a prosthetic device to relieve pain or to restore function. Common sites of arthroplasty are the hip, shoulder, knee, and elbow. Reasons for arthroplasty include a broken hip (total hip replacement) or arthritis.
- **Arthrodesis**: surgical fusing (joining) of two joint surfaces, making them permanently immobile. This procedure was once commonly performed to relieve joint pain. With improved arthroplasty procedures, however, arthrodesis is now less common.
- **Synovectomy**: surgical removal of the synovial membrane surrounding a joint. It prevents recurrent inflammation, thus reducing joint pain and further joint destruction.
- **Laminectomy**: surgical removal of a portion of a vertebra, exposing the spinal cord. It is usually performed to facilitate the removal of any source of pressure on the spinal cord (i.e., to remove bone fragments from spinal cord injury; to remove tumor from the spinal cord).
- **Spinal fusion**: grafting of bone from another area of the body into the disk interspace after a surgical procedure on the spine (e.g., laminectomy). After spinal fusion, mobility at the point of the fusion is lost.
- **Carpal tunnel repair**: a surgical procedure in which the median nerve is decompressed by the transection of surrounding ligaments. It is performed when the manifestations of carpal tunnel syndrome are severe, with progressive sensory loss in the fingers and hand.

■ PSYCHOSOCIAL ISSUES IN CONDITIONS OF THE MUSCULOSKELETAL SYSTEM

Psychological Issues

Emotional needs of individuals with musculoskeletal conditions often relate to prolonged dependence on others, the long-term nature of the condition, and uncertainty about the ability to resume regular responsibilities and activities. Restrictions on mobility and natural movements because of casts, braces, or traction or because of pain, limb irregularity, or absence of a limb is, for many individuals, unbearable. Depending on the extent of immobility, there may be a sense of powerlessness leading to anger, hostility, and, later, depression. If the musculoskeletal condition necessitates giving up some valued activity permanently, depression may deepen. Some individuals who have a strong athletic identity may fail to disclose their condition, continuing the activity even though it may cause additional damage.

Prolonged pain associated with many musculoskeletal system conditions consumes energy and may contribute to increased self-centeredness and dependence, as pain becomes the central issue in the lives of individuals experiencing it. Discomfort, as well as the restriction of mobility, can contribute to irritability, discouragement, and depression. Pain perception is related not only to various personality factors, but also to factors such as worker's compensation, litigation, or other benefits that may decrease individuals' motivation to reduce pain or restore function. As activities become limited owing to pain, individuals may enter into a vicious cycle in which they become demoralized and isolated, causing them to further restrict their activity (Guite, Logan, Sherry, & Rose, 2007).

Individuals who are planning to undergo musculoskeletal surgery may experience a mixture of fear and anticipation regarding the extent to which the surgery will restore lost function. Those having repeated surgery, such as a second joint replacement for arthritis, or continuing interventions for management of osteomyelitis may lose patience and hope.

Individuals with chronic conditions of the musculoskeletal system may force themselves to do more than they comfortably can because of fear being a burden to others. Inability to maintain previous activity levels may cause continued frustration. The unpredictability of conditions that are characterized by remissions and exacerbations (e.g., rheumatoid arthritis) may also be a source of tension.

Irregularities of limbs or posture associated with many musculoskeletal conditions, such as rheumatoid arthritis, ankylosing spondylitis, osteoporosis, or amputation, may lead to altered body image. Most individuals react to any body image change with anxiety and fear of rejection. The value and subjective meaning of appearance can influence individuals' reactions to the alteration of appearance such that concerns about acceptance of family, friends, and acquaintances can preoccupy their thoughts.

Activities and Participation

Although many conditions of the musculoskeletal system require only short-term intervention and impose only temporary restrictions on activity, some conditions require lifelong adaptation and significant lifestyle changes. In some conditions, such as osteoporosis, fear of fracture may lead to limitation of activity, which can in turn affect quality of life and contribute to depression (Kotz, Deleger, Cohen, Kamigaki, & Kurata, 2004). Restrictions on body movement resulting from a loss of muscle strength, irregularity of joints, or pain may alter the individual's activities of daily living, social activities, and recreational activities. Individuals may need to learn new ambulation

and transfer techniques and find alternatives to activities that place undue stress on joints. In addition, it may be necessary to install grab bars and safety rails in the home to provide stability and prevent falls.

Conditions affecting the ankles or the feet may require wearing of special shoes for protection of the joints and for comfort. Sitting while performing many tasks, such as meal preparation, may save wear and tear on weight-bearing joints. Conditions affecting joints of the hands, such as rheumatoid arthritis, may require use of assistive devices, such as hooks, zipper pulls, special openers, or other self-help aids, if individuals are to perform activities of daily living independently. Adaptive handles for combs and brushes may be of help for grooming. Soft lead pencils and felt-tipped pens may be useful for decreasing pressure on finger joints when writing.

At home, work centers may be established where all the items needed for a specific task are kept within easy reach. It may be necessary to lower tables and cabinets so that individuals with a musculoskeletal condition may be seated while they work and to raise beds, toilet seats, and chairs so that sitting and arising are easier. Organizing and planning daily tasks can help to reduce strain and fatigue.

Dietary modifications may be necessary in some conditions of the musculoskeletal system. Obesity places extra strain on joints; consequently, if obesity is an issue, a weight-reduction diet may be prescribed. Specific conditions, such as gout, may also require dietary modifications. Individuals with pain in or structural irregularity of the hands and those who have undergone upper-extremity amputation may need special adaptive eating utensils for activities such as cutting meat.

Many conditions of the musculoskeletal system require some form of therapeutic exercise to maintain joint function, restore strength and/or joint motion, or prevent structural irregularities. Such exercise programs must be incorporated into the daily routine. Conditions such as rheumatoid arthritis may require that individuals follow a pattern of specified rest periods during the day.

Most conditions of the musculoskeletal system do not hamper sexual activity. Nevertheless, pain, structural irregularities, decreased range of motion of joints, or alteration in body image may affect sexual function. Positioning may be difficult or painful, as in the case of rheumatoid arthritis or low back pain. In some instances, medications used for management of musculoskeletal conditions can affect sexual function. Steroids prescribed for a number of musculoskeletal conditions may decrease libido, and pain may inhibit sexual desire.

Because conditions of the musculoskeletal system can impair mobility and because in some cases individuals must depend on others for assistance, support and understanding of family and friends are paramount. Reassurance that physical changes or deformities are unimportant can be valuable to individuals' self-esteem and confidence, although such reassurance by family and friends is not always forthcoming.

Depending on the extent of discomfort, limitation of motion, and structural irregularity, individuals may be unable to perform all of their previous tasks, making it necessary for other family members to share household chores and duties. Their willingness or reluctance to accept necessary alterations in home life can affect how individuals adjust to their condition. When work or social activities are significantly altered by the individual's musculoskeletal condition, social identity may be altered. Role changes may be a source of stress. In some instances, if friendships initially developed around specific activities that now must be altered because of the condition, individuals may feel a sense of social isolation and "no longer fitting in."

When mobility is altered as a result of a musculoskeletal condition, it may be necessary to plan vacations around the condition. Other manifestations of the musculoskeletal condition may also need to be considered when planning vacations. Individuals with systemic lupus erythematosus may have to avoid hot, sunny beaches, whereas individuals with other musculoskeletal conditions may need to avoid colder climates. Individuals who are experiencing severe pain may be reluctant to venture on vacation at all.

Family and friends may have difficulty in coping with the feelings of hostility, frustration, or irritability expressed by individuals because of pain or increased dependency. Others may view these individuals as demanding, manipulative, and difficult. Depending on pre-morbid functioning of the family and the degree and quality of communication between family members, family dynamics can represent an increased source of tension.

Individuals with musculoskeletal conditions, especially those involving ongoing pain, are especially vulnerable to unorthodox, unproven "miracle cures." Although alternative and complementary practices have a place in management of musculoskeletal conditions (Pelletier, Astin, & Haskell, 1999), some unscrupulous individuals seek to take advantage of individuals' vulnerability by marketing and selling methods that are of dubious value. In addition to the expense, many fraudulent measures have dangerous side effects that, in some instances, can be fatal. Even if there are no side effects, individuals may use these methods in place of recommended interventions, thereby losing the therapeutic effects of conventional interventions. When complementary and alternative methods are used by individuals to treat musculoskeletal conditions, the safety of the method and the legitimacy of the individual providing it should always be determined before use.

■ VOCATIONAL ISSUES IN CONDITIONS OF THE MUSCULOSKELETAL SYSTEM

Restrictions associated with work-related musculoskeletal conditions are an increasing problem. Although many individuals with work-related injuries eventually return to their jobs, a substantial number of individuals do not (Turner et al., 2004). The functional consequences of musculoskeletal conditions are a multifactorial problem extending beyond the condition itself; that is, they are also the result of the workplace, the healthcare system, and the compensation system (Loisel et al., 2005).

The impact of a particular musculoskeletal condition on vocational function depends on the type of job previously held, individual factors related to job history and motivation, and the specific condition (Rahman, Ambler, Underwood, & Shipley, 2004). The amount of sitting, bending, stooping, or lifting that the job requires must be considered. Modification of the work environment, such as raising or lowering of worktables or chairs, may be necessary. Generally, it is important that individuals return to work and daily activities as soon as possible to maintain good work habits.

Injured-worker programs and work-hardening programs have grown in popularity as means to help individuals return to work. These programs use a systemic approach of case management, evaluation, and other interventions that prepares workers for successful and safe reentry into the workforce after injury (Schonstein, Kenny, Keating, & Koes, 2003; Weir & Nielson, 2001).

In injured-worker programs, individuals' physical capacity or level of function is evaluated as they progress through a graded series of job simulation tasks. Evaluation provides objective data regarding individuals' physical and functional capacity so that goals and a management plan can be established. Services are provided on an outpatient basis. Work-tolerance screening focuses on individuals' musculoskeletal strength, endurance, speed, and flexibility. Functional capacity evaluation documents individuals' ability to return to work from a physical, behavioral, and ergonomic perspective.

Work conditioning (work hardening) prepares individuals to return to competitive employment (Johnson, Archer-Heese, Caron-Powles, & Dowson, 2001). Its goal is to increase work tolerance, increase work rate, help individuals learn to control manifestations of their condition, increase confidence and proficiency, and teach individuals to use work adaptations and assistive devices. Such a program is highly structured and, in addition to including simulated or real work tasks, instills expectations for the real-world environment, such as promptness, attendance, and appropriate dress.

Assistive devices such as crutches, walkers, or canes may make ambulation slower and more difficult. In addition, the use of such devices makes it difficult—if not impossible—to carry objects from one point to another.

Rheumatoid arthritis, ankylosing spondylitis, systemic lupus erythematosus, and a number of other connective tissue conditions are progressive in nature and often follow an unpredictable course. Although not all individuals with these conditions experience severe functional consequences, ongoing care and evaluation are necessary. When remissions and exacerbations are associated with the condition, there may be unexpected periods of exacerbation in which work is missed. Individuals may need to avoid overexertion, stress, and fatigue, which may in turn necessitate altered or shortened work schedules to accommodate periods of rest.

Overuse of damaged joints should be avoided. For example, individuals with osteoarthritis of the knees should avoid excessive walking; those with carpal tunnel syndrome should avoid repetitive activities with the hands. Structural irregularity of joints not only may interfere with occupational function, but also may be potentially embarrassing to the individual in personal interactions at work. Occasionally, barriers such as financial disincentives, the status of legal claims, and other compensation protocols can interfere with effective rehabilitation of individuals with musculoskeletal conditions. Individuals may be hesitant to learn new skills or use devices that help them to maintain independence if, in so doing, they imperil possible financial benefits or are expected to return to a work environment they did not or will not enjoy.

CASE STUDIES

Case 1

Ms. M. is an office manager in a private physician's office. In addition to managing the office staff, she sits at her desk working on the computer for most of the day. Ms. M. recently began experiencing lower back pain, which became worse when she lifted a box she was attempting to move to a different location. Although she has had a number of tests, no specific cause for the back pain has been identified. Her pain has continued over the last three months to the extent that Ms. M. states she is unable to be at work most of the time.

1. Which specific information about M.'s condition should be considered when assessing her capacity for continuing her employment?
2. Is Ms. M.'s current job a good choice for employment given her current medical condition? Why or why not?
3. Which types of interventions might Ms. M. find helpful?

Case 2

Mr. U., a 19-year-old factory worker, was injured in a machinery accident at work and, as a result, experienced traumatic amputation of his left leg above the knee. His job at the factory involved operating a labeling machine. Mr. U. has received a permanent prosthesis and is ready to consider returning to work.

1. Which factors in addition to his injury would contribute to Mr. U.'s effective rehabilitation?
2. What other sources of referral might be helpful to Mr. U. in his rehabilitation?
3. Are there special adaptive devices or job modifications that might be helpful to Mr. U. if he chooses to go back to the factory?
4. Which environmental factors might you consider when helping Mr. U. with rehabilitation plan?

■ REFERENCES

Abeles, A. M., Pillinger, M. H., Solitar, B. M., & Abeles, M. (2007). Narrative review: The pathophysiology of fibromyalgia. *Annals of Internal Medicine, 146,* 726–734.

ACR Ad Hoc Committee on Neuropsychiatric lupus nomenclature. (1999). The American College of Rheumatology nomenclature and case definitions for neuropsychiatric lupus syndromes. *Arthritis & Rheumatism, 42,* 599–608.

Adams, N., Poole, H., & Richardson, C. (2006). Psychological approaches to chronic pain management: Part 1. *Journal of Clinical Nursing, 15,* 290–300.

Adams, N., & Sim, J. (2005). Rehabilitation approaches in fibromyalgia. *Disability & Rehabilitation. 27*(12), 711–723.

Allaire, S. H., Li, W., & LaValley, M. P. (2003). Work barriers experienced and job accommodations used by persons with arthritis and other rheumatic diseases. *Rehabilitation Counseling Bulletin, 46*(3), 147–156.

American College of Rheumatology Subcommittee on Rheumatoid Arthritis Guidelines. (2002). Guidelines for the management of rheumatoid arthritis: 2002 update. *Arthritis and Rheumatism, 46,* 328–346.

Aminoff, M. J. (2004). Mechanical and other lesions of the spine, nerve roots, and spinal cord. In L. Goldman & D. Ausiello (Eds.), *Cecil textbook of medicine* (22nd ed., pp. 2230–2239). Philadelphia: W. B. Saunders.

Amputee Coalition of America. (2000). *First step: A guide for adapting to limb loss.* Knoxville, TN: National Limb Loss Information Center.

Barzel, U. S. (2007). Osteoporosis. In R. E. Rakel & E. T. Bope (Eds.), *Conn's current therapy* (pp. 714–718). Philadelphia: W. B. Saunders.

Bennett, R. M. (2004). Fibromyalgia. In L. Goldman & D. Ausiello (Eds.), *Cecil textbook of medicine* (22nd ed., pp. 1710–1713). Philadelphia: W. B. Saunders.

Blank-Reid, C. (2003). Traumatic amputations: Unkind cuts. *Nursing, 33*(7), 48–51.

Boisset, M., & Fitzcharles, M. A. (1994). Alternative medicine use by rheumatology patients in a universal health care setting. *Rheumatology, 21,* 148.

Boskey, A. L. (2001). Musculoskeletal disorders and orthopedic conditions. *Journal of the American Medical Association, 285*(5), 619–623.

Boulware, D. W. (2004). Bursitis, tendonitis, and other periarticular disorders. In L. Goldman & D. Ausiello (Eds.), *Cecil textbook of medicine* (22nd ed., pp. 1641–1644). Philadelphia: W. B. Saunders.

Brause, B.D. (2004). Osteomyelitis. In: L. Goldman & D. Ausiello (Eds). *Cecil Textbook of Medicine* (22nd ed., pp 1827–1829). Philadelphia: W. B. Saunders.

Breban, M. (2007). Ankylosing spondylitis. In R. E. Rakel & E. T. Bope. (Eds.), *Conn's current therapy* (pp. 1141–1143). Philadelphia: W. B. Saunders.

Brown, R. E., & Wu, T. Y. (2003). Use of "spare parts" in mutilated upper extremity injuries. *Hand Clinics, 19*(1), 73–87, vi.

Bussell, M. H. (Ed.). (2000). *New developments in prosthetics and orthotics.* Philadelphia: W. B. Saunders.

Calhoun, J. H., Laughlin, R. T., Mader, J. T., & Maher, L. (1998). Osteomyelitis: Diagnosis, staging, management. *Patient Care, 32*(2), 93–94, 99–102, 105–106, 109.

Carr, E. (2007). Barriers to effective pain management, *Journal of Perioperative Practice, 17*(5), 200–208.

Chen, C. E., Ko, J. Y., Fu, T. H., & Wang, C. J. (2004). Results of chronic osteomyelitis of the femur treated with hyperbaric oxygen: A preliminary report. *Chang Gung Medical Journal, 27*(2), 91–97.

Chuan, J. J., & Taylor, K. (2007). Common sports injuries. In R. E. Rakel & B. T. Bope (Eds.), *Conn's current therapy,* (pp. 1162–1167). Philadelphia: W. B. Saunders.

Clauw, D. J. (2000). Treating fibromyalgia: Science vs. art. *American Family Physician, 62*(7), 1492–1495.

Colburn, K. K. (2007). Bursitis, tendonitis, myofascial pain, and fibromyalgia. In R. E. Rakel & B. T. Bope (Eds.), *Conn's current therapy.* (pp. 1148–1152). Philadelphia: W. B. Saunders.

Cornell, T. (2004). Ankylosing spondylitis: An overview. *Professional Nurse, 19*(8), 431–432.

Daigeler, A., Fansa, H., & Schneider, W. (2003). Orthotopic and heterotopic lower leg reimplantation: Evaluation of seven patients. *Journal of Bone and Joint Surgery* (Br), *85*(4), 554–558.

Deyo, R. A. (1998, August). Low-back pain. *Scientific American,* 49–53.

Deyo, R. A., Nachemson, A., & Mirza, S. K. (2004). Spinal-fusion surgery: The case for restraint. *New England Journal of Medicine, 350*(7), 722–726.

Deyo, R. A., and Weinstein, J. N. (2001). Low back pain. *New England Journal of Medicine, 344*(5), 363–370.

Douglass, A. B. (2007). Pain. In R. E. Rakel & E. T. Bope (Eds.), *Conn's current therapy* (pp 1–5). Philadelphia: W. B. Saunders.

Ehrlich, G. E. (2007). Osteoarthritis. In R. E. Rakel & E. T. Bope. (Eds.) *Conn's current Therapy.* (pp. 1153–1157). Philadelphia: W. B. Saunders.

Finkkelstein, J.S. (2004). Osteoporosis. In: L. Goldman & D. Ausiello (Eds., pp. 1547–1555). *Cecil Textbook of Medicine* (22nd ed). Philadelphia: W. B. Saunders.

Foley, K. M. (2003). Opioids and chronic neuropathic pain. *New England Journal of Medicine, 348*(13), 1279–1281.

Friel, K., Domholdt, & Smith, D. G. (2005). Physical and functional measures related to low back pain in individuals with lower-limb amputation: An exploratory pilot study. *Journal of Rehabilitation Research & Development, 42*(2), 155–166.

Gallagher, P. (2004). Introduction to the special issue on psychosocial perspectives on amputation and prosthetics. *Disability and Rehabilitation, 26*(14/15), 827–830.

Gallagher, P. & MacLachlan, M. (1999). Psychological adjustment and coping in adults with prosthetic limbs. *Behavioral Medicine, 25*(3), 117–124.

Giffords, E. D. (2003). Understanding and managing systemic lupus erythematosus (SLE). *Social Work and Health Care, 37*(4), 57–72.

Glajchen, M. (2001). Chronic pain: Treatment barriers and strategies for clinical practice. *Journal of the American Board of Family Practice, 14*(3), 211–218.

Griffin, J. W. (2004). Peripheral neuropathies. In L. Goldman & D. Ausiello (Eds)., *Cecil textbook of medicine.* (22nd ed., pp. 2379–2387). Philadelphia: W. B. Saunders.

Guite, J. W., Logan, D. E., Sherry, D. D., & Rose, J. B. (2007). Adolescent self-perception: Associations with chronic musculoskeletal pain and functional disability. *Journal of Pain.* Retrieved October 9, 2007, from www.sciencedirect.com

Hanley, M. A., Jensen, M. P., Ehde, D. M., Hoffman, A. J., Patterson, D. R., & Robinson. L. R., (2004). Psychosocial predictors of long-term adjustment to lower-limb amputation and phantom limb pain. *Disability and Rehabilitation, 26*(14/15), 882–893.

Harpham, W. S. (2001). Alternative therapies for curing cancer: What do patients want? What do patients need? *Cancer Journal for Clinicians, 51*, 131–136.

Hawker, G. A., Wright, J. G., Coyte, P. C., et al. (2000). Differences between men and women in the rate of use of hip and knee arthroplasty. *New England Journal of Medicine, 342*(14), 1016–1022.

Heesch, K. C., Miller, Y. D., & Brown, W. J. (2007). Relationship between physical activity and stiff or painful joints in mid-aged women and older women: A 3-year prospective study. *Arthritis Research & Therapy, 9*(2), 1–15.

Retrieved April 18, 2007, from http://arthritis-research.com/content/9/2R34.

Herbert, J. S., & Ashworth, N. L. (2006). Predictors of return to work following traumatic work-related lower extremity amputation. *Disability and Rehabilitation, 28*(10), 613–618.

Ide, M. (2004). Sexuality in persons with limb amputation: A meaningful discussion of re-integration. *Disability and Rehabilitation, 26(14/15),* 939–943.

Inman, R. D. (2004). The spondyloarthropathies. In L. Goldman & D. Ausiello (Eds.), *Cecil textbook of medicine* (22nd ed., pp. 1654–1660). Philadelphia: W. B. Saunders.

Johnson, L. S., Archer-Heese, G., Caron-Powles, D. L., & Dowson, T. M. (2001). Work hardening: Outdated fad or effective intervention? *Work, 16*(3), 235–243.

Johnson, L. M., Zautra, A. J., & Davis, M. C. (2006). The role of illness uncertainty on coping with fibromyalgia symptoms. *Health Psychology, 25*(6), 696–703.

Kolasinski, S. L. (2001, April 15). Complementary and alternative therapies for rheumatic disease. *Hospital Practice,* 31–39.

Kooijman, C. M., Dijkstra, P. U., Geertzen, A. E., Elzinga, A., & van der Schans, C. P. (2000). Phantom pain and phantom sensations in upper limb amputees: An epidemiological study. *Pain, 87,* 33–41.

Kotz, K., Deleger, S., Cohen, R., Kamigaki, A. & Kurata, J. (2004). Osteoporosis and health-related quality-of-life outcomes in the Alameda County study population. *Preventing Chronic Disease, 1*(1), 1–8.

Kranke, P., Bennett, M., Roeckl-Wiedmann, I., & Debus, S. (2004). Hyperbaric oxygen therapy for chronic wounds. *Cochrane Database System Review, 2,* CD004123.

Kvien, T. K. (2004). Epidemiology and burden of illness of rheumatoid arthritis. *Pharmacoeconomics, 22*(2 suppl), 1–12.

Kyle, R.A. & Rajkumar, S. V. (2007). Multiple myeloma. In: R. E. Rakel & E. T. Bope (Eds.), *Conn's current therapy* (pp. 546–551). Philadelphia: W. B. Saunders.

Lazzarini, L. (2007). Osteomyelitis. In R. E. Rakel & E. T. Bope (Eds.), *Conn's current therapy* (pp 1159–1162). Philadelphia: W. B. Saunders.

Loisel, P., Falardeau, M., Baril, R., José-Durand, M., Langley, A., Sauvé, S., et al., (2005). The values underlying team decision-making in work rehabilitation for musculoskeletal disorders. *Disability and Rehabilitation, 27*(10), 561–569.

Longley, K. (2006). Fibromyalgia: Aetiology, diagnosis, symptoms and management. *British Journal of Nursing, 15*(13), 729–733.

Maher, H. K. (2007). Carpal tunnel syndrome: An update. *AAOHN Journal, 55*(5), 216.

Marcus, R. (2000). Musculoskeletal health and the older adult. *Journal of Rehabilitation Research and Development, 37*(2), 245–254.

Martens, M. P., Hewett, J. E., Parker, J. C., Smarr, K. L., Ge, B., Slaughter, J. R., et al. (2006). Development of a shortened center for epidemiological studies depression scale for assessment of depression in rheumatoid arthritis. *Rehabilitation Psychology, 51*(2), 135–139.

Massey, P. B. (2007). Reduction of fibromyalgia symptoms through intravenous nutrient therapy: Results of a pilot clinical trial. *Alternative Therapies, 13*(3), 32–34.

Max, M. B. (2004). Pain. In L. Goldman & D. Ausiello (Eds.), *Cecil textbook of medicine* (22nd ed., pp. 138–145). Philadelphia: W. B. Saunders.

McCann, M. T. (2007). Spine pain. In R. E. Rakel & E. T. Bope (Eds.), *Conn's current therapy* (pp. 40–45). Philadelphia: W. B. Saunders.

Meunier, P. J., Roux, C., Seeman, E., Ortolani, S., Badurski, J. E., Spector, T. D.,et al. (2004). The effects of strontium ranelate on the risk of vertebral fracture in women with postmenopausal osteoporosis. *New England Journal of Medicine, 350*(5), 459–468.

Meyer, T. M. (2003). Psychological aspects of mutilating hand injuries. *Hand Clinics, 19*(1), 41–49.

Mikulus T. R., & O'Dell, J. (2000). The changing face of rheumatoid arthritis therapy: Results of serial surveys. *Arthritis and Rheumatism, 43,* 464–465.

Millea, P. J., & Holloway, R. L. (2000). Treating fibromyalgia. *American Family Physician, 62*(7), 1575–1582.

Molton, I. R., Jensen, M. P., Ehde, D. M., & Smith, D. G. (2007). Phantom limb pain and pain interference in adults with lower extremity amputation: The moderating effects of age. *Rehabilitation Psychology, 52*(3), 272–279.

Moreland L. W., & O'Dell, J. R. (2002). Glucocorticoids and rheumatoid arthritis: Back to the future. *Arthritis and Rheumatism, 46,* 2553–2563.

O'Dell, J. R. (2004a) Rheumatoid arthritis. In L. Goldman & D. Ausiello (Eds.), *Cecil Textbook of Medicine* (22nd ed., pp. 1644–1654). Philadelphia: W. B. Saunders.

O'Dell, J. R. (2004b). Therapeutic strategies for rheumatoid arthritis. *New England Journal of Medicine, 350*(25), 2591–2599.

Oliver, S. (2007). Best practice in treatment of patients with rheumatoid arthritis. *Nursing Standard, 21*(42), 47–56.

Pelletier, K. R., Astin, J. A., & Haskell, W. L. (1999). Current trends in the integration and reimbursement of complementry and alternative medicine by managed care organizations (MCOs) and insurance providers: 1998 update and cohort analysis. *American Journal of health Promotion, 14*(2), 125–133.

Portenoy, R. K. (1994). Opioid therapy for nonmalignant pain: Current status. In H. L. Fields & J. C. Liebeskind (Eds.), Progress in pain research and management, Vol. 1. Pharmacological approaches to the treatment of chronic pain; new concepts and critical issues: *The Bristol-Myers Squibb Symposium on Pain Research.* (pp 247–287). Seattle: IASP Press.

Prestwood, K. M., & Raisz, L. G. (2002). Prevention and treatment of osteoporosis. *Clinical Cornerstone, 4*(6), 31–41.

Proehl, J. A. (2004). Accidental amputation. *American Journal of Nursing, 104*(2), 50–53.

Rahman, A., Ambler, G., Underwood, M. R., & Shipley, M. E. (2004). Important determinants of self-efficacy in patients with chronic musculoskeletal pain. *Journal of Rheumatology, 31*(6), 1187–1192.

Rajan, M., & Kerr, H. (2000). Rheumatology. *British Medical Journal, 321(7265),* 882–886.

Resch, K. L., Hill, S., & Ernst, E. (1997). Use of complementary therapies by individuals with "arthritis" *Clinical Rheumatology, 16,* 391.

Richardson, C., Adams, N., & Poole, H. (2006). Psychological approaches for the nursing management of chronic pain: Part 2. *Journal of Clinical Nursing, 15,* 1196–1202.

Ritz, E., & Mann, J. F. E. (2000). Disparities in the use of total joint arthroplasty. *New England Journal of Medicine, 342*(14), 1043–1045.

Rowbotham, M. C. (2004). Specific pain syndromes. In L. Goldman & D. Ausiello (Eds.), *Cecil textbook of medicine* (22nd ed., pp. 2222–2224). Philadelphia: W. B. Saunders.

Ruiz-Irastorza, G., Khamashta, M. A., Castellino, G., & Hughes, G. R. (1999). Systemic lupus erythematosus. *Lancet, 357,* 1027–1032.

Schedler, M. (2006). Pain: Six degrees of separation. *Reviews on Systemic Enzymes, 4*(4), 1–2.

Schlesinger, N., & Schumacher, H. R. Jr. (2001). Gout: Can management be improved? *Current Opinions in Rheumatology, 13,* 240–244.

Schnitzer, T. J., & Lane, N. E. (2004). Osteoarthritis. In L. Goldman & D. Ausiello (Eds.), *Cecil textbook of medicine* (22nd ed., pp. 1698–1702) Philadelphia: W. B. Saunders.

Schonstein, E., Kenny, D. T., Keating, J., & Koes, B. W. (2003). Work conditioning, work hardening and functional restoration for workers with back and neck pain. *Cochrane Database System Review, 1,* CD001822.

Schrager, S. (2004). Osteoporosis in women with disabilities. *Journal of Women's Health, 13*(4), 431–437.

Schur, P. H. (2004). Systemic lupus erythematosus. In L. Goldman & D. Ausiello (Eds.), *Cecil textbook of medicine* (22nd ed., pp. 1660–1670). Philadelphia: W. B. Saunders.

Shanahan, J. C., & St. Clair, E. W. (2007). In R. E. Rakel & E. T. Bope (Eds.), *Conn's current therapy* (pp. 1131–1137). Philadelphia: W. B. Saunders.

Simmons, B. P., & Borsch, J. P. (2006). Hands: Strategies for strong pain-free hands. *Harvard Health Report, 1,* 39.

Smith, S. M., Kress, T. A. H., & William, M. (2000). Hand/wrist disorders among sign language communicators. *American Annals of the Deaf, 145*(1), 22–25.

Sohng, K. Y. (2003). Effects of self-management course for patients with systemic lupus erythematosus. *Journal of Advanced Nursing, 42*(5), 479–486.

Solomon, D. H., Finkelstein, J. S., Katz, J. N., Mogun, H., & Avorn, J. (2003). Underuse of osteoporosis medications in elderly patients with fractures. *American Journal of Medicine,*
11(5), 398–400.

Steinmehl, E. (2006). Help for hurting hands. *Health, 20*(6), 112.

Stucki, G., Cieza, A., Geyh, S., et al. (2004). ICF core sets for rheumatoid arthritis. *Journal of Rehabilitation Medicine, 44* (suppl), 87–93.

Sugihara, A., Watanabe, H., Oohashi, M., et al. (2004). The effect of hyperbaric oxygen therapy on the bout of treatment for soft tissue infections. *Journal of Infection, 48*(4), 330–333.

Swann, J. (2007a). Rheumatoid arthritis: When the body rebels against itself. *Nursing & Residential Care, 9*(5), 222–224.

Swann, J. (2007b). Rheumatoid arthritis: Coping strategies. *Nursing & Residential Care, 9*(6), 269–272.

Swinkels, A., & Dolan, P. (2004). Spinal position sense and disease progression in ankylosing spondylitis: A longitudinal study. *Spine, 29*(11), 1240–1245.

Terkeltaub, R. A. (2003). Gout. *New England Journal of Medicine, 349*(17), 1647–1655.

Terkeltaub, R. A. (2004). Gout. In L. Goldman & D. Ausiello (Eds.), *Cecil textbook of medicine* (22nd ed., pp. 1702–1710). Philadelphia: W. B. Saunders.

Trethewey, P. (2004). Systemic lupus erythematosus. *Dimensions of Critical Care* Nursing, *23*(3), 111–115.

Turner, J. A., Franklin, G., Fulton-Kehoe, D., Egan, K., Wickizer, T. M., Lymp, J. F., et al., (2004). Prediction of chronic disability in work-related musculoskeletal disorders: A prospective, population-based study. *BMC Musculoskeletal Disorders, 5*(1), 14.

van Velzen, J. M., van Bennekom, C., van der Woude, L. H. V., & Houdijk, H. (2006). Physical capacity and walking ability after lower limb amputation: A systematic review. *Clinical Rehabilitation, 20,* 999–1016.

Varga, J., Manzi, S. M., & Lakos, G. (2007). Connective tissue disorders. In R. E. Rakel & E.T. Bope (Eds.), *Conn's current therapy* (pp. 936–944). Philadelphia: W. B. Saunders.

Vas, J., Aguilar, I., Perea-Milla, E., & Méndez, C. (2007). Effectiveness of acupuncture and related techniques in treating non-oncological pain in primary healthcare: An audit. *Acupuncture in Medicine, 25*(1-2), 41–46.

Vecchio, P. C. (1994). Attitudes to alternative medicine by rheumatology outpatient attenders. *Journal of Rheumaology, 21,* 145.

Walsh, J. D., Blanchard, E. B., Kremer, J. M., & Blanchard, C. G. (1999). The psychosocial effects of rheumatoid arthritis on the patient and the well partner. *Behaviour Research and Therapy, 37,* 259–271.

Weir, R., & Nielson, W. R. (2001). Interventions for disability management. *Clinical Journal of Pain, 17*(4 suppl), S128–S132.

Werner, R. A. (2006). Evaluation of work-related carpal tunnel syndrome. *Journal of Occupational Rehabilitation, 16,* 207–222.

Wiberg, M., Hazari, A., Ljungberg, C., Pettersson, K., Backman, C., Nordh, E., et al. (2003). Sensory recovery after hand reimplantation: A clinical, morphological, and neurophysiological study in humans. *Scandinavian Journal of Plastic and Reconstructive Surgery and Hand Surgery, 37*(3), 163–173.

Wilhelmi, B. J., Lee, W. P., Pagensteert, G. I., & May, J. W, Jr. (2003). Reimplantation in the mutilated hand. *Hand Clinics, 19*(1), 89–120.

Wilson, B. A. Jr. (1998). *A primer on limb prosthetics.* Springfield, IL: C. C. Thomas.

Wortmann, R. I. (2002). Gout and hyperuricemia. *Current Opinions in Rheumatology, 14,* 281–286.

Yildiz, S., Kiralp, M. Z., Akin, A., et al. (2004). A new treatment modality for fibromyalgia syndrome: hyperbaric oxygen therapy. *Journal of Internal Medicine Residents, 32*(3), 263–267.

Chapter 17

Skin Disorders, Burns, and Facial Disfigurement

■ STRUCTURE AND FUNCTION OF THE SKIN

The skin is the largest organ of the body. It has a number of functions:

- Protection of the body's inner structures from microorganisms, drying, and trauma
- Regulation of body temperature through evaporation of perspiration for cooling and constriction of superficial blood vessels to conserve heat
- Excretion of water and electrolytes through perspiration
- Sensory perception of touch, pressure, and pain

The skin consists of two layers: the epidermis and the dermis (see Figure 17-1). The outer layer of the skin (**epidermis**) protects the deeper tissues from drying, from invasion by organisms, and from trauma. The epidermis has several layers. The deepest layer of the epidermis constantly produces new cells, which are pushed to the surface of the skin; there they die, are shed, and are replaced by new cells. Cells called *melanocytes* contain the skin pigment melanin, which is responsible for skin color. Dark-skinned people have more melanin than do light-skinned people.

The inner layer of skin (**dermis**) lies beneath the epidermis. It contains blood vessels, nerves, lymphatics, hair follicles, and sebaceous and sweat glands, as well as various types of cells that promote wound healing. The dermis also contains major sensory fibers responsible for distinguishing pain, touch, heat, and cold.

With the exception of the palms of the hands and the soles of the feet, hair follicles are located in the dermis throughout the body; although they are more numerous in some areas, such as the scalp, axilla, and pubic area. Hairs are continually falling out and being replaced by new ones. When this process is excessive, thinning or baldness results.

Sebaceous glands, contained within the dermis and surrounding hair follicles, produce an oily substance called *sebum* that protects the skin from excessive dryness. *Sweat glands*, also located in the dermis, are present all over the body, but are concentrated in the axilla, forehead, palms of the hands, and soles of the feet. They produce perspiration, which aids in regulation of the body temperature as well as excretion of water and electrolytes. When the environment is warm, evaporation of perspiration cools the body. When the environment is cool, constriction of superficial blood vessels conserves body warmth.

Interfacing with the dermis at its lower level is a **subcutaneous** (under the skin) layer of fat, called adipose tissue. This subcutaneous fat not only provides insulation for the body, but also gives shape and contour to the body over bone.

■ PSYCHOSOCIAL AND VOCATIONAL IMPACT OF SKIN CONDITIONS

The skin is readily visible. Its condition determines to a great extent how individuals appear to the world. Skin conditions, although not generally life-threatening, can have an adverse effect on quality of life, restricting work, social, family, leisure, and sexual activities (Lamberg, 1997; Morgan, McCreedy, Simpson, & Hay, 1997). Healthy skin is correlated with higher self-esteem and better self-image. A skin disorder that may seem trivial to others can have a major psychological impact on the individual who experiences it. Society places great emphasis on appearance, and appearance often helps to determine how individuals interact with society. Not only does society place a high value on clear, healthy skin, but skin disorders are sometimes perceived as being associated with uncleanliness or contagion.

Even though few skin conditions are actually contagious, people may avoid contact with individuals with skin conditions because of fear that the condition is contagious. Emotional responses to disfiguring skin conditions involve not only a negative effect on individuals' self-image but also adverse effects on interpersonal relationships and stigmatization imposed by society. Individuals with obvious skin disease or scarring due to burns or trauma may experience stares, expressions of revulsions, or avoidance by others so that they become social outcasts. Individuals with disfiguring skin conditions may experience significant secondary psychological symptoms including depression, social phobia, or paranoia. Psychological implications of skin conditions may extend to all domains of individuals' lives, including the workplace.

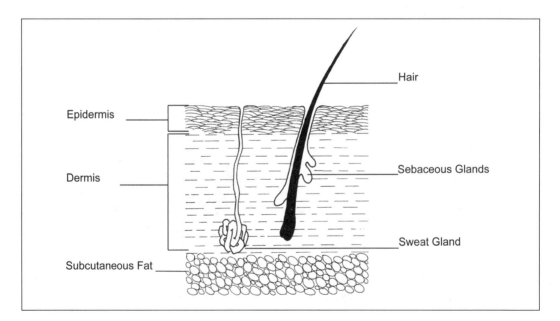

Figure 17-1   The skin

■ SKIN CONDITIONS

Because the skin is in constant contact with the environment, it is vulnerable to injury and irritation. It is also vulnerable to changes in the internal body environment and may provide visible evidence of systemic conditions, such as lupus erythematosus (see Chapter 16). Emotional factors can also precipitate or contribute to disorders of the skin. Skin disorders may be localized or may involve the entire body. They may cause mild discomfort or severe pain and disfigurement.

Dermatitis

The general term **dermatitis** describes a superficial inflammation of the skin. *Atopic dermatitis* is a chronic inflammatory skin condition involving a complex interrelationship of genetic, psychological, immunologic, and environmental factors (Chamlin, 2007). Although it is more common in childhood, it can be a lifelong condition. Depending on its location, atopic dermatitis can affect appearance, especially if on the face. Constant scratching of the skin can cause tenderness and bleeding. If the skin's protective outer layers crack, individuals are also at risk of infection. Treatment is directed toward correcting skin dryness, controlling the itch, and preventing infection.

Eczema is a type of dermatitis characterized by redness (**erythema**), swelling (**edema**), and itching (**pruritus**). In addition to treating the general dryness and controlling the itching, topical steroids are sometimes applied in cases of eczema.

Treatment of atophic dermatitis includes avoidance of prolonged contact with hot water (i.e., taking lukewarm showers rather than long, hot baths), avoidance of drying soaps, and use of moisturizers on the skin. Medications such as antihistamines or steroid creams and ointments may be used to control itching; however, prolonged use of steroid medications is contraindicated due to potential side effects.

New medications called topical immunomodulators are also used. In severe cases, phototherapy (light therapy) or photochemotherapy (combination of ultraviolet light and special medication) may be used.

Contact dermatitis is a localized skin inflammation that results from contact with a specific substance. The symptoms occur at the site of contact. The offending substance may produce a localized allergic response (*allergic contact dermatitis*) as a result of a previous exposure, or the substance may be a primary irritant that causes a nonallergic skin reaction (*irritant contact dermatitis*) following exposure (Schalock & Zug, 2007). Common causes of localized allergic contact dermatitis include chemicals, dyes, cosmetics, and industrial agents. Alkalis, acids, metals, salts, solvents, and various dusts may cause irritant dermatitis. Usually only the skin that comes into contact with the substance is involved, so the area of skin affected is rather clearly demarcated. Symptoms generally disappear when contact with the offending agent is avoided. In addition to localized allergic reactions, individuals can experience generalized allergic reactions as described next.

Allergic Reactions

An **allergy** is a hypersensitivity to a specific substance or substances. Some individuals experience allergic reactions after exposure to certain substances that cause an immune response within the body. Their sensitization to the substance may take days or weeks to occur. Once the response has been established, the next contact with the substance produces allergic symptoms.

Allergic responses may be external or systemic. External allergic reactions consist of symptoms such as hives (**urticaria**), redness, swelling, itching, or rash. Systemic allergic responses, usually caused by allergic reactions to medication or certain foods, may include skin manifestations in addition to generalized body symptoms, some of which can seriously compromise respiratory function. The treatment of allergy is usually directed toward avoiding contact with the offending agent, reducing sensitivity to the substance if contact cannot be avoided, or reducing or eliminating the symptoms associated with the allergic response.

Psoriasis

Psoriasis is a chronic inflammatory disease in which there is greatly accelerated epidermal cell turnover. As a result of the rapid formation of these cells, individuals develop noticeable skin lesions. There are several variations of psoriasis, which are categorized as localized or generalized depending on the severity of the condition and its overall impact on the individual's quality of life and well-being (Pardasani, Feldman, & Clark, 2000). Some studies have indicated that impairment in quality of life for individuals with psoriasis may be greater than the effects on quality of life produced by other conditions such as rheumatoid arthritis or cancer (Christopher, 2001).

Plaque psoriasis is characterized by plaques of erythema (redness), covered with silvery scales, which tend to shed. Patches or plaques may occur on localized areas, such as the elbows and knees, lower back and the scalp, or they can cover the entire body. In some instances, individuals develop *pustular psoriasis*, in which small pustules are spread over the body and, in some instances can lead to systemic infection. Some individuals with psoriasis develop *psoriatic arthritis*, which causes aching and disfigurement of joints.

Although the primary cause of psoriasis remains unknown, it is considered a genetically influenced, immune-mediated chronic disorder (Lee & Koo, 2007; Pardasani, Feldman, & Clark, 2000). Psoriasis may be triggered by a combination of genetic, systemic, or environmental factors. It is characterized by periods of **remission** (when symptoms become better) and periods of **exacerbation** (when symptoms become worse) of varying frequency and duration. Thus the course of the psoriasis is often unpredictable and can improve or get worse for no obvious reason. Emotional stress and anxiety may aggravate the condition. Climate change or warm temperatures also tend to make the condition worse. For many individuals, psoriasis may improve in the summer but become worse in the winter (Schon & Henning Boehncke, 2005).

Treatment of Psoriasis

There is no known cure for psoriasis, so treatment is directed toward control of the condition. The goal of treatment is to suppress the immune-mediated response, which causes symptoms. Any aggravating factors should be identified and removed if possible. Given that injury to the skin can trigger flare-ups, trauma to the skin should be avoided as much as possible.

Treatment depends on the severity of the condition. Psoriasis can be treated with topical agents; if symptoms do not respond to such topical treatment, then psorisis may be treated with a systemic agent. If individuals' condition is limited, most *dermatologists* (physicians who specialize in diagnosis and treatment of conditions of the skin) initially treat psoriasis with a topical steroid. There are seven potency levels of topical steroids, and the strength prescribed depends on the area to be treated and the thickness of plaques. For example, a weaker strength of steroid would be applied to the face. Topical steroids are applied one to three times per day with the aim of increasing immune activity locally. Emollients are often used in combination with topical steroids to increase their efficacy.

Although relatively safe with few systemic side effects, topical steroids cannot be used indefinitely. If applications are applied too frequently or if too strong an agent is used, **atrophy** (shrinkage) or thinning of the skin can occur. Long-term use of steroids can lead to *tachyphylaxis,* a condition in which the body becomes immune to the effects of the medication because of repeated use.

Topical steroids can also be used in combination with other agents, such as vitamin D analogs or topical retinoids. Combination therapy allows lower doses of individual agents to be used, helping to minimize side effects and maximize efficacy.

Older, but still effective topical treatments include use of coal tar preparations or anthralin, a cream most often used to treat scalp psoriasis. Coal tar can be formulated into shampoos, gels, or solutions for soaking. Although its mechanism of action is not clear, coal tar seems to reduce inflammation. Coal tar preparations are inexpensive but can be messy to use, staining both skin and clothing. Anthralin can also stain skin, clothing, and bedding. Because of some reports linking coal tar to cancer, some countries and states prohibit the sale of coal tar.

Individuals with moderate to severe psoriasis may use any of the previously mentioned treatments in conjunction with phototherapy, which can lead to remission of psoriasis. In phototherapy, individuals come to the physician's office and spend several minutes in a light booth where they receive a regulated dose of ultraviolet light; both ultraviolet B and ultraviolet A are used The light causes a decrease in activity of the immune system. Ultraviolet B therapy can be either broadband or narrowband. The dose of light is based on the individual's skin type and the minimal dose that produces redness (**erythema**). When combined with other topical or systemic medications, care must be taken not to increase individuals' **photosensitivity** (sensitivity to light), which could result in burns.

Some individuals do not respond to phototherapy or may be unable to receive it (e.g.,

because of the distance between the treatment facility and their home, or because of their work schedule). In these instances, systemic medications may be used instead. Medications such as methotrexate, aceitretin, or cyclosporine may all be used to treat moderate to severe psoriasis. While all three of these agents are effective, they have side effects—liver damage, renal damage, increased blood lipids, and bone marrow suppression—that require frequent blood monitoring (Lebwohl, 2000). Other side effects may include hypertension and dryness of the skin and mucous membranes. In addition, the medications can be *teratogenic* (causing fetal abnormalities), so they should not be used when there is a chance of pregnancy.

The newest treatment options for psoriasis are biological drugs. This class of medications includes substances derived from living material that are injected or given intravenously. They act at the cellular level and affect various targets in the immune system that are involved in pathophysiology of psoriasis. Biological agents have been shown to have equal or better efficacy than older systemic treatments of psoriasis, and they appear to have few side effects. A major limitation to their use is their expense, as they can cost as much as $1000 per month.

Psychosocial Impact of Psoriasis

Psoriasis ranges from a cosmetically annoying condition to a physically disabling and disfiguring condition. It does not affect the individual's general health, but the psychological and social stigma associated with an obvious unsightly skin disease may cause frustration and despair. Psoriasis can cause difficulty with work performance, problems with social rejection, sexual dysfunction, and depression. Itching may be mild or severe and can cause loss of sleep and general fatigue, which can contribute to irritability. The condition can be a burden in terms of the financial and time resources required to deal with it, can interfere with work, and can disrupt the individual's lifestyle. Although psoriasis is not infectious, it may be a source of stares, embarrassing questions or comments, or outright avoidance of the individual by others. The prognosis depends on the extent and the severity of the disease. In general, the earlier the disease begins, the more severe its manifestations.

Infections of the Skin

A number of organisms, including bacteria, fungi, parasites, or viruses, may infect the skin. Infection may be the primary cause of a skin disorder, or it may be a secondary condition associated with another skin disorder. The degree and length of disability associated with infections of the skin depend on the type and severity of the infection. Effective therapy requires the proper identification of the causative organisms and treatment appropriate to those particular organisms.

Acne

Acne is the most commonly encountered skin condition. It results from interaction between bacteria in the skin, excess oil production, and hormones. The face, neck, and trunk of the body are the body parts most frequently affected. Although acne is most common in adolescence, some individuals—especially women—have acne that continues into young adulthood. Acne in itself is not frequently thought of as a disabling condition, but it can have a devastating effect on the individual's self-image and self-esteem. The goal of treatment of acne is to prevent the clogging of hair follicles, reduce inflammation, mitigate infection, and minimize scarring. Treatment usually consists of topical application of medication and, occasionally, systemic medication in severe or prolonged cases. In some instances individuals with severe scarring from acne may

choose to have cosmetic procedures such as resurfacing or dermabrasion (a procedure in which scars, wrinkles, or other skin blemishes are worn away) to diminish the scarring once their acne is no longer active.

Herpes Zoster (Shingles)

Herpes zoster (also called *shingles*) is a reactivation of the virus that caused chickenpox in individuals at a younger age. After the individual has had chickenpox, the virus remains dormant in the nervous system. When the individual's immune system becomes weakened because of aging, or because of medical conditions such as organ transplantation, cancer, or HIV infections, the virus can become reactivated. **Vesicules** (fluid-filled blisters) erupt along a peripheral sensory nerve route. The blisters, which form a band along the nerve, are usually located on the trunk of the body, causing pain, itching, burning, and tenderness along the nerve route. Although vesicles usually appear on the trunk of the body, they may also affect the face and eye. Pain in the affected area may be severe. The condition may last up to a month. The reactivated virus is contagious, so individuals who have never had chickenpox or who have never been immunized against chickenpox should avoid contact with individuals with herpes zoster.

Treatment of Herpes Zoster

The goal of treatment for herpes zoster is to relieve pain, reduce potential complications, and shorten the duration of the outbreak. Antiviral medication, administered either orally or intravenously, is often required. Steroids or anti-inflammatory medication may also be used. Pain accompanying herpes zoster is often treated with analgesics.

Herpes zoster usually has no residual effects. Complications of the condition can include prolonged pain at the site of the skin lesion even after lesions have subsided. Other complications may include scarring, which may be quite disfiguring if it involves the facial area. If the eye is affected, another complication may consist of ulceration, which could result in blindness.

Skin Cancers

Cancer of the skin occurs more frequently than does cancer of any other organ. Because *basal cell carcinoma* is directly visible, it can be diagnosed earlier and, therefore, has a high cure rate. *Malignant melanoma*, a cancer originating in the melanocytes (cells containing skin pigment), is a more dangerous and potentially fatal type of skin cancer because it spreads rapidly into deeper skin layers and metastasizes to other body organs (see Chapter 18). Because of the seriousness of the condition, surgical removal of the melanoma itself, as well as large portions of surrounding tissue, may be necessary to eradicate the cancer. This procedure may lead to significant deformity, depending on the location.

■ GENERAL DIAGNOSTIC PROCEDURES FOR CONDITIONS OF THE SKIN

Biopsy

Biopsy consists of removal of a specific tissue specimen for microscopic examination. Biopsies are performed to diagnose a variety of conditions, including skin cancer and many other types of skin lesions. This relatively simple procedure can be performed on an outpatient basis.

Scrapings, Cultures, and Smears

Scales of a skin lesion may be gently scraped from the surface of the skin and examined under a microscope. If there is an *exudate* (fluid or matter from tissue), a sample is removed with a swab and implanted in a *culture medium*,

where it is later examined for growth of organisms. In other instances, the exudate is placed on a slide and examined immediately under the microscope; this procedure is known as a *smear*.

Patch Tests

To identify the substances that are responsible for allergic reactions, *patch tests* may be performed. Small amounts of various substances that are suspected of causing the reaction are applied to the skin, and the area is later examined for possible reactions.

■ GENERAL TREATMENT OF CONDITIONS OF THE SKIN

Medications

Many skin conditions are treated with topical medications that are applied directly to the skin surface (topical application) in the form of lotions, creams, ointments, or powders. The type of medication chosen depends on the cause of the skin condition. For example, antifungals are used for fungal infections, antibiotics or antibacterials for bacterial infections, and antivirals for viral infections. Topical antipruritics may be applied to reduce the discomfort due to itching. Topical corticosteroids are sometimes prescribed to reduce local inflammatory responses.

Because topical medications can have side effects, prolonged use or overuse of medications such as corticosteroids should be avoided. Some skin conditions may be treated with systemic medications (medications that are injected or taken orally to be carried throughout the body), such as antibiotics and corticosteroids. Although corticosteroids can produce dramatic improvement, they also have serious potential side effects. Consequently, the use of corticosteroids requires careful monitoring by a physician.

Dressings and Therapeutic Baths or Soaks

Treatment of skin conditions in which there is excessive skin scaling or in which crusts have formed over lesions may include wet soaks or therapeutic baths to reduce the drying effects of air, relieve discomfort, or enhance the removal of scales and crusts so that healing may take place. In some instances, dressings are applied to skin lesions to protect the skin from injury and infection from the environment.

Light Treatment (Phototherapy)

Artificial light sources may be used for localized or generalized treatments of various skin conditions. Light therapies are frequently accompanied by therapeutic baths or soaks, or they may be used in combination with topical medication to potentiate its effect.

Dermabrasion

Dermabrasion consists of buffing, or abrading, the top surface of the skin so as to reduce scarring.

Chemical Face Peeling

Chemical face peeling involves a controlled chemical burn that destroys the upper layer of the skin. It is generally done for cosmetic purposes to remove fine lines or blemishes, but it can also be helpful in the treatment of acne and precancerous growths. Individuals with chemical face peeling should avoid the sun and be aware that the skin will not tan evenly.

Plastic and Reconstructive Surgery

Plastic and reconstructive surgery is a branch of surgery involving correction of deformity, restoration of function of parts of the body, or enhancement of physical appearance. It plays an important part in rehabilitation, not only to improve healing and establish or reestablish function, but also to enhance individuals' self-image and minimize limitations.

Plastic surgery is, of course, important in cases involving conditions of the skin. Nevertheless, plastic surgeons do not limit surgery to only one body part, but rather use concepts and techniques of plastic surgery on many parts of the body. For example, plastic surgery may be used to minimize or correct congenital anomalies such as cleft lip or cleft palate. It may be used to restore function lost due to **contractures** (tightening of tissue around a joint, which then limits range of motion). It may be used to correct deformity and restore function after a hand injury or to promote healing and correct deformity caused from complications such as **decubitus ulcer** (pressure sores which are caused by immobility and lack of blood supply to tissue such that tissue death occurs). Plastic and reconstructive surgery may also be used to correct deformities that occur secondary to a variety of medical conditions or their treatment, such as in cases of cancer in which a large portion of tissue has been removed or deformity results.

Plastic and reconstructive surgery can help to restore function and minimize disfigurement, thereby assisting individuals' adjustment to their condition and reentry into the workplace and the community. The extent to which reentry is possible varies from individual to individual and depends on the part of the body affected, the extent of limitations that remain, and the person's own psychological characteristics.

■ BURNS

The most traumatic of all skin injuries is that caused by burns (Balasubramani, Kumar, & Babu, 2001). Any tissue injury resulting from direct heat, flame, chemicals, radiation, or electrical current is termed a *burn*. Treatment and prognosis of individuals with burns depend on the cause or type of burn, depth of burn, and the amount of body surface that has been burned.

Types of Burn Injuries

Thermal Burns

The most common type of burns is *thermal burns*, which are caused by fire, hot liquids, or direct contact with a hot surface. In addition to causing direct injury to the skin, thermal burns can cause severe damage to underlying structures if the heat is intense or the exposure is prolonged.

Chemical Burns

Chemical burns result from direct contact with strong acids (e.g., sulfuric acid), alkaline agents (e.g., lye), gases (e.g., mustard gas), or other chemicals that cause tissue death. The extent of injury from chemical burns depends on the duration of the contact, the concentration or strength of the chemical, and the amount of tissue exposed to the chemical source. Some chemicals cause burns directly through the production of physiologic changes in the tissue with which they come into contact; other chemicals cause burns indirectly through the heat produced by their chemical reaction with the skin. In some instances, chemicals can cause freeze burns.

Freeze Injuries

Freeze injuries, such as frostbite, are also treated as if they were burns. In addition to frostbite, chemicals such as propane or freon can cause burn injuries.

Radiation Burns

The degree of damage caused by a *radiation burn* depends on the dose of radiation received. Sources of radiation burns may include ultraviolet radiation, such as that from the sun, and ionizing radiation, such as that from nuclear materials and x-rays. Localized skin reactions to low doses of radiation may cause discomfort, but usually heal spontaneously. Larger doses of local radiation may damage underlying tissues and organs, requiring more extensive treatment.

Electrical Burns

Electrical burns result from direct contact with electrical current or lightning. Injuries from electrical burns range from local tissue damage to sudden death because of cardiac arrest. The effects of electricity on tissue depend on the current, the voltage, the type of current (e.g., direct or alternating), and the duration of contact. *Flash burns*, or low-voltage electrical injuries, often result in greater disability that may include cognitive or behavioral changes as well as chronic pain. *High-tension injuries* (more than 1000 volts) often result in amputation, larger areas of damage, or death (Latenser, 2007).

Because the entry point of the electric current may be relatively small, electrical burns may appear to have caused little external damage. However, extensive internal damage may result as the current travels through the body tissues, damaging nerves, blood vessels, and other major organs. The electrical current may also interfere with the electrical activity of the heart, causing the heart to stop (*cardiac arrest*). Electrical burns are generally full-thickness burns and hence are associated with severe post-burn disabilities, which may include multiple amputations necessitated by damage to blood vessels, nerves, bones, or muscle resulting from the injury. If clothing of the individual caught on fire as a result of exposure to the electricity source, thermal burns may also be present.

Individuals with electrical burns may experience secondary injuries such as fractures, dislocations, or spinal cord injury because of falls associated with the injury or some sensorineural hearing loss, which generally improves over time. In some instances, however, there may be delayed damage. For instance, high-voltage electrical injuries can be associated with cataracts (see Chapter 5) that form three or more years after injury (Pruitt, 2004).

Lightning injuries may be classified as mild, moderate, or severe. Being struck by lightning can, of course, be fatal; even so, a number of people survive. In mild cases, individuals may appear dazed and confused, having only mild physical injury. In more severe cases, individuals may experience sensory organ damage, such as rupture of the tympanic membrane in the ear or cataract formation in the eye, which may not show up for weeks, months, or years after the incident. If cardiac arrest occurred and the individual experienced **hypoxia** (decreased oxygen) before resuscitation could occur, there may be brain damage or a seizure disorder may develop. People who survive lightning injury may also have residual effects of insomnia or other sleep disturbances, anxiety, or reduced fine intellectual function.

Inhalation Injury

Inhalation injury to the respiratory tract is caused by inhalation of steam, toxic gases, or vapors. Individuals with inhalation injury experience cough, increasing hoarseness, shortness of breath, anxiety, and wheezing. Inhalation of noxious gases alone may lead to brain injury or death. Direct injury to the respiratory tract may also cause swelling, compromising the patency of the airway. Treatment usually involves administrating 100% oxygen and maintaining an open airway (Nelson & Thompson, 1998). Inhalation injuries may sometimes necessitate **tracheostomy** (surgical opening into the trachea) to assist with breathing.

Burn Depth

The degree of tissue damage caused by a burn varies with the source of the burn, but several other factors can affect burn severity as well. One such factor is the burn depth. Burn depth depends on the temperature of the burning agent and the length of exposure. Burn injuries may consist of only one burn depth, or a combination of different burn depths may be present.

Burn depth is typically divided into four categories.

- **Superficial (first-degree) burn**: a burn that affects only the epidermis (outer layer of the skin). The skin becomes reddened and painful, but no underlying structures are damaged.
- **Partial-thickness (second-degree) burn**: a burn that affects both the epidermis and the dermis. The skin is reddened and blisters erupt, providing a portal of entry for organisms that can cause infection at the burn site. Second-degree burns are very painful owing to the stimulation of sensitive nerve endings in this layer of the skin.
- **Full-thickness (third-degree) burn**: a burn that destroys the dermis and epidermis, as well as skin appendages, such as hair follicles, sebaceous glands, and sweat glands. There is little pain, because nerve endings have been destroyed. Full-thickness burns cannot heal spontaneously and are more susceptible to infection.
- **Fourth-degree burn**: a burn in which tissue damage extends to the underlying subcutaneous fat, muscle, or bone.

In addition to the source of the burn and the burn depth, the percentage of body surface affected determines the severity of the burn. A commonly used method of calculating the amount of body surface injured is the **Rule of**

Nines, in which the body is graphically divided into areas that represent a different percentage of the total body surface (see Figure 17-2).

A more accurate method of estimating the total body surface burn is the *Lund and Browder method*. Recognizing that body proportions are different in children and adults, this method calculates the surface area of different body parts according to age. The chart used in the Lund and Browder model lists various body sections and the percentage of body surface each section represents for ages ranging from one year of age to adult. Each burned area is given percentage points based on the age of the individual; points are then added to estimate the total area of the body surface burned.

Burn Severity

The location of the burn also affects burn severity. For example, persons with burns to the upper body, especially the head and neck, may be prone to respiratory complications because of possible smoke inhalation, heat damage to the respiratory structures, exposure to toxic by-products of combustion of material such as synthetic material used in home furnishings, or restriction of air passages due to swelling caused by the injury. For electrical burns, points of contact and the pathway that the current followed through the body are important considerations in determining the severity of tissue damage. Individuals' age and medical history are important considerations as well. Individuals who are very young or very

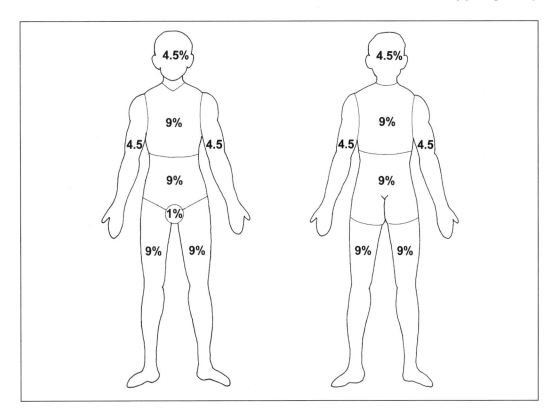

Figure 17-2   Rule of Nines

old are most vulnerable to the effects and complications of burns. Preexisting debilitating systemic conditions, such as heart disease, diabetes, lung disease, or chronic abuse of drugs or alcohol, can further complicate recovery and severely affect recovery and prognosis.

Individuals experience a systemic response after major burns. Severe burns disrupt the body's internal balance. Because of tissue injury, plasma seeps from blood vessels into surrounding tissues, causing swelling and decreasing the amount of fluid in the general circulation. As a result, the body's general homeostasis (equilibrium) is lost, which can affect all body systems. A second danger that negatively affects prognosis for individuals with burns is infection, especially for those with partial-thickness or full-thickness burns. Individuals with burns may experience severe **pruritus** (itching) for up to a year after the injury.

Depending on the extent and location of the burn, individuals may experience a variety of disabilities. For example, burns involving the hand may result in loss or contracture of the fingers, limiting joint motion. Severe burns of a leg may impair ambulation or necessitate amputation. Burns around the head and face may involve loss of vision or loss of nose, ears, or hair. Other causes of disfigurement may include *Keloid scars*, large rope-like configurations of scar tissue that form on the skin surface and that are out of proportion to the amount of scar tissue normally expected for wound healing. Keloid scars may continue to grow over time, leading to additional disfigurement. These cannot be readily removed, because additional keloid scarring may be stimulated by surgical intervention. In some instances radiation may be used to help reduce scarring.

Burn Treatment

Individuals who have experienced burns undergo dramatic physiologic and metabolic

changes over the course of the injury, which includes continuing changes as the process evolves (Demling & Gates, 2004). The type of treatment used for burns depends on the severity of the injury.

Burns may also be combined with other injuries if they were associated with a vehicle accident or explosion. Although individuals with minor burns and no complications may be treated at home, those with moderate or severe burns require hospitalization. Most individuals who have been moderately or severely burned are transferred to a hospital that has a specialized burn center. Burn centers are specially equipped to provided multifaceted care for individuals with moderate to severe burn injuries. The staff specialize in burn care and are trained to use a multidisciplinary approach. Professionals working in the burn unit may include physicians, nurses, psychologists, psychiatrists, social workers, and rehabilitation counselors. Although the amount of time individuals with burns spend in the hospital varies with the extent, degree, and location of the burn; the presence of any inhalation injury; and the individual's general condition prior to the burn injury, a rule of thumb is one day of hospitalization for every 1% of body surface area burned. During the acute phase of injury, treatment of moderate or severe burns is directed toward stabilizing individuals' general condition, restoring fluid balance, and preventing complications. The major task for the individual during this phase is survival. The greater the surface area of the body burned and the greater the degree of the burn, the greater the risk of complications.

A major complication of burn injury is infection, which, unless controlled, can result in widespread infection throughout the body (**sepsis**). Therefore, during the acute phase, the **eschar** (charred, dead tissue) may be **debrided** (removed) to reduce the risk of infection and to promote wound healing. Debridement can usually be done at the bedside. As it involves clipping away dead tissue, it is relatively painless. Burn wound excision, by contrast, involves removal of the burn in preparation for skin grafting. As excision is extremely painful, this procedure is almost always performed in the operating room. This practice stands in contrast to practice of the past, when painful and stressful debridements—rather than surgical excisions—were done on a daily basis, oftentimes in a whirlpool bath.

Because individuals who have been severely burned are vulnerable to infection, precautions must be taken to prevent them from being exposed to harmful organisms. The greatest danger comes from organisms within the individual's own body. Even so, some burn units may maintain a relatively sterile environment in which individuals with severe burns are placed in a room with a special air filtration system to screen out harmful organisms.

In some burn units, persons who provide care may wear caps, gowns, and masks to protect individuals with burns from infection. Visitors may be restricted or, when allowed to visit, may be asked to wear masks and gowns. As a result, individuals with burns may experience an increased sense of social isolation. Because of the stress imposed by these restrictions, and because of the growing evidence that risk of infection from outside sources is minimal, some burn units now restrict the environment much less so that caps and gowns are not worn by personnel or visitors, and the time frame for visiting is more liberal.

Nutritional needs of individuals with severe burns are great. In the early post-burn period, individuals may lose up to one pound or more per day. A high caloric intake is, therefore, essential to meet the increased energy requirements during the post-burn period. In individuals with larger burns, it is usually necessary to supply extra calories either via a tube in the esophagus or, rarely, intravenously. The preference for feeding in the intestine (known as *enteral feedings*) is due to the substantial infec-

tious complications associated with intravenous feedings (known as *parenteral nutrition*).

Burn wounds are treated in different ways. Sometimes they are treated with an exposure method in which no dressing or covering is applied to the wound. In these instances, more sterile conditions are essential to prevent infection. In other instances, the wound may not be covered, but topical medication, such as silver sulfadiazine to inhibit bacterial growth, may be applied. In some cases, burn wounds are covered with dressings that are changed daily. Methods of treatment depend on the type and extent of the burn wound, as well as on the general philosophy of the burn unit in which individuals are being treated.

Individuals with severe burns require daily hygiene to deter infection. Individuals may be asked to wash daily with antimicrobial soap as they would at home. Individuals may also need surgical debridements, in which necrotic tissue is cut away to prevent organisms from collecting and growing on the dead tissue.

Certain parts of the body require special care when burned. When the hands, arms, legs, or neck have been burned, special care is necessary to prevent the loss of function due to scarring or contracture (fixation of a joint in a position of nonfunction). In some cases, affected joints may be splinted in a position of function to prevent formation of contracture. Facial burns may not only cause disfigurement, but can also damage the ears or eyes. Ear burns can lead to loss of cartilage and edema resulting in infection. Regardless of the part of the body affected, every effort must be made to prevent complications that could further interfere with function.

After the acute phase of treatment, *grafting procedures* usually begin. A *graft* is tissue that is transplanted to a part of the body to repair an injury or defect. Biologic dressings may be used to cover a burn wound temporarily and prepare it for grafting. The types of biologic dressings include the following:

- **Xenograft** (heterograft): a graft taken from another species. Porcine (pig skin) grafts are often used for burn wounds.
- **Homograft** (allograft): a graft taken from the same species, but not the same person. Homografts may be taken from a living donor or from a cadaver skin bank. Another type of homograft is *amnion*, which consists of placental membrane.
- **Biosynthetic graft:** a graft that has been chemically manufactured. Synthetic skin substitutes are viable alternatives as temporary wound coverings. Such material is semitransparent and sterile. It adheres to the wound and prevents infection, and can also help in debridement. A biosynthetic graft is left in place for 3 to 4 weeks and gradually separates from the wound as new skin is formed.

It is often necessary to change biologic dressings every several days. Such dressings can decrease the amount of pain individuals experience by covering nerve endings. They also help to prevent infection until permanent grafting occurs, or until the wound heals. Most biologic dressings are changed every 2 to 5 days to prevent the body from rejecting the graft.

When the burn wound appears healthy, a skin graft is applied. An **autograft** is a section of the individual's own skin that has been removed from an uninvolved site. Depending on the size of the graft needed, the same donor site may be used repeatedly. A *split-thickness graft* consists of the epidermis and part of the dermis and occurs as one of two types. The first type, a *sheet graft*, is a single layer. The second type, *mesh graft*, is a graft in which many little slits have been made to allow it to expand and cover a larger area. A *full-thickness graft*, which includes the epidermis and the dermis from the donor site, may be used for reconstruction.

The graft area may be bandaged or not, depending again on the area involved as well as the philosophy of the burn unit. The grafted part of the body should be kept immobilized. If the graft is on an extremity, a splint may be applied to prevent movement, which could disrupt the graft. Extremities that are splinted should be maintained in a functional position for maximum benefit during immobilization and to prevent additional disability from contractures from occurring. When lower extremities are involved, the legs may be kept elevated and wrapped in Ace wraps or pressure garments to reduce swelling and subsequent rupture of small blood vessels. Elastic hose may also be worn when the individual is up. If the individual's face has received a graft, strenuous exercise, which could disrupt the graft, should be avoided.

When larger quantities of tissue are needed, a *flap* may be used. A flap is a tissue in which one area remains attached to the donor site and, consequently, has its own blood supply. The free end of the flap is then placed over the injury, sutured into place, and allowed to heal. Because flaps maintain their own blood supply, there may be better cosmetic results than with grafts, which may not maintain natural skin color.

The healing burn area may be compressed with elastic dressings to prevent or decrease the formation of **hypertrophic** (overgrowth) scarring (Richter, 2005). Special elasticized garments, commonly called pressure garments, such as gloves, vests, face masks, or neck garments, are available to be worn continually over the body part for a year or more to prevent this type of scar formation (see Figure 17-3). The garments are customized to fit the specific body part involved.

Individuals may be required to wear compression garments for one to two years after the initial injury. Such garments must be worn 23 hours per day. Because they are unattractive and are hot and uncomfortable, individuals may have a difficult time adjusting emotionally to this phase of treatment. If contractures have occurred as a result of the burn, physical therapy may be necessary to return mobility to a joint. When the measures are unsuccessful or if the contracture is severe, surgical intervention may be necessary.

Many individuals with severe burns require reconstructive or plastic surgery after the wound has healed, especially if there has been severe deformity or disfigurement. Such surgical interventions may be performed to reconstruct a body part, such as the nose or the ear, or to remove hypertrophic scar tissue. Many of these procedures take place over a number of years after the initial burn injury.

Corrective cosmetics (camouflage therapy) can also be used for skin discoloration or to minimize scars or suture lines. Corrective cosmetics differ from standard make-up in that they provide heavier coverage and adhere better to the skin (LeRoy, 2000).

If individuals with severe burns experience major hair loss, wigs or toupees may also be worn. In some instances surgical placement of hair plugs may be used for scalp hair replacement, as well as surgical hair plants for eyebrows if the eyebrows are missing.

Long-Term Disability for Individuals with Burn Injury

Individuals with burn injury may experience long-term consequences that affect their ability to function (Sliwa, Heinemann, & Semik, 2005). Conditions affecting the skin may include hypertrophic scars that result not only in aesthetic deformity, but also dry skin that causes itching and may interfere with sleep, as well as skin areas that are susceptible to injury, cold, and sun exposure (Sheridan, Schulz, Ryan, & McGinnis, 2004). Orthopedic conditions, including amputations or contractures of extremities, resulting from burns may

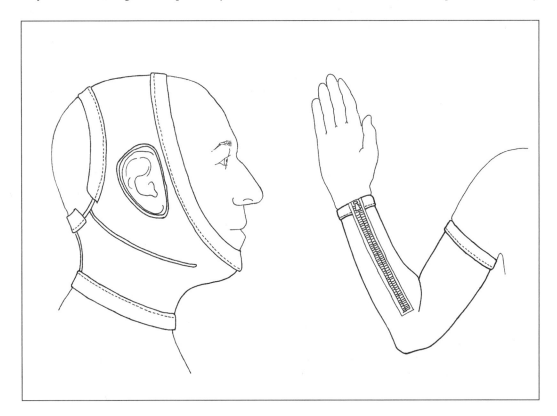

Figure 17-3   Pressure garments

affect mobility, and if upper extremities are affected, dexterity. After burn injury, individuals may also experience post-traumatic stress syndrome, depression, or sleep disorders, all of which can affect function. In addition, there may be preexisting disability that contributed to the burn injury, such as substance abuse or psychiatric disorder, that will further compound rehabilitation (Sheridan et al., 2004).

Personal/Psychological Issues in Burn Injury

The burn experience can be both physically and emotionally devastating. It threatens the integrity of both the physical and psychological identity of affected individuals (McQuaid, Barton, & Campbell, 2000). Burn scars are cosmetically disfiguring and force individuals to deal with alterations in body appearance. In addition to the traumatic nature of the burn accident, individuals must undergo painful treatment, which may induce even more emotional and psychological responses.

Responses to burn injury vary with the individual's premorbid personality traits, the characteristics of the burn injury, and the psychological meaning of the injury to the individual (Gilboa, 2001). Individuals who have been scarred or disfigured by burns must make psychological and physiologic adjustments not only to their disfigurement, but also to the immediate injury and to the long-term course of hospitalization and treatment. The suddenness of the injury itself produces a primary emotional stress. The impact of the injury is heightened by a variety of other situational factors, such as the separation from family, friends, and other sources of gratification; the experience of pain; the disruption of future life plans; and the threat to the sense of desirability and attractiveness to others. Recovery of individuals with severe burns is long and

can be dehumanizing. In the initial stage of burn recovery, individuals frequently experience anxiety both due to the traumatic nature of the injury and the loss of independence, as well as from treatments, which are painful, and fear of death.

During this stage of recovery, individuals may become agitated and hostile. They may experience sleep disruption and deprivation, increasing irritability. As recovery progresses and individuals become more aware of their circumstances, they may regress, becoming overly dependent. Loss of independence, fear of disfigurement, and exposure to continuing painful treatments and procedures produce a constant source of stress. In addition to the disfiguring and painful aspects of burns, many people face stress due to occupational loss, and consequently, fears regarding their financial future.

Treatment of burns often involves isolation, pain, multiple operations, and procedures that take place over an extended period of time. Depression is prevalent in individuals who have been burned (Van Loey & Van Son, 2003). It frequently results from feelings of helplessness and grief over loss of function or appearance. Looking at the injury for the first time can be a traumatic event for which individuals need reassurance and optimism as well as a realistic view of their injury and potential for recovery (Birdsall & Weinberg, 2001).

Individuals in a burn unit are subjected to numerous painful treatments and procedures, and they may feel isolated. They may perceive that they have little power over what is done to them and for them, which can be frightening and frustrating. They may feel a loss of both personal and social satisfaction, as well as an alteration in their relationships with others. As already mentioned, anxiety is a common psychological response to burns. Individuals with burns may be apprehensive—and realistically so, because of the painful procedures that they must endure. For some, the pain associated with the treatment procedures is a reminder of the initial injury, a notion increasing anxiety and intensifying pain (Yu & Dimsdale, 1999). Reactions may become generalized so that, even after the treatment period, individuals continue to experience anxiety about unknown or unrecognized dangers.

Because burns are frequently associated with accidents, depending on the circumstances, individuals may experience anger, guilt, regret, or resentment. If the accident was caused by the negligence or actions of others, individuals who were burned may experience hostility and anger. If the accident was caused by their own actions or if others were also injured as a result, self-blame and guilt may intensify individuals' reaction to their injury.

As individuals begin to think about the future after the immediate burn treatment period, psychological responses may be characterized by false hopes and magical optimism, particularly when skin grafting and reconstruction begin. Changes associated with burns may require the individual to acquire a new sense of self that is much different from the earlier one (Brewster, Bennett, & Gamelli, 2006). Individuals may have unrealistic expectations about the results of surgery or deny that there will be a permanent deformity. When continuing disfigurement and/or limitations become apparent, they may again sink into a state of depression and withdrawal before gradually adjusting to their condition.

Discharge from the hospital does not mark the end of the stress that individuals with burns experience. It is difficult psychologically for individuals who have been disfigured by burns to reenter the community, where they may be subjected to pity and curiosity of strangers as well as stares and insensitive remarks. Individuals may test family and friends with unusual requests or with behaviors designed to get attention. Adjusting to the reactions of others, dealing with social stigma, and realistically accepting limitations are important psychological issues with which the individual with burns must deal.

Activities/Participation Issues after Burn Injury

Improved survival rates of individuals with burn injury have made restoration and independence possible for growing numbers of burn survivors (Spires, Bowden, Ahrns, & Wahl, 2005). Issues that arise in everyday activities in relation to burns depend on the extent, nature, and location of the burn itself. For example, severe burns of the hands can result in contracture of the hands and fingers, necessitating the use of assistive devices for the activities of daily living. Burns to the face that result in loss of vision may also make it necessary to use adaptive devices (see Chapter 19).

The sexuality of individuals with burns is often a neglected part of treatment and rehabilitation. Sexual concerns are important during acute treatment in the burn unit as well as during discharge and ongoing rehabilitation. Sexuality encompasses much more than sexual activity or genital function: It encompasses the whole person and is an important part of identity, self-image, and self-concept. The disfiguring nature of burn injury can challenge individuals' view of themselves as sexual beings and can affect their adjustment and adaptation.

Individuals who have been burned severely often require a series of reconstructive operations over several years. Thus frequent hospitalizations may interrupt work and home activities. Relationships may be altered because of absences from the social environment necessitated by these repeated hospitalizations. Increased dependence and length of hospitalization due to burns can disrupt relationships within the family as well as other social relationships. Friends and family may be shocked at the sudden change in an individual's appearance after a burn injury.

Depending on the circumstances of the accident, family members and friends may feel anger, guilt, or resentment, which can be manifested in a variety of ways. In an attempt to make sense of the tragedy and its aftermath, family members, friends, and co-workers may focus on the question of responsibility for the accident. Those who were present at the time of the injury may feel that they should have done more or that they were to blame. Others may wonder why they escaped the same type of injury. These feelings may affect reactions to the individual and further social interactions with him or her. Families may grieve for the image they once had of the individual or they may grieve for the potential they feel the individual had that will now not be realized. Family reactions can range from over-solicitude to emotional withdrawal. Concerns about financial considerations and altered social roles may cause additional family stress.

Support groups and/or burn camps which help individuals face the challenges of their burn injury and treatment and allow individuals and their families to share common concerns may be helpful (Gaskell, 2007). Groups such as the National Phoenix Society, for example, can assist individuals and their families to cope with the ongoing difficulties of returning to society.

Vocational Issues in Burn Injury

The ability of individuals who have been burned to return to their former occupation depends not only on the occupation itself, but also on the extent and location of the burn. Many individuals are able to return to employment within 6 months of injury. At times, the main factor in determining how successful individuals can be in returning to their former position is the attitudes of others in the workplace. Acceptance of the burn survivor in the workplace by fellow employees may be difficult for a variety of reasons. If the injury was work related, depending on the circumstances, co-workers may feel guilty, causing them to alter their approach to the individual. Others may feel uncomfortable because of the individual's appearance and avoid contact with him or her. In some instances, even though individuals who have been severely burned may not consider themselves disabled, they may be perceived as such by others because of their appearance.

Emotional stress on the part of co-workers can preclude the individual's effective reentry at the workplace. Employers may not have confidence in individuals' ability to return to the former job or may be concerned about others' reaction to individuals with burns if disfigurement has occured. Considerable intervention with co-workers and employers is sometimes necessary to provide a smoother transition for individuals returning to work after burn injury. Those with severe burns that necessitate extensive reconstructive surgery may require intermittent hospitalizations over a 1- to 2-year period after the initial injury. Disruption to work activity associated with hospitalizations should be considered before individuals return to regular employment. Those who have other disabilities resulting from burns, such as the loss of a limb or the loss of vision, have the vocational limitations noted for those with the same disability due to other causes (see the specific related chapters). Contracture as a result of burns may also limit mobility and, if the hands are involved, manual dexterity.

Individuals who must wear compression garments to prevent hypertrophic scarring may need to avoid extremely warm work environments because of the excessive warmth of the garment. Those who wear compression gloves also have decreased manual dexterity. A facial mask may be a cosmetic disability if dealing with the public is a requirement of the occupation. The degree to which cosmetic appearance due to the burn itself is a factor in employment depends on the individual, the occupation, and the employer.

Skin that has been grafted may be more sensitive than normal skin. Consequently, grafts should not be exposed to extremes of temperature. If individuals are exposed to the sun, they should use sunscreen and wear sun-protective clothing. Because burns may have destroyed sweat glands, individuals' ability to regulate body temperature may be altered. In addition, there may be less fat insulation at burned areas than in healthy normal tissue, which affects the individual's ability to tolerate extremes of temperature. Extremely dry climates may exacerbate the itching that may be associated with the new skin growth of skin grafts. A more humid environment may be desirable.

Other residual problems from burns may also affect the appropriateness of the work environment. For example, individuals who have experienced altered lung function as a result of inhalation injury should avoid work settings characterized by air pollution or exposure to smoke and dust. Individuals with burns to the lower extremities may have difficulty in standing for prolonged periods and may need more sedentary employment.

■ PSYCHOSOCIAL AND VOCATIONAL ISSUES IN CONDITIONS OF THE SKIN

Personal/Psychological Issues

The skin, which is exposed and, therefore, readily observable, determines to a great extent an individual's appearance to others, and it is through personal appearance that others build an image of the individual. Individuals, in turn, observe the reactions of others and incorporate them into their own self-image. Consequently, conditions affecting the skin can have considerable impact on individuals' perception and attitudes. Disease or injury affecting the face may be particularly devastating. More than any other body part, the face is tied to personal identity. Although clothing can cover other body parts, the face is left exposed so that disfigurement is readily observable. Our society places considerable emphasis on a clear, radiant appearance. When disease or injury mars this image, it is not surprising that the psychological impact on the affected individuals is considerable.

Acute skin conditions may be treated and prevented. Chronic skin conditions require ongoing treatment or intervention. Stress affects some skin conditions, and individuals with these conditions may need to learn ways to reduce the amount of stress in their environment or to alter their reaction to stress.

Activities/Participation

Necessary changes in lifestyle resulting from skin conditions depend on the severity of the condition and on the extent and circumstances of the disability. Skin conditions resulting from exposure to or contact with certain substances within the environment make it necessary to avoid those substances. The discomfort associated with some skin conditions, such as itching, may affect daily activities to some degree. If special baths or dressings are required, these treatments must be provided for within the daily routine. In the case of burns, if compression garments are worn, or if individuals have cosmetic prosthesis or make-up that needs to be applied, extra time is needed on a daily basis to prepare for the day.

Although conditions of the skin may not affect sexual function directly, society places considerable importance on physical attractiveness, especially when related to issues of sexuality. Consequently, skin disease or disfigurement (particularly of the face), as well as the reactions of others may alter individuals' feelings of desirability. Anxiety or depression that accompanies skin conditions may further disrupt sexual function.

Disease or injury to the skin may isolate individuals perhaps more than any other condition. Some people, because they associate skin diseases with uncleanliness and contagiousness, may avoid individuals with skin disorders even though these associations are unfounded. Because of these reactions of others, individuals with skin disease or injury may become very sensitive. Having experienced stares or other negative reactions, they may develop an accentuated state of awareness and assume that others are focusing totally on their appearance. They may become extremely self-conscious and withdraw from social contact.

Visible disabilities provoke greater discrimination and social stigma than do invisible disabilities. Physical attractiveness is highly valued in our society, where attractiveness is viewed as a salable commodity. Skin conditions, especially if they involve the face, may evoke even more profound responses from others. People may feel uneasy in the presence of individuals with disfigurement or deformity and uncertain as to what to do or say. In social settings, individuals with deformity or disfigurement due to a skin condition or injury may encounter staring, feelings of pity, or repulsion. These reactions may cause individuals to limit or avoid social activities or to restrict their social interactions with others.

Vocational Issues

Most individuals with skin conditions continue in their regular line of employment, although individuals whose skin conditions are precipitated or exacerbated by exposure to substances in the work environment may require special considerations in choice of employment. In these instances, alterations in the work site or precautions in the performance of certain work-related activities may be necessary. If stress precipitates or exacerbates the skin condition, measures to decrease stress at the work site or to improve the individual's reaction to stress should also be taken. In some instances, it may be necessary to alter the work site.

Because skin cancer appears to be related to exposure to the sun, those who work outside should take precautions to avoid excessive exposure, such as wearing protective clothing or sun shields. Those who have had skin cancer or who have a propensity toward it should take additional precautions to avoid direct exposure to the sun as much as possible. Likewise, individuals who are being treated with medications that cause photosensitivity, or individuals who have new skin grafts, may need to avoid the sun.

Attitudes of employers and co-workers may create barriers to employment for individuals with skin conditions, especially when the condition alters their appearance considerably. Co-workers may fear contagion or may be uncomfortable because of the individual's appearance. Consequently, education and strategies to alleviate misperceptions may be an important factor in facilitating the individual's successful reentry or continuation in the work setting.

CASE STUDIES

Case 1

Mr. L., a 25-year-old man who worked as an insurance agent, was severely burned during a family outing when a camp stove exploded. The burns affected more than 50% of Mr. L.'s body, including his legs, shoulders, face, neck, chin, and ears as well as some of his scalp. After undergoing a number of cosmetic surgeries, he has regained full mobility of extremities, but has significant facial scarring. Mr. L. has a Bachelor of Science degree in business. Prior to his injury he was engaged; however, since his injury, his fiancé has broken off the engagement. Mr. L. is currently living with his parents. You have been asked to work with Mr. L. to discuss his vocational rehabilitation plans.

1. Which specific issues related to the accident is it important to address?
2. Which other issues might be important to consider in Mr. L.'s case?
3. What additional medical information may you need in working with Mr. L. on his vocational rehabilitation plan?

Case 2

Ms. G. was involved in an auto accident that resulted in her car catching on fire. A bystander pulled Ms. G. out of the car, but she experienced significant smoke inhalation, severe burns of her hands, and second-degree burns of her chest. As a result of the burns to her hand, Ms. G.'s thumbs and index fingers were amputated. She is 45 years old and has worked as a waitress most of her life. She has a high school education. Her husband is a coal miner. She has two children.

1. Which specific issues regarding Ms. G.'s injury would you consider?
2. How do the specific injuries Ms. G. received affect her rehabilitation potential?
3. What additional medical information might you need in working with Ms. G.?
4. Which vocational options may be feasible for Ms. G.?

■ REFERENCES

Balasubramani, M., Kumar, T. R., & Babu, M. (2001). Skin substitutes: A review. *Burns, 27*(5), 534–544.

Birdsall, C., & Weinberg, K. (2001). Adult patients looking at their burn injuries for the first time. *Journal of Burn Care Rehabilitation, 22*(5), 360–364.

Brewster, L. P., Bennett, B. K., & Gamelli, R. L. (2006). Application of rehabilitation ethics to a selected burn patient population's perspective. *Journal of the American College of Surgeons, 203,* 766–771.

Chamlin, S. L. (2007). Atopic dermatitis. In R. E. Rakel & E. T. Bope (Eds.), *Conn's current therapy* (pp. 1001–1004). Philadelphia, Saunders.

Christopher, E. (2001). Psoriasis: Epidemiology and clinical spectrum. *Clinical Experimental Dermatology, 26,* 314–320.

Demling, R. H., & Gates, J. D. (2004). Medical aspects of trauma and burn care. In L. Goldman & D. Ausiello (Eds.), *Cecil textbook of medicine* (22nd ed., pp. 642–649). Philadelphia: W. B. Saunders.

Gaskell, S. L. (2007). The challenge of evaluating rehabilitative activity holidays for burn-injured children: Qualitative and quantitative outcome data from a burns camp over a five-year period. *Developmental Neurorehabilitation, 10*(2), 149–160.

Gilboa, D. (2001). Long-term psychosocial adjustment after burn injury. *Burns, 4,* 335–341.

Lamberg, L. (1997). Dermatologic disorders diminish quality of life. *Journal of the American Medical Association, 277*(21), 1663.

Latenser, B. A. (2007). Burn treatment guidelines. In R. E. Rakel & E. T. Bope (Eds.), *Conn's current therapy* (pp. 931–934). Philadelphia: W. B. Saunders.

Lebwohl, M. (2000). Psoriasis treatment options continue to grow. *Dermatology Times, 21*(11), 14–16.

Lee, C. S., & Koo, J. (2007). Papulosquamous disorders. In R. E. Rakel & E. T. Bope (Eds.), *Conn's current therapy* (pp. 931–934). Philadelphia: W. B. Saunders.

LeRoy, L. (2000). Camouflage therapy. *Dermatology Nursing, 12*(6), 415–419.

McQuaid, D., Barton, J., & Campbell, E. A. (2000). Body image issues for children and adolescents with burns. *Journal of Burn Care Rehabilitation, 21*(3), 194–198.

Morgan, M., McCreedy, R., Simpson, J., & Hay, R. J. (1997). Dermatology quality of life scales: A measure of the impact of skin diseases. *British Journal of Dermatology, 136,* 202–206.

Nelson, L. A., and Thompson, D. D. (1998). Burn injury. *Plastic Surgical Nursing, 18*(3), 159–169.

Pardasani, A. G., Feldman, S. R., & Clark, A. R. (2000). Treatment of psoriasis: An algorithm-based approach for primary care physicians. *American Family Physician, 61*(3), 725–732.

Pruitt, B. A. (2004). Electric injury. In L. Goldman & D. Ausiello (Eds.), *Cecil textbook of medicine* (22nd ed., pp. 640–642). Philadelphia: W. B. Saunders.

Richter E. F. III. (2005). Burn injuries. In H. H. Zaretsky, E. F. Richter III, & M. G. Eisenberg (Eds.), *Medical aspects of disability* (3rd ed., pp. 151–157). New York: Springer.

Schalock, P. C., & Zug, K. A. (2007). Contact dermatitis. In R. E. Rakel & E. T. Bope (Eds.), *Conn's current therapy* (pp. 1013–1015). Philadelphia: W. B. Saunders.

Schon, M. D., & Henning Boehncke, N. (2005). Psoriasis. *New England Journal of Medicine, 352*(18), 1899–1912.

Sheridan, R. L., Schulz, J. T., Ryan, C. M., & McGinnis, P. J. (2004). Case 6-2004: A 35-year-old woman with extensive, deep burns from a nightclub fire. *New England Journal of Medicine, 350*(8), 810–821.

Sliwa, J. A., Heinemann, A., & Semik, P. (2005). Inpatient rehabilitation following burn injury: Patient demographics and functional outcomes. *Archives of Physical Medicine Rehabilitation, 86,* 1920–1923.

Spires, M. C., Bowden, M. L., Ahrns, K. S., & Wahl, W. L. (2005). Impact of an inpatient rehabilitation facility on functional outcome and length of stay of burn survivors. *Journal of Burn Care Rehabilitation, 26,* 532–538.

Van Loey, N. E., & Van Son, M. J. (2003). Psychopathology and psychological problems in patients with burn scars: Epidemiology and management. *American Journal of Clinical Dermatology, 4*(4), 245–272.

Yu, B. H., & Dimsdale, J. E. (1999). Posttraumatic stress disorder in patients with burn injuries. *Journal of Burn Care Rehabilitation, 20*(5), 426–433.

Chapter 18

Cancers

■ STRUCTURE AND FUNCTION OF THE CELL

The basic unit of all living things is the **cell**. The human body contains approximately 75 trillion cells. Although different types of cells perform different functions, all cells have certain basic characteristics in common. All cells require nutrition and oxygen to live, and almost all cells have the ability to reproduce. Reproduction of cells is a controlled process in which cells die and form at an approximately equal rate in adults, maintaining a balance in the number of cells present at any time. The precise way in which cell growth and reproduction are regulated within the human body is unknown. Some cells, such as those that make up the layers of the skin or the lining of the intestine, grow and reproduce frequently. Other cells, such as those that make up the musculature of the gastrointestinal tract, may not reproduce for years. Cells that make up neurons, the functional units of the nervous system, do not reproduce at all. Similarly, little is known about the mechanism that controls the number of each specific cell type that is produced.

Different types of cells make up different parts of body tissue. Cells are named for their different characteristics. For example, *epithelial cells* are found in the skin, the lining of body organs (e.g., the lining of the intestine), and glandular tissue (e.g., the breast or prostate). Blood vessels, lymph vessels, and other lymph tissue are composed of *endothelial cells*. Different types of cells are also found in muscle, nerve, bone, and other tissues in the body.

Every cell contains *DNA* (genetic material that is the blueprint for all the body's structures). *Genes*, which are composed of DNA, carry hereditary information about all characteristics of the organism. Although each cell contains all the genes for a particular organism, it uses only particular genes. This discrimination in the use of genes is the basis for different cell types. Genes determine how cells grow, as well as when or whether the cells divide to form new cells. Before cells can reproduce, however, genes must reproduce themselves. After genes reproduce, the cell divides, forming another cell identical to itself. It is through this systematic, organized reproduction of cells that continuity of life is maintained.

■ DEVELOPMENT OF CANCER

Cancer is not one condition, but rather many conditions. More than 100 types of cancers are distinguished. Cancers can arise from any type of cell and are classified according to the cell of origin. Most frequently, the term "tumor" is assumed to be synonymous with "cancer"; however, not all tumors are cancerous. A

tumor, also called a neoplasm, is a new and irregular growth of cells that serves no useful function and may interfere with healthy tissue function. The reason for the proliferation of cells is often unknown.

Tumors may be **benign** (noncancerous). Although benign tumors may disturb body function by exerting pressure on surrounding tissues, thereby preventing surrounding organs from obtaining a sufficient blood supply, they usually grow slowly, do not invade surrounding tissue, remain localized, and do not recur once removed. Generally, cells in benign tumors closely resemble regular cells in the tissue from which they multiplied.

Malignant tumors, by contrast, are capable of destructive growth and have the ability to invade surrounding tissues and move to other parts of the body. Malignant tumors are cancerous tumors.

Cancer develops when there has been an alteration (*mutation*) in the DNA within the regular cell. As a result, the control mechanism that regulates cell reproduction is lost. Because the reproduction of cancer cells is uncontrolled, they reproduce more rapidly than exceeds the rate at which the regular cells in the tissue die. Some of the more virulent cancer cells are often described as *anaplastic*, meaning that their appearance takes on irregular characteristics so that they are less differentiated than are the regular cells from which they are derived.

The original site of cancer cell reproduction is called the *primary site*, sometimes referred to as the *primary tumor*. Cancer cells do not remain confined to the original site, but rather extend into and invade surrounding tissues as they reproduce. In addition, cancer cells are less adhesive than are regular cells. Selected cancer cells may break off from the original cluster, enter the bloodstream or the lymph system, and travel to other parts of the body, where they begin another irregular pattern of reproduction. The movement of cancer cells from the original site to another part of the body is called **metastasis**. Cancer cell reproduction at this additional site is called a *secondary tumor*, meaning that metastasis has occurred and that the secondary tumor is not the original site of cancer growth.

Cancer cells compete with regular cells for nutrients. Reproduction of cancer cells is not well regulated, and some cancer cells reproduce at a more rapid rate than do regular cells. Eventually, available nutrients are taken from the regular cells to nourish the cancer cells.

■ CAUSES OF CANCER

The exact cause of cancer is unknown. Many causes probably exist, and it may be necessary for a variety of factors to be present in order for cancer to develop. Although specific causes are unknown, several factors are known to increase the risk of cancer (Blot, 2004):

- Radiation
- Some chemicals and pollutants
- Alcohol
- Diet
- Smoking and tobacco use
- Some viruses
- Chronic physical irritation to a body part
- Ultraviolet rays (sun)
- Hereditary predisposition

Chemicals or other substances that are thought to cause cancer are called **carcinogens.** Some carcinogens may be present in the environment, but not readily evident. Individuals may be exposed to carcinogens within the environment or workplace for a number of years before cancer develops. Some substances may not be carcinogenic in themselves, but may serve as co-carcinogens, promoting tumor formation in combination with other carcinogenic agents. Other factors, such as hormonal secretion, diet, and stress, have been implicated as potential factors in the development of or propensity for cancer, but the specific mechanisms that contribute to this relationship are unknown.

■ TYPES OF CANCERS

Any type of cell in the body may be the source of cancer. Cancers are named for the type of tissue from which they originated. Some common types of cancers and the corresponding tissue from which they arise are described here:

- **Carcinoma**: cancer of the epithelial cells
- **Sarcoma**: cancer of the bone, muscle, or other connective tissue
- **Lymphoma**: cancer of the lymphatic system
- **Leukemia**: cancer of blood cells or blood precursor cells
- **Melanoma:** cancer of the pigment-producing cells, usually of the skin

Because the specific behavior of cancer cells depends on the type of cell from which they originated, no generalizations can be made about cancer. Each type of cancer may progress at a different rate and may respond to different types of intervention in different ways. Consequently, classification of cancer is important in determining both management and prognosis.

■ STAGING AND GRADING OF CANCER

When cancer is diagnosed, it is important to determine not only the cancer type, but also the extent to which cancer cells have spread. This process is called **staging.** Staging of all cancers not only helps physicians determine the **prognosis** (prediction of the course and outcome of the condition), but also helps to determine the type of intervention that is most appropriate.

The most common system for staging today is the *TNM system*, which classifies cancer according to tumor size, node involvement, and metastasis. The letter *T* stands for *tumor*; *N*, for *node*; and *M*, for *metastasis*. When there is no evidence of a primary tumor, the stage is defined as T0. If cancer cells are present but have not invaded surrounding lymph nodes, the stage is defined as Tis (previously called in situ). As the tumor increases in size, it may be staged from T1 to T4, depending on the tumor size and involvement. When there is no lymph node involvement, the N staging is N0. If cancer cells extend beyond the initial tissue site and involve the lymph nodes in the surrounding area, however, the stage is either N1, N2, or N3 (previously called regional involvement), depending on the degree of involvement and the irregularity of nodes. If the cancer cells remain at the original site, even though the surrounding tissues and lymph nodes are involved, the M staging is M0. When cancer cells have metastasized to another area of the body, staging is either M1, M2, or M3, depending on the extent of the metastasis.

Histologic studies and *grading* are laboratory procedures in which the type and structure of cancer cells are determined microscopically. Histological grading is based on the appearance of cells and the degree of differentiation. Cells are graded as follows:

- Grade I: mild dysplasia (cells are slightly different from regular cells)
- Grade II: moderate dysplasia (cells are more irregular)
- Grade III: severe dysplasia (cells are very irregular and poorly differentiated)
- Grade IV: anaplasia (cells are immature and undifferentiated; cells of origin are difficult to determine)

A **pathologist** (a physician who specializes in the diagnosis of abnormal changes in tissues) examines the cells under a microscope to determine their type and the extent to which they differ from their regular precursors. The histologic type of cell and the grading of the cell are important in the determination of the interventions instituted *and* the prognosis. Individuals with tumor cells that are *well differentiated* (more similar to the cell of origin, with a more organized structure) may have a better prognosis, for example, than do an individuals with tumor cells that are considered anaplastic (containing more irregularities in structure).

■ GENERAL DIAGNOSTIC PROCEDURES IN CANCER

In general, the earlier the diagnosis of cancer, the better the prognosis. Some cancers grow and invade surrounding tissue without causing physical manifestations; These cancers are called *occult malignancies*. Tests and procedures used to detect irregularities before manifestations develop are called cancer screening procedures. When manifestations occur or when screening procedures have positive or suspicious results, additional diagnostic testing is necessary.

Radiographic Procedures (X-Ray)

In addition to conventional x-rays, *computed axial tomography* (CAT scan), *magnetic resonance imaging* (MRI), *ultrasound*, and, occasionally, arteriography may be helpful in identifying an irregularity in anatomic structure or the presence of a tumor. *Mammography* is a soft-tissue radiographic examination of the breast that is frequently used as both a screening procedure and a diagnostic procedure because it can reveal cancerous lesions before they can be detected by direct examination of the breast. Although these tests are important in identifying irregularities, they are rarely used alone in the diagnosis of cancer. A positive diagnosis requires microscopic examination of the tumor cells (histologic testing).

Diagnostic Surgery

In some instances, surgery may be done to confirm or rule out the presence of cancer. Depending on the size and location of the tumor, the surgical procedure may be relatively minor, such as the removal of an external wart or polyp, or a major intervention, such as *exploratory laparotomy* (the surgical opening of the abdomen for the purpose of investigation).

Regardless of the type of diagnostic surgery performed, an accurate diagnosis of cancer can be made only after a microscopic examination of the tissue. For such an examination, a **biopsy** is performed to remove a small portion of tissue from the body. Biopsies may be done by inserting a needle into the tumor and removing some cells through the needle (*needle biopsy*). They may also be done by making an incision and removing a portion of the tumor (*incisional biopsy*). The type of biopsy done depends on the size and location of the tumor.

Cytology

The study of cells that have been scraped from tissue surrounding the area of interest is called *cytology*. Perhaps the best-known example of diagnostic cytology is the *Papanicolaou smear (Pap smear)*. Cells from sputum specimens that have been coughed up from the lungs and other types of fluids may also be examined through diagnostic cytology.

Endoscopy

An endoscopic examination involves the insertion of a tubular device into a hollow organ or cavity to visualize the inside of the structure directly. This procedure may be done through a natural body opening or through a small incision. Examples of endoscopic examinations are bronchoscopy (see Chapter 14), sigmoidoscopy, gastroscopy and esophagoscopy (see Chapter 12), and laryngoscopy (examination of the larynx or vocal cords). Endoscopy is also used as a method for obtaining a tissue sample from the internal structure for a histologic examination.

Nuclear Medicine

In nuclear medicine, small amounts of radioactive materials are used for diagnostic procedures, and somewhat larger amounts are used for the management of conditions. In the diagnosis of cancer, nuclear medicine procedures may be used for the detection and staging of cancers in the thyroid glands, liver, and bone. They may also be used to detect the presence of metastases.

Laboratory Tests

Although laboratory tests per se may not be diagnostic for cancer, results of such tests may indicate impaired physiologic function that is a result of the cancer, such as the anemia or altered white blood cell count associated with leukemia. In some instances, laboratory tests are used for screening purposes. For example, both alpha-fetoprotein and carcinoembryonic antigens are usually found in embryonic and fetal tissues, but disappear after birth. In later life, however, tumors may produce these substances. Consequently, elevated levels of either substance in adults may be an indication of certain types of cancers or other conditions.

■ GENERAL MANAGEMENT OF CANCER

Many modalities are available to prevent, control, or cure cancer. Management modalities can be classified as follows:

- Surgery
- Chemotherapy
- Radiation (external or internal)
- Biological (immunotherapy, hormone therapy, gene therapy)
- Bone marrow transplantation

These interventions may be used alone or in combination. Many therapies involve multiple approaches rather than one. When interventions consist of several different types of therapy, management is said to be *multimodal*.

A number of factors are considered when deciding which procedures are best for the management of a particular cancer. A major consideration is the *type of cancer* itself. Because different cancers grow at different rates, metastasize to different spots, and react differently to various forms of intervention, the histologic type of cancer is a major determinant in management decisions. The *stage of cancer* is also considered. The extent to which cancer has invaded surrounding tissues and the presence of any metastases determine how aggressive and what type of intervention should be instituted. Tumor location and its relationship to other vital organs determine the accessibility of the tumor for removal.

The goal of cancer management also influences the type of intervention used. Goals for management of cancer can include any of these:

- Cure
- Extension of life
- Prevention of metastasis
- Palliation

In terms of cancer management, cure is usually defined as no evidence of cancer for 5 years after intervention, indicating a regular life expectancy for the individual. Management for the prevention of metastasis, also called adjuvant therapy, is directed toward eliminating cancer that, although not detectable and not symptomatic, may be present and may cause a recurrence of cancer. Palliative therapy is directed toward the relief of manifestations or complications of cancer, such as obstruction or severe pain, rather than toward cure.

Factors related to the individual with cancer must also be taken into consideration. Manifestations of other conditions unrelated to the cancer, the cancer itself, or age may compromise individuals' ability to withstand certain interventions. In some cases, individuals may feel that the benefits of some forms of cancer therapy are not worth the risks and side effects; consequently, individuals may refuse the recommended interventions.

Cancer may be managed with systemically or local interventions. Often, management of cancer consists of a combination of the two. Cancer may be managed surgically, chemically (chemotherapy), with radiation, or with other means—separately or in combination.

Surgical Procedures

Usually directed toward the local management of cancer, surgical procedures may be preventive, curative, palliative, or reconstructive (Sausville & Longo, 2007). **Preventive** surgery may be performed when precancerous or suspicious lesions are found. For example, a mole or polyp that, although not malignant, has a high probability of becoming malignant in the future may be removed. **Curative** surgery is generally more extensive. It may involve not only the tumor, but also an organ or surrounding tissue. Depending on the size and location of the tumor, curative surgery can affect subsequent function only minimally, can impair function severely, or can cause permanent disfigurement. **Palliative** surgery is directed toward reducing the size or retarding the growth of the tumor, or relieving severe discomfort associated with the presence of the tumor. In all instances, the goal of palliative surgery is to prolong or increase the quality of life rather than to cure the cancer. *Reconstructive surgery* is directed toward restoring maximal function or correcting disfigurement.

Surgical procedures used in management of cancer may be considered simple or radical.

Simple surgical procedures usually involve removal of the tumor, while surrounding structures and organs remain intact. **Radical** surgical procedures are more extensive. In radical surgery not only is the tumor removed, but some underlying tissue (e.g., muscle or organ) is removed as well. Radical surgery often results in alteration in function or appearance to some degree.

With advances of medical techniques, less radical procedures are now being performed. Surgery now might include *laser surgery* or *cryosurgery* (using low temperatures to devitalize or destroy cells).

Chemotherapy

Chemotherapy alone is often curative in many cancers; and in others cancers, adjuvant chemotherapy used in conjunction with other therapies can augment the survival benefit of those other therapies (Green, 2004). Antineoplastic medications (chemical agents that destroy cancer cells) are used in the systemic management of cancer. These agents may be used alone or in conjunction with other forms of therapy, such as surgery and radiation. This type of therapy, called chemotherapy, can be used for cure, prevention, or palliation. In general, chemotherapeutic agents affect the growth and reproduction of cancer cells.

A number of antineoplastic medications are used in the management of cancer (Freidenbergs, Grunwald, & Kaplan, 2005). Although these medications are different and may be administered differently, most affect rapidly dividing cells. Unfortunately, in addition to destroying and damaging cancer cells, these medications can damage regular cells that grow rapidly, such as the cells of the hair follicles, skin, lining of the gastrointestinal tract, and bone marrow. As a result of the vulnerability of these cells, the toxic side effects of chemotherapy may include hair loss (**alope-cia**), loss of appetite, nausea, vomiting, diarrhea, fatigue, and suppression of bone marrow function. The altered bone marrow function may interfere with the production of various components of blood. Therefore, individuals undergoing chemotherapy may develop anemia, may bruise easily because of decreased blood clotting ability, and may be highly susceptible to infection because they have fewer white blood cells.

Chemotherapeutic agents may be given intravenously, intramuscularly, subcutaneously, orally, or topically. In other instances, high concentrations of chemotherapeutic agents may be injected directly into a body cavity, such as the bladder or the peritoneal cavity, to manage localized tumors. Interventions may be instituted on either an outpatient basis or an inpatient basis.

Chemotherapeutic regimens vary with the agent and the cancer. Some regimens are given daily; others are given for 1 day every 3 to 8 weeks. Some individuals may use a portable device (*infusion pump*) that pumps small amounts of the chemotherapeutic agent constantly into a vein (*infusion therapy*). In some instances, because the chemotherapeutic agent is administered in small doses over time, toxic side effects may be reduced. This type of intervention delivers the maximal dosage of the medication to the tumor site and may result in fewer systemic side effects. New agents called **chemoprotectants** (drugs that protect the body against cancer medications), which ameliorate the toxic effects of drugs used in chemotherapy at higher doses, have been developed as well.

Not all individuals who receive chemotherapy experience all possible side effects. Those who do not have severe side effects can, for the most part, continue their daily activities. No special precautions are necessary, with the exception of avoiding exposure to individuals with colds or flu because resistance may be lowered during chemotherapy.

Radiation Therapy

Radiation therapy can be curative for some types of cancers while enabling individuals to preserve organ or tissue structure and function (Bertino & Hait, 2004). With radiation therapy, high-energy rays are used to damage cancer cells and prevent them from growing and reproducing. This technique may be used to cure cancer, to relieve manifestations, or to keep cancer under control.

Radiation therapy may be delivered externally or internally. During external radiation therapy, a machine beams high-energy rays to the cancer so that the maximum effect of the radiation takes place in the tumor itself within the body. Even though the radiation penetrates the skin and underlying tissue, it does minimal damage to these structures. Internal radiation therapy involves inserting small amounts of radioactive material into the body, a procedure called *brachytherapy*.

Several types of internal radiation are distinguished. With intracavity therapy, a radioactive substance is placed in a body cavity for a period of approximately 24 to 72 hours and then removed; for example, a radioactive implant may be placed into the vagina for the management of cervical cancer. With interstitial therapy, a radioactive substance is placed into needles, beads, or seeds and implanted directly into the tumor. The interstitial implant may be removed after a specific period of time, or it may be left in place permanently, depending on the half-life of the radioactive source.

Like chemotherapy, radiation therapy can affect growth and reproduction of regular cells, resulting in potentially toxic side effects.

The number of regular cells exposed to the radiation, the dosage of radiation, the part of the body receiving radiation therapy, and unique characteristics of the individual determine the side effects experienced. These side effects may appear either immediately or some weeks or months after the radiation therapy was administered. Some individuals experience generalized manifestations similar to those of radiation sickness: nausea, vomiting, loss of appetite, fatigue, and headache. Other individuals may experience side effects specific to the area irradiated, such as sore throat if the head or neck has been irradiated, or localized skin reactions, such as radiation burn. Like chemotherapy, radiation therapy may cause bone marrow depression, resulting in anemia, lowered resistance to infection, and possibly hemorrhage.

Biological Therapies

Immunotherapy

A newer approach to the management of cancer is *immunotherapy*. Because human cancer cells express cancer-associated antigens, the goal of immunotherapy is to strengthen the individual's own immune system so that it recognizes cancer cells as foreign objects and destroys them (Rosenberg, 2004). Thus the body's own immune system is enhanced to fight cancer cells.

Immunotherapeutic agents can also help to increase the susceptibility of cancer cells to the *cytotoxic agents* (chemicals that are detrimental to or destroy cells). Many immunologic approaches to cancer management are already being used, including the interferons and interleukin-2. Interferon is thought to enhance the actions of cell-killing cells that attack and destroy cancer cells. It also slows cell division and suppresses tumor growth (Sherwood, 2007). Another example of immunotherapy involves administration of bacille Calmette-Guérin (BCG), which is used in the management of superficial bladder cancer.

Hormone Therapy

Adjuvant *hormone therapy* can be used to increase the benefits of chemotherapy in cancers that are hormone dependent (such as certain breast cancers that are estrogen dependent and prostate cancers that are androgen dependent). Hormones are not used to kill cancer cells, but rather to keep the cancer cells from growing, so that individuals remain in remission for extended periods of time. Hormone preparations work by blocking hormone receptors so that the cancer cells cannot use estrogen or androgen.

Gene Therapy

Gene therapy in the management of cancer is currently in its infancy. This type of therapy works by actually modifying the genetic structure of the cancer cell to suppress or inhibit tumor growth.

Bone Marrow Transplantation

Bone marrow transplantation is performed when the escalation of chemotherapy (chemical substances or drugs used to manage cancer) may result in a cure of the cancer, but the dosage would be lethal to the individual's bone marrow. In addition, bone marrow transplants seem to have an antitumor effect on their own, aside from chemotherapy, which can enhance effectiveness of cancer management. Bone marrow transplants are used for a variety of cancers including leukemias, Hodgkin's and non-Hodgkin's lymphomas, multiple myeloma, and breast cancer.

The goal of bone marrow transplantation is to provide healthy cells that can differentiate into blood cells to replace deficient or pathologic cells. The transplanted cells have the ability to completely replace and produce all red blood cells, platelets, T lymphocytes, and B lymphocytes (see Chapter 10) as well as other marrow **stem cells** (cells that can reproduce and differentiate into other types of cells).

In preparation for bone marrow transplantation, individuals receive large doses of radiation and/or chemotherapy that eradicate any viable marrow, kill tumor cells, and suppress the immune system to reduce the chance of rejection of the transplant. As a result of the the immune system suppression, however, individuals receiving a transplant are highly susceptible to infection. After after the individual receives an infusion of cells from the donor, the person's bone marrow regenerates using the new cells.

Taking bone marrow from the donor is a surgical procedure in which marrow is removed from the *iliac crests* (hip bone) while the donor is under spinal or general anesthesia. *Allogenic transplants* (taken from another individual) have the advantage of not risking contamination with cancer cells, but have the disadvantage of having a higher incidence of transplant rejection, or *graft-versus-host disease* (GVHD), in which the transplanted cells attack cells of individuals who received them. To minimize the chance of rejection or GVHD, the more closely matched the donor is to the individual, the better. Identical twins are the most compatible donors.

Individuals can also receive *autologous transplants* (cells taken from their own body). With autologous transplants, cells are removed from the individual prior to irradiation or chemotherapy, frozen, and then thawed and reinfused. The advantage of autologous infusions is that they avoid the risk of rejection or GVHD. The disadvantage is that there is risk of contamination with tumor cells from the individual's body. Also, autologous transplants lack the extra antitumor effect that is seen with allogenic transplants.

In addition to being found in the bone marrow, stem cells circulate in the peripheral blood and may be used for transplant. Peripheral stem cell transplantation is a procedure by which cells are removed from the peripheral blood, thereby avoiding a surgical procedure. For autologous transplants, this procedure may be used if the individual is too debilitated to withstand a surgical procedure. The disadvantage of autologous transplant is, once again, the risk of contamination with other cancer cells.

For allogenic transplant, although the donor is able to avoid a surgical procedure, the recipient may run a greater risk of rejection of the transplant or GVHD because he or she receives a larger number of T cells from the donor. The most critical period is 2 to 4 weeks after the bone marrow transplantation. Because of the immunosuppression that occurs prior to surgery, individuals may have an increased susceptibility to infections for as long as 3 months after the transplant. In addition, because immunosuppressive therapy drastically reduces the components in the blood that control bleeding, complications such as hemorrhage may arise.

■ COMMON CANCERS AND SPECIFIC TYPES OF CANCER MANAGEMENT

The diagnostic procedures, interventions used in cancer management, and functional limitations associated with cancer differ depending on the anatomic site involved. In many instances, a combination of interventions, including surgery, chemotherapy, and irradiation, is used. In the management of cancer in its very early stages, surgery alone may be sufficient.

Cancer of the Gastrointestinal Tract

Management of cancer of the gastrointestinal tract or accessory organs often involves the removal or major resection of the organs involved. Because manifestations of cancers of the esophagus, stomach, liver, and pancreas frequently become evident only late in the course of the disease, interventions may be directed toward palliation rather than cure (Macdonald, 2006).

Surgical management for cancer of the mouth may include removal of the tumor as well as removal of the nearby lymph glands to determine whether cancer has spread. If cancer has spread to the neck or other tissues, more radical surgery may be indicated, resulting in facial deformity or disfigurement because of the amount of tissue removed. If the tongue has been partially removed, speech may be affected. Reconstructive surgery may be required later to minimize these effects.

Cancer of the esophagus has been linked to smoking or gastroesophageal reflux disease (Terry, Lagergren, Ye, Nyren, & Wolk, 2000; Wu, Wan, & Bernstein, 2001; Brown et al., 2001). Other risks include obesity (Lagergren, Bergstrom, Adami, & Nyren, 2000) and Barrett's esophagus (Shaheen & Ranshoff, 2002), in which irregular tissue extends from the opening of the stomach into the esophagus. Management of cancer of the esophagus may consist of radiotherapy with or without chemotherapy or surgery.

When esophageal cancer is localized, the affected part of the esophagus may be removed and reattached to the remaining part of the esophagus (Enzinger & Mayer, 2003). When the cancer is more severe, **esophagectomy** (removal of the esophagus) may be necessary. If the individual has the esophagus removed, an artificial opening must be made into the stomach, with a tube inserted through which liquid feedings can be taken. After the feeding, the opening is then "plugged" to prevent leakage. After removal of the esophagus, individuals lose the ability to eat or drink through the mouth. Obviously, the ramifications of this type of surgery may influence individuals' willingness to have surgical versus other forms of interventions for their cancer.

Cancer of the stomach varies with geographic location of individuals affected. For instance, some countries have a higher incidence of stomach cancers than others. Risk factors for developing cancer of the stomach include environmental factors (including dietary intake and cigarette smoking); genetic factors; and predisposing conditions (e.g., chronic peptic ulcer, chronic gastritis) (Rustgi, 2004). Both diagnosis and interventions to treat stomach cancer have been greatly enhanced by the advent of endoscopic ultrasonography. Management of stomach cancer usually consists of surgical resection of the stomach and chemotherapy (Rustgi, 2004).

Cancer can occur in either the small intestine or the large intestine. Cancer of the large bowel or rectum (*colorectal cancer*) is one of the most lethal type of cancers in the Western world (DuBois, 2004). Management of colorectal cancer usually involves both surgical removal of the tumor and some resection of the colon itself, carried out through an incision in the abdomen (Pappas & Jacobs, 2004). In many instances, the cancerous part of the bowel can be removed and the two remaining ends joined together (**anastomosis**), enabling the individual to retain regular bowel function. When this is not possible, a colostomy may be performed (see Chapter 12).

Cancer of the Larynx

Although many structures in the head and neck can be a site of cancer, one of the most common cancers of the head and neck is cancer of the **larynx** (voice box). Smoking and alcohol are two leading risk factors for laryngeal cancer and are synergistic in their effects (Syrjänen, 2007; Posner, 2004; Wu et al., 2001). Some occupations also appear to have increased risk owing to secondary toxic exposures.

Manifestations of Cancer of the Larynx

The larynx contains the vocal cords. The most common symptom in cancer of the larynx is alteration in voice quality or hoarseness. Other manifestations may include **dysphagia** (difficulty in swallowing) and cough.

Diagnosis of Cancer of the Larynx

Diagnostic procedures used to identify problems of the larynx include *laryngoscopy*, in which a hollow tube is inserted into the larynx so that the physician can inspect the structures of the larynx and assess the function of the vocal cords.

Management of Cancer of the Larynx

Although management of cancer of the larynx depends on a number of factors, it usually involves irradiation, surgery, or a combination of the two. Although traditionally management of advanced cancer of the larynx involved total removal of the larynx, nonsurgical approaches involving chemotherapy and radiation are now frequently used instead of surgery in many cases (Forastiere et al., 2003). When the tumor is small (stage T1 or T2, N0 and M0), radiation alone may be used rather than surgery to eradicate the tumor (Vokes & Stenson, 2003). Laser interventions, which destroy the tumor by intense light beams, may also be used to manage cancer of the larynx in its early stages. If the tumor is discovered early, before there has been extensive involvement of the surrounding tissues, it may be necessary to remove only part of the larynx. This procedure is called a subtotal (partial) laryngectomy. Both subtotal laryngectomy and laser intervention can preserve the capacity for regular speech, although they may affect voice quality to some degree.

When the cancer is more advanced, it may be necessary to remove the larynx completely (**laryngectomy**).Usually, individuals who have undergone this type of surgery are unable to breathe or speak by regular mechanisms. After the larynx has been removed, the trachea is no longer connected either to the nasopharynx or to the nasal passages (see Chapter 14). The surgeon creates a permanent opening called a **tracheostomy** in the individual's neck and trachea, and the individual breathes through this opening (laryngeostoma) rather than through the nose and mouth (see Figure 18-1). Although able to eat and drink as usual, individuals must breathe, cough, and sneeze through the tracheostomy. The sense of smell, and consequently taste, is diminished because air flows through the opening in the neck instead of through the nose.

Psychosocial Issues in Cancer of the Larynx

Consequences of head and neck cancer, and cancer of the larynx in particular, can permanently alter individuals' physical, psychological, social, emotional, nutritional, and communicative functioning (Eadie & Doyle, 2005). The psychosocial and vocational effects of laryngectomy can be profound. A healthy voice is critical for effectiveness at work as well as in personal and social interactions (Zeitels & Healy, 2003). Individuals immediately lose the ability to make vocal sounds for speech as well as the audible sounds of laughter or crying. Consequently, physicians attempt to preserve as much of the larynx as possible (Lewin, 2005). When this is not possible, individuals must learn new techniques for speaking (Dobbins, Gunson, Bale, Neary, Ingrams, & Brown, 2005).

Attempts to improve the ability to speak after interventions for laryngeal cancer have

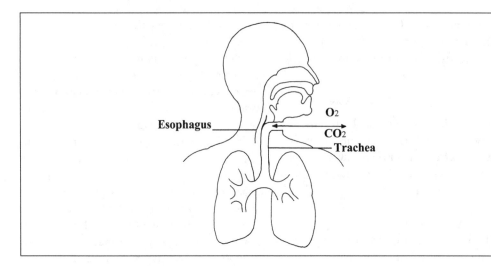

Figure 18-1   Tracheostomy

been successful. Surgical techniques have evolved so that much of the larynx can be spared and does not have to be totally removed. Also, improved methods of voice rehabilitation after total laryngectomy have been developed. Three types of voice rehabilitation techniques after total laryngectomy are utilized:

- Tracheo-esophageal (shunt speech)
- Esophageal speech
- Electromechanical speech

In tracheo-esophageal techniques, a **fistula** (a passageway from one structure to another) is surgically constructed between the trachea and the esophagus with a small prosthesis being placed in the fistula (Hancock, Houghton, Van As-Brooks, & Coman, 2005). Closing the tracheostomy with the hand or fingers moves air from the trachea to the esophagus, creating a *pseudovoice*. As a result, individuals are able to produce lung-powered speech of better quality than previously accomplished with other methods such as esophageal speech. The prosthesis in the fistula prevents food and liquid from entering the airway when the individuals is eating. A limitation of the fistula is the need for periodic removal of the prosthesis for cleaning and replacement, and the need to use one hand to occlude the tracheostomy during speech. Special valves that fit into the opening are available so that the need for manual coverage of the opening is eliminated. During regular breathing, the valve remains open; however, when individuals begin to speak, because of increased expiratory pressure, the valve closes.

Esophageal speech is a technique of speaking that involves trapping air in the esophagus and gradually releasing it at the top of the esophagus to produce a pseudovoice. If sounds produced by esophageal speech are too soft to be heard, a personal amplifier-speaker may be used to increase sound volume. Given that the air capacity of the upper esophagus is considerably less than that of the lungs, esophageal speech is typically limited in rate, volume, and duration.

Electrolaryngeal speech is another speech alternative that may be used by individuals with laryngectomy. It utilizes a battery-powered vibratory device called an artificial larynx. Several types are available; however, most are electronic, battery-operated devices that are held against the throat to produce sound.

Although the artificial larynx is relatively easy to use, the speech produced in this way has a mechanical, monotone sound that some individuals find objectionable.

Regardless of the type of speech alternative individuals use, speech–language pathologists are usually consulted for evaluation and possible interventions based on individuals' specific voice issues. Speech–language pathologists assess factors that affect voice production, identify any problem behaviors, and plan interventions to rectify the problem.

When individuals have a total laryngectomy, they must also adjust to the visible opening in the neck, the laryngeostoma. Any disfigurement, especially when related to a visible area, may damage individuals' self-concept and self-image. For cosmetic purposes, individuals may wear a scarf or other covering loosely around the neck. This covering also helps to keep dust and dirt out of the opening. Another type of covering available is a foam filter, which keeps moisture loss to a minimum, as well as preventing hair, shaving cream, or other particles from falling into the trachea during routine daily hygiene. Because the opening leads directly into the trachea and lungs, individuals must avoid activities such as swimming and water sports in which water could enter the opening. For showering, special laryngectomy shower collars that prevent water from running into the airway are available. With a laryngeostoma, individuals no longer have the benefit of having air humidified as it passes through the upper airway passages. Consequently, they may need to run a humidifier, especially at night, to keep the trachea moist.

Because the quality of speech is altered, individuals who have undergone laryngectomy may avoid social situations in which they have to speak, because they perceive their altered speech as distasteful and embarrassing. Although individuals can carry out most activities of daily living as usual, some may notice a decreased ability to lift heavy objects, because they cannot close the tracheostomy to build up internal pressure, as those without tracheostomy can do by compressing their lips and holding their breath. Individuals who have had a total laryngectomy should always carry an identification card or wear a medical identification bracelet to inform emergency personnel that they are a total neck breather

Vocational Issues in Cancer of the Larynx

Although only a few jobs may prove difficult for individuals after a laryngectomy, individuals may not return to work because of fear of rejection by fellow workers or because of employers' misconceptions about their ability to perform (Cady, 2002). Those jobs performed in environments with extreme heat or cold, or those that expose individuals to extreme dust or fumes, should probably be avoided. Although the physical aspects of laryngectomy may not affect individuals' ability to work, the impact that use of alternative modes of speech may have on employment can be striking, especially if individuals' use of voice is a necessary component of work. Employers and co-workers may also view individuals as being less socially acceptable because of their speech and, therefore, avoid interactions. Social support from friends, family, or participation in peer support groups such as the Lost Chord Club can help significantly in the adjustment process.

Cancer of the Lung

Lung cancer is one of the leading causes of cancer death in the United States and accounts for more than 80% of cancers diagnosed in this country (Miller, 2004). Occupational exposure to carcinogens accounts for approximately 15% of all lung cancer cases (Cleary, Gorenstein, & Omenn, 1996). When exposure is associated with tobacco use, however, the risk of development of lung cancer increases dramatically (Miller, 2004).

Lung cancer can be found in a variety of cell types with varied rates of growth, with some types being slow growing and other types being much more aggressive. Manifestations are often not apparent until lung cancer has reached an advanced stage. Lung cancer is usually diagnosed through chest x-ray, CT scan, bronchoscopy, or biopsy.

Management of lung cancer may be surgical, with removal or resection of the lung, or it may consist of radiation therapy, chemotherapy, or a combination of those approaches. When used in the management of lung cancer, radiation therapy is usually for palliation, rarely for cure. For individuals with a type of lung cancer called small-cell carcinoma, chemotherapy is generally the intervention of choice. If surgical intervention is used for lung cancer, the primary aim is to remove the total tumor.

The extent of the surgery depends on the cancer and its location in the lung. Removal of an entire lung is called a **pneumonectomy**; the removal of only one lobe of the lung is called a **lobectomy**. A segmental resection is a surgical procedure in which a segment of the lung is removed. After having a portion of the lung removed, individuals may need to limit their physical activity to some degree, depending on the amount of lung removed and the functional capacity remaining.

Given that cigarette smoking is frequently linked to lung cancer, emphysema may also coexist, further limiting respiratory capacity and, consequently, physical activity.

Cancer of the Musculoskeletal System

Musculoskeletal cancers frequently result in the amputation of an extremity (see Chapter 16). For some types of bone cancers, it may be possible to remove only a section of bone and to avoid amputating the whole extremity. In some instances, bone cancers may be reduced by chemotherapy and then controlled by radiotherapy.

Cancer of the Urinary System

Cancer can develop in any organ of the urinary system, but the most frequent site of cancer in the urinary tract is the bladder. There is a high correlation between bladder cancer and cigarette smoking (Vogelzang, 2004; Droller, 1998).

The most common symptom of bladder cancer is **hematuria** (blood in the urine). When bladder cancer is suspected, the individual generally undergoes a procedure called cystoscopy in which a tube called a cystoscope is inserted into the bladder, enabling the physician to visualize the inner surface of the bladder and to take a biopsy for laboratory examination.

Bladder cancer is generally classified as superficial (in which the cancer cells are confined to the lining of the bladder) or invasive (in which the cancer cells have penetrated other tissues). Although cancer of the bladder may be managed in a variety of ways, depending on the stage and type of cancer involved, the most common intervention for invasive cancer is radical **cystectomy**, a procedure in which the total bladder is surgically removed. Removal of the whole bladder necessitates surgical reconstruction to provide a means for urinary drainage, a procedure called *urinary diversion*. Although removal of the bladder once affected quality of life for individuals, because of major advances in urinary diversion, radical cystectomy is now a more acceptable option. Continent urinary diversions allow individuals to avoid external collection devices and permit minimal change in body image with only a small **stoma** (opening) in the abdomen.

When the total bladder is removed, an artificial reservoir for collection of urine must be substituted. Several types of reservoirs may be used. If the entire lower urinary system is removed, including the **urethra** (a tubular structure through which urine is excreted from the bladder to the outside of the body through the urinary meatus), an internal reservoir is constructed with an opening through which a catheter can be inserted for urinary drainage to the outside of the body. If the bladder alone is removed, leaving the urethra intact, a reservoir may still be constructed, but the individual will be able to continue to excrete urine through the urethra and almost-normal urination may be possible.

In some cases, only a portion of the bladder may be removed. The removal of a portion of the bladder may greatly diminish the capacity of the bladder, leading to a need to urinate more frequently.

Another procedure for urinary diversion is *cutaneous ureterostomy*, in which the ureters are brought through the abdomen to the outside of the body, where they drain directly into a bag attached to the outside of the abdomen. A urostomy bag is worn over the opening to collect urine.

Yet another urinary diversion procedure is an *ileal conduit*, which involves removing a segment of small intestine (the ileum) and reconnecting the two remaining ends of bowel. Ureters are then connected to one end of the loop of small intestine that has been removed, and the other end of the loop of small intestine is brought to the outside of the abdomen to form an opening through which urine can drain. In such a case, there is no voluntary control over the drainage of urine through the opening of either the cutaneous ureterostomy or the ileal conduit.

Less common types of urinary diversion include *ureterosigmoidostomy*, in which the ureters (tubes that drain urine from the kidneys to the bladder) are connected to the colon so that urine is excreted through the rectum.

Because urine mixes with the contents of the colon, bowel movements are liquid, and frequent evacuation of stool is necessary. Because of the potential contamination of the urinary system by organisms of the colon, a major complication of this type of urinary diversion is chronic pyelonephritis (see Chapter 15).

When cancer of the bladder is superficial, the cancer may be managed with bacille Calmette-Guérin (BCG), a form of immunotherapy in which the body's own immune system is stimulated to respond to and fight the cancer cells. This therapy consists of instilling the BCG vaccine into the bladder. When superficial cancer of the bladder is more advanced, chemotherapy may also be used.

Cancer of the kidney may necessitate removal of the kidney (**nephrectomy**). When both kidneys are involved, a portion of one kidney may be left intact so that the person maintains renal function. If both kidneys must be completely removed, individuals must be placed on regular dialysis (see Chapter 15).

Cancer of the Brain or Spinal Cord

When malignant tumors of the brain are small and accessible, and if they have not invaded surrounding tissue, they may be surgically removed, followed by interventions with chemotherapy or radiation. If there are no complications from surgery, individuals may be able to return to active life. Some individuals experience neurological deficits after surgery (see Chapters 3 and 4). At other times, the tumor may be embedded in the brain, or may be located in a part of the brain that is inaccessible, so that surgery is not possible without considerable risk to the individual. In these instances, chemotherapy or radiation therapy alone may be instituted as a means of control or palliation. The degree or type of limitation that results from a malignant brain tumor depends on the type of cancer, its size, and its location within the brain as well as any residues that might be experienced from surgery.

Cancers develop less often in the spinal cord than in the brain. Manifestations of a spinal cord tumor may be similar to those experienced with a spinal cord injury, including paralysis (see Chapter 4). Spinal cord tumors are usually managed surgically, with irradiation and chemotherapy playing roles as adjunct therapies.

Lymphomas

The lymphatic system is a connection of lymph nodes and vessels in which a clear fluid called lymph circulates through the body. The lymphatic system acts to fight infection and contributes to the body's immune system (see Chapter 10). Cancers of the lymphatic system are called lymphomas.

There are two classifications of lymphomas:

- Hodgkin's disease
- Non-Hodgkin's lymphoma

Hodgkin's Disease

Hodgkin's disease is a malignant condition of the lymphatic system that primarily affects the lymph nodes (Portlock & Yahalom, 2004). The cause of Hodgkin's disease is unknown, but it is described as a chronic, progressive condition in which irregular cells gradually replace the regular cells within the lymph nodes. Many individuals with Hodgkin's disease are **asymptomatic** (have no manifestations) or have only peripheral **lymphadenopathy** (enlargement of lymph nodes).

Hodgkin's disease is usually diagnosed through an excisional biopsy of an affected lymph node. Bone marrow is rarely affected; however, a bone marrow biopsy may also be performed.

Although many individuals' condition is advanced at the time of diagnosis, advances in interventions for management of Hodgkin's disease have made it mostly curable (DeVita, 2003). Management of Hodgkin's disease varies with the stage at which it is diagnosed. Radiation therapy is usually used in the early stages of the condition, and chemotherapeutic agents are often used in the later stages. In the late stage of the condition, a variety of chemotherapeutic agents may be used in combination to manage the condition. Because of the severe toxic effects of this intervention, individuals may have manifestations of nausea and vomiting, bone marrow suppression, and **peripheral neuropathy** (changes of sensation in the extremities). When Hodgkin's disease is found in the early stages and interventions are instituted promptly, it has a high rate of remission, and individuals with this condition have an excellent prognosis.

Non-Hodgkin's Lymphoma

Non-Hodgkin's lymphoma involves the proliferation of the lymph cells that are usually disseminated throughout the body. Diagnosis is made through examination of tissue that has been removed. Often bone marrow biopsy is also done because bone marrow involvement is likely.

Unlike persons with Hodgkin's disease, most individuals with non-Hodgkin's lymphoma are in advanced stages of the condition before diagnosis is made. The most common symptom is generalized **lymphadenopathy** (enlargement of the lymph nodes) (Bierman, Harris, & Armitage, 2004). The condition may be low grade, meaning that it progresses slowly, or it may be aggressive high grade, meaning that it progresses rapidly and can be fatal in months. Individuals with high-grade non-Hodgkin's lymphoma generally have manifestations of unexplained weight loss or unexplained fever. Non-Hodgkin's lymphoma is usually managed with radiation therapy in the early stages, and chemotherapy in conjunction with radiation therapy in the later stages, with possible bone marrow transplant.

Multiple Myeloma

Multiple myeloma is a slowly progressive cancer in which uncontrolled reproduction of irregular plasma cells leads to the destruction of the bone marrow and extends into the bone. Bone marrow produces red blood cells, white blood cells, and platelets, which control blood clotting. As the bone marrow is destroyed, individuals with multiple myeloma may experience either anemia or bleeding. The first symptom of multiple myeloma is often bone pain, which may be concentrated in the back. Bone destruction can also lead to **pathologic fractures** (fractures that occur because of conditions affecting the bone rather than from injury) and spinal cord compression.

Diagnosis of multiple myeloma may be based on blood tests, radiologic examination of the skeletal system to identify bone destruction, or biopsy of the bone marrow itself. Chemotherapy and, at times, radiation therapy are the major interventions used.

Because inactivity results in additional breakdown of bone, emphasis is placed on helping individuals remain active. Prognosis depends on the stage of the cancer when diagnosed; however, multiple myeloma is not currently curable.

Leukemia

Cancers of tissues in which blood is formed are called leukemias. A number of types of leukemias exist. Leukemia can be classified as acute or chronic.

Acute Leukemia

In most instances, there is no known cause of *acute leukemia*. Nevertheless exposure to radiation, occupational exposure to certain chemicals, viruses, and genetic links have all been cited as possible contributing factors (Appelbaum, 2004). In acute leukemia, there is proliferation of malignantly transformed stem cells (cells from which other cells originate) in the bone marrow that suppresses growth and differentiation of regular blood cells. Many irregular, immature white blood cells are released into the circulatory system. As a result, individuals with acute leukemia frequently experience anemia, **neutropenia** (small numbers of mature white blood cells), and **thrombocytopenia** (irregular number of platelets). They may also experience fatigue, headache, susceptibility to infection, and bruising or hemorrhage.

Acute leukemia is a rapidly progressing condition, so interventions are usually instituted immediately. The goal of intervention is to induce complete remission. Management usually consists of chemotherapy and, in some cases, bone marrow transplantation.

Chronic Leukemia

Chronic leukemia encompasses a broad spectrum of conditions and involves overproduction of white blood cells causing **splenomegaly** (enlargement of the spleen) (Keating & Kantarjian, 2004). Individuals often do not show any manifestations initially, so that the condition is first discovered through blood tests during a routine physical examination or medical consultation because of another problem. When manifestations are present, individuals often have fatigue or weight loss.

Chronic leukemia is an unpredictable condition. In some individuals it may progress slowly so that they live with the condition for decades, often dying from other causes; in other individuals, the condition requires frequent and multiple forms of therapy and can result in death within a few years (Rai and Chiorazzi, 2003). Although there are few or no manifestations in the early stages of the leukemia, if it progresses individuals may experience headaches, bone pain, joint pain, or fever. Diagnosis is based on results of blood tests and presence of an enlarged spleen.

Immediate management of chronic leukemia is usually not necessary unless complications occur. Initial management may consist of oral medication to control the irregular blood cell proliferation. Later interventions may consist of medications such as interferon or other types of chemotherapy.

Cancer of the Breast

Breast cancer is the most common cancer affecting women in the United States (Muss, 2004). As with other types of cancer, early diagnosis of breast cancer is most predictive of prognosis and cure (Punglia, Morrow, Winer, & Harris, 2007; Fletcher & Elmore, 2003). Regular breast self-examination and mammography can lead to early detection, thereby permitting early intervention. The primary management options for breast cancer are selected based on the stage of the cancer at the time of diagnosis. Interventions may be local, regional, or systemic. Local/regional control usually involves surgery.

Traditionally, management of breast cancer involved removal of the entire breast (**mastectomy**) through either simple mastectomy or radical mastectomy; in the latter procedure, the entire breast and its underlying tissue, including muscle and lymph nodes, are removed. Studies have shown, however, that modified procedures in many cases are just as effective in preventing metastasis or improving survival. These alternative surgical techniques may include the following options:

- *Lumpectomy*: (removal of the cancerous lesion itself and a small amount of surrounding breast tissue)
- Partial or *segmental mastectomy*: removal of a quadrant of the breast

The appropriateness of using more conservative surgical techniques that preserve as much of the breast tissue as possible depends on the size and location of the tumor. In many instances, regardless of the type of surgery,

radiation therapy and chemotherapy are used as adjunct therapies (Burstein, Polyak, Wong, Lester, & Kaelin, 2004).

Depending on the extent of surgery, individuals may experience some limitation in arm motion on the affected side. They may engage in physical therapy or other exercises to gain mobility and range of motion gradually. Lymphedema (swelling due to blockage of the lymph system), in which there is a swelling of the arm on the side of the mastectomy, may also occur—usually when the lymph nodes have been removed and the circulation of lymph fluid is slowed. Individuals may also have increased susceptibility to infection on the operative side.

Breast Reconstruction

Recent advances in cosmetic surgery have made breast reconstruction a viable option for some individuals. Breast reconstruction that uses implants or tissue transfer (involving movement or transfer of tissue from another part of the body) has become more common in the last few years. Prior to the advent of such breast reconstruction techniques, women had few choices but to wear an external prosthesis, which could be cumbersome and uncomfortable during physical activity, and which was not easily incorporated into the woman's body image.

The entire breast may be reconstructed (a procedure that may require two or more operations over several months' time) or, if there is sufficient chest muscle and the skin remaining after the removal of the tumor is of good quality, a prosthesis may be inserted into a pocket created under the chest muscle. In some instances, immediate breast reconstruction occurs at the time of the original surgery, which ameliorates the experience of breast loss. When the amount of muscle and tissue remaining is insufficient for breast reconstruction, other surgical procedures may be performed in which tissues from other parts of the body are used in the reconstruction of the breast. In some cases, tissue expanders may be used. Tissue expanders are adjustable implants filled with a salt solution that are inflated to stretch tissue after mastectomy. These implants may be temporary or permanent.

When breast reconstruction is not an option or when the individual chooses not to have such a procedure, a permanent breast form called a prosthesis may be used. Breast forms vary in weight and are matched to the size and contour of the remaining breast. Breast prostheses are sold in surgical supply stores, or they may be available in the lingerie departments of large department stores.

Psychosocial Issues in Breast Cancer

Like other cancers, breast cancer frequently produces complex psychological changes that involve altered sense of self and changes in relationships (Turner, Kelly, Swanson, Allison, & Wetzig, 2005). The psychological implications of breast cancer can be devastating for some women. The emotional impact of the loss of breast tissue varies from individual to individual. Not only are there concerns associated with the cancer itself, but also concerns regarding changes in appearance. Breast cancer poses a dual threat, in the form of risk to life as well as threat to female self-image. The deformity that may be associated with loss of breast tissue is a constant reminder of a life-threatening condition. As a sexually associated structure and societally valued symbol of attractiveness, the breast is also closely linked to a woman's self-esteem.

The Reach to Recovery program of the American Cancer Society was established in 1969 as a means to help women adjust to breast cancer. In this program, volunteers who have fully recovered from breast cancer visit the individual and answer questions, provide tips, and offer encouragement. Breast cancer support groups have also been found helpful by some individuals.

Gynecologic Cancer

Types of Gynecologic Cancer

Gynecologic cancers include cancer of the ovary, uterus, or cervix, or the external genitalia. Regular screenings can be important in early recognition of gynecologic cancers and, consequently, early intervention and cure.

Ovarian cancer, an insidious condition, generally shows no early detectable manifestations and has, therefore, often metastasized by the time the cancer is diagnosed. When ovarian cancer is diagnosed, surgery is always required, and probably chemotherapy after surgery.

Cancer of the cervix (the neck of the uterus, opening into the vagina) is detected through regular Pap screening—a type of test in which cancer cells can be identified microscopically. Although a variety of causes of cervical cancer have been suggested, recent findings have suggested that infection with the human papillomavirus (HPV) is a critical factor (Baden, Curfman, Morrisey, & Drazen, 2007). In an attempt to reduce the risk of cervical cancer, an HPV vaccine has been developed to prevent cancer induced by this virus, although how and when the vaccine should be used, and how effective it might be remain a topic of debate (Baden et al., 2007).

Early-stage cervical cancer usually has no manifestations, so regular screening is important for finding the cancer early. If cervical cancer is untreated, it can invade other organs and metastasize. In the case of early-stage disease, and especially if the woman wants to preserve fertility, the cancerous portion of the cervix may be excised, leaving the uterus. If the cancer is more advanced, both the cervix and the uterus are removed (total hysterectomy).

Cancer of the uterus is the most common gynecologic cancer (Molpus & Jones, 2004).

Cancer of the endometrium (lining of the uterus) is diagnosed by biopsy of the endometrium. Early manifestations of endometrial cancer consist of abnormal uterine bleeding. Management usually consists of hysterectomy with accompanying **oophorectomy** (removal of the ovaries).

There are generally no physical limitations associated with gynecologic cancer and its management. However, individuals with advanced cancer, and those who undergo chemotherapy or radiation therapy in combination with surgery, may experience fatigue and other side effects related to the therapy itself.

Psychosocial Issues in Gynecologic Cancer

In addition to the stress caused by having a diagnosis of cancer, the psychological issues associated with gynecologic surgery may cause some individuals significant distress. Gynecologic surgery because of cancer may produce changes in perception of body image, fertility, or sexuality. Removal of reproductive organs may have emotional and psychological consequences on the perception of sexual function, which affects the relationship with the woman's partner. Although surgery such as hysterectomy typically does not impair sexual function, considerable misinformation may surround gynecological surgery and can cause concern for the woman and her significant other. In instances where the cancer involves the external genitalia and necessitates its removal, the disfigurement and threat to body image may also produce significant emotional distress. Providing the individual and her partner with accurate information about the surgery and its implications can help to alleviate problems.

Cancer of the Prostate

The *prostate* is a gland that surrounds the urethra in males and secretes fluid, which bathes and nourishes human semen. Prostate can-

cer may be detected through screening techniques, including physical examination and blood tests for prostate-specific antigen (PSA) (Small, 2004). Other manifestations that individuals may experience are difficulties in urination owing to bladder outlet obstruction.

Another condition, *benign prostatic hypertrophy (BPH)*, although not a malignancy, may cause similar problems. Consequently, biopsy of the prostate is generally needed to confirm a diagnosis of cancer.

Interventions, as with other types of cancer, are determined mainly by staging of the cancer. Radical proctectomy, in which the prostate gland is removed, may be performed; however, cryotherapy, in which the prostate is frozen with liquid nitrogen so that tissue **necrosis** (death) occurs, is also used in case of prostate cancer. Individuals may also have adjunctive therapy, such as hormone therapy or radiation therapy. Complications of surgery in some individuals with prostate cancer include impotence and incontinence.

Skin Cancers

Skin cancer is the uncontrolled growth and reproduction of irregular skin cells. Most skin cancers, if detected and treated early, can be cured. The number one risk factor associated with skin cancer is overexposure to the sun. Individuals with fair skin are at greater risk than individuals with darker skin. Prevention of skin cancer involves protecting oneself from ultraviolet exposure, using sunscreen, covering skin with clothing, and minimizing outdoor activities when the sun is the strongest.

Several types of skin cancer are distinguished. *Basal cell cancers* are the most common type of skin cancer and originate in the layer of cells that form the base between the **epidermis** (the top layer of skin cells) and the **dermis** (the lower level of skin cells) (see Chapter 17). Less common are *squamous cell cancers*, which originate in the uppermost layers of skin. Both types of skin cancer usually do not spread and are easily cured if interventions—usually removal—are instituted promptly.

The most serious type of skin cancer is *malignant melanoma*, a cancer that originates from the melanocytes, the cells that produce the skin's pigment or color. Malignant melanoma spreads quickly and is more frequently fatal. Therapy for melanoma is primarily surgical (Schuchter, 2004).

■ PSYCHOSOCIAL ISSUES IN CANCER

Psychological Issues

Regardless of the type of cancer or the type of intervention instituted, psychological issues arise in all individuals with cancer. Reactions to the diagnosis of cancer vary according to the individual and often depend not only on the type and extent of the cancer, but also on the individual's own particular situation and coping skills.

Despite advances of management interventions, the word "cancer" still generates fear in many individuals and is stigmatizing for others. Individuals often perceive cancer as a threat to their mortality and their future, no matter what the actual prognosis. Individuals may fear loss of relationships, independence, job, integrity of the body and its functions, and life. Diagnosis of cancer may also be a symbol of vulnerability, loss of control, or helplessness. Even when the prognosis is good, fear of recurrence lingers with many individuals. When disfigurement owing to surgical procedures accompanies the diagnosis of cancer, adjustment to the altered self-image tends to cause further stress and anxiety.

Many individuals with cancer are emotionally overwhelmed when they first learn their diagnosis. Their initial reactions may include depression, irritability, fear, withdrawal, anger and hostility, or denial. Over time, they may come to accept their condition and try to make whatever adaptations are necessary to proceed with life.

Individuals who are younger when diagnosed with cancer may experience greater psychological distress. Body image may be more greatly affected, education and career paths may need to be postponed, and economic and social independence may be thwarted. The cost of interventions may be prohibitive for young adults who have not had an opportunity to establish a financially secure base. Forming or maintaining intimate relationships may also be made more difficult because of the diagnosis, regardless of the prognosis.

Coping with cancer is not static, but rather is a dynamic process, evolving over time (Livneh, 2000). Through each clinical stage of cancer, individuals utilize different coping skills to learn how to live with a potentially life-threatening condition. Reactions of individuals during each phase can determine their level of functioning at each phase as well as their adherence to the medical protocol.

Holland (1989) described four phases of coping during the clinical course of cancer. Individuals with cancer experience different concerns and different psychological reactions at each phase.

The first phase occurs when manifestations are initially identified. During this time individuals may experience anxiety, which can serve as motivation to seek medical attention or, if the anxiety is too great, may lead to denial of manifestations, thereby delaying diagnosis and subsequent interventions.

The second phase is described as the period during which a definitive diagnosis of cancer is made. Depending on their premorbid perceptions of cancer, individuals may experience significant emotional distress or display an attitude of problem solving and determination to do whatever is necessary for cure.

The third phase involves the interventions and adjuvant therapy. During this phase, individuals may express positive feelings of empowerment in actively participating in management of the cancer, or they may experience feelings of hopelessness and doom.

During the fourth phase, when the interventions are complete, individuals may be in remission (free from cancer manifestations). During this time, they may have feelings of uncertainty regarding the possibility of recurrence of the cancer or development of another cancer at a future date. In this last clinical phase, individuals may have feelings of vulnerability and uncertainty about future plans or feelings of confidence and optimism about working toward goals for the future.

In some instances, individuals may minimize the seriousness of the illness in an attempt to assimilate its impact and to marshal the resources and coping skills needed to deal with the perceived threat. Clarifying ambiguity and uncertainty while permitting denial is at times a difficult balance for all concerned. Some individuals cope by finding a general purpose or meaning to the illness that establishes a framework for events experienced. Other individuals gain a sense of control by seeking as much information as possible about their cancer and its management. Information can be an important tool in reducing anxiety, but it must be acquired at a rate that is manageable for the individual (Leydon, 2000). As a result of increased cancer survival rates, the quality of the individual's life and involvement in management decisions has become a central issue for health care providers and the individual with the condition alike.

Coping with cancer is an ongoing effort in which the individual reacts to the condition and its implications. Issues for individuals vary across a lifetime, as each life stage has its own opportunities and limitations. Individuals' reactions are influenced by outside forces as well as by their own intrinsic capabilities. Living with the fear of recurrence may promote stress and anxiety (Longo, 2007; McGrath, 1999). Individuals may need help in coping with distress caused by the therapy used to manage their cancer. The uncertainty of not knowing when or if the cancer will recur, or if a new malignancy will develop, can be a constant source of apprehension. Individuals may exhibit a wide spectrum of adaptive responses that may change over the course of the condition or over time.

Activities and Participation

The extent to which cancer affects individuals' everyday activities depends on the type and location of the cancer and its management. Side effects of radiation therapy or chemotherapy, such as nausea, loss of appetite, or fatigue, may affect daily activities during interventions or for a short time after they are instituted. Certain surgical procedures for various types of cancer may also affect individuals' lifestyles to some degree. For example, amputation, colostomy, and laryngectomy all require some adaptation of certain daily tasks.

The effects of cancer on sexuality differ from person to person. Some individuals experience no difficulty with sexual functioning. Others experience a decrease in sexual desire because of fatigue, pain, depression, or anxiety. Some forms of cancer and its management may have direct impact on sexual activity; for example, surgery may directly affect the organs of sexual function. In addition, surgery may have indirect effects on sexual activity if it alters individuals' physical appearance, thereby influencing their body image and self-esteem. Regardless of whether cancer directly or indirectly affects individuals' ability to engage in sexual intercourse, the need for closeness and demonstration of affection, such as hugging, touching, or kissing, is usually unchanged.

Despite public education about the new medical advances that have rendered many cancers curable, the general public—and perhaps even family and friends of individuals with cancer—may still hold the unfounded belief that "cancer" is a synonym for "death." Such misconceptions may lead to the emotional withdrawal of friends and acquaintances as they attempt to lessen the impact of loss before it occurs.

Acquaintances may avoid individuals with cancer because the diagnosis reminds them of their own mortality and because it engenders unpleasant feelings. The physical changes that occur because of surgery or other interventions may make friends or family uncomfortable and may contribute to aversion and further avoidance of individuals with cancer. Others may have the mistaken notion that cancer is contagious and avoid close physical contact with individuals or shun them altogether.

Just as alienation may result from the diagnosis of cancer, so may overprotection and enforced dependency, both of which erode individuals' sense of self-esteem and control. Family and friends may feel the need to protect individuals, as well as themselves, from the realities of cancer. Family members may not share their feelings and concerns, creating tension within the family group. As a result, the impact of the condition and the associated emotions may be denied. The individual with cancer, in an effort to avoid alienation or rejection, may also conceal his or her true emotions.

Challenges that confront family members of individuals with cancer are shaped by the type of cancer, the extent of the cancer, the type of intervention implemented, the quality of the family relationship prior to diagnosis, and concurrent stressors they may be experiencing (Sherman & Simonton, 2001). Because cancer may change over time—being characterized by remissions, relapses, need for additional interventions, or just unpredictability—individuals' place and role in the family may evolve, requiring different approaches over time (Moulton, 2000).

The extent to which cancer affects social activities depends not only on the attitudes and acceptance of the individuals involved, but also on physical factors such as pain and fatigue. Considerations, including time spent at the hospital and time associated with various interventions, may supercede social and family activities. Special provisions that encourage individuals with cancer to participate in social activities can decrease the disruption and the sense of conflict felt by these individuals and their families over time.

■ VOCATIONAL ISSUES IN CANCER

There have been a number of reports of employment discrimination and lack of rehabilitation services for persons with cancer (Conti, 1995; Feldman, 1987; Hoffman, 1991). One report cited a survey that found that workers with cancer were fired or laid off five times as often as other workers (Arnold, 1999). Not only can the economic implications of cancer be great, but work also takes on particular importance as a symbol of self-esteem, self-sufficiency, and an affirmation of life.

As with other conditions, the most significant barriers to employment after diagnosis of cancer may be the attitudes of employers and fellow workers, who may have the same misperceptions about cancer that some other social groups have. Attitudes of hopelessness related to a diagnosis of cancer may be expressed in employers' reluctance to allow individuals with cancer to return to work, their unwillingness to make concessions for any associated limitations, or their rejection of special aspects of interventions for cancer management. In some instances, employers and co-workers may view cancer as a contagious condition. Employers may also express concern about the ability of these individuals to perform the same work-related tasks for which they had been responsible prior to diagnosis, and some may view cancer survivors as a potential economic burden rather than as productive employees.

Although courts have argued about the status of cancer survivors under the Americans with Disabilities Act (ADA), some have agreed that ADA provides important legal rights for individuals with cancer (Hodges, 1999). As courts continue to discuss the definition of disability, educating and informing employers and individuals with cancer about the protections that ADA provides is an important step in advocacy and in helping individuals obtain or maintain employment for which they are qualified and that they desire (Arnold, 1999).

Vocational planning requires an awareness of the attitudes and prejudice that may exist in the work setting, as well as a specific knowledge about the condition and its management requirements, individuals' functional limitations, and demands of the work setting. Because of the variability of the limitations and prognosis with the type and location of cancer, the importance of short-term versus long-term planning should be considered. The variability of the limitations experienced and the prognosis for morbidity and life expectancy vary with the type and location of the cancer. Therefore, the type of plan, and the determination of whether short-term or long-term planning is most feasible, depend to a great extent on these factors. It is also necessary to understand the multidimensional impact of the diagnosis of cancer on the individual and the family. The degree to which individuals' former employment is still suitable takes many variables into account and must be examined realistically in the context of the demands and implications of returning to the former work setting, as well as the individual's own particular strengths and limitations.

CASE STUDIES

Case 1

Ms. E. has her own wallpaper-hanging business. She is 42 years old, is divorced, and has no children. Her most recent mammogram showed a mass in her right breast. Upon biopsy, the mass was found to be malignant. The physician recommended partial removal of a quadrant of the breast followed by chemotherapy. Ms. E. is concerned about her ability to maintain her wallpapering business. She does most of the wallpaper hanging herself, with only minimal assistance from a helper she has hired on a part-time basis.

1. Which factors related to Ms. E.'s condition would it be important to consider when evaluating her ability to continue in her line of work?
2. Which psychosocial factors might be important to address in Ms. E.'s rehabilitation plan?
3. Which types of services or assistive devices might be helpful to assist Ms. E.?

Case 2

Mr. M. is a 56-year-old truck driver. He has been a heavy user of tobacco and alcohol for the last 40 years. After he had experienced consistent hoarseness for more than a year, he was evaluated by a physician and found to have cancer of the larynx. Subsequently, Mr. M. had a laryngectomy.

1. Which specific issues related to Mr. M.'s laryngectomy would you consider when assessing his rehabilitation potential?
2. Which limitations would Mr. M. experience after his laryngectomy?
3. Is it feasible for Mr. M. to continue in his current line of employment? If so, which specific factors might it be important to consider?
4. Are there specific accommodations or assistive devices that may be helpful to Mr. M.?

■ REFERENCES

Appelbaum, F. R. (2004). The acute leukemias. In L. Goldman & D. Ausiello (Eds.), *Cecil textbook of medicine* (22nd ed., pp. 1161–1166)). Philadelphia: W. B. Saunders.

Arnold, K. (1999). Americans with Disabilities Act: Do cancer patients qualify as disabled? *Journal of the National Cancer Institute, 91*(10), 822–825.

Baden, L. R., Curfman, G. D., Morrissey, S., & Drazen, J. M. (2007). Human papillomavirus vaccine: Opportunity and challenge. *New England Journal of Medicine, 356*(19), 1990–1991.

Bertino, J. R. & Hat, W. (2004). Principles of cancer therapy. In L. Goldman & D. Ausiello (Eds.), *Cecil textbook of medicine* (22nd ed. pp. 1137–1150). Philadelphia: W. B. Saunders.

Bierman, P. J., Harris, N. L., & Armitage, J. O. (2004). In L. Goldman & D. Ausiello (Eds.), *Cecil textbook of medicine* (22nd ed., pp. 1174–1184). Philadelphia: W. B. Saunders.

Blot, W. J. (2004). Epidemiology of cancer. In L. Goldman & D. Ausiello (Eds.), *Cecil textbook of medicine* (22nd ed., pp. 1116–1120). Philadelphia: W. B. Saunders.

Brown, L. M., Hoover, R., Silverman, D., et al. (2001). Excess incidence of squamous cell esophageal cancer among US black men: Role of social class and other risk factors. *American Journal of Epidemiology, 153*, 114–122.

Burstein, H. J., Polyak, K., Wong, J. S., Lester, S. C., & Kaelin, C. M. (2004). Ductal carcinoma in situ of the breast. *New England Journal of Medicine, 350*(14), 1430–1441.

Cady, J. (2002). Laryngectomy: Beyond loss of voice—Caring for the patient as a whole. *Clinical Journal of Oncology Nursing, 6*(6), 1–5.

Cleary, J., Gorenstein, L. A., & Omenn, G. S. (1996, September 15). Lung cancer: Prevention is the best cure. *Patient Care,* 35–36; 39; 42; 45–47; 51–52; 55; 59–60; 62; 67.

Conti, J. V. (1995). Job discrimination against people with cancer history. *Journal of Applied Rehabilitation Counseling, 26*(2), 12–16.

DeVita, V. (2003). Hodgkin's disease: Clinical trials and travails. *New England Journal of Medicine, 348*(24), 2375–2376.

Dobbins, M., Gunson, J., Bale, S., Neary, M., Ingrams, D., & Brown, M. (2005). Improving patient care and quality of life after laryngectomy/glossectomy. *British Journal of Nursing, 14*(12), 634–640.

Droller, M. J. (1998). Bladder cancer: State of the art care. *CA: A Cancer Journal for Clinicians, 48*(5), 269–284.

DuBois, R. N. (2004). Neoplasms of the large and small intestine. In L. Goldman & D. Ausiello (Eds.), *Cecil textbook of medicine* (22nd ed., pp. 1121–1220). Philadelphia: W. B. Saunders.

Eadie, T. L., & Doyle, P. C. (2005). Quality of life in male tracheoesophageal (TE) speakers. *Journal of Rehabilitation Research & Development, 42*(1), 115–124.

Enzinger, P. C., & Mayer, R. J. (2003). Esophageal cancer. *New England Journal of Medicine, 349*(23), 2241–2252.

Feldman, F. L. (1987). The return to work: The question of workability. *Proceedings of the Workshop on Employment Insurance, and the Patient with Cancer* (pp. 27–35). New York: American Cancer Society.

Fletcher, S. W., & Elmore, J. G. (2003). Mammographic screening for breast cancer. *New England Journal of Medicine, 348*(17), 1672–1679.

Forastiere, A. A., Goepfert, H., Maor, M., Pajak, T. F., Weber, R., Morrison, W., et al. (2003). Concurrent chemotherapy and radiotherapy for organ preservation in advanced laryngeal cancer. *New England Journal of Medicine, 349*(22), 2091–2098.

Freidenbergs, I., Grunwald I., & Kaplan, E. (2005). Cancers. In H. H. Zaretsky, E. F. Richter III, & M. G. Eisenberg (Eds.), *Medical aspects of disability* (3rd ed., pp. 159–178). New York: Springer.

Green, M. R. (2004). Targeting targeted therapy. *New England Journal of Medicine, 350*(21), 2191–2195.

Hancock, K., Houghton, B., Van As-Brooks, C. J., & Coman, W. (2005). First clinical experience with a new non-indwelling voice prosthesis (Provox NID) for voice rehabilitation after total laryngectomy. *Acta Oto-Laryngologia, 125*, 981–990.

Hodges, A. C. (1999). The Americans with Disabilities Act: Legal protection for the employment of the cancer patient. *Legal Information Network for Cancer.* Retrieved June 7, 2004, from http://www.cancerline.org/adact.html.

Hoffman, B. (1991). Employment discrimination: Another hurdle for cancer survivors. *Cancer Investigation, 9,* 589–595.

Holland, J. C. (1989). Clinical course of cancer. In J. C. Holland & J. H. Rowlands (Eds.), *Handbook of psychooncology: Psychological care of the patient with cancer* (pp. 75–100). New York: Oxford University Press.

Keating, M. J., & Kantarjian, H. (2004). The chronic leukemia's. In L. Goldman & D. Ausiello (Eds.), *Cecil textbook of medicine* (22nd ed., pp. 1150–1161). Philadelphia: W. B. Saunders.

Lagergren, J., Bergstrom, R., Adami, H. O., & Nyren, O. (2000). Association between medications that relax the lower esophageal sphincter and risk for esophageal adenocarcinoma. *Annals of Internal Medicine, 133,* 165–175.

Lewin, J. (2005). Patients with head and neck cancer: Treatment selections and effects on functional outcomes. *ASHA Leader, 10*(5), 9–11.

Leydon, G. M. (2000). Cancer patients' information needs and information seeking behavior: In depth interview study. *British Medical Journal, 320(7239),* 909–913.

Livneh, H. (2000). Psychosocial adaptation to cancer: The role of coping strategies. *Journal of Rehabilitation, 66*(2), 40–49.

Longo, D. L. (2007). Approach to the patient with cancer. In *Harrison's internal medicine: Part 5, oncology and hematology; Section 1, neoplastic disorders.* New York: McGraw-Hill. http://www.accessmedicine.com/content.aspx?aID=60411.

Macdonald, J. S. (2006). Gastric cancer: New therapeutic options. *New England Journal of Medicine, 355*(1), 76–79.

McGrath, P. (1999). Posttraumatic stress and the experience of cancer: A literature review. *Journal of Rehabilitation, 65,* 17–23.

Miller, Y. E. (2004). Lung cancer and other pulmonary neoplasms. In L. Goldman & D. Ausiello (Eds.), *Cecil textbook of medicine* (22nd ed., pp. 1201–1208). Philadelphia: W.B. Saunders.

Molpus, K. L. & Jones H. W. III. (2004). Gynecologic cancers. In L. Goldman & D. Ausiello (Eds.), *Cecil textbook of medicine* (22nd ed., pp. 1238–1241). Philadelphia: W. B. Saunders.

Moulton, G. (2000). Cancer survivor issues are all in the family. *Journal of the National Cancer Institute, 92*(2), 101–103.

Muss, H. B. (2004). Breast cancer and differential diagnosis of benign lesions. In L. Goldman & D. Ausiello (Eds.), *Cecil textbook of medicine* (22nd ed., pp. 1230–1238). Philadelphia: W. B. Saunders.

Pappas, T. N., & Jacobs, D. O. (2004). Laparoscopic resection for colon cancer: The end of the beginning? *New England Journal of Medicine, 350*(20), 2091–2092.

Portlock, C. S. & Yahalom, J. (2004). Hodgkin's disease. In L. Goldman & D. Ausiello (Eds.), *Cecil textbook of medicine* (22nd ed., pp. 1166–1173). Philadelphia: W. B. Saunders.

Posner, M. (2004). Head and neck cancer. In L. Goldman & D. Ausiello (Eds.), *Cecil textbook of medicine* (22nd ed., pp. 1195–1201). Philadelphia: W. B. Saunders.

Punglia, R. S., Morrow, M., Winer, E. P., & Harris, J. R. (2007). Local therapy and survival in breast cancer. *New England Journal of Medicine, 356*(23), 2399–2405.

Rai, K., & Chiorazzi, N. (2003). Determining the clinical course and outcome in chronic lymphocytic leukemia. *New England Journal of Medicine, 348*(18), 1797–1799.

Rosenberg, S. A. (2004). Shedding light on immunotherapy for cancer. *New England Journal of Medicine, 350*(14), 1461–1463.

Rustgi, A. K. (2004). Neoplasms of the stomach. In L. Goldman & D. Ausiello (Eds.), *Cecil textbook of medicine* (22nd ed., pp. 1208–1211). Philadelphia: W. B. Saunders.

Sausville, E. A., & Longo, D. L. (2007). Principles of cancer treatment: Surgery, chemotherapy, and biologic therapy. In *Harrison's internal medicine: Part 5, oncology and hematology; Section 1, neoplastic disorders.* New York: McGraw Hill. http://www.accessmedicine.com/content.aspx?aID=61153.

Schuchter, L. (2004). Melanoma and nonmelanoma skin cancers. In L. Goldman & D. Ausiello (Eds.), *Cecil textbook of medicine* (22nd ed., pp. 1248–1253). Philadelphia: W. B. Saunders.

Shaheen, N. & Ransohoff, D. F. (2002). Gastroesophageal reflux, Barrett esophagus, and esophageal cancer: Scientific review. *Journal of the American Medical Association, 287,* 1972–1981.

Sherman, A. C. & Simonton, S. (2001). Coping with cancer in the family. *The Family Journal: Counseling and Therapy for Couples and Families, 9*(2), 193–200.

Sherwood, L. (2007). *Human physiology.* Belmont, CA: Thomson Brooks/Cole.

Small, E. J. (2004). Prostate cancer. In L. Goldman & D. Ausiello (Eds.), *Cecil textbook of medicine* (22nd ed., pp. 1243–1248). Philadelphia: W. B. Saunders.

Syrjänen, S. (2007). Human papillomaviruses in head and neck carcinomas. *New England Journal of Medicine, 356(19),* 1993–1995.

Terry, P., Lagergren, J., Ye, W., Nyren, O., & Wolk, A. (2000). Antioxidants and cancers of the esophagus and gastric cardia. *International Journal of Cancer, 87,* 750–754.

Turner, J., Kelly, B., Swanson, C., Allison, R., & Wetzig, N. (2005). Psychosocial impact of newly diagnosed advanced breast cancer. *Psycho-Oncology, 14,* 396–407.

Vogelzang, N. J. (2004). Tumors of the kidney, bladder, ureters, and renal pelvis. In L. Goldman & D. Ausiello (Eds.), *Cecil textbook of medicine* (22nd ed., pp. 1226–1230). Philadelphia: W. B. Saunders.

Vokes, E. E., & Stenson, K. M. (2003). Therapeutic options for laryngeal cancer. *New England Journal of Medicine, 349*(22), 2087–2089.

Wu, A. H., Wan, P., & Bernstein, L. (2001). A multiethnic population-based study of smoking, alcohol and body size and risk of adenocarcinoma of the stomach and esophagus (United States). *Cancer Causes Control, 12,* 721–732.

Zeitels, S. M., & Healy, G. B. (2003). Laryngology and phonosurgery. *New England Journal of Medicine, 349*(9), 882–892.

Chapter 19

Assistive Technology

■ INTRODUCTION

Individuals with disability now live more independently in their communities than ever before. Changes in social philosophy as well as changes in policy and legislation have contributed greatly to this phenomenon (Peterson & Rosenthal, 2005a). The new *International Classification of Functioning, Disability, and Health* (ICF; World Health Organization, 2001) is a system that promotes use of universal classifications of function in conjunction with diagnostic information (Bruyére & Peterson, 2005). As a classification system, it de-emphasizes limitations associated with disability, focusing instead on functional capacities with regard to psychosocial and environmental factors. The ICF also proposes a model of functioning and disability that suggests a changing and reciprocal relationship exists among disability, personal factors, and the environment (Peterson & Rosenthal, 2005b). In other words, it emphasizes what people do on a daily basis rather than focusing on what they have the ability to do (Scherer & Glueckauf, 2005).

Renewed emphasis on the importance of participation by individuals with disability in society at large has contributed greatly to increased inclusion. However, development of new assistive devices, which facilitate independent activities and employment, has also been a major factor in expanding inclusion (Berry & Ignash, 2003). Focus on helping individuals not only achieve greater functional capacity, but also increase their ability to perform in the context of their environment and personal goals is an important component in the overall rehabilitation process (Blair, 2000; Kroll, Beatty, & Bingham, 2003). Assistive technology enables individuals to participate and be involved in activities of daily living as well to fulfill roles within the context of their particular life situation (Scherer, Sax, & Glueckauf, 2005).

■ DEFINING ASSISTIVE TECHNOLOGY

Everybody uses assistive technology in a broad sense. Informally, assistive technology can be thought off as any tool, apparatus, device, or machine used by a person to accomplish some practical task or purpose in a home, work, or recreational setting (Blake & Bodine, 2002; King, 1999). For instance, use of a calculator to balance a checkbook, a telephone to link with colleagues, and a computer to play computer games are examples of assistive technology used by the general population.

Individuals with disability have long used assistive technology in some form for specific need. Use of wheelchairs, Braille watches, and hearing aids are common examples; however, these devices were often used in keeping with the medical model, rather than being the result of individual choice (Mendelsohn & Fox, 2002). The importance of assistive technology matched to the needs of the individual became more important through ensuing legislation. The Americans with Disabilities Act (ADA), which was enacted in 1990, established the right of individuals with disability to receive reasonable accommodations that would enable them to perform essential job functions. The role and importance of assistive technology for individuals with disability were affirmed with the signing into law of the Assistive Technology Act of 1998, which was reauthorized in 2004.

The Assistive Technology Act of 2004 defines assistive technology as follows:

> Any item, piece of equipment, or product system, whether acquired commercially off the shelf, modified, or customized, that is used to increase, maintain, or improve functional capabilities of individuals with disabilities (Assistive Technology Act, 2004).

Types of Assistive Devices

Assistive devices may be "high tech" (devices that are technologically complex, require precise operations, and involve sophisticated materials). Alternatively; they may be "low tech" (devices that are made from readily available materials and are simple, inexpensive, and easy to use). The type of assistive technology used should depend on the preferences, needs, and goals of the individual using the device.

Assistive technology enables people to achieve personal goals and to move toward future achievements, as well as to gain and maintain employment and to be independent in activities of daily living and in society. Tech-nology plays an important role in rehabilitation in that it increases the functional capacity of individuals with disabilities. The development of new technologies has made the home, education, and work environments more accessible for persons with disability and has increased their social, educational, and employment opportunities (Berry & Ignash, 2003).

Proliferation of technology, however, can also make it difficult to ensure that, as devices are developed, they truly meet the needs of the individuals for whom they are intended (Blair, 2000; Kroll, et al., 2003). It is always important to ascertain whether the assistive device chosen for a specific disability is most appropriate to the individual's needs and is reasonably priced. Whether devices are used for picking up mail at the mailbox, getting the newspaper from the driveway, or participating in an adventure vacation such as mountain climbing, assistive technology will only be as effective as its ability to meet the needs and goals of the specific individual who uses it.

Individuals' use of assistive technology and the types of devices used may change over time or as individuals' age. If individuals have a progressive disability, different assistive devices may be needed over the course of the condition to accommodate additional limitations. In other instances, different devices may be required because an individual's lifestyle has changed. Human circumstances are not static, so flexibility must be maintained in evaluating the continuing and changing needs of individuals.

Assistive devices vary in complexity. Whereas some devices are relatively easy to use, others require considerable training and practice before they can be used effectively. The most effective assistive device is one that individuals are comfortable using and that meets their own particular needs. Technological devices, especially if they are high tech, may be intimidating to some individuals. Anxiety or insecurity about the ability to use a device may cause individuals to avoid using it or to abandon it. The more sophisticated the device, the more complicated it may be to use. Consequently, assistive devices should be "user friendly."

Assistive technology and its associated services, if they are to be applied effectively, must be viewed within the context of the life of the individual. Having technology available does not necessarily mean that the resulting assistive device will be useful or that it will be used. Many factors aside from availability are relevant (Hasselbring & Glaser, 2000).

Other Types of Assistive Devices

Prostheses

Assistive devices help individuals with disabilities obtain greater functional capacity and independence in some way. Prosthetic devices provide replacement of a body part or function. For example, prosthetic legs assist individuals to stand, walk, and run. Neuroprosthetic arms with implanted or skin-surface electrodes can assist individuals with grasping, holding, and carrying tasks.

Some assistive devices may be used for cosmetic purposes, such as a prosthetic external ear, which may have limited functional use but can be important to the individual's willingness to participate in social interactions. In other instances, assistive devices help prevent complications that may interfere with an individual's functional capacity. For example, pressure sores are a major complication for individuals with limited mobility or lack of sensation and can result in extended hospital stays, time off from work, and substantial cost. Devices to prevent pressure sores from occurring, although not directly related to function, help individuals achieve their full functional capacity.

Service Animals

Although not "devices" per se, service animals can greatly enhance individuals' functional capacity in home, work, or social environments. Although dogs are most often used, simian aides can also be used for a variety of tasks, such as retrieving items that have been dropped, obtaining items that they have been instructed to retrieve, opening doors, and replacing or storing items in their appropriate place.

Guide dogs can help individuals with visual impairments increase their mobility. Service dogs for individuals with hearing impairments can alert individuals to sounds that require action, such as a baby crying or a doorbell ringing. Larger dogs may assist individuals in wheelchairs to obtain greater mobility by helping to pull a wheelchair when greater propulsion is needed.

Individuals with disabilities should be actively involved in choosing their assistive devices and in assessing the devices' effectiveness. Devices can range from simple do-it-yourself items, such as a paint can opener to help when there is reduced hand strength or low-tech devices such as canes or crutches (Allen, 2001), to sophisticated computer software for individuals with cognitive impairments (Hasselbring & Glaser, 2000). Regardless of the potential sophistication of adaptive devices, the most effective device will still be one that individuals are willing and able to use in their own environment to meet their specific needs. Consequently, before any device is selected, it is important to consider the individual's specific goals and tasks within a given environment, psychosocial incentives and disincentives, personal characteristics, and abilities and preferences (Blair, 2000).

■ USES OF ASSISTIVE TECHNOLOGY

Assistive devices are used to increase independence, save time and energy, and prevent injury. The type and use of assistive technology depend on the needs of the individual. Some common uses are listed here:

- Mobility, postural control, and transfers
- Transportation
- Self-help/personal care needs
- Home management/safety
- Communication/sensory needs
- Recreation
- Cognitive/memory/learning needs
- Workplace modification
- Accessibility

Mobility, Postural Control, and Transfers

Mobility refers to the ability to move within and around the immediate environment as well as the ability to travel to other destinations away from home. Mobility aids vary greatly in their type and use (Chen, Chen, Chen, & Lin, 2003). They can be used to help someone move in bed, get on or off a toilet, move around the home or neighborhood, or get to school, work, or areas for recreation.

Some devices are designed to assist individuals with seating or positioning. They enable individuals to maintain postural control, manage pressure and comfort, or to provide postural accommodation.

Both low-tech aids, such as transfer boards, canes, or walkers, and high-tech aids, such as manual or power wheelchairs, scooters, or GPS devices, are used to help individuals achieve mobility and move from location to location. Microcomputer-controlled powered wheelchairs and powered wheelchairs with puff–sip controls provide increased mobility to individuals with severe disabilities. New technological advances may provide wheelchairs that have instrumentation to alert users that they are too close to objects or that decrease power when there is an object in the path (Galvin & Scherer, 1996). Different wheeled mobility devices may be needed for the same individual. Some individuals may require one type of wheelchair for indoor use and another type for sports or outdoor use. Lifts and stairway guides also increase individuals' mobility both in the home and away from home.

Transportation

Transportation is another important mobility need, both for getting to work and for achieving increased independence. Adapted personal vehicles, which include hand controls and steering devices to accommodate the needs of individuals with limited use of one or more extremities, may enable individuals to drive standard motor vehicles. Van conversions and buses that have been adapted to include wheelchair lifts enable individuals to carry wheelchairs or scooters, which can then be used at their point of destination.

The sophistication of assistive technology related to transportation will continue to be enhanced in the future. Without public awareness, however, environmental constraints may remain a barrier to full adaptation. Wheeled mobility aids and transportation aids are maximally effective only when the environment accommodates their use. Both adaptive devices and environmental modification are necessary for individuals to reach their full independent living and work potential.

Self-Help/Personal Care Needs

Assistive technology for self-help or personal care needs facilitates completion of tasks of daily living such as eating, drinking, brushing hair, brushing teeth, putting on clothes, dressing, bathing, toileting, or tying shoes. These devises are generally low-tech aids. Although they are usually less expensive, they are nevertheless vital to independence and to reaching goals in other areas (Thyberg, Hass, Nordenskiod, & Skogh, 2004). Such a device may be as simple as an item purchased from a hardware store, or it can be specially manufactured to meet a specific need. Examples of devices that may be helpful for self-care include modified eating utensils, electric toothbrushes, button hooks, sock guides, zipper aids, and support bars or rails.

The task to be performed and the environments in which the device is to be used determine the type of device needed for activities of daily living. Individuals' needs may change as they move to different environments. For example, devices used in the home for activities of daily living may not be appropriate on a business trip. The appropriateness of each device should be considered in the context of the setting in which it is to be used.

Home Management/Safety

A variety of devices used by individuals *without disability* also help to increase the functional capacity of individuals *with disability*. Devices such as microwave ovens, electric can openers, and other electronic devices may be convenience items for people without disability, yet can significantly increase the functional capacity and independence of people with disability. The increasing sophistication of computers, robotics, and other electronic devices may also offer more functional independence in activities of daily living for persons with disabilities in the future.

Assistive technology for home management or safety includes devices that help with tasks such as cooking, cleaning, turning lamps on or off, locking/unlocking and opening doors, hearing the doorbell, writing checks, hearing a smoke alarm, or being aware of danger. Signaling and alerting devices, bottle and can openers, modified lighting, and automated closet adapters are examples of assistive technology that may increase individual's ability to function more independently in the home (LoPresti, Brienza, Angelo, & Gilbertson, 2003).

Communication/Sensory Needs

Communication is a complex activity involving perception and integration of information. It includes speaking, writing, reading, hearing, signing, and other nonverbal means of communicating. Communication is vital to a number of tasks many people take for granted, such as talking to others, being able to hear or talk on the phone, making appointments, sending e-mails, or being able to explain a medical problem to a physician. Assistive devices to aid in communication currently range from low-tech devices such as books and pencils to high-tech aids, such as augmentative and alternative communication (AAC) devices (Neumann, Hinterberger, Kaiser, Leins, Birbaumer, & Kubler, 2004). Whether individuals use low-tech or high-tech devices, a certain degree of cognitive and motor ability as well as training is required.

Communication devices can be either manual or electronic. Examples of manual devices include communication boards, which contain line drawings, pictures, symbols, or other systems in which individuals spell out messages or indicate phrases to another person. Electronic systems are often computer based and may filter or manipulate vocalizations or provide synthesized speech, such as an electronic voice-output communication aid (VOCA). VOCAs are computerized devices that produce synthetic or digitized speech output when activated. Individuals then point to visual-graphic symbols, which are used to represent messages. Because these devices provide speech output, they are more easily integrated into everyday environments with unfamiliar people (Miranda, 2001). Other types of devices that aid in communication include computer hardware and software applications that provide writing assistance, speech-generating devices, and the artificial larynx.

Because of the complexity of communication and the varying capabilities and needs of individuals in different situations, no one type of device is appropriate for everyone. The selection of assistive technology to aid in communication is based on a systematic analysis of the individual's characteristics and environmental demands. In addition, a trial period of use is often necessary to determine how easily the individual is able to use the device and how well it meets the individual's needs (Sigafoos, O'Reilly, Ganz, Lancioni, & Schlosser, 2005). The device chosen to augment or enhance communication must be one that meets the specifications of the individual who will be using it. Because communication is such an individual and personal function, the individual using a device is best qualified to evaluate whether it improves communication outcomes.

Communication devices are also available for individuals who need to increase their functional capacity in sensory areas, including sight, hearing, touch, taste, or smell (Sokol-McKay, Buskirk, & Whittaker, 2003). Assistive devices to increase functional capacity in these areas may range from simple to complex. Examples of simple devices include eyeglasses, magnifiers, or a bath thermometer to prevent burns. Examples of more complex devices include voice recognition computers and optical-to-vibrotactile prostheses that make it possible for individuals who are blind to distinguish patterns of stimulation, enabling them to discriminate between certain properties of three-dimensional space.

Assistive devices for individuals who are deaf or hard of hearing may use amplification, vibrotactile prompts, or visual cues. Assistive devices such as hearing aids and telecommunication display devices can help individuals who are deaf or hard of hearing to function more easily in a hearing world.

Recreation

Recreational activities may range from gardening, playing cards, or reading to watching television, riding a bicycle, or climbing a mountain. The assistive devices needed for recreational activates vary with individual need, interest, and ability. Technology developers have already created sports equipment that enables athletes without disability to achieve far greater feats than previously had been expected. Some of the same types of technology have since been applied to recreational devices for individuals with disabilities, giving them a new freedom not previously enjoyed by members of earlier generations.

The sophistication of the technology used for recreational equipment varies with the activity. The technology needed for assisting individuals in card playing is much different from that needed for helping individuals in downhill skiing. Not all individuals want to pursue the same type of recreation they enjoyed prior to their disability, but some will certainly embrace the opportunity to continue. Frequently, the major barrier to continuing the recreational activities of their choice is the bias of those around them, who may believe that certain activities are inappropriate for individuals with disability.

Cognitive/Memory and Learning Needs

Cognitive and learning disability may be either a primary disability or a secondary disability. Whether the disability is acquired, such as with traumatic brain injury; a result of brain deterioration, such as in dementia; or a congenital disability, such as intellectual disability, the individual's functional capacity is complex and unique and may change over time. In addition, when cognitive disability exists, other areas of function, such as motor or behavioral function, memory, or learning are frequently affected as well. Assistive technology can enhance performance of functional tasks as well as mitigate to some extent the behavioral, memory, or learning problems, that may accompany some cognitive disabilities (Scherer, 2005; Hammel, 2003).

Memory function, regardless of the cause, can impair individuals' quality of life and their ability to function independently. Although many techniques that have been utilized to increase memory performance, such improvement is often short-lived. A number of external devices of systems that serve as memory enhancements have been developed. Some assistive devices permit the user to record and play back messages; others are used as reminders, such as voice-activated reminder calendars. Both can be of help to individuals with memory problems.

Because the needs of individuals with cognitive disability may be so complex and multifactorial, matching the individual to the appropriate assistive device can present quite a challenge. An assistive device designed to address one area of function may negatively affect other aspects of the individual's need. For example, individuals may use a small portable device to assist with memory, but the operation of the device may be impossible because of motor difficulty the individual also experiences. In addition, very sophisticated devices may be adequate for assisting an individual to achieve greater functional capacity in some areas, but the individual may not have the cognitive capacity to learn to operate it.

Workplace Modification

The American with Disabilities Act assured that reasonable accommodation would be afforded to individuals with disability so that qualified individuals with disability could be employed. "Reasonable accommodation" was defined as a modification of a work site or job that did not impose financial hardship on the employer. The intent of job or workplace modification was to increase individuals' functional capacity and, thereby, to enhance their ability to perform the job.

Additional assistive devices may not be needed in the workplace if appropriate environmental accommodations can be made. For some individuals, modification of the environment through better lighting, air-temperature control, or removal of obstacles through architectural modifications or restructuring of the job may be all that is necessary to enable them to achieve functional capacity.

In other instances, finding alternative ways to perform a job function or modifying existing devices may produce the same result. When assistive technology is needed, the necessary devices may be either low tech, such as reachers or extenders, or high tech, such as robotics (O'Day, Palsbo, Dhont, & Scheer, 2002).

Although computer technology can help individuals increase their functional capacity, some disabilities make computer use difficult, such that other assistive devices may be needed to enhance computer use. For instance, head controls or other adaptive computer aids can provide an alternative means to computer access (Fichten, Barile, Asuncion, & Fossey, 2000). Software has also been developed that automatically adjusts to the needs of the particular individual, especially if the disability limits head or neck or movement of the upper extremities (LoPresti & Brienza, 2004). Control mechanisms or switches may also be used to operate computers or communication aids, thereby increasing functional capacity.

When assistive devices are needed in the workplace, as in other settings, the type of device is determined by the specific need and the individual's preference. As in other areas of the individual's life, high-tech devices are not always the most appropriate or effective way to meet an individual's need or to increase his or her ability to perform a specific function effectively. Focusing on individuals' ability (rather than their disability) and including them in the process of determining what is needed are the most useful approaches to determining which, if any, adaptive devices will be beneficial.

Accessibility

Accessibility can involve more than architectural structure. Assistive devices for use in the environment may also increase individuals' ability to function within their environment. Simple examples are a Braille labeler to help in identifying items, a talking location indicator, and verbal announcement of bus stops or elevator floors.

■ INDIVIDUAL ASSESSMENT

Individuals' physical and psychosocial environments both affect the usefulness of an assistive device. Consequently, the characteristics of the environment must always be considered (Blair, 2000; Hammel, 2003). Both the type and number of assistive devices needed will vary. Few people function in only one setting. Thus individuals with disabilities may require specific devices for activities of daily living, different devices to be used at work, and still other devices to be used in social and recreational settings.

People with similar disabilities may not require the same type or the same number of assistive devices. The type of assistive device needed depends on where the equipment will be used, the tasks and activities required in each environment, and the extent to which tasks would be enhanced by the use of the device. Architectural accessibility and the amount of environmental support needed for the use of an assistive device are important considerations as well. The physical environment in which the assistive device is to be operated must be assessed, and obstacles that could interfere with the device's use must be identified. Sometimes environmental modification alone may increase the individual's ability to function. As society becomes increasingly aware of the need for universal design so that environments are more accessible for all individuals, design may change so that many of today's physical barriers no longer exist in the future.

In addition to the physical environment, the psychosocial environment affects the usefulness of assistive devices. The amount of support and encouragement individuals receive from others in their environment may be a major determinant of the degree to which an assistive device is used.

The cultural environment in which individuals function also plays a major role in the type of device obtained and the extent to which it is used. For example, not all individuals who are deaf or hard of hearing believe that they need to compensate for their decreased auditory function. Many of these individuals have a strong cultural identity within the Deaf community and may not be receptive to many of the technological advances that are currently available or that may become available in the future.

A thorough assessment of the individual's preferences and needs must be conducted before any assistive device is obtained. If one type of device is inadequate to meet an individual's needs, it should not be assumed that no viable alternatives exist. Likewise, it should not be assumed that all individuals with the same disability will require the same type of device. Although it is likely that individuals with severe disability will require high-technology devices, it should not automatically be assumed that individuals want that type of device or that other devices could not be equally useful.

Although access to consumer-responsible assistive devices and services is federally mandated, individuals differ in their needs, values, perspectives, motivations, and expectations—all of which can affect the use of assistive devices. All assistive devices should be matched to unique individual's capabilities and temperament. The success of adaptive devices is often determined by the degree to which those devices match individuals' values and perspectives rather than the potential usefulness of any particular device for day-to-day activities.

■ SUPPORTS AND BARRIERS TO USING ASSISTIVE TECHNOLOGY

Assistive technology, whether high tech or low tech, is only as useful as the extent to which it meets the needs and goals of the individual for whom it was designed. One barrier that prevents some individuals from using certain types of assistive technology successfully is the amount of energy or work required to use it. Sometimes this problem may be remedied by a simple adjustment to the device, such as changing the location of a control. In other instances, because of the complexity of the device or the mechanics involved in its effective use, modifications cannot be made. When devices are too hard to operate, user motivation and success rates diminish (King, 1999).

Just as physical effort may reduce motivation and success in using assistive technology, so may the amount of cognitive effort required. The more obvious the purpose of the device and the method required to use it, the less cognitive effort is needed to operate it. The more thought individuals need to put into the use of a device, or the more problem solving that is required for its effective use, the less effective the device will be.

The amount of time required to use assistive technology and the degree to which it meets the purpose for which it is designed may also affect use of the device. Devices that require a number of steps, as well as devices that are slow to respond to command, are less likely to meet the individual's needs than are devices that take relatively few steps to use and respond to commands immediately.

The cosmetic appearance of the device may affect user motivation as well. Appearance is important to everyone. Individuals with disability may become even more sensitized to the appearance of such devices and what the devices communicate about them to others; specifically, they may feel they should not appear disabled to others. For instance, an individual who is already in a wheelchair and now requires a hearing aid, rather than looking at the hearing aid as a way of increasing functional capacity may fear that it signals to others that the person is in a state of deterioration and decreased ability. Devices that are designed to have a more visually appealing appearance are more likely to be utilized than those devices that are perceived by the individual to communicate negative images to others in the environment (King, 1999).

Cultural differences can also have a profound impact on the extent to which assistive technology is incorporated into the individual's life. The individual's culture, language, beliefs, and customs must be taken into account when selecting a device. Related to the individual's culture is his or her philosophy of chronic illness and disability, rehabilitation, and inclusion into society. Individuals may have cultural objections to certain types of technology; these beliefs and preferences must be taken into account before assistive devices are provided.

Lastly, assistive devices must be durable and easily repaired. All mechanical or electrical devices can malfunction. The more complex the device, the more prone it may be to malfunction, and usually the more complicated and expensive the repairs. If an assistive device must be shipped to a manufacturer for repair, the turnaround time for repair should be relative short, or a loaner device should be available if the individual is to continue to be motivated to use the device. Likewise, cost of repair must be taken into account.

■ APPRAISAL OF ASSISTIVE DEVICES AND ALTERNATIVES

As new technologies become available, more choices of assistive devices will be offered to meet specific needs. Oddly enough, the large number of choices available may make it more difficult to choose the device best suited to the individual. Assistive devices must be assessed realistically. It is important that performance claims made by the manufacturer be substantiated by research. New devices on the market should have been appropriately evaluated, and performance results, safety data, and durability information should be readily available.

One should also assess the degree to which an assistive device can be upgraded or expanded as new technology becomes available to accommodate new features. In some instances, compatibility with other assistive devices may be important to determine. The initial cost of the assistive device, its maintenance costs, the availability of resources for repair and associated costs, and the costs of replacement should all be assessed.

It is also important to consider the degree to which a device accurately reflects an individual's preferences, lifestyle, and values. The simplicity of less elaborate assistive devices should be weighed against the sometimes greater functionality of more elaborate devices in the context of the specific needs of the individual. Whether a device is portable may determine whether an individual can use the device in more than one setting. The degree to which assistance is needed to learn to use a device and the extent to which the device can be used independently are other factors that affect utilization.

Although emphasis is placed on the degree to which a device increases functional capacity or quality of life, the aesthetics of the device cannot be ignored. The appearance of a device, its ease of use, and the disruption associated with its use in certain settings can determine individuals' willingness to use it. If individuals feel conspicuous using a device, believe it is stigmatizing, or feel that it interferes with social interaction, the device may be abandoned.

The physical and cognitive abilities needed to use an assistive device also are important considerations. Ergonomic aspects of the technology, as well as individuals' ability to learn to use a device and maintain it, should be explored. The best assistive device is not always the most expensive option. Locating the best assistive device requires closely examining the costs and benefits of the device (as opposed to just the available alternatives) and then matching the device to the individual's specific needs and resources.

To maximize the effectiveness of assistive devices, professionals working with individuals with disability need to have comprehensive knowledge of the disability and its limitations (Kroll & Neri, 2003; Wehman, Wilson, Parent, Sherron-Targett, & McKinley, 2000), a good understanding of the multiple consequences of access barriers and barriers to service delivery (Bingham & Beatty, 2003; Neri & Kroll, 2003), and a knowledge of bureaucratic structure that could interfere with appropriate service delivery (Darrah, Magil-Evans, & Adkins, 2002; O'Day et al., 2002). Most of all, professionals need to involve the individuals with disability in the decision about assistive devices and ask those individuals how they can best help them meet their goals and achieve maximum function and independence.

■ PSYCHOSOCIAL ISSUES

The usefulness of a device in helping individuals achieve their goals and functional capacity may be compromised if a number of psychosocial issues are not taken into consideration.

Stigma

Stigma—that is the feeling of being devalued by others—is a common experience for many individuals with disability (Parette & Scherer, 2004). Additional stigma may be experienced with assistive technology usage (Zimmer & Chappell, 1999). An individual using an assistive device may feel the device increases the visibility of the disability, calling attention to it, emphasizing loss of functional capacity and increased vulnerability (Luborsky, 1993). Some individuals may believe that use of an assistive device brings about heightened evaluation and scrutiny of them in social settings, such that they feel an increased sense of alienation and isolation. As a result, use of these devices may affect individuals' self-image and result in lowered self-esteem if they perceive that others are treating them differently and that social interactions are negatively affected by the device. Rather than experience increased stigma, individuals may elect not to use the device at all, even though it could increase their functional capacity.

Aesthetics

Linked to self-image and self-esteem is the appearance of the assistive technology. The aesthetic qualities of the device may also determine the degree to which the device is used. Products that are designed to be more attractive and aesthetically pleasing may increase individuals' willingness to use them.

Cultural Factors

Varying cultural values, belief systems, and family structures can significantly influence the extent to which assistive technology is incorporated into an individual's life. Disability in general, and assistive technology in particular, may be viewed very differently by different cultures, and even in different subcultures embedded within a larger culture. Cultural philosophy regarding health and illness, their meaning, and the process of healing may have much to do with the success or failure of interventions to introduce assistive technology.

The culture of individuals may affect not only how they accept and adjust to their disability, but also their willingness to use assistive technology to increase functional capacity. Independence for an individual with disability may not be viewed as important in some cultures in which it is expected that family and community will meet the needs of the individual. A high-tech device may be viewed as an extravagance and a luxury rather than as a useful tool needed to increase functional capacity. Use of an assistive device may have social consequences for individuals from different cultures. No matter how useful the device may appear to be in helping the individual increase function, unless cultural factors are considered, interest in and acceptance of assistive technology may not be sufficient to bring about positive outcomes regarding its use.

Age

Chronological age and developmental stage influence individuals' adaptation to chronic illness and disability and can also affect individuals' receptivity to and acceptance of assistive technology designed to help them achieve greater functional capacity. Although each individual is unique, age does, to some extent, define life tasks, expectations, and physical and mental preparedness of individuals in various stages of the life span. Although the degree and type of disability individuals experience contribute to the rate of use of assistive technology, the age of the individual and the tasks associated with his or her life stage may also significantly affect the type of assistive technology needed and the extent to which it is used. Older adults with the same disability and same limitations may have different assistive technology needs than do younger adults.

■ THE FUTURE OF ASSISTIVE TECHNOLOGY

The ability of assistive technology to increase functional capacity of individuals with disability is expanding rapidly. Further development and use of assistive technology will be affected by several factors:

- The shift from institutional care to community based services
- Movement from the medical model of disability to a social model

- Increased roles for individuals with disability in selection and application of assistive technology (Cook, 2002)

The emphasis on helping individuals with chronic illness or disability function in their everyday life in the community in accordance with their goals will influence the type of assistive technology utilized as well as the development of new technologies. Increased consideration is being given to the cultural and social effects of assistive technology. In addition, technology developers are investigating economic factors and means to increase accessibility. The concept of universal design emphasizes the creation of products and environments that are amenable to use by all people. It implies that environmental demands on all abilities should be minimized. Seven basic principles underlie universal design:

1. Equitable use
2. Flexible use
3. Simple and intuitive use
4. Perceptible information
5. Tolerance for error
6. Low physical effort
7. Size and space for approach and use (Follette Story, 2001)

Equitable use refers to products that are useful and marketable to people with diverse abilities. Not only is the design appealing to all users, but everyone can use the product in the same way so that individuals aren't segregated or stigmatized by its use. Rather than requiring separate facilities for individuals with disabilities (such as toilet stalls), universal design provides ways of accommodating all people, regardless of their disability status. Curb cuts are an example of a design that is helpful to everyone crossing the street, from those with a stroller, to those in a wheelchair.

Flexibility implies that the product accommodates a wide range of individual preferences and abilities. Individuals are provided with a choice in method of use. Elevators or automatic doors are examples of assistive technology that offer options and accommodate individual abilities. Sensor-activated faucets that have hands-free operation is another example of a design that provides flexibility in use.

Simple, intuitive design eliminates unnecessary complexity. Such a design is easy to understand regardless of the user's experience, knowledge, or language skills. Devices are able to accommodate a wide range of literacy and language skills and follow a predictable and intuitive mode of use. As an example, kitchen blenders with high-contrast on/off switches require no training and are relatively easy to use.

Perceptible information refers to effective communication of necessary information regardless of the individual's sensory abilities or the ambient conditions. Examples include use of different modes for presentation of essential information, such as using pictures, verbal, or tactile modes, or providing compatibility with a variety of devices used by individuals who have sensory limitations.

Tolerance for error refers to designs that minimize hazards and the adverse consequences of accidents or unintended actions. For instance, arranging furniture to minimize hazards, providing warnings of potential hazards, or providing fail-safe features are all examples of this principle of universal design.

Low physical effort implies that the design can be used efficiently and comfortably with a minimum of sustained physical effort and with a minimum of fatigue. Lever door handles, as an example, do not require pinching, twisting, or grasping.

Other examples include rocker light switches and sensor-activated doors that promote ease of performance, which can be beneficial to everyone.

The last principle—size and space for approach and use—refers to products that are designed so that approach, reach, manipulation, and use are appropriate regardless of body size. Examples include showers without thresholds, cabinets that may be used by seated or standing users, and accommodations in hand or grip size.

Making products and environments more usable by a wider range of individuals will reduce the currently higher cost of specialized products and the need for special environmental modifications. When individuals without disability and individuals with disability use the same products, the stigma once associated with use of special products is decreased. Products that are universally designed are also usually more aesthetically pleasing which contributes to decreased stigma and enhanced motivation for use (Fozard, Rietsema, Bourna, & Graafmans, 2000).

■ REFERENCES

Allen, S. M. (2001). Canes, crutches and home care services: The interplay of human and technological assistance. *Center of Home Care Policy Briefs, Fall* (4), 1–6.

Americans with Disabilities Act of 1990. P.L. 101–336.

Assistive Technology Act of 1998. P.L. 105–394.

Assistive Technology Act of 2004. P.L. 108–364.

Berry, B. E., & Ignash, S. (2003). Assistive technology: Providing independence for individuals with disabilities. *Rehabilitation Nursing, 28*(1), 6–14.

Bingham, S. S., & Beatty, P. W. (2003). Rates of access to assistive equipment and medical rehabilitation services among people with disabilities. *Disability Rehabilitation, 25*(9), 487–490.

Blair, M. E. (2000). Assistive technology: What and how for persons with spinal cord injury. *SCI Nursing, 17*(3), 110–118.

Blake, D. J., & Bodine, C. (2002). An overview of assistive technology for persons with multiple sclerosis. *Journal of Rehabilitation Research and Development, 39*(2), 299–312.

Bruyére, S. M., & Peterson, D. B. (2005). Introduction to the special section on International Classification of Functioning, Disability and Health (ICF): Implications for rehabilitation psychology. *Rehabilitation Psychology, 50,* 103–104.

Chen, Y. L., Chen, S. C., Chen, W. L., & Lin, J. F. (2003). A head oriented wheelchair for people with disabilities. *Disability Rehabilitation, 25*(6), 249–253.

Cook, A. M. (2002). Future directions in assistive technologies. In M. Scherer (Ed.), *Assistive technology: Matching device and consumer for successful rehabilitation* (pp. 269–280). Washington, DC: American Psychological Association.

Darrah, J., Magil-Evans, J., & Adkins, R. (2002). How well are we doing? Families of adolescents or young adults with cerebral palsy share their perceptions of service delivery. *Disability Rehabilitation, 24*(10), 542–549.

Fichten, C. S., Barile, M., Asuncion, J. V., & Fossey, M. E. (2000). What government, agencies, and organizations can do to improve access to computers for postsecondary students with disabilities: Recommendations based on Canadian empirical data. *International Journal of Rehabilitation Research, 23*(3), 191–199.

Follette Story, M. (2001). Principles of universal design. In W. F. E. Preiser & E. Ostroff (Eds.), *Universal design handbook*. New York: McGraw-Hill.

Fozard, J. L., Rietsema, J., Bourna, H., & Graafmans, J. A. (2000). Gerontechnology: Creating enabling environments for the challenges and opportunities of aging. *Educational Gerontology, 26,* 331–345.

Galvin, J. C., & Scherer, M. J. (1996). *Evaluating, selecting, and using appropriate assistive technology*. Gaithersburg, MD: Aspen.

Hammel, J. (2003). Technology and the environment: Supportive resource or barrier for people with developmental disabilities? *Nursing Clinics of North America, 38*(2), 331–349.

Hasselbring, T. S., & Glaser, C. H. (2000). Use of computer technology to help students with special needs. *Future Child, 10*(2), 102–122.

King, T. W. (1999). *Assistive technology: Essential human factors*. Boston, MA: Allyn and Bacon.

Kroll, T., Beatty, P. W., & Bingham, S. (2003). Primary care satisfaction among adults with physical disabilities: The role of patient-provider communication. *Managed Care Quarterly,* *11*(1), 11–19.

Kroll, T., & Neri, M. T. (2003). Experiences with care coordination among people with cerebral palsy, multiple sclerosis, or spinal cord injury. *Disability Rehabilitation, 25*(19), 1106–1114.

LoPresti, E. F., & Brienza, D. M. (2004). Adaptive software for head-operated computer controls. *IEEE Transactions on Neural System Rehabilitation Engineering, 12*(1), 102–111.

LoPresti, E. F., Brienza, D. M., Angelo, J., & Gilbertson, L. (2003). Neck range of motion and use of computer head controls. *Journal of Rehabilitation Research and Development, 40*(3), 199–211.

Luborsky, M. R. (1993). Sociocultural factors shaping technology usage: Fulfilling the promise. *Technology and Disability, 2*(1), 71–78.

Mendelsohn, S., & Fox, H. R. (2002). Evolving legislation and public policy related to disability and assistive technology. In M.J. Scherer (Ed.), *Assistive technology: Matching device and consumer for successful rehabilitation.* Washington, DC: American Psychological Association, 17–28.

Miranda, P. (2001). Autism, augmentative communication, and assistive technology: What do we really know. *Focus on Autism and Other Developmental Disabilities, 16*(3), 141–151.

Neri, J. T., & Kroll, T. (2003). Understanding the consequences of access barriers to health care: Experiences of adults with disabilities. *Disability Rehabilitation, 25*(2), 85–96.

Neumann, N., Hinterberger, T., Kaiser, J., Leins, U., Birbaumer, N., & Kubler, A. (2004). Automatic processing of self-regulation of slow cortical potentials: Evidence from brain-computer communication in paralyzed patients. *Clinical Neurophysiology, 115*(3), 628–635.

O'Day, B., Palsbo, S. E., Dhont, K. K., & Scheer, J. (2002). Health plan selection criteria by people with impaired mobility. *Medical Care, 40*(9), 725–728.

Parette, P., & Scherer, M. (2004). Assistive technology use and stigma. *Education and Training in Developmental Disabilities, 39*(3), 217–226.

Peterson, D. B., & Rosenthal, D. A. (2005a). The International Classification of Functioning, Disability and Health (ICF) as an allegory for history and systems in rehabilitation education. *Rehabilitation Education, 19(2 & 3),* 95–104.

Peterson, D. B., & Rosenthal, D. A. (2005b). The International Classification of Functioning, Disability and Health (ICF): A primer for rehabilitation educators. *Rehabilitation Education, 19 (2 & 3),* 81–94.

Scherer, M. J. (2005). Assessing the benefits of using assistive technologies and other supports for thinking, remembering, and learning. *Disability and Rehabilitation, 27*(13), 731–739.

Scherer, M. J., & Glueckauf, R. L. (2005). Assessing the benefits of assistive technologies for activities and participation. *Rehabilitation Psychology, 50*(2), 132–141.

Scherer, M. J., Sax, C. L., Glueckauf, R. L. (2005). Activities and participation: The need to include assistive technology in rehabilitation counselor education. *Rehabilitation Education, 19*(2), 177–190.

Sigafoos, J., O'Reilly, M., Ganz, J. B., Lancioni, G. E., & Schlosser, R. W. (2005). Supporting self-determination in AAC interventions by assessing preference for communication devices. *Technology and Disability 17,* 143–153.

Sokol-McKay, D., Buskirk, K., & Whittaker, P. (2003). Adaptive low-vision and blindness techniques for blood glucose monitoring. *Diabetes Education, 29*(4), 614–618.

Thyberg, I., Hass, U. A., Nordenskiod, U., & Skogh, T. (2004). Survey of the use and effect of assistive devices in patients with early rheumatoid arthritis: A two-year follow-up of women and men. *Arthritis and Rheumatism, 51*(3), 413–421.

Wehman, P., Wilson, K., Parent, W., Sherron-Tagett, P., & McKinley, W. (2000). Employment satisfaction of individuals with spinal cord injury. *American Journal of Physical Medicine and Rehabilitation, 79*(2), 161–169.

World Health Organization. (2001). *International Classification of Functioning, Disability, and Health: ICF.* Geneva: Author

Zimmer, Z., & Chappell, N.L. (1999). Receptivity to new technology among older adults. *Disability and Rehabilitation, 21,* 222–230.

Chapter 20

Financing, Delivery, and Allocation for Rehabilitation Services in the United States

By Michael Landry, PhD

According to the National Coalition on Health Care and other organizations such as Kaiser Family Foundation, healthcare spending in the United States continues to rise at an alarming pace (NCHC, 2007; Kaiser Family Foundation, 2007). The United States spent an estimated $2 trillion on health care in 2005, which represented 16% of the gross domestic roduct (GDP) (Catlin, Cowan, & Heffler et al., 2006; Catlin, Cowan, Heffler, & Washington, 2007). Borger et al. (2006) have projected that by 2015 these figures will rise to $4 trillion when they will account for 20% of GDP. Despite these escalating costs, it is not yet clear what proportion of this amount is spent on rehabilitation services. Nevertheless, it is quickly becoming clear that the demand for rehabilitation services is increasing because of a multitude of factors such as an aging population, increasing public expectations, and vastly improved morbidity and mortality.

The U.S. Department of Labor has predicted that the demand for health professionals in areas such as rehabilitation counseling, occupational therapy, and physical will grow at a faster pace than the average of all other occupations in the next decades (U.S. Department of Labor, 2007). Rehabilitation disciplines are growing at this rapid pace due to an increasing demand for rehabilitation services across the continuum of care, from hospitals and institutions to the home and community sectors. As the rehabilitation industry continues along this aggressive expansion trajectory, it will be increasingly important for counselors and clinicians to understand the structure of the U.S. health care system. It has been reported that despite the growing need or demand, access to rehabilitation services remains particularly problematic (Steffanilla, 1999; Landry, Jaglal, Wodchis, Cooper & Cott, in press), therefore, knowing the basic structure of health care can facilitate access and advocacy on behalf of clients.

This chapter reviews the structure of rehabilitation services in the United States along three dimensions: funding, delivery, and allocation.

■ FUNDING

A wide array of private (out-of-pocket, private insurance, and employer-based insurance) and public (government) funding arrangements for health and rehabilitation services exists in the United States. However, the Organization for Economic Cooperation and Development (OECD) has reported that the United States has the lowest proportion of public spending to overall health care spending among the 30 wealthiest countries. On the other hand, the public share of overall spending in the United Kingdom and Canada is 85.5% and 69.8% respectively (OECD, 2006). Approximately 44.7% of all U.S. healthcare spending in 2004 came from the public sources, mostly from federal and state governments.

Private Financing

There are three main types of private financing for health services:

- Out-of-pocket expenditures
- Private direct-purchase insurance plan
- Employer-based insurance plans

Out-of-Pocket (OOP) payment for services is a means of direct purchasing of a service. Within this structure, clients pay directly from their account for services rendered by the physician, hospital, or rehabilitation provider. Unfortunately, the costs of purchasing health services—especially required by catastrophic injuries with a long hospital inpatient stay can be particularly significant. Himmelstein, Thorne, and Woolhandler (2005) have reported that half of all bankruptcies in the United States are related to unexpected medical expenses.

The U.S. Census Bureau defines private health insurance as a "health plan provided through an employer or union or purchased by an individual from a private health insurance company" (U.S. Census Bureau, 2007). There are two primary divisions in this case:

- Employer-based insurance plans
- Direct-purchase insurance plans

Employer-based insurance plans consist of health insurance plans offered through an individual's employer, or a spouse's or relative's employer. A direct-purchase insurance plan is health insurance purchased by an individual from a private company.

In direct-purchase plan, the individual purchases (usually by paying a monthly premium) an insurance policy against healthcare costs. The subscriber or beneficiary must also be aware of the following costs:

- *Deductibles*: the amount that must be paid prior to the insurance company paying its portion
- *Co-payments*: an amount the beneficiary must pay to the provider per transaction
- *Uncovered services*: services that are not insured by the policy

In recent years, the premiums associated with these private insurance plans have increased dramatically. Sandstrom, Lohman, and Bramble (2003) have suggested that such growth is based on economic reasons, such as inflation; demographic change, including expanding demand for health services among the "baby boomer" generation; and systems changes, such as increased administrative bureaucracy.

Employer-based insurance plans are similar to direct-purchase plans. They are the most significant insurance plans that are purchased by an employer on behalf of the employee. To deal with increasing premium costs, some employers choose to self-insure, meaning that they do not contribute to purchase a policy from a private insurance company on behalf of their employees, but rather establish their own plan to insure employees. Finally, some employers choose not to provide any insurance at all to their employees as a way of reducing costs.

Public Financing

Public funding or financing of health services includes plans funded by federal, state, and local governments. In general, public financing involves heavy statutory and regulatory authority.

Medicare

Medicare is the largest and most influential healthcare program in the United States. This federal program underwrites the healthcare costs for people 65 and older. It also finances services for people who are younger than 65, but who nevertheless qualify for Medicare because they have long-term disabilities, and persons at any age with end-stage renal disease. Individuals covered by Medicare must pay both premiums and deductibles, which are based on income and types of services. Medicare has four distinctive parts: Parts A, B, C, and D. Following is a brief review of Medicare; more detailed information can be found at the U.S. Department of Health and Human Services website (http://www.medicare.gov).

Medicare Part A

Medicare Part A is hospital insurance that covers the individuals who qualify for inpatient hospital care, short-term skilled nursing, skilled rehabilitation facility care, home health care, and hospice. The benefits include basic room and board, along with all medically necessary services; rehabilitation services in these settings must be authorized. The individual must pay deductibles on these services.

The skilled nursing facility benefit and the home health care benefit are to some degree based on the need for rehabilitation services such as occupational therapy and physical therapy, as the intent of these benefits is improvement in function following a hospital stay. The home healthcare benefit is based on home confinement and the need for rehabilitation services. Hospice benefits are provided to beneficiaries diagnosed with terminal illness; they include nursing, social services, and counseling.

Medicare Part B

Medicare Part B is supplemental medical insurance that finances services outside hospitals such as outpatient care, home health service, and medical equipment including orthotics and prosthetics. Individuals qualify for Medicare Part B if they are older than 65 years, are spouses of beneficiaries, have a disability, or have end-stage renal disease.

Medicare Part B will fund rehabilitation services in skilled rehabilitation facilities such as outpatient settings, including private practices and hospitals. The beneficiary must pay an annual deductible to receive Part B benefits.

Medicare Part C

Medicare Part C was established by the Balanced Budget Act of 1997. Medicare Part C is a blending of Part A and Part B, where the services are generally provided through a managed care organization such as a health maintenance organization (HMO).

Medicare Part D

Medicare Part D provides optional prescription drug coverage for eligible beneficiaries, who must pay a monthly premium for this benefit. This coverage may help lower prescription drug costs and protect beneficiaries against higher future costs. Insurance companies operate these plans, which are offered by private companies that have been approved through the Medicare program.

Medicaid

Medicaid is administered at the state level and is available to eligible low-income individuals and families. Eligibility criteria are complex, but generally include families with dependent children, the aged, blind individuals, and persons with disabilities who are in financial need. Unlike with Medicare, Medicaid beneficiaries must qualify by demonstrating level of need based on income, assets, and life circumstances. Because this program is run at the state level, eligibility criteria vary from state to state, but overall they are means tested. In general, the following groups satisfy these criteria:

- Families who meet states' Aid to Families with Dependent Children (AFDC) eligibility requirements,
- Pregnant women and children younger than age 6 with a family income at or below 133% of the federal poverty level
- Children ages 6 to 19 in a household with family income up to 100% of the federal poverty level
- Caretakers (relatives or legal guardians) who take care of children younger than age 18 (or age 19 if still in high school)
- Recipients of Supplemental Security Income (SSI)
- People living in medical institutions who have monthly income up to 300% of the SSI income standard

According to the Centers for Medicare and Medicaid Services (CMS), each individual state's Medicaid program offers the same set of basic services (Table 20-1). States may also receive matching funds from the federal government to provide certain optional services (Table 20-2).

State Children's Health Insurance Program

The *State Children's Health Insurance Program (SCHIP)* is a program administered at the state level that provides health care to low-income children whose parents do not qualify for Medicaid. States choose from four different options in designing SCHIP benefit packages. For instance, each state may offer *benchmark coverage* [i.e. packages equivalent to either the Federal Employees' Health Benefit Package (FEHBP), or the Blue Cross Blue Shield plan in the state], *benchmark equivalent coverage* (i.e., packages proven to be equivalent to benchmark coverage by a qualified actuary), *existing state-based comprehensive coverage* (i.e., packages equivalent to the pre-SCHIP programs run by Florida, New York, and Pennsylvania), or *Secretary-approved coverage* (i.e., state-designed

---

Table 20-1   Basic Services Offered through Medicaid

1. Inpatient hospital services
2. Outpatient hospital services
3. Prenatal care
4. Vaccines for children
5. Physician services
6. Nursing facility services for persons aged 21 or older
7. Family planning services and supplies
8. Rural health clinic services
9. Home health care for persons eligible for skilled-nursing services
10. Laboratory and x-ray services
11. Pediatric and family nurse practitioner services
12. Nurse-midwife services
13. Federally qualified health-center services, and ambulatory services of an FQHC that would be available in other settings
14. Early and periodic screening, diagnostic, and treatment services for children under age 21 years

Table 20-2   Optional Services Offered through Medicaid

1. Diagnostic services
2. Clinic services
3. Intermediate care facilities for persons with mental disease
4. Prescribed drugs and prosthetic devices
5. Optometrist services and eyeglasses
6. Nursing facility services for children under age 21 years
7. Transportation services
8. Rehabilitation and physical therapy services
9. Home and community-based care to certain persons with chronic impairments

packages requiring approval by the U.S. Department of Health and Human Services).

Each state's SCHIP program insures inpatient, outpatient, and emergency care, along with some specialist care. States are required to provide "well-baby" and "well-child" visits, as well as immunizations. Almost all states cover mental health and substance abuse services. Dental services are optional under SCHIP, but are required by Medicaid.

Veterans Affairs

The Department of Veterans Affairs (VA) operates the largest healthcare system in the world and provides medical assistance to eligible veterans of the U.S. Armed Forces. To be eligible for VA services, an individual must meet program eligibility. Once eligibility is established, beneficiaries may be insured for inpatient/outpatient care, prescription drugs, physicians' services, mental health care, home health and hospice, rehabilitation therapy, and prosthetics and orthotics. Further detailed information regarding the VA coverage can be accessed directly from its website (www.va.gov).

Indian Health Service

Indian Health Service (IHS) is a health care program through which the Department of Health and Human Services provides medical assistance to eligible Native Americans at IHS facilities. For further information regarding

eligibility and types of services funded, visit the IHS website (www.ihs.gov).

■ DELIVERY

The second definitional dimension of health systems is *delivery*. Individual providers (i.e., physical therapists, occupational therapists, and speech language pathologists) usually work within some type of provider organization (i.e., hospitals, home care agencies, private firms). A tremendous political debate has focused on how delivery should be structured. In particular, it is important to appreciate the ownership structure, and the issues surrounding the implications of delivery by *public, private not-for-profit (NFP)* or *private for-profit (FP)* providers.

Controversy surrounds the role of the FP and NFP sectors in healthcare delivery. On the one hand, advocates of FP delivery generally state that FP can deliver higher-quality and more efficient services than NFP providers. On the other hand, opponents argue that FP delivery costs more than the NFP sector, suggesting that one of the cost drivers in the FP sector is administration costs. Devereaux et al. (2002) have reported that death rates are higher in FP hospitals, that private FP hospitals have higher costs of care than NFP hospitals in the United States, and that, if Canada were to introduce FP hospitals, it could result in an additional $3.6 billion in government healthcare spending annually.

In terms of quality, Himmelstein, Woolhandler, Hellander, and Wolfe (1999) have reported that the quality of care is better in the NFP sector as opposed to the FP sector. Furthermore, Devereaux et al. (2002) confirmed what Relman and Rennie (1980) previously reported: U.S.-based hemodialysis care provided in FP centers is associated with a statistically higher risk of mortality as compared to NFP care. Similar findings were reported by Garg et al. (1999) in the delivery of kidney transplantation. Although not all parties fully agree, it appears that, on balance, the literature reports that the NFP sector may be more cost-effective and have better clinical outcomes than the FP sector.

The literature is somewhat divided in determining the degree to which the FP sector performs better than the NFP sector. For instance, Vaillancourt and Linder (2003) performed a systematic review of the literature and reported that, of 149 published studies, 59% determined that the NFP performed better, 29% found no difference, and 12% found that the FP performed better. The outcomes measure used to determine performance was loosely defined as "access," "quality," and "cost-effectiveness" across a variety of models of delivery, ranging from HMOs to dialysis centers to nursing homes, to name only a few. There are no published reports that have evaluated this phenomenon in physical therapy services delivery in hospitals or in the community, or between NFP or FP providers.

Managed Care

Managed care is a model of health care in which the financing and delivery of medical care are conducted through a coordinated and integrated system of selected physicians and hospitals that provide comprehensive services to individuals enrolled in a specific healthcare plan. The goal of managed care is to control unnecessary costs and use of health care while still providing good access to high-quality health care. The terms *managed care organization (MCO)* and *health maintenance organizations (HMO)* are used to describe healthcare plans that deliver specific services to a group of individuals on a prepaid basis. HMOs are managed care organizations whose premise is that future medical problems can be avoided through preventive measures. Consequently, routine medical checkups and health promotion activities are encouraged. HMOs operate in designated services areas. If the individual travels outside the service area, coverage is guaranteed only for life-threatening emergencies.

Point-of-service plans (POSs) are another kind of healthcare plan gathered under the managed care umbrella. In POSs, certain characteristic of HMOs are combined with traditional indemnity plans in which physicians are reimbursed for services provided or in which individuals covered in the plans are reimbursed for money spent on services. This type of plan provides individuals with the option at each "point of service" to choose a provider covered under the plan or to choose another individual outside the plan.

Precise definitions of managed care are difficult because market forces shape this concept, so it is continually being modified. Although initially implemented as a cost-containment strategy, managed care has since assumed a greater responsibility for improving the quality of health care delivered to enrolled members. Identifying appropriate treatment, including the type, duration, and location, through case management has become a crucial aspect of services.

A variety of managed care organizations exist. The *staff-model HMO* is a system in which the organization owns the facility in which enrolled individuals receive services, and healthcare providers are employees of the organization. This model provides the HMO with more control over services rendered.

The *group-model HMO* is a system in which physicians in one or more groups of practice form partnerships or corporations. This group, in turn, negotiates a flat rate to be paid to the group by an HMO. Healthcare providers in the group are then responsible for paying employees, paying for hospital care, and paying for care provided by specialists outside the group. The network model is similar to the group model except that a network of group practices contact with an MCO.

The *Individual Practice Association* (IPA) model enables individual physicians to be associated with an HMO without being under direct contract or being direct employees of the organization. Physicians in the IPA can deliver services to individuals who are in the specific HMO plan as well to those not in the plan.

In the *direct-contract model*, physicians contract directly with the HMO. A *preferred provider organization* (PPO) is a predetermined group of healthcare providers who have agreed to follow specific practice guidelines and accept a specific amount for services. *Provider-sponsored organizations (PSOs)* consist of groups of healthcare providers who have established their own providers, clinics, hospitals, or other facilities that provide care.

According to Sandstrom et al. (2003), there are three basic tenets of managed care:

- Limited access to the universe of providers
- Payment mechanisms that reward efficiency
- Enhanced quality through improved monitoring

In all of these cases, the key principles are to reduce unnecessary services and to maximize the efficiency of services when needed. This theory holds that if these objectives can be maintained, costs of health services delivery can be reduced while improving quality of care.

Robinson (2001) reported that managed care has been an economic success, but a political failure as a strategy because it "gives with one hand, while taking away with the other." This point has been hotly debated and been found to be unacceptable to the general population in the United States. The reported financial success came in the form of return on investment for shareholders within the profit model that was facilitated by the U.S. Congress's passage of the 1973 *Health Maintenance Organization Act,* which stated that HMOs could legally control costs by rationing care (Bloche & Jacobson, 2000). The political failure occurred because of the perceived inequalities that existed between groups as well as the suspect motives behind some clinical decision making. Furthermore, Robinson (2001) reports that within the past decade, healthcare cost control through managed care has "lost" political votes, while increasing healthcare spending has "won" votes. It is also known that MCOs are relaxing the gatekeeping processes as well as decreasing the use of utilization reviews. Thus it can be concluded that the nature of managed care is shifting as the consumer of the services becomes more involved and empowered in the decision-making process.

■ ALLOCATION

The third and final dimension that defines health systems is *allocation*. This term refers to the incentive structures set up to operationalize how monies flow from the *payer* to the *provider* of services. Saltman and von Otter (1992) and many others, such as Hollander et al. (1998) and Saltman and Figueras (1998), have indicated that allocation mechanisms are part of a continuum from a fully planned system to a fully market-driven system (Figure 20-1).

At one end of this continuum are centrally planned models wherein clients follow money. In this situation, all financing of services is fully controlled by a central agency under a global or capped budget. In such single-payer models, the incentives may be to provide fewer services. At the other extreme is the fully market driven model wherein money is controlled by clients. In this kind of *volume-* or *service-based model*, there may be an incentive to provide more services because the provider stands to increase revenues from doing so. Under the planned models of the allocation continuum, individuals are entitled to have equal access to services; at the other end of the continuum, services move away from being an entitlement and into an arena wherein access may be determined to a greater degree by levels of available funding.

Along this continuum are a series of other allocation options. For instance, *regionally planned models* of financing indicate a situation where a demographic area sets its priorities

and allocates funds to align with such priorities. *Capped budgets*, also called *bundles payments*, can be based on either the organization or the client. For instance, with a capped budget, an organization might receive a basket of payment to fund (and possible deliver) services. Such an allocation system may control prices paid, but have no controls over the volumes of services provided or the number of individual clients who may require services.

In another approach, such payments can be related to the individual person or client in. *Diagnosis-related group (DRG)* funding classification is one such form of allocation that falls along this continuum. DRG is a case-mix funding system that groups together clients who have similar clinical diagnoses and who should presumably be similar in their consumption of resources (i.e., all postoperative hip replacement clients within a certain demographics should have similar resource utilization trends). This system is used primarily in the United States as a method of funding

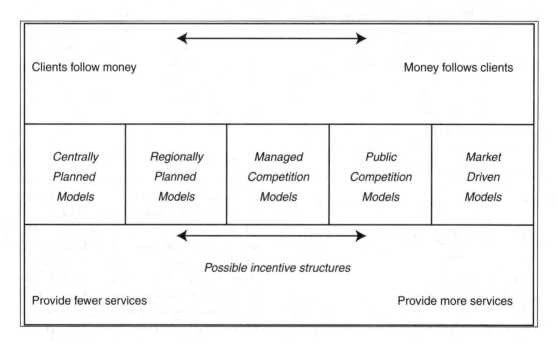

Figure 20-1   Allocation Models within Health Systems.

hospitals. In this case, the funding agency would allow for a basket payment to provide services for specific conditions or diagnosis, and the provider would then use this funding to deliver services.

Recognizing that economic incentives are tempered by other factors, including professionalism and ethical practice, the incentive structures that are built into each of these models may be different. For instance, at the "clients follow money" end of the continuum, where global or capped budgets exist, the incentives for the provider might be to reduce services as a way of controlling overall costs. At the "money follows clients" end of the continuum, where service- or volume-based systems exist, the provider incentive might be to deliver more services, as cost controls are much less visible.

■ METHODS OF PAYMENT AND INHERENT INCENTIVES

There a number of ways in which to transfer financing from the payer to the provider. Providers may be reimbursed in any of the following ways:

- Fee-for-service
- Per visit
- Per episode
- Capitation

Fee-for-Service Payment

In a *fee-for-service (FFS)* system, the provider is paid a specific amount for each type or unit of service provided. A fee schedule is generally used to determine the overall cost of an episode of care or visit. For instance, if an individual receives services A, B, and C during a particular visit to a provider, that provider will invoice the client a total amount by adding the cost of each service or product. If the provider charged a specified amount per unit of time, the client would also be invoiced

based on the time spent with the provider. The provider's financial incentive within an FFS structure is to maximize delivery of care so as to maximize the provider's revenue potential. As Evans (1984) has noted, the possibility for providers to inadvertently have a direct influence over demand creates a situation of "supplier-induced demand."

Per Visit Payment

With *per visit payment*, the cost of a particular visit to the provider is set to a predetermined amount irrespective of the time spent with the provider or the basket of services that were provided in that visit. The financial incentive for the provider in this case is to provide the least amount of time or services because there is no financial incentive for "topping up." Some would also argue that there is no incentive to provide high-quality and effective service.

Per-Episode Payment

In the *per-episode payment* framework, providers are given a one-time payment for services rendered for individuals with specific diagnoses or conditions. This allocation methodology is generally reserved for large institutions that are providing highly complex, medically based services to specific DRGs. The incentive within this allocation mechanism is for the provider to access only noncomplicated DRGs—for instance, providing surgical procedures to individuals with few comorbidities who are in generally good health. Policy analysts colloquially term this process "cherry picking" meaning that the provider has a financial incentive to care for only a certain type of client.

Capitation

The capitation mechanism applies to a group of individuals who are within the eligible network. In a capitated environment, a provider is given regular payment (either on a monthly or a yearly basis) to provide all services to those who are on the roster with that provider. In general, this mechanism is used with MCOs that expect that, if there is a large enough group of enrollees, the risk of utilization will be spread across them in such a way as to provide a financial incentive. The financial risk to the provider is the greatest with this type of allocation mechanism.

■ ISSUES OF MANAGED CARE FOR INDIVIDUALS WITH CHRONIC ILLNESS OR DISABILITY

One underlying concept for MCOs is the importance of disease management and cost containment. *Disease management* is defined as comprehensive treatment of medical conditions, including prevention of disease or disability, and diagnosis, treatment, and management of disease and disability when they occur. The primary aim of managed care, however, is to reduce costs and the amount of services used.

Individuals with chronic illness and disability have complex medical needs requiring extensive healthcare services (Cutler, Rosen, & Vijan, 2006), and they often require the services of a multidisciplinary team using multiple strategies. Consequently, the managed care model may not always be adequate to meet these complex needs.

Medicaid and Medicare are federal programs for funding the health care for many people with disabilities. Increasingly, however, these programs are being administered through managed care plans. Of course, many services necessary for individuals with chronic illness or disability are expensive. To control costs, managed care plans may attempt to minimize the utilization of medical services, including by restricting benefits to individuals with chronic illness or disability.

Although managed care may have some positive benefits for individuals with chronic illness and disability, such as care coordination, prevention practices, and low cost of the medications that are managed via a formulary, it also has some notable limitations (Grabois & Young, 2001):

- Delay in getting appointments or test results
- Denial of referral to specialists
- Inaccessibility of equipment in managed care facilities
- Inadequate skill of physicians in managed care facilities to treat specific chronic illness or disability
- Need for specific approval by an MCO before the most effective medication for treatment of a condition can be obtained if the drug is not listed in the plan's formulary
- Limited services for assistive devices

Managed care was first implemented in the healthcare industry, but its principles are now being applied to other services. This trend's effects on individuals with chronic illness and disability could be profound.

Because individuals with chronic illness or disability may also experience medical complications and need a variety of allied services, such as home care, personal assistants, or consultation with medical specialists, costs can be further increased for these individuals. For specific disabilities, some restriction of service is included in many managed care plans. For instance, although all managed care plans offer treatment for substance abuse and dependence, varying limits and restrictions on that care apply. Likewise, managed care plans cover treatment of psychiatric disability, albeit with limits and restrictions. Specifically, the number of visits to a mental health provider may be limited.

The number of Medicaid recipients in managed care plans has risen dramatically in the past few years (Health Care Financing Administration, 1994). It is evident that the cost of care for individuals with severe disability poses challenge for a system such as managed care, which emphasizes cost control. Many of the formulas used to determine appropriate services are based on the average needs of individuals without disability, rather than on the needs of persons with severe disability or chronic illness. Managing the care of individuals with chronic illness and disability requires a commitment of financial resources that many managed care plans cannot or will not make. Consequently, the needs of individuals with chronic illness or disability may not always be identified and, if identified, may not be adequately served.

■ CONCLUSION

This chapter has reviewed the basic structure of health care in the United States. As always, however, "the devil is in the details." The intricacies of funding, delivery, and allocation vary widely across state borders. As such it will be essential for rehabilitation counselors and clinicians to develop a fuller understanding of these mechanisms in their particular jurisdiction.

■ REFERENCES

Bloche, M. G., & Jacobson, P. D. (2000). The Supreme Court and bedside rationing. *Journal of the American Medical Association.* 284(21), 2776–2779.

Borger, C., Smith, C., Truffer, C., et al. (2006 February 22). Health spending projections through 2015: Changes on the horizon. *Health Affairs,* Web Exclusive W61.

Catlin, A., Cowan, C., Heffler, S., & Washington, B. (2007), National health spending 2005: The slowdown continues. *Health Affairs, 26*(1), 142–153.

Catlin, A., Cowan, S. C., Heffler, S., et al. (2006). National health spending in 2005. *Health Affairs, 26*(1), 142–153.

Cutler, M. C., Rosen, A. B., & Vijan, S. (2006). The value of medical spending in the United States, 1960–2000. *New England Journal of Medicine, 335,* 920–927.

Devereaux, P. J., Choi, P. T. L., Lachetti, C., et al. (2002). A systematic review and meta-analysis of studies comparing mortality rates of private for-profit and private not-for-profit hospitals. *Canadian Medical Association Journal, 166*(11), 1399–1406.

Evans, R. G. (1984). *Strained mercy: The economics of Canadian health care.* Toronto, ON: Butterworth.

Garg, P. P., Frick, K. D., Diner-West, M., & Powe, N. R. (1999). Effect of the ownership of dialysis facilites on patients' survival and referral for transplantation. *New England Journal of Medicine, 341*(22), 1653–1660.

Grabois, E., & Young, M. E. (2001). Managed care experiences of persons with disabilities. *Journal of Rehabilitation, 67*(3), 13–19.

Health Care Financing Administration. (1994). The Medicare and Medicaid statistical supplemental of the heal care financial review. HFCA Publication # 03374. Washington, DC: Author.

Himmelstein, D. E., Thorne W. D., & Woolhandler, S. (2005 February 2). Illness and injury as contributors to bankruptcy. Health Affairs, Web Exclusive W5-63.

Himmelstein, D. E., Woolhandler, S., Hellander, I., & Wolfe, S. M. (1999). Quality of care in investor-owned vs. not-for-profit HMOs. *Journal of the American Medical Association, 282*(2), 159–163.

Hollander, M. J., Deber, R. B., Jacobs, P. (1998). A critical review of models of resources allocation and reimbursement in health care: A report prepared for the Ontario Ministry of Health. Victoria, BC: Canadian Policy Research Networks.

Kaiser Family Foundation. (2007). Health care spending in the United States and OECD. http://www.kff.org/insurance/snapshot/chcm010307oth.cfm.

Landry, M. D., Jaglal, S. B., Wodchis, W. P., Cooper, N. S., & Cott, C. A. (in press). Rehabilitation services following total joint replacements in Ontario, Canada: Can "prehabilitation" programs mediate an increasing demand? *International Journal of Rehabilitation Research.*

National Coalition on Health Care (NCHC). (2007). Health insurance costs. http://www. nchc.org/facts/cost.shtml.

Organization for Economic Cooperation and Development (OECD). (2006). Health statistics. http://www.oecd.org/topicstatsportal/ 0,2647,en_2825_495642_1_1_1_1_1,00.html.

Relman, A. S., & Rennie, D. (1980). Treatment of end-stage renal disease: Free but not equal. *New England Journal of Medicine, 303,* 9996-9998.

Robinson, J. C. (2001). The end of managed care. *Journal of the American Medical Association. 285*(20), 2622-2628.

Saltman, R. B., & von Otter, C. (1992). *Planned markets and public competition: Strategic reform in Northern European health systems.* Philadelphia: Open University Press.

Saltman, R. B., & Figueras, J. (1998). Analyzing the evidence on European health care reforms. *Health Affairs, 17*(2), 85-108.

Sandstrom, R. W., Lohman, H., & Bramble, J. D. (2003). *Health services: Policy and systems for therapists.* Upper Saddle River, NJ: Prentice Hall.

Steffanilla, T. (1999). Referral and access to physical therapy services. In K. A. Curtis (Ed.), *The physical therapist's guide to health care, 2*(17). Thorofare, NJ: Slack.

U.S. Census Bureau. (2007). Health insurance. http://www.census.gov/hhes/www/hlthins/ hlthinstypes.html.

U.S. Department of Labor. (2007). Bureau of Labor Statistics. http://www.bls.gov/oco/ ocos080.htm.

Vaillancourt R. P., & Linder, S. H. (2003). Two decades of research comparing for profit and nonprofit health provider performance in the United States. *Social Science Quarterly, 84*(2), 219-241.

Medical Terminology

All professions and sciences have their own terminology that give speed, precision, and economy to communication. Medicine is no exception. Medical terms can often seem like a foreign language. Nevertheless, nonmedical professionals working with individuals with chronic illness or disability need to become familiar with commonly used terms so that they can communicate with medical providers and have a better understanding of information contained within medical reports and records. Although each medical term could be looked up in a medical dictionary, the process would be time consuming. Memorizing some commonly used terms can be helpful, but it is unrealistic to memorize all terms with which you may come in contact. Consequently, becoming familiar with prefixes and suffixes commonly found in medical terminology can help you translate unfamiliar terms and provides a framework from which you may be able to figure out a general meaning of a term. Following are common prefixes and suffixes, along with some general terms that are frequently encountered.

■ PREFIXES

Prefix	Meaning
adeno	glandular
angio	vessel
ankyl	crooked, growing, together
anti	against
arthro	joint
bi	double, twice
bili	bile
brachy	short
brady	slow
broncho	bronchi
cardio	heart
cephalo	head
cervico	neck
chole	gall, bile
cholecyst	gallbladder
chondro	cartilage
circum	around
craneo	skull
cysto	bladder
derma	skin
dis	negative

dors	back	myelo	bone marrow, spinal cord
duodeno	duodenum		
dys	difficult, painful	myo	muscle
ect	outside	narco	numbness
endo	inside	neo	new, recent
entero	intestine	nephro	kidney
eryth	red	neuro	nerve
ferro	iron	non	not
fibro	fibers	nos	disease
fore	before, in front of	ocul	eye
galacto	milk	odonto	tooth
gastro	stomach	oligo	few, little
gingive	gums	ophth, optic	eye
glyco	sugar	os	mouth
gyneco	female	oss, osteo	bone
hemato	blood	oto	ear
hemi	half	pan	all
hemo	blood	path	disease
hepato	liver	peri	around
histo	tissue	pharyng	pharynx
homo	same	phlebo	vein
hydro	water	photo	light
hyper	increased	pneumo	lung
hypo	decreased	pod	foot
hystero	uterus	post	after
iatr	physician	pre	before
idio	peculiar	procto	anus, rectum
inter	between	pseudo	false
intra	within	psych	the mind
jejuno	jejunum	pto	fall
laryngo	larynx	pyelo	kidney
latero	side	pyo	pus
leuko	white	pyro	fever
lipo	fat	quadri	four
lithio	stone	radio	radiation
macro	big, large	recto	rectum
mal	bad, poor, abnormal	retro	backward
masto/mammo	breast	rhino	nose
mega	great, large	sacro	sacrum
melan	black	salpingo	fallopian tube
meso	middle	sclero	hard or hardening
micro	small	skeleto	skeleton
mono	single	sten	narrow
muco	mucus	stomato	mouth
multi	many	sub	under, beneath

super, supra	above, extreme
tachy	fast
thermo	heat
thoraco	chest
thromb	clot
uretero	ureter
vaso	vessel

■ SUFFIXES

Suffix	Meaning
algia	pain
ase	enzyme
cele	tumor, swelling
centesis	to puncture
cide	causing disease
cyte	cell
dynia	pain
ectasis	dilation
ectomy	excision
emesis	vomiting
emia	blood
esthesia	sensation
gram	tracing, mark
graphy	record, picture
iasis	condition, pathological state
itis	inflammation
kinesis	motion
lithiasis	stones
lysis	breakdown
mania	madness
megaly	enlargement
norexia	appetite
odynia	pain
ology	science or study of
oma	tumor
osis	disease
ostomy	new opening
otomy	incision, cutting
pathy	sickness, disease
penia	lack
pepsia	digestion
pexy	fixation
phage	ingesting

phylaxis	protection
plasty	repair
plegia	paralysis
ptosis	prolapse
rhagia	hemorrhage
rhea	flow, discharge
sclerosis	hardness
scopy	visually examine
sect	cut
statis	halt
stenosis	narrowing
uria	urine

■ TERMINOLOGY RELATED TO POSITION AND DIRECTION

Term	Meaning
anterior	before or in front
distal	far away from
dorsal	pertaining to the back
inferior	below
lateral	to the side
medial	to the center
palmar	pertaining to the palm of the hand
plantar	pertaining to the sole of the foot
posterior	behind or in back
prone	lying face down
proximal	nearest to
superior	above
supine	lying face upward
volar	pertaining to the front or abdominal surface

■ TERMINOLOGY RELATING TO BODY AREAS

Term	Meaning
carpal	pertaining to the wrist
cervical	pertaining to the seven vertebrae in the neck
costal	pertaining to the ribs
cranial	pertaining to the skull

femoral	pertaining to the thigh
frontal	pertaining to the front
pelvic	pertaining to the pelvis
sternal	pertaining to the sternum or breastbone
thoracic	pertaining to the 12 vertebrae in the upper portion of the back; chest cavity

■ PREFIXES OF QUANTITY

Prefix	Meaning
ambi	both
bi	two
di	two
hemi	half
mono	one
multi	many
olig	few
poly	many
tri	three
uni	one

GENERAL TERMS

complication: disease concurrent with another disease

diagnosis: determination of or naming of a disease

disease: structural or functional change within the body judged to be abnormal

etiology: study of the cause of disease; also, the cause of a disease

history: written description of symptoms in medical record

idiopathic: cause unknown

incidence: measure of the number of individuals newly diagnosed with a specific condition

manifestation: signs, symptoms, laboratory abnormalities

morbidity: rate of disease or proportion of diseased persons living in a given locality; frequency of occurrence of a condition within a population

mortality: proportion of deaths to the population of a region; the death rate from a particular condition; measure of the number of people dying from a condition in a given period of time

pathogenesis: development of disease; sequence of events that lead from cause to structural abnormalities and finally to manifestations of disease

pathology: study of disease

prevalance: number of people with a disease at any given point in time

prognosis: probable outcome of a disease

signs: physical observations made by the person examining an individual

symptoms: evidence of disease as perceived by the individual experiencing it

syndrome: cluster of findings associated with a disease

Glossary of Medical Terms

abduction movement of a body part away from the midline of the body

abductor muscle that moves a limb laterally, away from the body

abrasion scraping or rubbing off of the skin

accommodation change in the shape of the lens to help the eye focus for near or far vision

achalasia type of dysphagia in which motility of the lower portion of the esophagus is decreased and food is unable to pass into the stomach efficiently

acoustic nerve auditory nerve; eighth cranial nerve

acoustic reflex movement of the muscles attached to the malleus and stapes as a response to intense sound

acquired hearing loss hearing loss occurring after birth or later in life

active exercise individual independent performance of a specified exercise regimen under the direction or supervision of a physical therapist

adaptation chemical process in which the eye adjusts to see in the dark

Addison's disease condition involving underproduction of hormones by the adrenal cortex

adduction movement of a body part toward the midline of the body

adductor muscle that moves a limb closer to the body

adenopathy enlargement of lymph nodes

afferent nerves peripheral nerves that carry messages to the central nervous system

agnosia inability to interpret sounds or visual images, or to distinguish objects by touch

agoraphobia fear of being in a situation or place from which it might be difficult or embarrassing to escape or in which no help may be available if a panic attack occurs

agranulocytosis marked reduction in the level of a specific type of leukocyte

akathisia extreme restlessness; inability to sit still for any length of time

akinesia complete or partial absence of movement

allergen substance that causes an allergic response

allergy hypersensitivity to a specific substance or substances from previous exposure

allograft graft taken from the same species but not the same person; homograft

alopecia hair loss

alveoli air sacs in lungs in which exchange of oxygen and carbon dioxide takes place

Alzheimer's disease progressive, degenerative type of dementia

amblyopia loss of sight or dimness of vision

amino acids building blocks of protein

amnesia loss of memory

amputation removal of a body part

amyotrophic lateral sclerosis progressive condition in which degeneration occurs of the nerve cells that convey impulses to initiate muscular contraction

anaphylaxis severe systemic reaction resulting from sensitivity to a foreign protein

anaplastic term to describe cancer cells that take on abnormal characteristics and become less differentiated than the normal cells from which they are derived

anasarca generalized edema

anastomosis connection of two tubular structures, through surgery or through a pathological process

anemia condition in which a reduction in the amount of hemoglobin or the number of red blood cells occurs

aneurysm blood-filled sac formed by a dilation of the walls of an artery or vein

angina pectoris chest pain

anhidrosis lack of sweating

ankylosing spondylitis systemic rheumatic disorder affecting the joints and ligaments of the spine

ankylosis immobility or fixation of a joint

anomia inability to name objects or remember names

anophthalmia congenital absence of the eye

anorexia appetite loss

anosmia loss of sense of smell

anosognosia one-sided neglect (e.g., condition in which individuals are unable to see objects on either the right or the left of the central field of vision)

anoxia lack of oxygen

antibody an immune substance produced within the body in response to a specific antigen

antigen a substance that causes the body to manufacture antibodies against a particular allergen

anuria condition in which the kidney is unable to excrete urine

aorta largest artery in the body

aortic semilunar valve valve through which blood is pumped from the heart into the general circulation

aphagia inability to swallow

aphasia inability to communicate through speech, writing, or signs due to brain dysfunction

apnea cessation of breathing

apraxia loss of ability to organize and sequence specific muscle movements to perform a task

apraxia of speech articulation disorder characterized by the inability to position and sequence the muscle movements involved in speech

arachnoid membrane middle, cobweb-appearing membrane that covers the brain and spinal cord

arrhythmia abnormality of the heart rhythm

arteriosclerosis thickening and loss of elasticity of arteries

arthritis joint inflammation

arthrocentesis aspiration of synovial fluid from a joint cavity

arthrodesis surgical fusing of two joint surfaces, making them permanently immobile

arthrogram radiographic study of a joint

arthroplasty surgical replacement, formation, or reformation of a joint

arthroscopy visualization of a joint through an arthroscope inserted into the joint

articulation coming together of two bones at a joint

ascites retention of fluid in the abdominal cavity

asphyxia suffocation due to decrease of oxygen and increase of carbon dioxide in the body

aspiration withdrawal of fluid or gas from a cavity by means of suction

aspiration pneumonia inflammation of the lung resulting from inhalation of foreign substances or chemical irritants

asthma chronic inflammatory disease of the airways

astigmatism distortion of the visual image resulting from an irregularity in the shape of the cornea or lens

asymptomatic without symptoms

ataxia impairment of muscle coordination

atelectasis collapse of the lung

atherosclerosis buildup of plaque on inner walls of blood vessels

athetosis slow, writhing, purposeless movement

atonic lacking normal tone or strength

atresia narrowing or closing of a normal opening; often congenital

atria two upper chambers of the heart

atrophy shrinkage

attention deficit/hyperactivity disorder condition that appears before age 7 that is characterized by inattention, hyperactivity, and impulsivity

aura warning (flash of light or other unusual sensation) before a seizure

auricle visible portion of the outer ear

autistic disorder disorder of brain function with behavioral consequences, including impairment in reciprocal social interactions and impairment in verbal and nonverbal communication

autograft graft from individual's own skin

autoimmune disease disease in which the immune system directs a response that attacks the body's own cells as if they were foreign substances

autonomic dysreflexia condition occurring in individuals with spinal cordinjury resulting from excessive neural discharge from the autonomic nervous system and characterized by sudden rise in blood pressure, profuse sweating, and headache

autonomic nervous system part of the peripheral nervous system that controls involuntary functions

axon process emerging from the neuron that conducts electrical impulses away from the cell body

bacteremia presence of bacteria in the bloodstream

basal ganglia gray matter imbedded within the white matter of the brain

benign noncancerous

bicuspid valve mitral valve of the heart

biliary term applying to the gallbladder, liver, and their ducts

binocular vision coordinated use of both eyes to produce a single image

biopsy removal of a small portion of tissue from the body so that it may beexamined microscopically (e.g., needle biopsy)

biosynthetic graft graft that has been chemically manufactured

blindness total loss of light perception

blood dyscrasias large group of disorders that affect the blood

body image individual's perception of his or her own physical appearance and physical function

bradycardia slow heartbeat

bradykinesia extreme slowness of movement

brain stem portion of central nervous system located at base of the brain between cerebrum and spinal cord

Broca's aphasia type of nonfluent aphasia characterized by misarticulation, laborious speech, hesitancy, and reduced vocabulary

Broca's area portion of the brain anterior to Wernicke's area and the major area of expressive function

bronchi branches leading from the trachea into the lungs

bronchiectasis dilation of the bronchi or bronchioles

bronchospasm tightening of small muscles around air passages

burr holes openings placed in the skull to relieve increased intracranial pressure

bursa sac that contains synovial fluid in the synovial joints

bursitis inflammation of the bursa

CABG coronary artery bypass graft

calculi stones

cancer cellular tumor; not one disease, but a broad term used to describe many diseases

candidiasis yeast infection

capillaries minute blood vessels connecting smallest arteries (arterioles) and veins (venules)

carbuncle a boil with infiltration into adjacent tissues

carcinogens chemicals or other substances that are thought to cause cancer

carcinoma cancer of the epithelial cells

cardiac tamponade severe constriction of the heart because of accumulation of fluid in the pericardial sac

cardiomegaly enlargement of the heart

cardiospasm achalasia

carpal tunnel repair surgical procedure indicated for carpal tunnel syndrome

carpal tunnel syndrome painful condition involving compression of the median nerve in the wrist

carriers individuals who harbor germs of a disease and transmit the disease to others, while remaining well themselves that creates form and maintains structure

cataract clouding or opacity of the lens of the eye

cell body portion of the neuron

central deafness hearing loss resulting from disorder of the auditory center of the brain

cerebellum portion of the brain located beneath the occipital lobe of the cerebrum

cerebral palsy developmental disability in which injury to the brain occurs during the fetal period, at birth, or in early childhood

cerebrospinal fluid fluid bathing the brain and spinal cord

cerebro vascular accident stroke

cerebrum largest portion of the brain

cerumen earwax

cervix neck of the uterus, opening into the vagina

cholecystectomy removal of the gallbladder

cholecystitis inflammation of the gallbladder

cholelithiasis gallstones

chorea jerky, involuntary movements

choreoathetosis abrupt, jerky movements

chronic bronchitis defined clinically as a condition in which a chronic productive cough persists on most days for a minimum of 3 months in the year for not less than 2 consecutive years

chronic obstructive pulmonary disease collection of diseases including emphysema, chronic bronchitis, and chronic asthma

cilia hairlike projections

circumduction circular movement

cirrhosis progressive disease of the liver in which liver function is altered because of fibrous changes in the structure of the liver

clonic pertaining to jerky movement of muscle

closed head injury injury in which the skull has not been broken

coccyx tailbone

cochlea chamber of the inner ear

colectomy removal of all or part of the colon

collateral circulation alternate blood supply routes

colon large intestine

colostomy surgical opening in the outer wall of the abdomen through which a portion of the large intestine is brought to the external surface for elimination of fecal material

coma state of unconsciousness

compulsions persistent actions

concussion mild to moderate head injury in which a loss of consciousness occurs, varying from a few minutes to 24 hours after the injury

conductive hearing loss damage, obstruction, or malformation in the external or middle ear that prevents sound waves from reaching the inner ear

confabulation making up experiences to fill memory gaps

congenital present at birth

congenital hearing loss hearing loss present at birth

conjunctiva membrane that lines the inner eyelid and covers the front part of the eye

conjunctivitis inflammation of the conjunctiva

contracture deformity in which a permanent contraction of a muscle occurs, resulting in the immobility of a joint

contusion soft tissue injury resulting from a blunt, diffuse blow in which the skin is not broken, nor are bones broken, but local hemorrhage occurs with associated bruising and damage to deep soft tissue under the skin

conversion disorder disorder in which physical function, often related to neurological function, is lost but no organic cause for the loss can be found

COPD chronic obstructive pulmonary disease

cor pulmonale right-sided heart failure

coronary angioplasty procedure to enlarge a narrowed coronary artery

coronary arteries vessels that carry blood directly to the myocardial muscle

coronary artery bypass graft procedure to relieve narrowing or constriction of coronary arteries

coronary artery disease condition in which arteries that supply blood directly to the myocardial muscle become narrowed or occluded

cortex gray matter that makes up the outer portion of the cerebrum

cranial nerves peripheral nerves that transmit messages directly to the brain

craniotomy surgical procedure in which the skull is opened to remove matter or to control bleeding

cranium skull; bony cover surrounding the brain

creatinine waste product eliminated by the kidney

Crohn's disease inflammation of segments of the small intestine

cross-tolerance demonstration of higher tolerances for related substances when tolerance for one substance has been developed

Curling's ulcer stress ulcer associated with burns

Cushing's disease condition involving overproduction of hormones by the adrenal cortex

Cushing's ulcer peptic ulcer associated with head injury

cyanosis bluish or gray appearance of skin resulting from lack of oxygen supply

cyclothymia mood disorder characterized by symptoms similar to those of bipolar disorders, with both hypomanic and depressive symptoms

cystic fibrosis hereditary condition in which mucus-secreting organs in the body become obstructed by abnormal, thick mucus, resulting in degeneration and scarring of the organs involved

cystitis inflammation of the bladder

cytology study of cells

deafness inability to discriminate conversational speech through the ear

debride remove dead tissue

decibels (dB) sound intensity or loudness

decubitus ulcers pressure sores

delusions false beliefs

dementia deterioration of cognitive abilities

dendrite process emerging from cell body of neuron that is involved in transmission of electrical impulses to the cell body

dental caries cavities

dermabrasion procedure in which scars, wrinkles, or other skin blemishes are worn away to diminish scarring

dermatitis superficial inflammation of the skin

dermis inner layer of skin lying beneath the epidermis

diabetes insipidus condition involving inadequate secretion of the antidiuretic hormone from the pituitary gland

diabetes mellitus chronic disorder of carbohydrate metabolism in which an imbalance of the supply of and demand for the hormone insulin occurs

dialysis artificial means to replace kidney function

diaphoresis excessive sweating

diaphragm muscular wall that separates abdominal cavity from thoracic cavity

diastole phase of heart activity when the heart is relaxed and the chambers are filling

diplopia double vision

disability limitation or restriction of activity that results from an impairment

discography radiographic study of the cervical or lumbar disks

diskectomy removal of a portion of a disk

dislocation displacement or separation of a bone from its normal joint position

distal farthest from the center of the body

diuresis increased urinary output

diverticulum small balloon-like sac or pouch

diverticulitis infection or inflammation of diverticula

diverticulosis presence of numerous diverticula in the intestinal wall

DNA genetic material that is the blueprint for all the body's structures

dormant inactive

dorsiflexion backward movement

dorsiflexor muscle that bends a body part backward

duodenum first part of the small intestine

duodenal ulcer peptic ulcer in the upper portion of the small intestine

dura mater outer membrane of the brain and spinal cord

dysarthria impairment in the coordination and accuracy of the movement of the lips, tongue, or other parts of the speech mechanism

dysgraphia impaired writing ability

dyskinesia abnormal involuntary movements

dyslexia inability to understand written words

dyspepsia indigestion

dysphagia difficulty in swallowing

dyspnea difficulty in breathing

dysrhythmia irregularity of heartbeat

dysthymia chronic condition characterized by symptoms similar to those experienced in major depression but in a lesser degree

dystonia abnormal muscle tone

dysuria painful urination

ecchymosis purplish discoloration at the site of injury resulting from bleeding under the skin

eczema acute or chronic inflammatory condition of the skin with any of a combination of symptoms, including vesicles, scales, crusts, and redness

edema presence of abnormally large amounts of fluid in tissue spaces

edematous swollen

efferent nerves peripheral nerves that carry impulses away from the central nervous system

electrolytes electrically charged particles that are important to many of the body's internal functions (e.g., sodium and potassium)

embolus foreign particle or blood clot that travels in the bloodstream until it lodges in a blood vessel too small to allow its passage

emotional lability condition in which emotional reactions are inappropriate for the situation and usually unpredictable

emphysema permanent enlargement of the alveoli resulting from overinflation of and destructive change in the alveolar walls

encephalitis inflammation of the brain

endarterectomy removal of plaque or clot in the carotid artery

endocarditis inflammation of the inner lining of the heart

endocardium lining of the inner surface of the heart

endometrium lining of the uterus

end-stage renal disease disease or damage to the kidney to the point that it ceases to function

epidermis outer layer of skin

epidural pertaining to the space between the dura and the skull

epiglottis flap at back of throat that closes over opening to trachea when food is swallowed

epilepsy chronic neurological condition in which neurons in the brain create abnormal electrical discharges that cause temporary loss of control over certain body functions

epistaxis nosebleed

erythema redness

erythrocytes red blood cells

eschar dead tissue resulting from burns

esophageal reflux backflow of stomach contents into the esophagus

esophageal varices dilated tortuous veins of the esophagus

esophagectomy removal of the esophagus

esophagitis inflammation of the esophagus

eustachian tube tube connecting the throat and the tympanic cavity of the middle ear

eversion outward-turning movement

exacerbation time period when symptoms become worse

exertional dyspnea shortness of breath with activity

exophthalmos abnormal protrusion of the eyeball

expiration expulsion of air from the lungs

extension straightening movement

extensor muscle that straightens a limb

factitious disorder condition in which individuals voluntarily produce psychological or physical symptoms because of a compulsive need to assume the sick role

feces solid waste from the body

fetal alcohol syndrome toxic effects of alcohol on developing fetus during pregnancy resulting in deformity of the infant

fibromyalgia cluster of signs and symptoms in which individuals experience diffuse aching, pain, and stiffness in muscles and/or joints

fibrosis formation of fibrous tissue

fistula opening between two tubular structures

flaccid limp

flat affect showing little emotional responsiveness

flexion bending movement

flexor muscle that bends a limb

fluent aphasia receptive or sensory aphasia

frontal lobe portion of the brain located in the front part of each hemisphere

functional disorder disorder that has no readily identifiable organic cause

fused joined

gastric ulcer ulcer in the stomach

gastritis inflammation of the stomach

gastroenterostomy surgical procedure in which the bottom of the stomach and small intestine are opened, and the two openings are connected to create a passage between the body of the stomach and the small intestine

gene unit of heredity that is composed of DNA and carries hereditary information about all characteristics of the organism

gingivitis inflammation of the gums

glaucoma increase in intraocular pressure

global aphasia limited ability to communicate

glomerular filtration process by which kidney removes waste products from the blood

glomerulonephritis inflammation of the glomeruli of the kidney

glomerulus small capillaries located in the nephron of the kidney

glycosuria glucose in the urine

goiter swelling of the neck resulting from enlargement of the thyroid gland

grading system used to describe the structure of cancer cells

gray matter nonmyelinated nerve fibers in central nervous system that receive, sort, and process nerve messages

Guillain-Barré syndrome acute and progressive condition characterized by muscular weakness usually beginning in the lower extremities and spreading upward

hallucinations sensory experiences without environmental stimuli

handicap disadvantage because of an impairment or disability that presents a barrier to fulfilling a role or reaching a goal

hearing impairment any degree and type of hearing disorder

hearing loss impairment in any part of the hearing system that interferes with hearing sound

hemarthrosis bleeding in the joint

hematemesis vomiting of blood

hematoma sac filled with accumulated blood

hematuria blood in the urine

hemianopsia loss of vision in half the visual field

hemiplegia paralysis on one side of the body

hemoglobin red pigmented protein that carries oxygen within the erythrocytes

hemolysis destruction of red blood cells

hemophilia chronic bleeding disorder characterized by a deficiency in or absence of one of the clotting factors

hemopoiesis process by which blood cells are formed

hemoptysis blood-streaked sputum

hemostasis cessation of bleeding from damaged vessels

hepatitis inflammation of the liver

hepatotoxin substance that is toxic to the liver

hernia (rupture) protrusion of an organ through the tissues in which it is normally contained

herniorrhaphy surgical procedure used to repair hernias

Hertz (Hz) sound frequency or pitch

heterograft graft taken from another species; xenograft

hiatal hernia protrusion of the stomach through an opening of the diaphragm and into the thoracic cavity

histology study of the structure of tissue

Hodgkin's disease chronic, progressive disease in which abnormal cells replace normal elements within the lymph nodes

homeostasis maintenance of an internal chemical balance within the body

homograft graft taken from the same species but not the same person; allograft

Huntington's chorea slowly progressive, hereditary disease of the central nervous system characterized by jerky, involuntary movements and intellectual deterioration

hydrocephalus buildup of fluid in the brain

hydronephrosis buildup of urine in the kidney resulting from backup of urine and blocked outflow

hyperalimentation nourishment through infusion of special nutritional solution into a large blood vessel

hyperbilirubinemia excess bilirubin in the blood

hypercapnia buildup of carbon dioxide

hyperglycemia accumulation of large amounts of glucose in the blood

hyperkalemia high levels of potassium in the blood

hyperopia farsightedness

hyperproliferation overgrowth of cells resulting from a tumor

hypertension high blood pressure

hyperthermia increased body temperature

hyperthyroidism overproduction of thyroid hormone

hypertonia exaggerated muscle tone

hypertrophic scars ropelike configurations of scar tissue that form on the skin surface

hypertrophy enlargement

hyperuricemia buildup of uric acid in the body

hypochondriasis type of somatoform disorder characterized by preoccupation with physical illness

hypoglycemia decreased sugar in the blood

hypothyroidism insufficient production of thyroid hormone

hypoxemia decreased level of oxygen in the blood

hypoxia decrease of oxygen

hysterectomy removal of the uterus

ileostomy portion of small intestine brought through surgical opening to the outside of the abdomen for drainage of fecal material

ileum last part of the small intestine

immune system complex organization of specialized cells and organs that distinguishes between self and nonself, defending the body against foreign mate-rials

immunosuppression suppression of the immune system

impairment loss or abnormality of function at the body system or organ level

in situ when referring to cancer, the state in which cancer cells are present but remain localized (i.e., they have not invaded the surrounding lymph nodes)

incisors teeth at the front of the mouth that provide a cutting action

incontinence loss of control of bladder or bowel

incus small bone in the middle ear

infarction death of tissue resulting from lack of blood supply

inflammatory bowel disease a group of disorders that cause inflammation and/ or ulceration in the lining of the bowel

inspiration breathing air into the lungs

intermittent claudication aching, cramping, or fatigue of muscles in the legs when walking

internal fixation placement of screws, pins, wires, rods, or other devices through the bone to hold bone fragments together

intracranial pressure increased pressure on the brain

intraocular pressure pressure within the eyeball

intravenous refers to an infusion directly into a vein

inversion inward-turning movement

iridotomy removal of a portion of the iris of the eye

irritable bowel syndrome chronic or intermittent condition of the gastrointestinal tract in which individuals experience spasms of the colon, diarrhea, and/or constipation, cramping, and abdominal pain

ischemia inadequate blood supply

jaundice yellowish appearance of the skin and whites of the eyes resulting from an excess level of bilirubin in the blood

jejunum middle section of the small intestine

joint place where two or more bones are bound together

keratoplasty plastic surgery of the cornea

keratotomy incision in the cornea

ketoacidosis condition caused by an excessive level of ketones in the blood that increases the acidity of the blood to toxic levels

ketone metabolic product of fat metabolism

ketoacidosis acidosis accompanied by a buildup of ketone bodies in the blood (diabetic coma)

ketosis buildup of ketone bodies in the blood

kidney failure diminished functioning of the kidney

kyphosis (hump back) permanent postural deformity of the back

labyrinth inner ear

labyrinthitis inflammation of the labyrinth of the inner ear

laceration injury involving a tear or cut in the skin and underlying tissues

laminectomy surgical removal of the posterior arch of a vertebra

language set of symbols combined in a certain way to convey concepts, ideas, and emotions

laparotomy surgical incision into the abdomen

laryngectomy surgical removal of the whole or a part of the larynx

laryngitis inflammation of the larynx

laryngostoma surgical opening in the neck through which the individual breathes

larynx voice box

legal blindness central visual acuity not exceeding 20/200 in the better eye with correcting lenses or central field of vision limited to an angle of no greater than 20 degrees

lens small transparent disk enclosed in a transparent capsule and located directly behind the iris of the eye

lethargy listlessness

leukemia cancer of the tissues in which blood is formed

leukocyte white blood cell

leukocytosis white blood cell proliferation

leukopenia abnormal decrease in the number of white blood cells

ligaments tough bands of fiber that connect bones at the joint site

litholapaxy crushing of a kidney stone in the bladder

lithotomy surgical procedure to remove kidney stones

lobectomy removal of a lobe (i.e., of the brain; of the lung)

loosening of associations no logical progression of thought and rapid shifting from one unrelated idea to another

lordosis swayback

low back pain pain in the lumbar or sacral region of the lower back

lymphadenopathy swollen lymph nodes

lymphatic system circulatory system separate from the general circulation and consisting of lymph vessels, lymph fluid, and lymph nodes

lymphedema swelling resulting from blockage in lymphatics

lymph fluid clear fluid that bathes the body's tissue

lymph nodes small glands of the immune system that are located throughout the body and act as filters

lymphocyte white blood cell

lymphoma cancer of the lymphatic system

macrophage phagocyte that ingests dead tissue

macula spot on the retina that is the area of most acute vision

macular degeneration degeneration of the macula of the eye

melanin skin pigment that is responsible for skin color

melanocytes cells containing the skin pigment melanin

malignancy cancerous growth

malignant cancerous, harmful, virulent

malignant melanoma cancer that originates in the cells that contain skin pigment

malingering producing symptoms intentionally for secondary gain

malleus small bone in the middle ear

mandible jaw bone

mastectomy amputation of the breast

mastoidectomy surgical procedure for the removal of infected mastoid air cells located in the mastoid process

mastoiditis infection of the mastoid cells within the mastoid process located in the skull

mastoid process bony prominence behind the outer ear

megaloblastic anemia presence of large abnormal red blood cells

melanoma cancer of the pigment-producing cells

melena passage of dark, tarry bowel movements, resulting from action of intestines on blood

Meniere's disease disorder of the inner ear that includes symptoms of dizziness, hearing loss, and ringing in the ears

meninges membranes covering the brain and spinal cord

meningitis inflammation of the meninges

meningocele type of spina bifida in which membranes surrounding the spinal cord push out through an opening in the spinal column

metastasis movement of cancer cells from their original site to another part of the body

microcephaly abnormal smallness of the head

micrographia reduction in handwriting size

microphage a small phagocyte that ingests bacteria

micturition urination

mitral valve valve between left atria and left ventricle of the heart

mixed hearing loss hearing loss involving both conductive hearing loss and sensorineural hearing loss

molars teeth at the back of the mouth that provide a grinding action

motor nerves peripheral nerves that carry impulses from the central nervous system to other parts of the body

multi-infarct dementia condition in which deficits in cognitive function result from small strokes in various locations of the brain

multiple myeloma cancer of plasma cells that is characterized by bone destruction

multiple sclerosis progressive disease of the central nervous system in which the myelin around message-carrying nerve fibers is destroyed in localized areas of the brain and spinal cord

mutation alteration or change of the DNA within the normal cell

myelin fatty sheath that surrounds the neuron

myelomeningocele most severe form of spina bifida

myocardial infarction death of a portion of the heart muscle

myocardium heart muscle

myopathy disease of the muscle

myopia nearsightedness

myositis inflammation of the muscle

myringoplasty type of tympanoplasty in which damaged eardrum is repaired

myringotomy incision into the eardrum to drain pus or fluid

necrosis tissue death

necrotic dead

neoplasm new and abnormal growth of cells that serve no useful function and may interfere with healthy tissue function

nephritis inflammation of the kidney

nephrolithotomy surgical entry into the renal calix

nephrosclerosis condition in which arteries of the kidney become thickened

nephrosis general term used to describe conditions, other than direct infection of the kidney itself, that damage thekidney

nephrotic syndrome collection of symptoms experienced in nephrosis

nerve bundle of fibers outside the central nervous system

neuroma bundle of nerve fibers

neuron functional unit of the nervoussystem

neuropathy general term to describe functional disturbances or changes in the nerves

neurotransmitter chemicals that help transmit nerve impulses between neurons

neutropenia small numbers of mature white blood cells

nocturnal dyspnea difficulty in breathing while lying down at night

nonfluent aphasia expressive or motor aphasia

non-Hodgkin's lymphoma proliferation of lymphoid cells that disseminate throughout the body

nystagmus involuntary eye movement

obsessions persistent thoughts

occipital lobe portion of the brain located in the posterior portion of each hemisphere

occult hidden

occupational lung disease group of lung disorders directly related to matter inhaled from the occupational environment

oliguria decreased production of urine

oophorectomy removal of the ovaries

open head injury injury in which the skull is broken or penetrated

open reduction surgical alignment of fractured bone

ophthalmologist physician who specializes in conditions and treatment of the eye

opportunistic infection infection that would not occur in individuals with normal immune system function

orthosis any mechanical device applied to the body to control motion of the joints and to control force or weight distribution on a body part

orthotist individual who constructs the orthosis to meet individual needs

ossicles small movable bones in the middle ear

osteoarthritis local joint disease associated with degeneration of a joint

osteomyelitis infection of the bone

osteophytes bone spurs

osteoporosis reduction in bone mass, causing bones to become weakened, fragile, and easily broken

otoacoustic emissions measured reflections in the outer ear of mechanical activity in the cochlea

otitis media infection of the middle ear

otolaryngologist physician who specializes in disorders of the ear and related structures

otosclerosis conductive hearing loss caused by fixing or hardening of the small bones in the middle ear that transmit sound impulses to the inner ear

ototoxic describes drugs or chemicals that destroy the hair cells of the inner ear or damage the eighth cranial nerve

oval window opening between the middle and inner ear

pain disorder preoccupation with pain that is severe enough to cause functional impairment in daily life

pain expression individual response to pain

pain threshold point at which sensation is perceived as pain

pain tolerance point at which individual finds pain unbearable

palliative giving temporary relief of symptoms but no cure

pallor pale-appearing skin

palpitations awareness of beating of the heart

pancreatitis inflammation of the pancreas

panic attack episode in which the individual has feelings of intense anxiety or terror, accompanied by a sense of impending doom

paracentesis puncture of a body cavity with the removal of fluid

paraparesis partial paralysis of the lower extremities

paraplegia paralysis of the lower extremities

parasympathetic nervous system part of the autonomic nervous system

paresthesia sensation of numbness or tingling in some part of the body

parietal lobe portion of the brain located in the middle of each hemisphere

Parkinson's disease slowly progressive disorder of the central nervous system involving extensive degenerative changes in the basal ganglia of the brain with associated loss of or decrease in levels of dopamine

parotitis inflammation of the parotid glands

passive exercise exercise of a body part by a therapist or by a mechanical device

pathologic fractures fractures that occur because of disease of the bone rather than from injury

pathologist physician who specializes in the diagnosis of abnormal changes in tissues

peptic ulcer disease chronic inflammatory condition characterized by ulcer formation in the esophagus, stomach, or duodenum

percussion manual tapping or vibration of the chest or other body cavity

percutaneous transluminal coronary angioplasty (PTCA) procedure to enlarge a narrowed coronary artery

perfusion blood supply to an organ

pericardial effusion accumulation of excessive fluid within the pericardial sac surrounding the heart

pericardiocentesis puncturing of the pericardium to drain accumulated fluid

pericarditis inflammation of the pericardium of the heart

pericardium outer covering of the heart

periodontal disease disease of the tissues that surround and support the teeth

periodontitis severe form of gum disease

periosteum tough outer covering of bone

peripheral near the outside or surface of the body

peripheral nervous system all nerves extending from the brain and spinal cord

peripheral neuropathy disease of the peripheral nerves

peripheral vascular insufficiency inadequate blood flow to or from the lower extremities

peristalsis rhythmic, muscular movements that move food through the digestive tract

peritoneum lining of the abdominalcavity

peritonitis inflammation of the peritoneum

pernicious anemia complication of surgical resection of the stomach

personality disorder disorder characterized by inflexible or maladaptive behaviors that impair interpersonal or occupational functioning

pervasive developmental disorders conditions in which impairment occurs in several areas of development, including social interaction and verbal and nonverbal communication or stereotypical behavior

phagocyte cell that destroys and ingests foreign material

phagocytosis the process of cells ingesting other cells and foreign objects

phantom limb pain chronic, severe pain sensation in the amputated extremity

phantom sensation sensation that the amputated extremity is still present

pharyngitis sore throat

pharynx throat

phlebitis inflammation of a vein

phlebotomy removal of quantities of blood to reduce plasma volume

phobia fear and anxiety related to specific situations, persons, or objects

photosensitive sensitive to the sun

pia mater inner membrane covering the brain and spinal cord

pinna visible portion of the outer ear

plasma watery, colorless fluid that makes up the liquid portion of the blood

pleura membrane lining the chest cavity

pneumonectomy removal of the lung

pneumothorax collapse of the lung resulting from air entering the thoracic cavity

poliomyelitis infectious disease that affects the nerve cells that control muscles

polycystic kidney disease hereditary disease characterized by the presence of many cysts in the kidneys

polycythemia increase in the number of red blood cells as well as in the concentration of hemoglobin within the blood

polycythemia vera form of polycythemia in which an overproduction of both red and white blood cells occurs

polydipsia excessive and constant thirst

polyuria excessive urination

postlingual hearing loss occurs after verbal language is obtained

posttraumatic stress disorder (PTSD) disorder that develops after experiencing or observing a traumatic or life-threatening event

postvocational hearing loss hearing loss that occurs after the individual has entered the work force

poverty of speech diminished use of the spoken word

prelingual hearing loss hearing loss that occurs before the individual acquires language, usually before the age of 3

presbycusis hearing loss resulting from aging

presbyopia loss of the ability of the lens to accommodate to near and far images

pressure sores decubitus ulcers

prevocational hearing loss hearing loss that occurs after acquiring language but before entering the work force

prognosis prediction of the course and outcome of the disease process

pronation downward-turning movement

prosthesis fabricated substitute for a missing part for activities, occupation, and cosmetic needs

prosthetist individual who specializes in making prosthetic devices

proteinuria protein in the urine

pruritus itching of the skin

psoriasis chronic inflammatory disease of the skin in which epidermal cells in the basal layer of the skin are formed too quickly

psychogenic pain pain that persists for months or years but has no readily identifiable organic cause

psychosis loss of contact with reality

PTCA percutaneous transluminal coronary angioplasty

pulmonary artery vessel carrying blood from the heart to the lungs

pulmonary edema collection of fluid in the lungs

purpura condition in which hemorrhage into the skin or other tissue occurs

purulent pertaining to pus-containing material

pyelolithotomy surgical entry into the pelvis of the kidney

pyelonephritis infection of the kidney

pyloroplasty widening the opening between the stomach and the small intestine

quadriplegia paralysis of all four extremities

radial deviation lateral movement of the hand inward toward the body

radiologist physician who specializes in radiographic procedures

radionuclide radioactive chemical

Raynaud's phenomenon spasms of the vessels in the fingers or toes that impair blood flow to those areas

recruitment hearing impairment characterized by an abnormal increase in the perception of loudness

reflex automatic response to stimuli

regurgitation backflow

remission period of weeks to years when symptoms subside

renal pertaining to the kidney

reticular formation groups of cells within the brain stem

reticulocyte newly formed red blood cells

retina innermost coat of the eye that receives images formed by the lens

retinitis pigmentosa slow, progressive loss of peripheral vision

retinopathy disease or disorder of the retina

rheumatic disease condition that produces symptoms that affect joints, connective tissues, and muscle

rheumatic fever condition caused by the body's immune response against a specific organism

rheumatic heart disease condition in which the body undergoes a type of al-lergic response that can cause heart damage

rheumatoid arthritis chronic, progressive, and systemic disorder characterized by inflammation and swelling of the synovial joints, resulting in pain, stiffness, and deformity

sarcoma cancer of the bone, muscle, or other connective tissue

sciatica syndrome of pain that radiates from the lower back into the hip and down the leg

sclera white part of the eye

scoliosis lateral S-shaped curvature of the spine

seizure temporary loss of control over certain body functions

self-concept an individual's perceptions and beliefs about his or her own strengths and weaknesses and beliefs about other people's perceptions of him or her

semicircular canals part of the vestibular system in the inner ear

sensorineural hearing loss hearing loss resulting from damage to nerve pathways that transmit nerve impulses or damage to areas of the brain in which sound is perceived

sensory nerves peripheral nerves that carry messages toward the central nervous system

sepsis widespread infection throughout the body

septicemia presence of toxins in the blood

sickle cell anemia severe anemia as a result of sickle cell disease; most severe form of sickle cell disease

sickle cell crisis manifestation of sickle cell disease in which blood flow to a body part becomes obstructed by rigid, sickled red cells

sickle cell disease a chronic hereditary disorder characterized by abnormal hemoglobin

sickle cell trait abnormal gene causing the hemoglobin abnormality in sickle cell disease

social phobia phobic disorder in which the individual fears situations that may result in ridicule or humiliation

somatic nerves peripheral nerves that innervate body structures that are under voluntary control

somatoform disorder experience of physical symptoms for which no organic cause can be found

spasticity increased muscle tone, causing stiffness and awkward movements

speech verbal expression of language concepts

spina bifida congenital disorder of the spinal column in which one or more vertebrae are left open

spina bifida occulta mildest form of spina bifida that does not involve damage to the spinal cord

spinal fusion the grafting of bone from another area of the body into the disk interspace after laminectomy

spinal nerves peripheral nerves that connect and transmit messages directly to the spinal cord

spleen organ composed of tissue that disposes of worn-out blood cells

splenectomy removal of the spleen

splenomegaly enlargement of the spleen

spondylolisthesis forward slipping of a vertebra

spondylolysis breakdown of a vertebra

sprain injury to a ligament and its attachment site because of overstress

staging system to describe the extent to which cancer cells have spread

stapedectomy surgical procedure in which the stapes is removed and replaced with a prosthesis

stapes small bone in the middle ear

stasis stagnation

status asthmaticus severe, prolonged attack of asthma

status epilepticus continuous, uncontrolled seizures

stem cells cells that have the potential to become any type of cell in the body

stenosis narrowing of a duct or canal (e.g., a blood vessel)

stoma artificial opening

stomatitis inflammation of the mouth

strabismus disorder in which the eyes cannot be directed to the same object or one eye deviates from the central tract

strain injury to the tendons and muscles resulting from overstretching or overuse

stress ulcer peptic ulcer that develops after an acute medical crisis

subarachnoid between the arachnoid membrane and inner membrane covering the brain

subcutaneous beneath the skin; oftens refers to fatty tissue

subdural pertaining to the space beneath the dura

subluxation partial separation of bone from the joint

supination upward-turning movement

sympathetic nervous system portion of the autonomic nervous system

synapse space between neurons where chemical transmission of electrical impulses takes place

syncope fainting

synovectomy surgical removal of the synovial membrane surrounding a joint

systemic lupus erythematosus autoimmune disease of unknown cause

systole contraction phase of the heart's work

tachycardia fast heartbeat

tamponade pathological compression of a part

tardive dyskinesia abnormal muscle movements as a side effect of antipsychotic drugs

temporal lobe portion of the brain located under the frontal and parietal lobes

tendinitis inflammation of a tendon

tendon band of tissue that connects muscle to bone

tenosynovitis inflammation of the tendon sheath

tetany involuntary contraction of the muscles

thalassemia group of inherited hemo-lytic anemias

thoracentesis removal of fluid from the thoracic cavity

thoracic refers to the chest

thorax chest cavity

thromboangiitis obliterans rare condition of small and medium-sized arteries of extremities in which blood flow is diminished to a body part

thrombocyte platelet

thrombocytopenia decrease in platelet number

thrombocytosis increase in platelet number

thrombophlebitis inflammation of a vein with clot formation

thrombus blood clot

thymus lymphoid organ lying in upper portion of chest that produces a hormone important in controlling development of lymphocytes

TIA transient ischemic attack

tinnitus ringing in the ears

tolerance with regard to substance use, body adaptation to the substance so that larger amounts of the substance are needed to produce the same effects

tonic rigid

tonometry measurement of pressure in the eye

tophi deposits of crystals in the joints

trachea windpipe

tracheostomy surgical opening into the trachea

trachoma chronic infectious disease of the conjunctiva and cornea

traction therapeutic method in which a mechanical or manual pull is used to restore or maintain the alignment of bones or to relieve pain and muscle spasm

transient ischemic attack (TIA) temporary blocking of cerebral arteries, causing slight temporary neurological deficits

traumatic brain injury injury to the brain from an external physical force to the head

tricuspid valve valve between right atrium and right ventricle of the heart

tuberculosis infectious disease caused by an organism called the tubercle bacillus

tumor new and abnormal growth of cells that serve no useful function and may interfere with healthy tissue function

tympanic cavity middle ear

tympanic membrane eardrum

tympanometry test of acoustic immittance in which the mobility or flexibility of the tympanic membrane are assessed by measuring how much sound energy is admitted into the ear as pressure is varied in the external auditory canal

tympanoplasty surgical procedure that involves the middle ear

ulcerative colitis inflammatory condition of the large intestine

ulnar deviation lateral movement of the hand away from the body

urea waste product eliminated by the kidney

uremia buildup of waste products (e.g., urea and creatinine) in the blood

ureterolithotomy surgical removal of stones from the ureter

ureterosigmoidostomy surgical procedure for urinary diversion in which the ureters are connected to the colon so that urine is excreted through the rectum

ureters tubes leading from the kidney draining into the bladder

urethra single tube leading from the bladder to the urinary meatus

urinary meatus outside opening through which urine is eliminated

urinary retention the inability to empty the bladder of urine

urinary tract collecting system for urine, including the ureters, bladder, andurethra

urticaria hives

vagotomy cutting of the vagal nerve

valvuloplasty procedure to dilate a narrowed or stenosed valve of the heart

varicose veins congestion of veins

vascular insufficiency inadequate blood and oxygen to a body part

vena cava large vessel carrying unoxygenated blood from general circulation to the right atrium of the heart

venesection removal of quantities of blood to reduce plasma volume

ventilation process by which gases are transported between the atmosphere and the alveoli

ventricles two lower chambers of the heart

vertebrae bony covering of the spinal cord

vertigo dizziness

vestibular system part of the inner ear that conducts impulses regarding body balance and movement

virus organism that cannot grow or reproduce outside of living cells

viscosity thickness

visual acuity ability to process visual detail; sharpness of vision

visual impairment any deviation of normal vision

visual spatial deficit deficiency in depth perception, judgment of distance, size, position, rate of movement, form, and relation of parts to wholes

vitrectomy removal of the vitreous humor in the eye

Wernicke's aphasia type of fluent aphasia in which effortless speech, relatively normal grammatical structure, and increased verbal output occur, but with reduced information content

Wernicke's area portion of the brain located over the temporal and parietal lobes and major area of receptive function

white matter myelinated fibers in central nervous system that conduct electrical impulses

withdrawal experience of physical symptoms when the amount of a substance is decreased or absent

xenograft graft taken from another species; heterograft

Medications

Prescription medications are an important aspect of treatment of many chronic conditions and many disabilities. For this reason, it is important to be familiar with major types of prescription drugs and their biological and behavioral effects.

At no time should a nonmedical person advise an individual to stop taking a prescription or to change the dosage prescribed by the physician. If there are questions or doubts about an individual's condition or an individual's reaction to a specific medication, a physician should be consulted.

▪ ROUTES OF ADMINISTRATION

Medications can be administered in a variety of ways. Knowing the different routes of administration can be helpful in planning effectively so that any special factors regarding medication that may affect an individual's rehabilitation plan can be considered. Routes by which medications can be administered are the following:

Oral

Ingested (swallowed)
Sublingual (under the tongue)
Buccal (on mucous membrane on the cheek or tongue)

Rectal

Suppository, inserted into the rectum
Liquid, given as a retention enema

Parenteral

Intravenous (into a vein)
Intradermal (into the skin)
Subcutaneous (into the fatty layer under the skin)
Intramuscular (into the muscle)

Other

Inhalation (breathing medication in)
Topical (on top of the skin)

▪ FACTORS INFLUENCING MEDICATION DOSAGE

For a medication to act therapeutically, it must be given in sufficient concentration to produce the desired effect. Dosage is based on individual differences among clients. These differences influence how the medication is metabolized and, therefore, absorbed. Factors that influence dosage and metabolism are the following:

1. **Age**. Children are generally more sensitive to drugs than adults and, therefore, generally require smaller doses.

2. **Body weight**. The ratio of body weight to the amount of drug taken determines the concentration of the drug within the body and, therefore, affects its potency.

3. **Time of administration**. Oral medications are absorbed more rapidly if the stomach and upper portion of the intestinal tract are free from food. However, drugs that irritate the stomach lining should be taken with food.

4. **Route of administration**. Medication injected directly into a vein has an immediate effect, whereas medication administered orally or injected into a muscle or subcutaneous tissue has a slower absorption rate, so it takes longer to reach a concentration in the body that will show an effect.

5. **Rate of excretion**. Some drugs build up in the body when they are not excreted or destroyed as fast as they are ingested. If a drug builds up in the body past a certain level of concentration, toxic symptoms can occur.

6. **Drug combinations**. Some drugs are given in combination with other drugs to enhance their action. Not all drugs are compatible when taken together, however, and some can seriously affect the action of other drugs. Consequently, it is important that the physician is aware of all medications an individual is taking, even those prescribed by other physicians.

7. **Pathology**. Certain diseases affect the absorption or excretion of different medications, rendering them ineffective or causing toxic symptoms.

8. **Allergies or other drug reactions**. Individuals are sometimes allergic to different medications or have an abnormal response to them. Once these medications are identified, individuals should be encouraged to inform physicians before other medications are prescribed of the names of the drugs along with the reactions experienced.

9. **Compliance**. A medication prescribed to treat a condition is only as effective as the client's ability or willingness to take the medication as prescribed.

■ METHODS OF CLASSIFYING MEDICATIONS

Drugs may be referred to in three ways:

1. **Chemical name.** This is the precise description of chemical constituents of the medication. An example of a chemical name is N-methyl-4-carbethoxypiperidine hydrochloride.

2. **Generic name.** This reflects the chemical name to which the drug belongs, but it is simpler. An example of a generic name is *meperidine*. Drugs prescribed by their generic name may be cheaper than those ordered by tradename, but they may not always have all the components of the trade-name counterpart.

3. **Trade name.** This represents the brand name of the drug. The trade name is registered, meaning the use of the name is restricted to the manufacturer, which is the legal owner of the name. There may be many trade names for the same generic drug. An example of a trade name is *Demerol*.

■ THERAPEUTIC CLASSIFICATION OF MEDICATIONS

Drugs can be placed into several categories based on the action or therapeutic effect they are expected to produce. These categories are called therapeutic classifications.

Category	Therapeutic Effect
Analgesic	Reduces pain

Antacid	Neutralizes stomach acid	Antiseptic	Inhibits growth of microorganisms
Antianxiety	Reduces symptoms of anxiety	Antispasmodic	Relieves muscle spasms
Antiarrhythmic	Corrects abnormal rhythm of the heart	Antithyroid	Blocks thyroid hormone production
Antibiotic	Kills or inhibits growth of microorganisms	Antitussive	Sedative to prevent cough
Anticoagulant	Lengthens the pro-thrombin time and helps to prevent clot formation	Antiviral	Kills or inhibits growth of virus
		Astringent	Causes contraction of tissue and halts discharge
Anticholinergic	Inhibits action of the involuntary nervous system	Bronchodilator	Opens airways to permit air to pass more freely in and out of the lungs
Anticonvulsant	Prevents convulsions or muscle spasm	Cardiotonic	Changes heart rhythm and rate and generally strengthens heart
Antidepressant	Psychic energizers used to treat depression	Cathartic	Relieves constipation
Antidiarrhetic	Prevents diarrhea	Cholinergic	Stimulates the effects of the parasympathetic nervous system
Antiemetic	Prevents nausea or vomiting		
Antifungal	Checks the growth of fungi	Corticosteroid	Produces dramatic short-term anti-inflammatory effects
Antihypertensive	Lowers blood pressure		
Antihistamine	Relieves symptoms of allergic reactions by preventing histamine action	Digestant	Supplements enzyme deficiency
		Digitalis preparation	Increases pumping action of the heart muscle
Anti-inflammatory	Reduces inflammatory reactions such as redness and swelling	Diuretic	Rids body of excess fluid
Antimicrobial (sulfonamide)	Inhibits growth of microorganisms	Expectorant	Thins mucus to help expectoration
Antineoplastic	Prevents growth and spread of cancerous cells	Histamine H_2 (receptor antagonist)	Blocks cells in the stomach lining from producing acid
Antipruritic	Relieves itching	Hypoglycemic agent	Oral medication that lowers blood sugar
Antipsychotic	Reduces psychotic symptoms and hallucinations	Immuno-suppressant	Blocks the body's natural response to foreign substances
Antipyretics	Reduces fever		

Laxative	Relieves constipation	Nitroglycerine	Dilates coronary arteries, enabling the heart muscle to receive more oxygen
L-dopa	Decreases symptoms of Parkinson's disease		
Muscle relaxant	Reduces abnormal movement; reduces excess muscle tightness		

Glossary of Diagnostic Procedures

alanine aminotransferase (ALT; formerly serum glutamic-pyruvic transaminase [SGPT]) blood test to identify liver disease

angiography (**arteriography**) injection of radiopaque contrast material into the arteries to visualize the vessels (see arteriography)

antinuclear antibodies (**ANA**) blood test that identifies the proteins or antibodies that are present with some autoimmune diseases

arteriogram (see arteriography)

arteriography (**angiography**) test performed to study the anatomy of vascular structures through injection of radiopaque material into the arteries; may be performed to evaluate vasculature of vessels of the kidney, adrenal gland, brain, heart, or lower extremities

arthrocentesis insertion of a needle into a joint cavity for removal of synovial fluid for examination

arthrography X-ray study of a joint in which contrast material is injected into a joint, the joint is moved through its range of motion, and X-ray films are taken

arthroscopy direct visualization of a joint through insertion of a small instrument called an arthroscope into the joint

aspartate aminotransferase (**AST; formerly serum glutamic-oxaloacetic transaminase** [**SGOT**]) blood test to measure enzyme levels to identify possible coronary occlusive heart disease or liver disease

audiometric testing noninvasive procedure involving measurement of the degree of hearing loss through an electronic device called an audiometer

barium enema (**lower GI series**) X-ray examination of the lower gastrointestinal tract

barium swallow (**upper GI series**) X-ray study of the upper gastrointestinal tract

biopsy removal of a specimen of tissue from a specified site for examination

bleeding time blood test used to measure the length of time it takes for bleeding to stop after a puncture wound; determines how quickly a platelet clot forms

blood urea nitrogen (**BUN**) blood test that measures the level of a waste product of protein metabolism (urea) in the blood; used to evaluate kidney function

bone marrow aspiration insertion of a needle into the marrow space of the bone and aspirating a small sample so it may be examined microscopically for various abnormalities in the number, size, and shape of the precursors of blood cells

bone scan intravenous injection of radio-isotopes that then concentrate in the bone, enabling the concentration to be measured by a special machine called a scanner, which produces a picture of the bone

bronchoscopy visual examination of the bronchial tubes through a long hollow tube inserted through the mouth and into the bronchus

caloric test test to measure vestibular nerve function

cardiac angiogram (see arteriography)

cardiac catheterization invasive procedure in which a catheter is passed into the vessel of an arm or leg and then threaded into the heart to study the chambers, valves, and blood supply of the heart and to measure internalpressures

cardiac stress test noninvasive exercise test that provides a graphic record of the heart's activity during forced exertion

chest roentgenography (**X-ray**) noninvasive radiographic procedure by which it is possible to visualize organs of the chest cavity on X-ray film

cholangiogram a study in which the bile ducts are visualized on X-ray film

cholecystography procedure in which the gallbladder is visualized on X-ray film to detect abnormalities, inflammation, or the presence of stones

complete blood count blood test that evaluates a variety of components of the blood

computed tomography (**CT scan, CAT scan**) special X-ray procedure that produces three-dimensional pictures of a cross-section of a body part

C-reactive protein test blood test used to identify inflammatory processes or tissue destruction

creatinine clearance test test that compares the level of creatinine in the blood and the amount of creatinine excreted in the urine over a specified period of time

cystoscopy insertion of a special tube called a cystoscope through the urethra into the bladder to directly visualize the bladder wall

differential blood test to measure the proportion of each type of white blood cell

digital venous subtraction angiography invasive procedure in which a catheter is inserted into a vein, a contrast medium is injected, and a series of X-rays of the blood vessels in the head and neck are taken and visualized on X-ray film

discography X-ray study of the cervical or lumbar disks

echocardiography noninvasive ultrasound procedure in which the size, motion, and composition of the heart and large vessels are recorded

electrocardiography (**ECG**) graphic representation of electrical activity of the heart muscle

electroencephalography (**EEG**) noninvasive procedure producing a graphic representation of the electrical activity of the brain

electromyography (**EMG**) procedure in which electrical activity of certain muscles is evaluated to diagnose certain muscle diseases

electronystagmography procedure to monitor eye movement

ELISA initial blood test to screen for HIV antibodies

endoscopy (see gastroscopy)

erythrocyte sedimentation rate (**ESR; sed rate**) blood test that measures the rate at which red blood cells settle in a special solution over a certain time period; detects tissue injury or inflammation

esophageal manoscopy (**manometry**) diagnostic procedure in which a catheter is placed through the individual's mouth into the esophagus to evaluate the function of the sphincter between the esophagus and the stomach

fasting blood sugar (**FBS**) blood test to measure the glucose level in the blood when the individual has had nothing to eat

fluorescein angiography test used to detect changes in the blood vessels of the retina

gastroscopy (**endoscopy**) diagnostic test in which a lighted, flexible tube called an endoscope or gastroscope is inserted through the mouth, into the esophagus, and into the stomach to enable the physician to visualize the walls of these organs

glucose tolerance test blood test in which the individual, after fasting, is given concentrated glucose to drink and then blood samples are drawn at 1-, 2-, and 3-hour intervals

gonioscopy examination of the internal structures of the eye

Halstead-Reitan Battery neuropsychological test battery

hematocrit blood test to measure the percentage or proportion of red blood cells in the plasma

hemoglobin blood test to evaluate the amount of hemoglobin content of erythrocytes

holter monitoring (**ambulatory electrocardiography; event recorder**) form of electrocardiography involving continuous recording of the heart's electrical activity; the individual wears the holter monitor externally

intravenous pyelogram (**IVP**) X-ray examination of the kidneys, ureters, and bladder in which a dye is injected into a vein in the arm and then X-rays are taken of the kidneys at intervals over approximately an hour to identify structural abnormalities as well as any prob-lems with passage of the dye through the urinary system

KUB (**kidney, ureters, and bladder roentgenography**) X-ray of the kidney, ureters, and bladder to determine the size, shape, and location of the structures

laparoscopy procedure in which a hollow tube called a laparoscope is inserted into a body cavity through a small incision and the contents of the body cavity are examined or surgical procedures are performed

laryngoscopy visual examination of the larynx through a tube called a laryngoscope that is inserted into the larynx; enables the physician to inspect the structure of the larynx as well as assess the function of the vocal cords

LE prep blood test that examines a specific cell in the blood; useful in diagnosis of systemic lupus erythematosus

lumbar puncture (**cerebrospinal fluid analysis, spinal tap**) insertion of a needle into the subarachnoid space of the spinal column at the lumbar area so that cerebrospinal fluid may be aspirated and studied through laboratory analysis

Luria-Nebraska Neuropsychological Battery neuropsychological test battery

magnetic resonance imaging (**MRI; nuclear magnetic resonance imaging** [**NMRI**]) noninvasive procedure in which rapid detailed pictures of body tissue are produced; involves no ionizing radiation, but rather the pictures are formulated when hydrogen atoms in a magnetic field are disturbed by radiofrequency signals

mean corpuscular hemoglobin concentration blood test that calculates the amount of hemoglobin in each red blood cell

mean corpuscular volume (**MCV**) blood test to calculate the volume of a single red blood cell

mental status examination structured interview used as screening instrument in assessing cognitive impairment

mini-mental state examination mental status test to evaluate orientation, memory, attention, and ability to write, name objects, copy a design, and follow verbal and written commands

Minnesota Multiphasic Personality Inventory (**MMPI**) objective personality test

myelography X-ray study of the spinal cord

nerve conduction velocity (electroneurography) procedure often performed in conjunction with electromyography; measures nerve activity at the nerve-muscle junction to assist in diagnosis of conditions that affect the peripheral nerves

neuropsychological tests procedures that are used to assess major functional areas of the brain

paracentesis procedure in which a needle is inserted into a body cavity to remove fluid

partial thromboplastin time (**PTT**) blood test to evaluate the special part of the clotting mechanism not evaluated by prothrombin time

patch test application to the skin of small amounts of various substances to identify allergic responses

platelet count blood test to measure number of platelets in the blood

positron emission transaxial tomography (**PET scan**) radionuclear study in which biochemical or metabolic activities of cells of body tissue are studied

postprandial blood sugar blood test in which the glucose level of the blood is measured several hours after eating

proctoscopy (see sigmoidoscopy)

prothrombin time (**PT**; **Pro Time**) blood test to measure the length of time that a blood sample takes to clot whencertain chemicals are added to it in the laboratory; tests for specific factors involved in clotting

pulmonary function tests procedures to assess the volume of air that can be taken in and expelled from the lungs as well as the ability to move air in and out of the lungs

radionuclide imaging intravenous injection of a radioactive substance that localizes in a body tissue so that multiple views of the structure can be taken with a special camera and the images can be evaluated

red blood cell count (**RBC**) measurement of the total number of red blood cells

reticulocyte count blood test to assess bone marrow function by measuring production of immature red blood cells

retrograde pyelogram procedure in which a small catheter is inserted through a tube that has been inserted into the bladder and then directed into the ureters to the pelvis of the kidney; dye is then injected through the catheter, and X-ray films are taken to visualize the structures and to detect any abnormalities

rheumatoid factor (**latex fixation; agglutination test**) blood test that determines whether an abnormal protein exists in the blood serum; assists in diagnosis of rheumatoid arthritis or other rheumatic diseases

Rorschach inkblot test projective personality test

serum creatinine measurement of the level of creatinine in the blood to evaluate kidney function

serum glutamic-oxaloacetic transaminase (**SGOT**) (see aspartate aminotransferase [AST])

serum glutamic-pyruvic transaminase (**SGPT**) (see alanine aminotransferase)

serum thyroxine (**T4**) blood test to measure level of thyroid hormone in the blood

Short Portable Mental Status Question-naire (SPMSQ) mental status test to assess orientation, personal history, remote memory, and calculation

sigmoidoscopy procedure involving direct visualization of the anus and rectum through a special instrument called a sigmoidoscope

sonography (ultrasonography) test in which sound waves passed into the body are converted to a visual image or photograph of a body structure

speech audiometry tests to measure the individual's ability to understand speech

Stanford Binet intelligence test

Thematic Apperception Test projective personality test

tonometry measurement of pressure of the eye

TSH blood test to measure level of thyroid-stimulating hormone (TSH) in the blood

tympanometry technique used to measure the amount of sound energy admitted into the middle ear

ultrasonography (see sonography)

urinalysis examination of urine under a microscope or through other laboratory procedures to evaluate the concentration, acidity, and presence of components such as protein, sugar, blood, bacteria, or other types of cells in the urine

urine culture laboratory examination of sterile urine to determine whether infection is present, and if so, to identify the infectious organism

venogram X-ray study in which dye is injected into veins of a body part andX-ray films are obtained at timed intervals to visualize the structure of the venous system

ventilation/perfusion scan (lung scan) radiographic procedure that measures transport of gases between the atmosphere and alveoli of the lung and/or the degree to which blood is passed through the vessels into the lungs

Wechsler Adult Intelligence Scale-Revised (WAIS-R) intelligence test

Wechsler Intelligence Scale for Children-Revised (WISC-R) intelligence test

Wechsler Preschool and Primary Scale of Intelligence (WPPI) intelligence test

Western blot blood test that is performed as confirmatory test for the HIV antibody

white blood cell count (WBC) measurement of the total number of white blood cells

Wood's light examination examination of the skin under an ultraviolet light to identify specific types of skin infections

Index

C

G